Handbook of Ophthalmology

Editor: Slade Decker

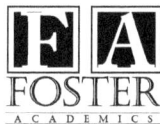

FOSTER
ACADEMICS

www.fosteracademics.com

Preface

Every book is initially just a concept; it takes months of research and hard work to give it the final shape in which the readers receive it. In its early stages, this book also went through rigorous reviewing. The notable contributions made by experts from across the globe were first molded into patterned chapters and then arranged in a sensibly sequential manner to bring out the best results.

Ophthalmology is the study of medicine which deals with the structure and the functioning of the eye along with its diseases. This field also encompasses the treatment of eye diseases with the strategic use of medications, laser therapy and surgery. Eye diseases are diagnosed through eye examinations and specialized tests such as ultrasonography, fluorescein angiography, etc. Cataract and macular degeneration are two common eye diseases. The clouding of the eye lens which results in decreased eye vision is known as cataract. Some of its symptoms include blurred vision, faded colours, trouble with bright lights, etc. Macular degeneration is an eye disorder in which the vision in the center of the visual field gets blurred or lost due to age. Ophthalmology is an upcoming field of medicine that has undergone rapid development over the past few decades. This book is a compilation of chapters that discuss the most vital concepts and emerging trends in the field of ophthalmology. It will help the readers in keeping pace with the rapid changes in this field.

It has been my immense pleasure to be a part of this project and to contribute my years of learning in such a meaningful form. I would like to take this opportunity to thank all the people who have been associated with the completion of this book at any step.

Editor

Investigation of the anti-cataractogenic mechanisms of curcumin through in vivo and in vitro studies

Jing Cao[1], Tao Wang[2] and Meng Wang[2*]

Abstract

Background: Cataract is the leading cause of blindness in elderly people worldwide, especially in developing countries. Studies to identify strategies that can prevent or retard cataract formation are urgently required. This study aimed to investigate the potential mechanism of the cytoprotective effects of curcumin in in vivo and in vitro experiments.

Methods: Male Wistar rats were randomly divided into three groups: the control group, the model group (administered 20 μmol/kg sodium selenite), and the curcumin group (pretreated with 75 mg/kg body weight curcumin 24 h prior to the administration of sodium selenite). The expression levels of heat shock protein 70 (HSP70), the activities of 8-hydroxy-2-deoxyguanosine (8-OHdG), catalase (CAT), malondialdehyde (MDA), superoxide dismutase (SOD), and glutathione peroxidase (GSH-Px) were assessed by using RT-PCR assay and ELISA. In addition, the cell viability, cell apoptosis, and cell cycle were assessed using a CCK-8 assay and flow cytometry in in vitro studies, followed by RT-PCR analysis to identify the mRNA expression levels of caspase 3, Bcl-2 associated X (Bax), B-cell lymphoma 2 (Bcl-2), cyclooxygenase (Cox-2), c-met, and Slug.

Results: Cataract was successfully established in rats of the model group and the curcumin group through intraperitoneal injection of sodium selenite. The expression levels of HSP70 and the activities of 8-OHdG and MDA in the curcumin group were decreased compared with those in the model group, whereas the activities of CAT, SOD, and GSH-Px were significantly higher than those in the model group ($P < 0.05$). In the in vitro studies, the cell viability and cell apoptosis significantly increased and decreased, respectively, in the curcumin group compared with the model group. Correspondingly, the mRNA expression of caspase-3, Bax, and Cox-2 was lower in the curcumin group than in the model group ($P < 0.05$).

Conclusions: This study suggested that curcumin attenuated selenite-induced cataract through the reduction of the intracellular production of reactive oxygen species and the protection of cells from oxidative damage.

Keywords: Curcumin, Cataract, Reactive oxygen, Cell viability, Cell apoptosis

Background

Cataract is the leading cause of blindness in elderly people worldwide, especially in developing countries [1]. It is estimated that blindness owing to age-related cataracts occurs in approximately 20 million people. At present, the gold standard for the treatment of cataract is the surgical replacement of the cloudy lens with an artificial lens when the cataracts cause problems in daily life [2]. However, the surgery is not an easily accessible treatment option in many countries, especially in low and middle-income countries. Moreover, cataract surgery can cause vision-related complications and risks, such as posterior capsule opacification, especially in infants and children, and place a significant burden on healthcare systems and patients' quality of life [3–5]. Although the surgical techniques and intraocular lens materials have advanced significantly in the last few decades, the outcomes have not substantially improved. Therefore, studies are urgently required to identify strategies that can prevent or retard cataract formation.

* Correspondence: wangmeng1985218@163.com
[2]Department of Ophthalmology, Linyi People's hospital of Shandong University, No. 27, Jiefang road, LinYi, Shandong 276003, China
Full list of author information is available at the end of the article

Although the nosogenesis of cataract is not clear, oxidative damage to the eye lens is thought to be an important mechanism in the initiation and progression of cataracts [6]. A series of highly reactive oxygen species (ROS), including superoxide anion ($O2^-$), nitric oxide (NO), hydroxyl radicals (OH-), and hydrogen peroxide (H_2O_2) has been proven to be implicated in different types of cataract formation [7]. Therefore, considerable efforts have been made to discover effective antioxidative pharmacological agents.

Curcumin, extracted from the rhizome of *Curcuma longa* Linn., is a natural polyphenol. It was first used as an antioxidant to prevent cataract formation in 1996 [8]. Since then, the study of curcumin as a potential anticataract agent has been one of the central areas of anticataract research [9–12]. Although curcumin has been studied for many years, evidenced-based research is still needed to clarify the biochemical roles in the prevention of cataract formation.

This study aimed to investigate the mechanisms involved in the potential use of curcumin to prevent cataract in in vivo and in vitro studies.

Methods

Curcumin and sodium selenite of commercially available analytical grades were purchased from Sigma China (Shanghai, China). The lens epithelial cells (LEC) of the HLEB-3 cell line were purchased from iCell Bioscience Inc. (Shanghai, China) and cultured in DMEM supplemented with 10% foetal bovine serum (FBS) in a humidified incubator maintained at 37 °C with an atmosphere of 5% CO_2.

Animals and treatments

Ten-day-old male Wistar rats with an average body weight of (25.4 ± 3.7) g were purchased from Shanghai SLAC Laboratory Animal Co., Ltd. (Shanghai, China). All rats were housed at room temperature of (25 ± 1) °C and subjected to a 12/12 h day/night cycle. The rats in all groups were fed a regular diet (Shanghai SLAC Laboratory Animal Co., Ltd., Shanghai, China) with distilled water ad libitum for a period of 2 weeks. The animal experiments were approved by the ethics committee of LinYi (LW2017003).

The rats were randomly allocated into three groups: the control group ($n = 6$), administered physiological saline; the model group (n = 6), administered sodium selenite (intraperitoneal injection with signal dose of 20 μmol/kg body weight sodium selenite) to induce cataract; and the curcumin group ($n = 6$), administered a curcumin pretreatment before sodium selenite (75 mg/kg body weight curcumin, orally administered 24 h before selenium administration), as described in previous studies [11, 13]. The eyes were examined every other day.

After treatment for 2 weeks, the rats were killed by cervical dislocation under anaesthesia and the lenses were dissected out, washed with ice-cold saline, and frozen at -70 °C until further use.

Biochemical examinations

A 10% homogenate was prepared in aqueous buffers of 0.1 M Tris-HCl (pH 7.4) and centrifuged at 10000 rpm at 4 °C for 30 min. The supernatant was isolated and used to test 8-oxo-deoxyguanosine (8-OHdG), malondialdehyde (MDA), catalase (CAT), superoxide dismutase (SOD), and glutathione peroxidase (GSH-Px) by using ELISA kits (Nanjing Jiancheng Biological Engineering Institute, Jiangsu, China) in accordance with the manufacturer's instructions.

Intracellular O_2^- concentration detection

The intracellular ROS concentration was detected in accordance with previous studies [14, 15]. Briefly, the cells in each group were stained with 5 μM DHE (dihydroethidium, Invitrogen Shanghai, China) at 37 °C in the dark for 30 min. Afterwards, the cells were examined by using a fluorescence activated cell sorter with excitation at 480–535 nm and emission at 590–610 nm.

Cell viability analysis

The HLEB-3 cells were seeded at a density of 1×10^4 cells/cm^2 in a 96-well plate, grown overnight, and then administered treatment as appropriate. The cells were treated with 200 μM H_2O_2 (H_2O_2 group), 200 μM H_2O_2 plus curcumin (0.2 mM in 2% acetonitrile solution, H_2O_2 + Curcumin group) for 24 h; cells without any treatment served as the control (Control group). The cell counting kit-8 (CCK-8) solution was then added to each well and incubated at 37 °C for 4 h. At the end of this treatment, absorbance was measured at 450 nm. The cell growth inhibition rate was calculated as described in reference [16]. The assay was repeated in triplicate.

Cell cycle and cell apoptosis assay

HLEB-3 cells were seeded in 6-well plates and treated with 200 μM H_2O_2 (H_2O_2 group), 200 μM H_2O_2 plus curcumin (0.2 mM in 2% acetonitrile solution, H_2O_2 + Curcumin group) for 24 h, and cells without any treatment served as the control. The cells were harvested, washed with phosphate-buffered saline (PBS), and stained with annexin V-FITC/PI (Becton Dickinson, Franklin Lakes, NJ, USA) at room temperature for 15 min. Subsequently, the cells were analysed by using flow cytometry.

For the cell cycle analysis, the three different treatments of HLEB-3 cells were applied for 48 h. Subsequently, the cells were harvested by trypsinisation, washed twice in PBS, and fixed in 70% ethanol at 4 °C overnight. The cells were then washed, resuspended in cold PBS, and treated with staining buffer at 37 °C in the dark for 30 min. The cell cycle was analysed by using flow cytometry.

Real-time PCR

Total RNA from the lenses or cells was extracted in each group by using Trizol reagent (Sigma). RT-PCR was performed as previously described [17]. The primers for heat shock protein (HSP70), caspase-3, Bcl-2 associated X (Bax), B-cell lymphoma 2 (Bcl-2), cyclooxygenase (Cox-2), c-met, and Slug are displayed in Table 1. The reactions were conducted in triplicate and the results are shown from three independent experiments.

Enzyme-linked immunosorbent assay (ELISA)

The protein expression levels of MDA, SOD, and CAT in the three treatment groups were measured by using individual ELISA kits in accordance with the manufacturer's instructions.

Statistical analysis

All data are expressed as the mean ± standard deviation. Comparisons between two groups were examined by Student's t test, computed by using GraphPad Prism (GraphPad Software, San Diego, CA, USA). A value of $P < 0.05$ was considered to indicate statistical significance.

Results

Construction of cataract model

After the injection of sodium selenite for 2 weeks, the lens of rats in the model group took on a white appearance and lost transparency; however, the transparency of rats in the curcumin group was improved compared with those in the model group.

Table 1 The sequences of primers for RT-PCR

Primer sequence (5'-3')	Gene
TTT CTG GCT CTC AGG GTG TT	HSP70-f
CTG TAC ACA GGG TGG CAG TG	HSP70-r
GACTTCGCCGAGATGTCCAGC	Bcl-2-f
CCGAACTCAAAGAAGGCCACAAT	Bcl-2-r
GTGCTATTGTGAGGCGGTTGT	Caspase 3-f
TCCATGTATGATCTTTGGTTC	Caspase 3-r
AGAAGGCTAAAGGAAACGAA	c-Met-f
GGACCGTCAAGAAGTAAATAAA	c-Met-r
CCCTGAGCATCTACGGTTTG	Cox-2-f
CAGTATTAGCCTGCTTGTCT	Cox-2-r
ATTTATGCAATAAGACCTATTCT	Slug-f
AGGCTCACATATTCCTTGTCACA	Slug-r
CTGACGGCAACTTCAACTGGG	Bax-f
GGAGTCTCACCCAACCACCCT	Bax-r

Determination of in vivo levels of HSP70, 8-OHdG, MDA, CAT, SOD, and GSH-Px

HSP70 levels in the lens were further determined by the RT-PCR analysis of each group. As shown in Fig. 1a, the HSP70 level in the model group was significantly higher than that in control group ($P < 0.05$); however, it was significantly reduced in the curcumin group, which suggested that curcumin could reverse some of the effect of selenite. To further investigate the effect of curcumin, the activities of 8-OHdG, MDA, CAT, SOD, and GSH-Px were measured by using ELISA assays. As shown in Fig. 1b–f, the activities of 8-OHdG and MDA significantly increased in the model group and the curcumin group compared with those in control group ($P < 0.05$). In addition, their expression levels were significantly lower in the curcumin group than those in model group ($P < 0.05$). The activities of CAT, SOD, and GSH-PX, showed an opposite trend in expression: a decrease in the model group and curcumin group was observed compared with those in the control group ($P < 0.05$). Similarly, their activities were higher in the curcumin group than in the model group ($P < 0.05$).

Evaluation of intracellular superoxide (O_2^-) level by DHE

To evaluate the concentration of ROS in each group, the quantified O_2^- level was determined by using fluorescent DHE. As shown in Fig. 2a, the O_2^- level, reflected by red fluorescence, was significantly higher in the model group ($P < 0.05$) compared with the control group, whereas it was much more suppressed in curcumin-treated cells than those in the model group ($P < 0.05$).

Cell viability and apoptosis analysis

Proliferation was examined in HLEB-3 cells treated with H_2O_2, H_2O_2 plus curcumin, and untreated HLEB-3 cells. The CCK-8 assay revealed that H_2O_2 treatment significantly decreased the viability of HLEB-3 cells ($P < 0.05$), whereas curcumin treatment partly reversed this decrease ($P < 0.05$, Fig. 2b).

The cell cycle analysis (Fig. 2c) indicated that the proportion of HLEB-3 cells in the G1 phase was significantly reduced in the model group and that curcumin could reverse this decrease ($P < 0.05$). Conversely, the proportion of HLEB-3 cells in the G2 phase was remarkably increased in the model group and decreased in the curcumin group ($P < 0.05$). The proportion of cells in the S phase was not significantly different between all three groups ($P > 0.05$).

Flow cytometry was used to determine cellular apoptosis in each group. As shown in Fig. 2d, H_2O_2 caused an increase in the number of dead HLEB-3 cells after treatment for 24 h (12.8% vs 27.2%). However, cell apoptosis in the H_2O_2 plus curcumin group was decreased (17.8%) compared with that in the H_2O_2 group.

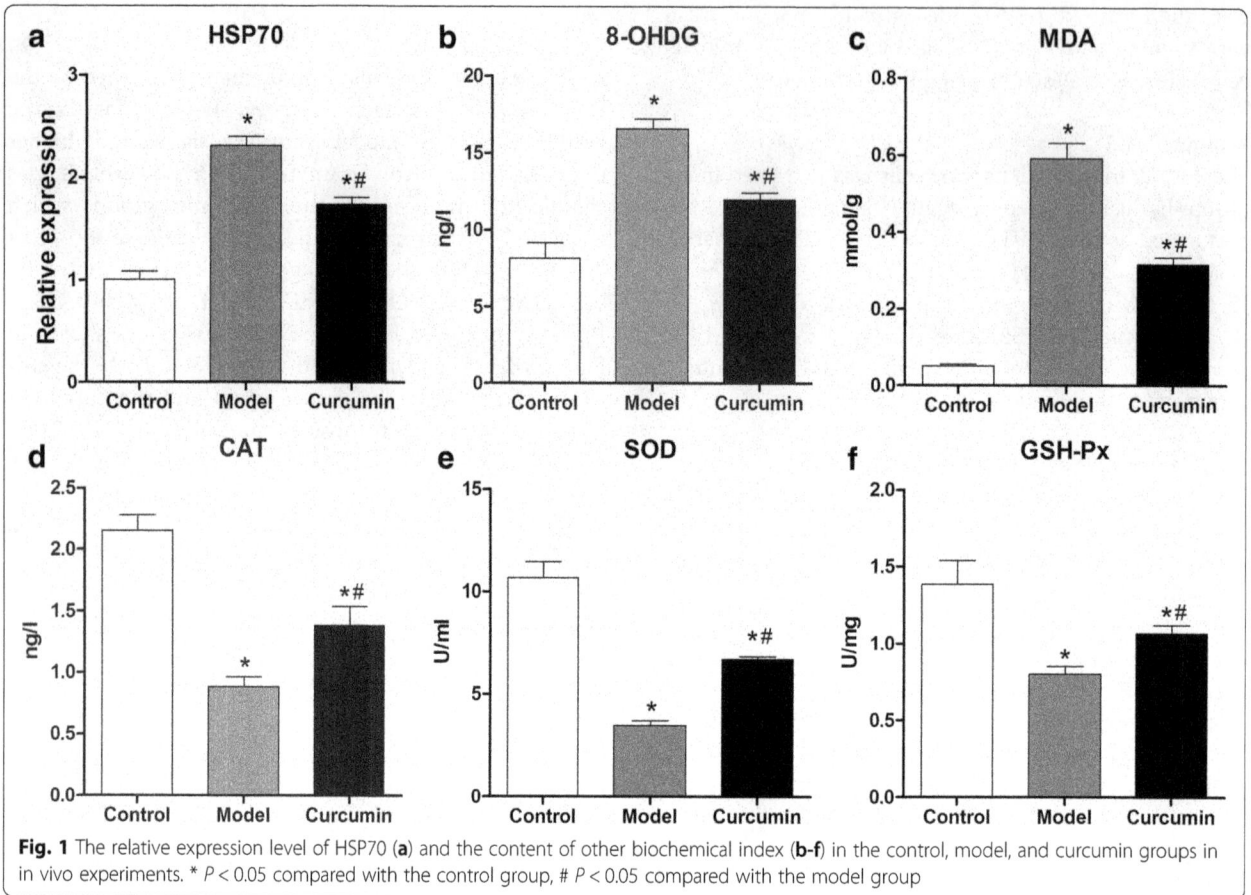

Fig. 1 The relative expression level of HSP70 (**a**) and the content of other biochemical index (**b-f**) in the control, model, and curcumin groups in in vivo experiments. * $P < 0.05$ compared with the control group, # $P < 0.05$ compared with the model group

In vitro *mRNA expression of caspase-3, Cox-2, Bax, Bcl-2, c-met, and Slug*

As shown in Fig. 3, the relative mRNA expression of caspase-3, Bax, and Cox-2 was significantly increased in the H_2O_2 group and the H_2O_2 + curcumin group compared with those in the control group ($P < 0.05$). In addition, curcumin treatment significantly decreased the expression levels of these genes compared with the H_2O_2 group ($P < 0.05$). The mRNA expression levels of c-met and Slug were increased in the H_2O_2 and H_2O_2 + curcumin groups, but the changes were not significant ($P > 0.05$).

Protein expression of MDA, SOD, and CAT

The protein expression of MDA, SOD, and CAT in the three treatment groups was determined by using ELISA. As shown in Fig. 4, MDA was significantly upregulated in the H_2O_2 group, whereas SOD and CAT were significantly downregulated in the H_2O_2 group ($P < 0.05$). In addition, curcumin treatment could reverse the effect of H_2O_2 on MDA, SOD, and CAT expression ($P < 0.05$).

Discussion

Cataract is the leading cause of blindness in the elderly people. Although surgery can be successfully used to

remove cataract, the rate of irreversible blindness caused by its complications is highly significant. Previous studies over the past few decades have neglected to screen natural compounds for the potential to ameliorate selenite-induced cataracts. In this study, we investigated the anti-cataractogenic activity of curcumin in in vivo and in vitro studies. The results showed that curcumin could reverse some of the effects of selenite through the regulation of the expression levels of HSP70 and the activities of reactive intermediates, including 8-OHdG, MDA, CAT, SOD, and GSH-Px. In addition, in vitro studies further suggested that curcumin could decrease the concentration of intracellular ROS and attenuate oxidative damage through the regulation of apoptosis-related genes.

The in vivo cataract model was established through the injection of selenium into the eye. This is a classical method for the creation of a cataract model [11, 13] and is used widely in the study of the pathogenesis of senile cataract and the effect of anti-cataract drugs [18]. The results showed that the eye lens isolated from rats injected with selenium took on a white appearance and decreased in transparency, whereas those from untreated rats did not. Interestingly, the administration of curcumin in the cataract model led to a decrease in selenite-

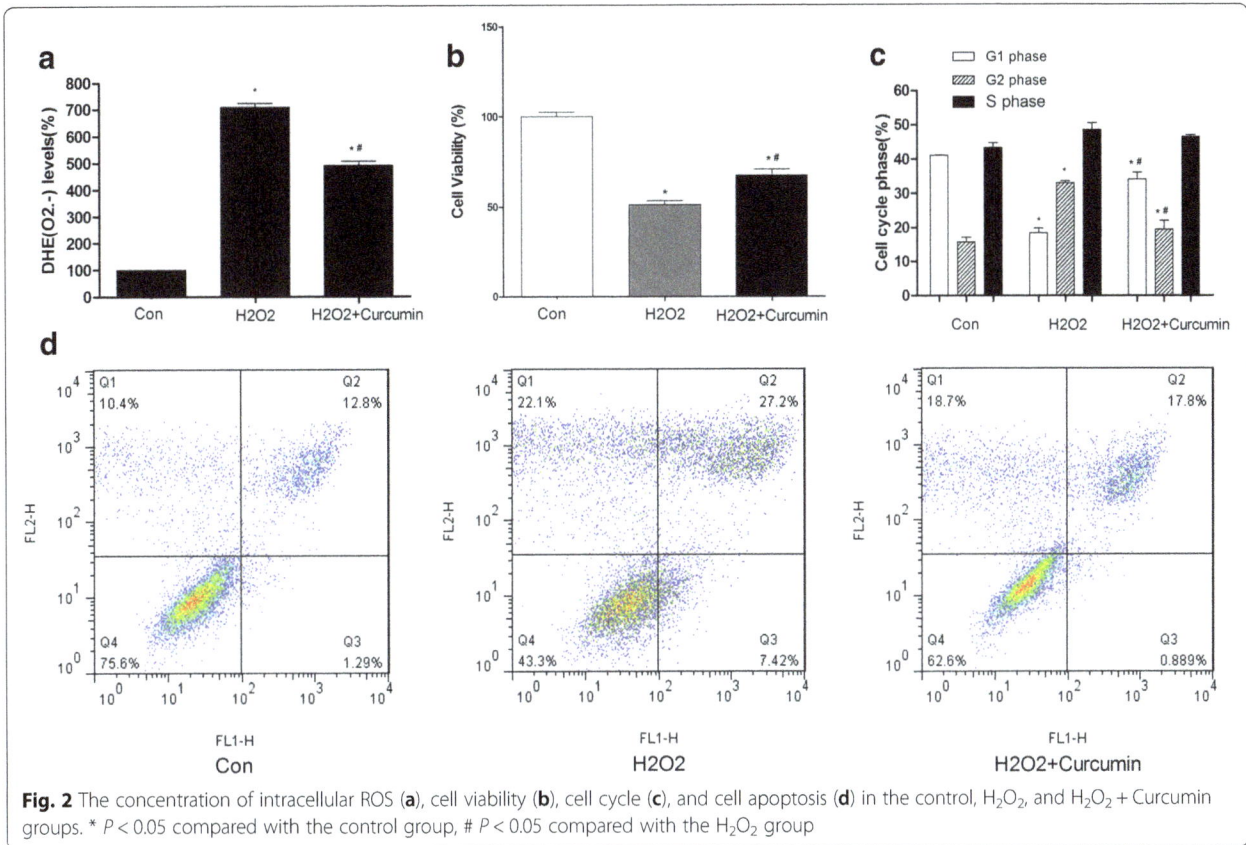

Fig. 2 The concentration of intracellular ROS (**a**), cell viability (**b**), cell cycle (**c**), and cell apoptosis (**d**) in the control, H_2O_2, and H_2O_2 + Curcumin groups. * $P < 0.05$ compared with the control group, # $P < 0.05$ compared with the H_2O_2 group

induced turbidity in the eye lens. These results were consistent with previous studies and indicated the successful establishment of the cataract models [19].

HSP70, a major member of the Hsp family, is crucial for the maintenance of normal lens microenvironments [20, 21]. It has been widely acknowledged that one of the major triggers factors for cataract formation is the accumulation of excessive free radical generation, which leads to further oxidative stress [22]. These free radicals may cause oxidative damage in the tissue of the anterior eye segment. The expression of HSP70 in the eye lens of rats exposed to selenium was significantly upregulated in our study. This result was consistent with those of Manikandan et al. [23]. Previous studies suggested that HSP70, HSP27, and HSP40 might play a role in the protection of the lens against a variety of stimulants, including oxidative damage, heat shock, and osmotic stress [21, 24, 25]. Interestingly, our results showed that HSP70 expression in the eye lenses of rats exposed to selenium was significantly upregulated and that curcumin could suppress this expression. We hypothesized that this was because HSP70 is a stress-induced protein and curcumin decreases the oxidative stress caused by an accumulation of free radicals; therefore, HSP70 expression was decreased in curcumin group. Correspondingly, the intracellular concentration of ROS was

significantly lower in curcumin-treated cells than in H_2O_2-treated cells in our study ($P < 0.05$).

In the present study, the activities of CAT, GSH-Px, and SOD were found to be significantly lower in the model group than in the control group in in vivo and in vitro experiments. However, this decrease was partly ameliorated by curcumin. Similarly, low levels of SOD were previously found in diabetic- and selenite-induced cataract models [26, 27], in which low levels of SOD caused irreversible lens damage. These results further supported the antioxidant properties of curcumin. As an end product of lipid peroxidation, MDA is considered to be a toxic compound in the eye owing to its high cross-linking ability with the lipid membrane [12, 28, 29]. Free radicals have the ability to cause lipid peroxidation, which lead to the loss of lens transparency and cataract formation [30]. A previous study demonstrated that thiobarbituric acid reactive substances, which are also the end products of lipid peroxidation, were increased by selenite-induced cataract. As the activity of MDA was decreased in the curcumin group compared with the model group, this study further demonstrated that curcumin could prevent selenite-induced cataractogenesis through a decrease in lipid peroxidation end products.

Reduced glutathione acts as the first line of defence against free radical-mediated damage. As an H_2O_2

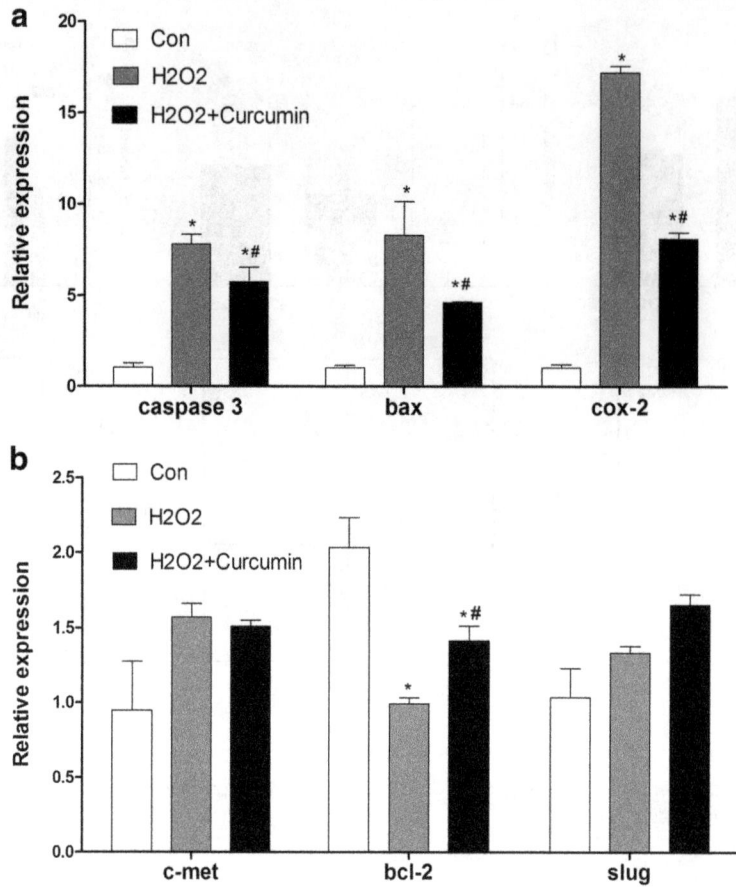

Fig. 3 The relative mRNA expression levels of caspase-3, Bax, Cox-2, c-met, Bcl-2 and Slug. * $P < 0.05$ compared with the control group, # $P < 0.05$ compared with the H_2O_2 group

scavenger, GSH-Px also acts as a membrane barrier for lipid peroxidation in the lens membrane. Studies have shown that glutathione deficiency leads to cataract in experimental animals [31] and our studies have shown that GSH-Px was reduced in the selenium-induced cataract model and increased in the curcumin group.

There are numerous studies that investigate the effect of curcumin on cataract. However, most have focused on the antioxidant effect of curcumin. In this study, we investigated the effect of curcumin on LEC apoptosis. As shown in Fig. 3, the cell viability was decreased in the model group and the percentage of apoptotic cells was increased compared with the control. However, those in

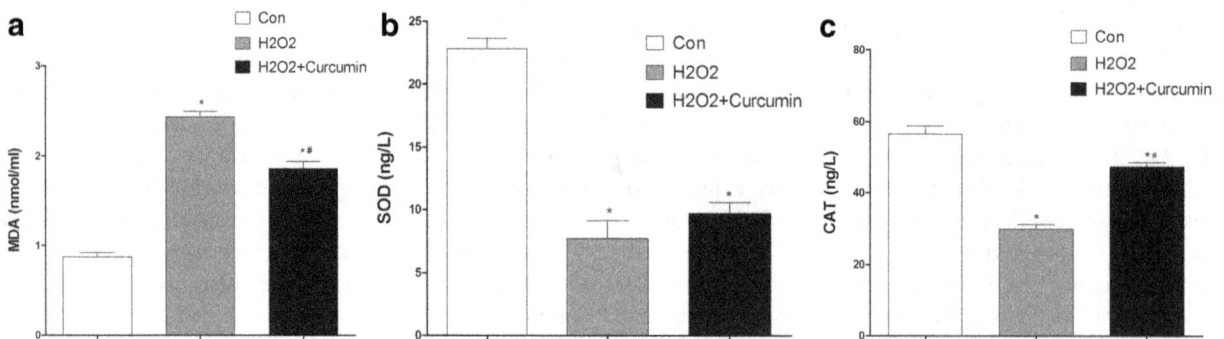

Fig. 4 The content of MDA, SOD, and CAT in the control, H_2O_2, and H_2O_2 + Curcumin groups. * $P < 0.05$ compared with the control group, # $P < 0.05$ compared with the H_2O_2 group

the curcumin group were increased and decreased, respectively. Through the analysis of the expression of apoptosis-related genes, we found that the expression levels of caspase-3, Bax, and Cox-2 were significantly upregulated in the model group and the curcumin group compared with those in the control group ($P < 0.05$). However, compared with the model group, the genes were significantly depressed in the curcumin group ($P < 0.05$). Bcl-2, as a repressor of apoptosis, showed the opposite trend.

The caspase cascade and the heterodimerisation of Bcl-2 family proteins are central components of programmed cell death. Bcl-2 family proteins play important roles in the activation of caspases [32]. Bcl-2 and Bax are two major proteins in the Bcl-2 family that repress apoptosis and promote apoptotic functions, respectively. Selenite caused cell apoptosis and when apoptosis occurred, the expression of Bcl-2 was reduced significantly, whereas the expression of Bax was increased in the model group. However, curcumin attenuated the occurrence of apoptosis through the downregulation of Bax and the upregulation of Bcl-2 expression. These data strongly indicated that the Bcl-2 family of proteins may be involved in the process of curcumin protection from ROS-induced oxidative damage.

The epithelial-mesenchymal transition (EMT) is the change in cell phenotype from an epithelial to a fibrocytic morphology. Previous studies suggested anterior LEC underwent EMT-like changes after cataract surgery [33], but these changes might lead to further complications of posterior capsule opacification. The expression of Cox-2 and Slug is a hallmark of the EMT [34]. In our study, the expression of Cox-2 is significantly upregulated in the model group. However, this expression was reduced to a large extent by curcumin. This was somewhat consistent with a previous study that discovered cataractous LEC underwent EMT expression of Cox-2 mRNA and protein, whereas normal LEC did not [35]. As curcumin significantly decreased the expression of Cox-2, we speculated that curcumin might be useful for the prevention of posterior capsule opacification. However, the expression of Slug was not significantly reduced by curcumin. In addition, the expression of c-met was also not significantly different among groups. The molecular mechanism of these changes warranted further investigations.

Conclusions

This study investigated the cytoprotective nature of curcumin in in vivo and in vitro experiments. The results showed that curcumin attenuated selenite-induced cataract through a reduction in the intracellular production of ROS and the protection of cells from oxidative damage. This study further suggested that curcumin might greatly reduce the occurrence of cataractogenesis as well as prevent posterior capsule opacification.

Abbreviations
8-OHdG: 8-Hydroxy-2-deoxyguanosine; Bax: Bcl-2 associated X; Bcl-2: B-cell lymphoma 2; CAT: Catalase; CCK-8: Cell counting kit-8; Cox-2: Cyclooxygenase; EMT: Epithelial-mesenchymal transition; FBS: Foetal bovine serum; GSH-Px: Glutathione peroxidase; H_2O_2: Hydrogen peroxide; HSP70: Heat shock protein; LEC: Lens epithelial cells; MDA: Malondialdehyde; NO: Nitric oxide; $O2^-$: Superoxide anion; OHs: Hydroxyl radicals; ROS: Reactive oxygen species; SOD: Superoxide dismutase

Acknowledgements
None.

Funding
None.

Authors' contributions
MW contributed to the conception and design of experiments and polished the manuscript. TW contributed to the execution of the experiments and the preparation of the manuscript. JC provided the curcumin and contributed to the analysis of data as well, as revision and preparation of the manuscript. All authors read and approved the final manuscript.

Competing interests
The authors declare that they have no competing interests.

Author details
[1]Department of pharmacy, Linyi People's hospital of Shandong University, LinYi 276003, China. [2]Department of Ophthalmology, Linyi People's hospital of Shandong University, No. 27, Jiefang road, LinYi, Shandong 276003, China.

References
1. Congdon NG, Friedman DS, Lietman T. Important causes of visual impairment in the world today. JAMA. 2003;290(15):2057–60.
2. Lamoureux EL, Fenwick E, Pesudovs K, Tan D. The impact of cataract surgery on quality of life. Curr Opin Ophthalmol. 2011;22(1):19–27.
3. Apple DJ, Solomon KD, Tetz MR, Assia EI, Holland EY, Legler UF, Tsai JC, Castaneda VE, Hoggatt JP, Kostick AM. Posterior capsule opacification. Surv Ophthalmol. 1992;37(2):73–116.
4. Apple DJ, Peng Q, Visessook N, Werner L, Pandey SK, Escobar-Gomez M, Ram J, Whiteside SB, Schoderbeck R, Ready EL, et al. Surgical prevention of posterior capsule opacification. Part 1: progress in eliminating this complication of cataract surgery. J Cataract Refract Surg. 2000;26(2):180–7.
5. Hodge WG. Posterior capsule opacification after cataract surgery. Ophthalmology. 1998;105(6):943–4.
6. Spector A. Review: oxidative stress and disease. J. Ocul. Pharmacol. Ther. official journal of the Association for Ocular Pharmacology and Therapeutics. 2000;16(2):193–201.
7. Babizhayev MA, Deyev AI, Linberg LF. Lipid peroxidation as a possible cause of cataract. Mech Ageing Dev. 1988;44(1):69–89.
8. Awasthi S, Srivatava SK, Piper JT, Singhal SS, Chaubey M, Awasthi YC. Curcumin protects against 4-hydroxy-2-trans-nonenal-induced cataract formation in rat lenses. Am J Clin Nutr. 1996;64(5):761–6.
9. Suryanarayana P, Krishnaswamy K, Reddy GB. Effect of curcumin on galactose-induced cataractogenesis in rats. Mol Vis. 2003;9:223–30.
10. Kumar PA, Suryanarayana P, Reddy PY, Reddy GB. Modulation of alpha-crystallin chaperone activity in diabetic rat lens by curcumin. Mol Vis. 2005; 11:561–8.
11. Padmaja S, Raju TN. Antioxidant effect of curcumin in selenium induced cataract of Wistar rats. Indian J Exp Biol. 2004;42(6):601–3.
12. Manikandan R, Thiagarajan R, Beulaja S, Chindhu S, Mariammal K, Sudhandiran G, Arumugam M. Anti-cataractogenic effect of curcumin and aminoguanidine against selenium-induced oxidative stress in the eye lens of Wistar rat pups: an in vitro study using isolated lens. Chem Biol Interact. 2009;181(2):202–9.

13. Doganay S, Borazan M, Iraz M, Cigremis Y. The effect of resveratrol in experimental cataract model formed by sodium selenite. Curr Eye Res. 2006; 31(2):147–53.

14. Pan Q, Liao X, Liu H, Wang Y, Chen Y, Zhao B, Lazartigues E, Yang Y, Ma X. MicroRNA-125a-5p alleviates the deleterious effects of ox-LDL on multiple functions of human brain microvessel endothelial cells. Am. J. Physiol. Cell Physiol. 2017;312(2):C119–30.

15. Tu LY, Bai HH, Cai JY, Deng SP. The mechanism of kaempferol induced apoptosis and inhibited proliferation in human cervical cancer SiHa cell: from macro to nano. Scanning. 2016;38(6):644–53.

16. Liu HZ, Xiao W, Gu YP, Tao YX, Zhang DY, Du H, Shang JH. Polysaccharide from Sepia Esculenta ink and cisplatin inhibit synergistically proliferation and metastasis of triple-negative breast cancer MDA-MB-231 cells. Iranian J. Basic Med. Sci. 2016;19(12):1292–8.

17. Mahmoud AM, Al-Alem U, Ali MM, Bosland MC. Genistein increases estrogen receptor beta expression in prostate cancer via reducing its promoter methylation. J Steroid Biochem Mol Biol. 2015;152:62–75.

18. Doganay S, Turkoz Y, Evereklioglu C, Er H, Bozaran M, Ozerol E. Use of caffeic acid phenethyl ester to prevent sodium-selenite-induced cataract in rat eyes. J Cataract Refract Surg. 2002;28(8):1457–62.

19. Liao JH, Huang YS, Lin YC, Huang FY, Wu SH, Wu TH. Anticataractogenesis mechanisms of Curcumin and a comparison of its degradation products: an in vitro study. J Agric Food Chem. 2016;64(10):2080–6.

20. Bagchi M, Katar M, Maisel H. Effect of exogenous stress on the tissue-cultured mouse lens epithelial cells. J Cell Biochem. 2002;86(2):302–6.

21. Dean DO, Kent CR, Tytell M. Constitutive and inducible heat shock protein 70 immunoreactivity in the normal rat eye. Invest Ophthalmol Vis Sci. 1999; 40(12):2952–62.

22. Spector A. Oxidative stress-induced cataract: mechanism of action. FASEB journal : official publication of the Federation of American Societies for Experimental Biology. 1995;9(12):1173–82.

23. Manikandan R, Beulaja M, Thiagarajan R, Arumugam M. Effect of curcumin on the modulation of alphaA- and alphaB-crystallin and heat shock protein 70 in selenium-induced cataractogenesis in Wistar rat pups. Mol Vis. 2011; 17:388–94.

24. de Jong WW, Hoekman WA, Mulders JW, Bloemendal H. Heat shock response of the rat lens. J Cell Biol. 1986;102(1):104–11.

25. Banh A, Vijayan MM, Sivak JG. Hsp70 in bovine lenses during temperature stress. Mol Vis. 2003;9:323–8.

26. Manikandan R, Thiagarajan R, Beulaja S, Sudhandiran G, Arumugam M. Effect of curcumin on selenite-induced cataractogenesis in Wistar rat pups. Curr Eye Res. 2010;35(2):122–9.

27. Lin D, Barnett M, Grauer L, Robben J, Jewell A, Takemoto L, Takemoto DJ. Expression of superoxide dismutase in whole lens prevents cataract formation. Mol Vis. 2005;11:853–8.

28. Wang K, Spector A. Alpha-crystallin can act as a chaperone under conditions of oxidative stress. Invest Ophthalmol Vis Sci. 1995;36(2):311–21.

29. Cekic S, Zlatanovic G, Cvetkovic T, Petrovic B. Oxidative stress in cataractogenesis. Bosn. J. Basic Med. Sci. 2010;10(3):265–9.

30. Yan H, Harding JJ. Glycation-induced inactivation and loss of antigenicity of catalase and superoxide dismutase. Biochem. J. 1997;328(Pt 2):599–605.

31. Fecondo JV, Augusteyn RC. Superoxide dismutase, catalase and glutathione peroxidase in the human cataractous lens. Exp Eye Res. 1983;36(1):15–23.

32. Vaux DL, Korsmeyer SJ. Cell death in development. Cell. 1999;96(2):245–54.

33. de Iongh RU, Wederell E, Lovicu FJ, McAvoy JW. Transforming growth factor-beta-induced epithelial-mesenchymal transition in the lens: a model for cataract formation. Cells Tissues Organs. 2005;179(1–2):43–55.

34. Medvedovic M, Tomlinson CR, Call MK, Grogg M, Tsonis PA. Gene expression and discovery during lens regeneration in mouse: regulation of epithelial to mesenchymal transition and lens differentiation. Mol Vis. 2006; 12:422–40.

35. Chandler HL, Barden CA, Lu P, Kusewitt DF, Colitz CM. Prevention of posterior capsular opacification through cyclooxygenase-2 inhibition. Mol Vis. 2007;13:677–91.

Clinical results of the open ring PMMA guider assisted capsulorrhexis in cataract surgery

Jee Hye Lee[1], Yong Eun Lee[2] and Choun-Ki Joo[1]* (iD)

Abstract

Background: To compare the results of continuous curvilinear capsulorrhexis(CCC) after application of an open ring-shaped guider compared with a free-hand procedure in eyes with cataracts.

Methods: This study comprised patients undergoing cataract surgery in Seoul St.Mary's Hospital, The Catholic University of Korea. Eyes were grouped depending on the capsulotomy method; CCC was performed by free-hand procedure on 94 eyes (free-hand group), and it was performed under the guidance after introduction of an open ring-shaped guider on consecutive 89 eyes (guided group). Horizontal and vertical diameter, area and circularity of capsulotomy were measured postoperatively at one day, two months and six months. Differences in parameters and the percentage of ideal capsulorrhexis were analyzed between the two groups.

Results: On the first postoperative day, the vertical diameter in the guided group (5.24 ± 0.16 mm) was significantly longer than that of the free-hand group (5.01 ± 0.65 mm, $P = 0.019$). The area of capsulotomy was larger in the guided group (21.55 ± 0.87 mm^2) than that of the free-hand group (20.34 ± 2.96 mm^2, $P < 0.001$). Circularity in the guided group (0.84 ± 0.03), was significantly greater than that of the free-hand group (0.69 ± 0.17, $P = 0.036$). Ideal capsulorrhexis was obtained in 60 eyes (67%) in the free-hand group and 81 eyes (86%) in the guided group.

Conclusions: After introduction of an open ring-shaped guider, CCC became larger and more circular with less anterior capsular contracture. The rate of acquiring ideal capsulorrhexis was higher in the guided group than it was in the free-hand group for six months after surgery.

Keywords: Continuous curvilinear capsulorrhexis(CCC), Open ring-shaped guider for CCC(ORGC), Ideal CCC

Background

Continuous curvilinear capsulorrhexis (CCC) is a standard technique in cataract surgery that is preferable to the can-opener capsulotomy [1]. CCC is essential for the safety of phacoemulsification and intraocular lens (IOL) implantation because it permits safe hydrodissection, cortical cleanup, and IOL centration while preventing posterior capsule opacification (PCO) [2, 3].

Previous studies suggest that the anterior capsulotomy size and circularity are important. If the capsulotomy is too small, fibrosis and hyperopic shift may ensue [4]. If the capsulotomy is too large or asymmetric, the IOL may be adversely affected by tilt, rotation, decentration, or posterior capsular opacification [5].

The ideal capsulorrhexis is a well-centered opening that perfectly overlaps the IOL optic by 360° [6]. This alignment ensures that the IOL contained in the capsular bag is close to the effective lens position (ELP) to avoid an inaccurate IOL power calculation [7]. When the capsular bag is close to the ELP, it prevents optic tilt, decentration, myopic shift, and capsular opacification due to symmetric contractile forces on the capsular bag that cause a shrink-wrap effect. Newer IOLs, including toric-, multifocal- and accommodating IOLs, are more sensitive to accurate positioning and would benefit from more reproducible sizing, shaping, and centration of the anterior capsulotomy.

* Correspondence: ckjoo@catholic.ac.kr
[1]Department of Ophthalmology & Visual Science, Seoul St. Mary's Hospital, The Catholic University of Korea, Seoul, South Korea
Full list of author information is available at the end of the article

Several methods that facilitate CCC completion have been invented. One of the widely used instruments is Wallace's circular corneal marker [8]. But this device provided only a rough guide outside the cornea. To resolve this problem, Suzuki et al. designed a marker that makes a semicircular mark directly on the lens capsule [9]. However, this marker was difficult to manipulate because of its metallic material and fixed semicircular design. The caliper proposed by Tassignon et al. is difficult to insert through a small corneal incision under 3.0 mm [10]. The VERUS ophthalmic caliper (Mile High Ophthalmics, Denver, CO) is a ring-shaped silicone device and has the enhanced lateral stability with micropatterning [11]. Also, Zepto precision pulse capsulotomy (Mynosys, Fremont, CA) which creates a capsulotomy automatically has been introduced and available on the market [12].

Recently, we reported a surgical technique using a new transparent open-ring guider made of PMMA to make a round, precise CCC with less radial tear [13]. Briefly, the open ring-shaped guider for CCC (ORGC, Lucid Co., Seoul, Korea) is a ring-shaped ruler with arc of 10° when opened. The ORGC is 0.125 mm thick with an internal diameter of 5.3 mm and an outer diameter of 5.8 mm (Fig. 1). It acts as a visual guide during the capsulorrhexis.

The purpose of our study was to compare the outcomes of CCC after application of an open ring-shaped guider compared with a free-hand procedure in eyes with cataracts.

Methods

This study was conducted by retrospective chart review from patients who had uneventful phacoemulsification and intraocular lens implantation. All of the surgeries were performed by the same surgeon (C-K.J) between 2012 and 2013 at Seoul St. Mary's Hospital. Written informed consent was obtained from all of the patients before their records were used. The study

complied with the institutional review board regulations at Seoul St. Mary's Hospital (CMC clinical research coordination center, study approval number: KCI2DISE0320), informed consent regulations, and the Declaration of Helsinki.

CCC was performed by free-hand procedure on 94 eyes (free-hand group). After introduction of an open ring-shaped guider, capsulorrhexis was performed under the guidance on consecutive 89 eyes (guided group). Each patient underwent complete ophthalmologic evaluation before surgery. Exclusion criteria included previous ocular surgery, trauma, active ocular disease which would affect post-operative visual acuity, poor pupil dilation, poor red reflex, or known zonule weakness.

The cataract severity was evaluated based on nuclear opacity using the lens opacities classification system (LOCS III). The axial length and K readings were measured using optical biometry (IOL Master, Carl Zeiss Meditec AG, Germany) before surgery. Phacoemulsification was performed under topical anesthesia with 4% lidocaine and 0.5% proparacaine hydrochloride (Alcaine; Alcon Laboratories, USA). A 2.2 mm clear corneal incision was made, and 1.4% sodium hyaluronate (Healon GV®; Advanced Medical Optics, USA) was injected into the anterior chamber. In the guided group, the surgeon picks up one end of the guider with forceps and turns the ORGC clockwise to insert it into the anterior chamber gently. After the guider is placed on the anterior capsule, the surgeon performed CCC along the internal border of the guider. In the free-hand group, without guidance, the surgeon made a round CCC targeted at a 5.3 mm diameter. Then the IOL forceps was used to remove the guider in a counterclockwise fashion through the corneal incision. Inserted IOLs were single-piece, monofocal, aspheric, hydrophobic acrylic lenses with 6 mm optic diameter (total diameter 13 mm) and 5° angulation (EC-1 YH PAL®, Aaren Scientific, Inc., USA).

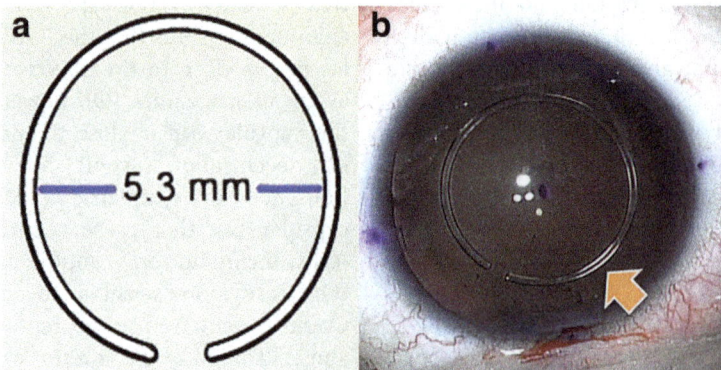

Fig. 1 a Open ring guider for CCC; inflexible polymethyl methacrylate caliper ring with an internal diameter of 5.3 mm. It is easy to insert into the eye because of its open-ring shape. b Open ring-shaped guider for continuous curvilinear capsulorrhexis (ORGC) (arrow) is inserted into the anterior chamber

Digital photographs under retro-illumination were used to analyze the size of capsulotomies. Photographs were taken during surgery, immediately after the CCC procedure, and postoperatively at 1 day, 2 months, and 6 months. Image J (National Institute of Health, Bethesda, MD, USA) was used to measure the diameter, area, and circularity of the images. The diameters of the capsulotomies were measured in relation to the incision site. The horizontal diameter refers to the diameter along the same axis as the incision (if a temporal incision was made, this would be nasal to temporal direction) and the vertical diameter is perpendicular to that axis. Circularity was calculated to determine if the capsulotomy shape was regular according to the following formula:

$$f_{circ} = \frac{4\pi A}{P^2}$$

(A = area, P = perimeter)

A circularity value of 1.0 indicates a perfect circle [14]. The percentage of ideal capsulorrhexis was also determined. Ideal capsulorrhexis is defined by a capsulotomy opening that completely overlaps the edge of the IOL optic at postoperative day one.

All data were analyzed using SPSS software (IBM SPSS Statistics version 19.0, Inc. Chicago, IL, USA). Student t-test and Chi-square test were used to compare the baseline characteristics of two groups. Mann-Whitney tests and Chi-square tests were used to compare the horizontal diameter, vertical diameter, area and circularity of the capsulotomy in the two groups. The significance level was set at $P < 0.05$ in all statistical analyses.

Results

A total of 183 eyes were assessed, with 89 eyes in the guided group and 94 eyes in the free-hand group. Preoperative mean axial length and k reading were 23.98 ± 2.76 mm, 46.56 ± 1.89 D in the free-hand group and 24.16 ± 2.48 mm, 44.16 ± 1.44 D in the guided group. Nuclear opacity grade was 2.98 ± 0.86 in the free-hand group and 3.14 ± 0.93 in the guided group. The differences between the two groups were not statistically significant with regard to age, sex, axial length, mean K reading, and cataract

severity before surgery (Table 1). Patients tolerated the surgery well and there were no intra- or postoperative complications. After 6 months, mean BCVA was LogMAR 0.36 ± 0.25 in free-hand group and LogMAR 0.31 ± 0.29 in guided group ($P = 0.14$).

Table 2 shows the mean and standard deviation values of capsulorrhexis parameters measured at 1 day postoperatively. The capsulotomies were not perfectly round and were slightly different from the intended diameter of 5.3 mm. The vertical diameter in the guided group was significantly longer than that in the free-hand group ($P = 0.019$), but the horizontal diameter was not significantly different across the two groups ($P > 0.05$). As a result, the area of capsulotomy (mm^2) was significantly larger in the guided group ($P < 0.001$). The circularity in the guided group was significantly better than in the free-hand group ($P = 0.036$). The percentage of ideal capsulorrhexis was 67% in the free-hand group and 86% in the guided group, which is statistically significant ($P = 0.011$).

The change of capsulotomy area according to the time course are shown as box plots in Fig. 2. The guided group showed a larger capsulotomy area with little variation than that of the free-hand group. During the first two postoperative months, the circularity decreased significantly in the free-hand group; however, no significant changes in circularity were found in the guided group ($P = 0.047$). Figure 3 shows a case of ideal capsulorrhexis, taken on postoperative day 1, illustrating complete overlap of the edge of the IOL optic.

Discussion

Manually constructing the anterior capsulorrhexis is technically challenging and is recognized as one of the most difficult aspects of cataract surgery to learn [15]. Free-hand capsulorrhexis is complicated by capsular tears in approximately 1% of cases [16]. Methods to improve manual capsulorrhexis using physical or virtual calipers have been developed [8, 10, 17]. However, all of these methods have their limitations. For example, Wallace's capsulotomy diameter mark, a reference ring that projects through the light source of the microscope to the anterior capsule, provides only a rough guidance. They tend to be affected by magnification or distortion

Table 1 Demographics of patients

Demographic	Free-hand group (n = 94)	Guided group (n = 89)
Age (y)	63.80 ± 9.48	64.08 ± 10.75
Sex (M:F)	43:51	41:48
Axial length (mm)	23.98 ± 2.76	24.16 ± 2.48
Inserted IOL	One-piece hydrophobic acrylic lens(EC-1YH PAL®)	
Mean K reading	46.56 ± 1.89	44.16 ± 1.44
Nuclear opacity (NO, LOCS III)	2.98 ± 0.86	3.14 ± 0.93

NO nuclear opalescence, *LOCS* lens opacities classification system

Table 2 Comparison of size, circularity, and rate of ideal capsulorrhexis postoperatively at 1 day

Parameter	Free-hand group	Guided group	P value
Parallel diameter (mm)	5.17 ± 0.40	5.24 ± 0.21	> 0.05*
Perpendicular diameter (mm)	5.01 ± 0.65	5.24 ± 0.16	0.019*
Area of capsulotomy (mm ^{2})	20.34 ± 2.96	21.55 ± 0.87	< 0.001*
Circularity of capsulotomy	0.69 ± 0.17	0.84 ± 0.03	0.036*
Ideal capsulorrhexis (%)	67	86	0.011†

*Mann-Whitney U test
†Chi-square test

caused by the cornea. The ring-shaped caliper proposed by Tassignon et al. can be deformed or damaged during insertion and removal. VERUS ophthalmic caliper has wider width comparing the ORGC which makes difficult to be used in patients with small pupil size.

Recently introduced femtosecond laser technology enables surgeons to create more uniform, accurate, and predictable anterior capsulotomy than that produced by manual capsulorrhexis [5, 16, 18–20]. Despite its perceived benefits, femtosecond laser-assisted cataract surgery is not widely used, even in high-volume refractive centers. This is largely due to the significant financial costs involved in its implementation [21].

Our results suggest that the guider helps a capsulorrhexis to have a good circularity and closer to the target diameter 5.3 mm. Although the horizontal diameter was not significantly different between the two groups, the vertical diameter in the guided group was significantly closer to the target diameter than in the free-hand group. There was a greater degree of variability in the free-hand group, as evidenced by the different standard deviations, for both area and circularity compared to the guided group.

For free-hand capsulorrhexis, the size of the CCC could potentially have a smaller vertical area because

this technique requires an uncomfortable pivot movement of the capsulotomy forceps through the small clear corneal incision site.

The accuracy and circularity of the capsulotomy size created by the guider were better at all time points measured after surgery. The CCC size decreased over time in both groups because of capsular contraction, although it was not statistically significant. Interestingly, the circularity of capsulorrhexis decreased significantly in the first 2 months postoperatively, only in the free-hand group. On the other hand, guided group maintained its circularity for postoperative 6 months.

We also analyzed the rate of ideal capsulorrhexis in two groups. With guider use, the surgeon can choose the exact location of the guider according to the limbus or dilated pupil center. In this study, the surgeon tried to place the guider between the center of limbus and dilated pupil, so the ideal capsulorrhexis rate was higher than free-hand group which was centered to the dilated pupil.

The major advantage of ideal capsulorrhexis is that it provides full control of lens epithelial cell proliferation, preventing posterior capsule opacification (PCO). Although we did not investigate the incidence of after-

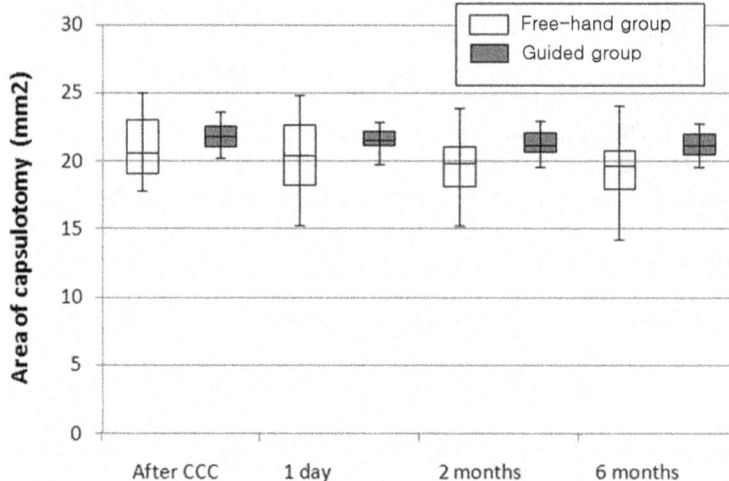

Fig. 2 Area of capsulotomy at different time point: after CCC, postoperative day one, day two and six months. The box is determined by the central mean, the 35th percentile, and the 75th percentile. The whiskers are determined by the 5th and 95th percentiles

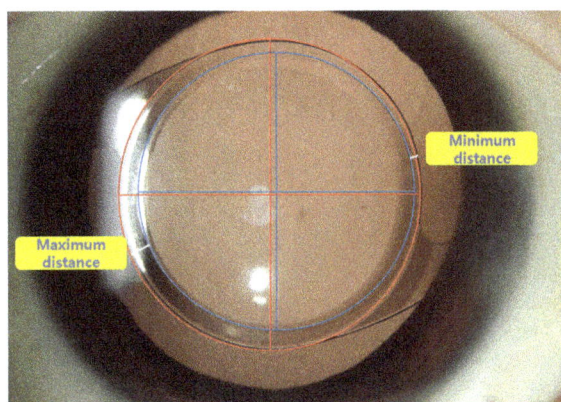
Fig. 3 Maximum and minimum distances between the edge of the capsulotomy and the edge of the IOL optic were calculated to determine capsulotomy- and IOL- overlap

cataract in this study, this technique is expected to reduce after-cataract.

Through evaluation of the maximum and minimum distances between the IOL optic and CCC edge, we found that there were no differences across the two groups. This observation may be because of two reasons. First, the size of CCC is much smaller in the free-hand group. In the free-hand group, both maximum and minimum distances were larger than guided group's distances. Second, if an ideal capsulorrhexis is made in the exact center of the capsular bag, the difference between maximum and minimum distances might be close to zero. These results mean that our capsulorrhexis was not made at real center of the lens capsule. Further study should be performed about the effect of using an ORGC guider on IOL centration.

A limitation of our study is that we analyzed patient charts retrospectively, which could have introduced selection bias. Although we used several IOL types, we selected only one IOL type to control the IOL's influence on the results.

Conclusions
We believe that the open ring-shaped guider for continuous curvilinear capsulorrhexis is a convenient and inexpensive tool that facilitates perfect capsulorrhexis shape and size and optimizes the outcome 6 months after the surgery.

Abbreviations
CCC: Continuous curvilinear capsulorrhexis; ELP: Effective lens position; IOL: Intraocular lens; ORGC: Open ring-shaped guider for CCC; PCO: Posterior capsule opacification

Authors' contributions
CK conceived of and designed the study. YE contributed to the drafting of the manuscript. JH contributed to the critical revision of the manuscript. All authors read and approved the final manuscript.

Competing interests
Dr. Joo is one of the inventors on the patent filed by the Catholic University of Korea covering details in this manuscript but the authors declare that they have no competing interests.

Author details
[1]Department of Ophthalmology & Visual Science, Seoul St. Mary's Hospital, The Catholic University of Korea, Seoul, South Korea. [2]The Ian eye center, Seoul, South Korea.

References
1. Gimbel HV, Neuhann T. Development, advantages, and methods of the continuous circular capsulorrhexis technique. J Cataract Refract Surg. 1990; 16(1):31–7.
2. Assia EI, Apple DJ, Tsai JC, Morgan RC. Mechanism of radial tear formation and extension after anterior capsulectomy. Ophthalmology. 1991;98(4):432–7.
3. Aasuri MK, Kompella VB, Majji AB. Risk factors for and management of dropped nucleus during phacoemulsification. J Cataract Refract Surg. 2001; 27(9):1428–32.
4. Sanders DR, Higginbotham RW, Opatowsky IE, Confino J. Hyperopic shift in refraction associated with implantation of the single-piece Collamer intraocular lens. J Cataract Refract Surg. 2006;32(12):2110–2.
5. Friedman NJ, Palanker DV, Schuele G, Andersen D, Marcellino G, Seibel BS, Batlle J, Feliz R, Talamo JH, Blumenkranz MS, Culbertson WW. Femtosecond laser capsulotomy. J Cataract Refract Surg. 2011;37(7):1189–98.
6. Joo CK, Shin JA, Kim JH. Capsular opening contraction after continuous curvilinear capsulorrhexis and intraocular lens implantation. J Cataract Refract Surg. 1996;22(5):585–90.
7. Cekic O, Batman C. The relationship between capsulorrhexis size and anterior chamber depth relation. Ophthalmic Surg Lasers. 1999;30(3):185–90.
8. Wallace RB 3rd. Capsulotomy diameter mark. J Cataract Refract Surg. 2003; 29(10):1866–8.
9. Suzuki H, Shiwa T, Oharazawa H, Takahashi H. Usefulness of a semicircular capsulotomy marker. J Nippon Med Sch. 2012;79(3):195–7.
10. Tassignon MJ, Rozema JJ, Gobin L. Ring-shaped caliper for better anterior capsulorrhexis sizing and centration. J Cataract Refract Surg. 2006;32(8):1253–5.
11. Kahook MY, Cionni RJ, Taravella MJ, Ang RE, Waite AN, Solomon JD, Uy HS. Continuous curvilinear capsulorrhexis performed with the VERUS ophthalmic caliper. J Refractive Surg. 2016;32(10):654–8.
12. Chang DF. Zepto precision pulse capsulotomy: a new automated and disposable capsulotomy technology. Indian J Ophthalmol. 2017;65(12):1411–4.
13. Lee YE, Joo CK. Open ring-shaped guider for circular continuous curvilinear capsulorrhexis during cataract surgery. J Cataract Refract Surg. 2015;41(7):1349–52.
14. Kranitz K, Takacs A, Mihaltz K, et al. Femtosecond laser capsulotomy and manual continuous curvilinear capsulorrhexis parameters and their effects on intraocular lens centration. J Refract Surg. 2011;27:558–63.
15. Dooley IJ, O'Brien PD. Subjective difficulty of each stage of phacoemulsification cataract surgery performed by basic surgical trainees. J Cataract Refract Surg. 2006;32(4):604–8.
16. Nagy Z, Takacs A, Filkorn T, Sarayba M. Initial clinical evaluation of an intraocular femtosecond laser in cataract surgery. J Refract Surg. 2009;25(12): 1053–60.
17. Dick HB, Pena-Aceves A, Manns M, Krummenauer F. New technology for sizing the continuous curvilinear capsulorrhexis: prospective trial. J Cataract Refract Surg. 2008;34(7):1136–44.
18. Kranitz K, Takacs A, Mihaltz K, Kovács I, Knorz MC, Nagy ZZ. Femtosecond laser capsulotomy and manual continuous curvilinear capsulorrhexis parameters and their effects on intraocular lens centration. J Refract Surg. 2011;27(8):558–63.
19. Nagy ZZ, Kranitz K, Takacs AI, Miháltz K, Kovács I, Knorz MC. Comparison of intraocular lens decentration parameters after femtosecond and manual capsulotomies. J Refract Surg. 2011;27(8):564–9.
20. Kranitz K, Mihaltz K, Sandor GL, Takacs A, Knorz MC, Nagy ZZ. Intraocular lens tilt and decentration measured by Scheimpflug camera following manual or femtosecond laser-created continuous circular capsulotomy. J Refract Surg. 2012;28(4):259–63.
21. Trikha S, Turnbull AM, Morris RJ, Anderson DF, Hossain P. The journey to femtosecond laser-assisted cataract surgery: new beginnings or a false dawn? Eye (Lond). 2013;27(4):461–73.

Effect of number and position of intraocular lens haptics on anterior capsule contraction: a randomized, prospective trial

Mihyun Choi[1], Marjorie Z. Lazo[2], Minji Kang[1], Jeehye Lee[1] and Choun-Ki Joo[1]* (iD)

Abstract

Background: The present study aimed to evaluate the degree of anterior capsule contraction (capsulorhexis contraction) with three different single-piece, hydrophilic acrylic intraocular lenses (IOLs).

Methods: Patients were prospectively randomized to be implanted with one of three types of IOLs during cataract surgery: the Ophtec Precizon (IOL A), the Lucid Korea Microflex (IOL B), and the Carl Zeiss Asphina (IOL C). One week, 2 weeks, and 6 months after surgery, the area of the anterior capsule opening was measured using digital retro-illumination images after dilation of the pupil. The data were then evaluated using POCOman software.

Results: The study included 236 eyes of 202 patients. The area of the anterior capsule opening reduced by 3.53 ± 3.31 mm (17.06% ± 15.99%) between 1 week and 2 months post-operatively in the IOL A group, by 0.62 ± 1.32 mm (2.87% ± 6.03%) in the IOL B group, and by 1.09 ± 1.53 mm (4.72% ± 6.10%) in the IOL C group. The IOL B group showed minimal anterior capsule contraction 2 months after surgery ($p < 0.001$).

Conclusions: IOLs with a four-plate haptic design (IOL B) showed more anterior capsular stability than those with a two-loop plate haptic (IOL A) or two-plate haptic (IOL C) design. The number and position of haptics in a capsular bag may affect anterior capsule contraction. We assume that supporting the zonules evenly may play a role in anterior capsular stability.

Keywords: Anterior capsule contraction syndrome, Anterior capsule of the lens, Capsulorhexis, Intraocular lens, Cataract surgery

Background

Anterior and posterior capsular opacification are still major complications of cataract surgery that occur due to the proliferation, migration, and differentiation of residual lens epithelial cells (LECs) [1, 2]. Contact with the intraocular lens (IOL) optic causes the LECs of the anterior lens capsule to undergo fibrosis, resulting in anterior capsule opacification (ACO) [1, 3]. This may in turn lead to contraction or retraction of the anterior capsule, and ultimately to a reduction in the free optic zone. Furthermore, anterior capsule contraction (ACC) may cause decentration of the IOL optic, as well as tilt of the IOL, and zonular stretching may lead to zonular rupture and subsequent dislocation of the IOL/capsular bag posteriorly [4–6].

The prevalence of posterior capsule opacification (PCO) has decreased due to technological and surgical improvements. Specifically, neodymium:yttrium-aluminum-garnet (Nd:YAG) laser capsulotomy is an effective PCO treatment option [7]. However, treatment can lead to further complications, including cystoid macular edema, IOL subluxation and damage, elevation of intraocular pressure, and retinal detachment [8, 9]. For these reasons, it remains important to prevent PCO. To do so, IOL manufacturers continuously modify IOL designs and materials, and ophthalmic

* Correspondence: ckjoo@catholic.ac.kr
[1]Department of Ophthalmology, College of Medicine, Seoul St. Mary's Hospital, The Catholic University of Korea, 222, Banpo-daero, Seocho-gu, Seoul 06591, Republic of Korea
Full list of author information is available at the end of the article

surgeons refine their surgical techniques to minimize the ACO and PCO risk.

Previous studies have reported that capsular fibrosis occurs 90–180 days after implantation [10], and the degree of ACC has been associated with many predictors, including individual, pathological, and surgical factors [11–13]. For instance, Hayashi et al. reported that the mean percentage reduction in the anterior capsule opening area was significantly greater in eyes with a silicone optic IOL than in eyes with an acrylic optic IOL. The same authors reported that the one-piece acrylic IOL appeared to withstand substantial postoperative capsular shrinkage, and that its optic and haptic design was not associated with ACC [3, 14]. In another study, Hayashi et al. observed no significant difference in ACC occurrence between acrylic IOLs with round-edge optics and those with sharp-edge optics [15]. Conversely, Sacu et al. reported that neither the material nor the haptic design of hydrophobic IOLs affected the occurrence of ACO or ACC [16]. A 2010 study found that greater ACC occurs after hydrophilic IOL implantation than after hydrophobic IOL implantation [17]. However, these studies only evaluated the material and edge type of the optics and the shape of the haptics, not the number and position of the haptics within the capsular bag. ACC occurs when the centripetal force of the anterior capsule opening margin (fibrotic change) differs from the centrifugal force of the capsular zonule [18, 19]. In this regard, to investigate whether the number and position of IOL haptics affected ACC, the present study evaluated the capsulorhexis aperture after implantation of three differently designed IOLs. The study also evaluated the rate of PCO for each IOL.

Methods

Patient recruitment, randomization, and intraocular lenses

This was a prospective, randomized study of patients who were to undergo cataract surgery at Seoul St. Mary's Hospital, Seoul, South Korea, between August 2016 and December 2016. Two-hundred thirty-six eyes of 202 patients were included. The study protocol followed the guidelines of the Declaration of Helsinki. Potential complications were explained to the patients in detail, and written informed consent was obtained before the study began. The inclusion criteria were (1) age over 55 years and under 75, (2) presence of age-related cataract, (3) axial length within the normal range (22–25.5 mm), and (4) dilated pupil larger than 8.0 mm in diameter. The exclusion criteria were histories of (1) ocular disease, (2) intraocular surgery, (3) laser treatment, (4) glaucoma, and (5) severe retinal pathology. Each patient underwent a complete ophthalmologic evaluation before their planned cataract surgery. During this evaluation, the status of the zonule was assessed. Specifically, 2.5% phenylephrine was instilled into the eyes of the patients; 30 min later, slit-lamp biomicroscopy was performed, with attention to lenticular centration or malposition, iris transillumination defects, pseudoexfoliation material on the anterior lens capsule or pupil margin, and phacodonesis (looseness that manifests as jiggling movements on the slit lamp). Patients with the following conditions known to affect ACC were also excluded: (1) retinitis pigmentosa, (2) diabetic retinopathy, (3) myotonic dystrophy, (4) uveitis, (5) old age (over 75 years), and (6) pseudoexfoliation syndrome [20].

Before the study began, a simple randomization was performed using Excel™ software (Version 2010; Microsoft). One of the following three randomly assigned IOLs was implanted during each patient's cataract surgery: Precizon IOL (OPHTEC; IOL A), Microflex IOL (Lucid Korea Inc.; IOL B), and CT Asphina 509 M IOL (Carl Zeiss; IOL C).

These three IOLs have different haptic designs, but all are made of acrylic material and are single-piece lenses (Table 1). All three have a hydrophilic acrylic characteristic, but the Asphina (IOL C) has hydrophobic surface properties. Each IOL has a different number and position of haptics. The Precizon (IOL A) has a two-loop plate haptic at a 180° interval around the optic, while the Microflex (IOL B) has a four-loop plate haptic at 96° and 84° intervals around the optic. The Asphina has a plate-shaped haptic (IOL C) at a 180° interval around the optic.

Surgical technique

The same experienced surgeon (C.K.J.) performed all cataract surgeries using a standard procedure. A 2.2-mm clear corneal incision was made, and 1.4% sodium hyaluronate (Healon GV) was injected into the anterior chamber to maintain the chamber's stability. To allow the area of the anterior capsule opening to be compared between groups after surgery, surgeons had to perform a continuous curvilinear capsulorhexis (CCC) with a specific size during each surgery. For this purpose, the Open Ring-shaped Guide for CCC [21] (ORGC; Lucid Korea, Inc.) was used. This is a ring-shaped ruler with an open 10° arc that guides targeted CCC size. The surgeon selected the size of the ORGC based on the IOL to be used. Specifically, an ORGC diameter of 5.2 mm was used with the Precizon, while a diameter of 5.4 mm was used with the Microflex and Asphina. The ORGC serves as a guideline for CCC, helping the surgeon to make an exact, symmetrical, 360-degree capsulorhexis–IOL overlap. The CCC was carefully performed using capsulorhexis forceps following the internal border of the guide. After thorough hydrodissection, phacoemulsification of the nucleus and aspiration of the residual

Table 1 Characteristics of the three types of acrylic intraocular lenses

	Precizon (IOL A)	Microflex (IOL B)	Asphina (IOL C)
Optic material	hydrophilic acrylic	hydrophilic acrylic	Hydrophilic acrylic (25%) with hydrophobic surface properties
Haptic material	hydrophilic acrylic	hydrophilic acrylic	Hydrophilic acrylic (25%) with hydrophobic surface properties
Optic diameter	6.0 mm	6.0 mm	6.0 mm
Overall length	12.5 mm	10.5 mm	11.0 mm
Haptic design	2 Plate loop design;sharp edged	4 Plate loop design; round-edged	2 Plate design(no loop);sharpedged
Haptic angulation	0°	5°	0°
Optic type	Biconvex	Biconvex	Biconvex
Sphericity	Aspheric	Spheric	Aspheric

cortex were performed using an Infiniti™ gravity-fluidics torsional phacoemulsification machine (Alcon Laboratories, Inc.). The folded IOLs were implanted in the bag with an injector. After IOL implantation, the ophthalmic viscoelastic device (OVD) was carefully removed from the anterior chamber and capsular bag by coaxial irrigation/aspiration (I/A). Specifically, OVD aspiration from the bag was facilitated by tilting the IOL slightly and positioning the I/A tip behind the IOL optic. Anterior capsule polishing, which can affect the residual LECs of the anterior capsule, *was not performed* [22]. There were no surgical complications leading to patient exclusion. Post-operative treatment consisted of prednisolone acetate (1.0%; Pred Forte®) and moxifloxacin (Vigamox®) eye drops 4 times a day for 1 month. Follow-up examinations were performed at 1 week (± 2 days), 2 months (± 14 days), and 6 months (± 1 month).

Assessment of anterior capsule opening size and posterior capsule opacification using standardized retro-illumination photography

At each follow-up visit, LogMAR visual acuity (corrected distance visual acuity [CDVA]) and refraction were tested, and a slit-lamp examination was performed. Patients received 2.5% phenylephrine at least 30 min before the digital retro-illumination images were taken.

The digital retro-illumination images were taken from the anterior and posterior capsule at each visit using a digital camera (Sony HDR-CX300) mounted on a modified Zeiss 30 slit lamp with an external light and flash light source [7]. The operator measured the area of the anterior capsule opening by analyzing the image of digital retro-illumination using POCOman software [23]; Fig. 1). PCO area and severity were also measured in the retro-illumination images using POCOman software. All measurements were repeated three times and performed by a single experienced technician. The average measurement was used in the statistical analysis. POCOman was introduced in 2004 as an objective and repeatable method that uses retro-illumination images to quantify PCO area and severity, as well as the area of the anterior capsule opening. Since the diameters of IOL optics were the same in each group, the actual area of the anterior capsule opening was calculated in proportion to the optic size. The POCOman software measures the area of the anterior capsule opening by the operator setting the opening area scale; this is done subjectively. The software can also analyze PCO by texture analysis to derive the percentage area and severity of PCO in a semiobjective manner by allowing the user to define the PCO within the automatically calculated image.

Statistical analysis

Statistical analysis was performed using IBM SPSS Statistics ver. 24.0 (IBM SPSS Statistics for Windows, Version 24.0., Armonk, NY, USA). Paired t-tests and Mann–Whitney U tests were used for pairwise comparisons. The Kruskal–Wallis test and one-way ANOVA were used to compare the three IOLs. All data were expressed as mean ± standard deviation. A *p*-value of less than 0.05 was considered statistically significant.

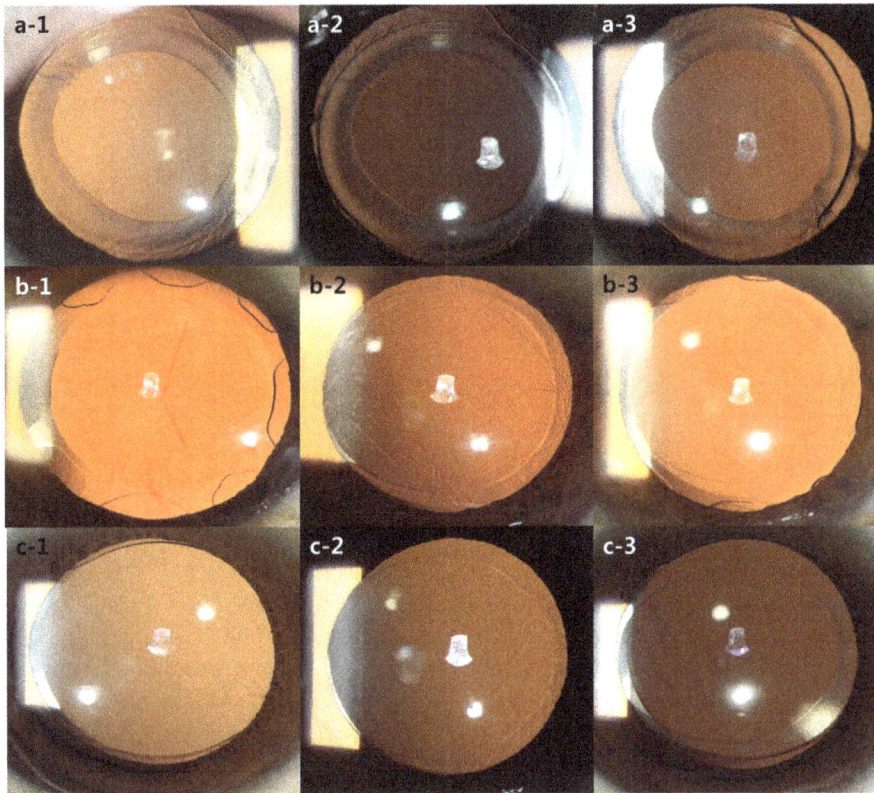

Fig. 1 Digital retro-illumination images of implanted (**a**) two-loop plate-haptic IOL, (**b**) 4-loop plate-haptic IOL, (**c**) plate-haptic IOL, at 1 week (1), 2 months (2) and 6 months (3) after surgery. (IOL = intraocular lens)

Results

Two hundred thirty-six eyes of 202 patients were included in the study. The mean age of the patients at surgery was 65.43 years ±9.41 (SD) (range 55–75 years). One-hundred thirty-eight (58.5%) were women and 98 (41.5%) were men. At the 6-month follow-up examination, 186 patients (92.1%) were examined. No adverse event occurred during this study.

Seventy-six eyes (67 patients) were implanted with the IOL A, 78 eyes (66 patients) with the IOL B, and 82 eyes (69 patients) with the IOL C. The average patient age in each group was 64.79 ± 10.22 years, 66.61 ± 9.2 years, and 64.40 ± 10.29 years, respectively ($p = 0.533$). The characteristics of the patients in the three groups are presented in Table 2. No significant differences were found regarding male-to-female ratio ($p = 0.106$), ratio of left to right eyes ($p = 0.301$), or axial length ($p = 0.438$) between the groups. Patients with diabetic retinopathy were excluded. However, those with diabetes alone, which is also known to affect ACC, were not excluded. Regardless, there was no significant difference in the proportion of diabetic patients among the three groups ($p = 0.643$; Table 2). The target diopter was calculated using the SRK-T formula as the predicted refractive error after cataract surgery. The IOL C group showed a more

myopic target than the IOL A and IOL B groups (-0.66 ± 0.91, -0.61 ± 0.84, and -1.01 ± 1.09, respectively; $p = 0.016$). However, there was no significant difference in the diopter of the implanted IOL ($p = 0.208$; Table 2).

Visual acuity

The pre-operative mean CDVA values were 0.25 ± 0.22 in the IOL A group, 0.34 ± 0.37 in the IOL B group, and 0.29 ± 0.33 in the IOL C group ($p = 0.17$). At the 2-month follow-up, the values were 0.05 ± 0.1, 0.05 ± 0.08, and 0.05 ± 0.14 ($p = 0.36$), respectively. At the 6-month follow-up, they were 0.04 ± 0.08, 0.06 ± 0.08, and 0.07 ± 0.11 ($p = 0.19$), respectively. There was no significant difference in CDVA among the three groups either before or after surgery.

Anterior capsule opening size

Table 3 summarizes the mean ($\pm$ SD) area of the anterior capsule opening in each of the three groups. The mean areas of the anterior capsule opening at 1 week, 2 weeks, and 6 months after surgery were 20.69 ± 1.50 mm^2, 17.17 ± 3.23 mm^2, and 17.01 ± 3.11 mm^2, respectively, in the IOL A group; 21.70 ± 0.86 mm^2, 21.07 ± 1.50 mm^2, and 20.48 ± 1.09 mm^2, respectively, in the IOL B group; and 21.43 ± 1.09 mm^2, 20.34 ± 1.60 mm^2, and $19.86 \pm$

Table 2 Patient Characteristics

	Precizon (IOL A)	Microflex (IOL B)	Asphina (IOL C)	P-value[a]
Eyes (n)	76	78	82	
Mean age(yr)	64.79 ± 10.22	66.61 ± 9.2	64.40 ± 10.29	0.533
Male/Female	28/48	34/44	36/46	0.106
DM (n)	5	7	7	0.643
OD/OS	33/42	36/42	48/34	0.301
Axial length (mm)	23.46 ± 3.11	23.92 ± 2.81	23.22 ± 2.75	0.438
CDVA before surgery(log MAR)	0.2 ± 0.16	0.35 ± 0.24	0.28 ± 0.31	0.501
Diopter (D) (range)	19.73 ± 3.53 (7.0 ~ 25.5)	20.26 ± 1.99 (16.5 ~ 25.0)	18.7 ± 3.51 (8.0~ 24.5)	0.208
Target (D) (range)	−0.66 ± 0.91 (− 2.78~ 0.04)	−0.61 ± 0.84 (− 2.99~ 0.06)	− 1.01 ± 1.09 (− 2.98 ~ 0.0)	0.016

[a] Kruskal Wallis test

1.58 mm^2, respectively, in IOL C group. The area of the anterior capsule opening decreased in all three groups from 1 week to 2 months after surgery, and from 2 months to 6 months after surgery. However, the reduction was greatest in the first 2 months after surgery (Fig. 2). The area of the anterior capsule opening after 1 week was smallest in the IOL A group, but no significant difference was observed among the three groups in this regard ($p = 0.068$; Table 3). At 2 and 6 months after surgery, the area of the anterior capsule opening was significantly smaller in eyes with an IOL A than in eyes with an IOL B or IOL C ($p < 0.001$). The reduction in the area of the anterior capsule opening between 1 week and 2 months after surgery was $3.53 ± 3.31$ mm^2 ($17.06\% ± 15.99\%$) in the IOL A group, $0.62 ± 1.32$ mm^2 ($2.87\% ± 6.03\%$) in the IOL B group, and $1.09 ± 1.53$ mm^2 ($4.72\% ± 6.10\%$) in the IOL C group (Fig. 3). Thus, the IOL A showed the lowest anterior capsular stability after surgery, while the IOL B showed the greatest anterior capsular stability ($p < 0.001$; Table 3). In addition, with regards to the ACC that occurred between 1 week and 2 months after surgery, the IOL B showed a smaller reduction in the area of the anterior capsular opening than did the IOL C, though this was not significant ($p = 0.093$; Fig. 3).

Posterior capsule opacification

Table 4 shows the calculated values for PCO in the three groups using the POCOman software. The mean PCO scores at 1 week, 2 months, and 6 months postoperatively were $6.51 ± 3.34$, $11.09 ± 6.81$, and $13.75 ± 7.49$, respectively in the IOL A group; $6.16 ± 3.87$, $27.23 ± 14.90$, and $43.26 ± 12.79$, respectively, in the IOL B group; and $6.46 ± 5.69$, $15.56 ± 8.18$, and $16.98 ± 5.48$, respectively, in the IOL C group. There was no difference among the three groups 1 week after surgery. However, at 2 and 6 months after surgery, PCO was more pronounced in the IOL B group ($p < 0.001$).

Change in refractive error

Table 5 shows the spherical equivalent (SE) value in each group at the post-operative follow up. As shown in Table 2, the pre-operative refractive targets differed among the three groups, and the IOL C group had a more myopic target. The mean changes in SE values between 1 week and 6 months after surgery were $0.18 ± 0.49$ in the IOL A group, $− 0.01 ± 0.84$ in the IOL B group, and $0.12 ± 0.47$ in the IOL C group ($p = 0.046$). The refractive outcome was most stable in the IOL B group. The IOL A and IOL B groups showed a hyperopic shift, and there was no significant difference between two groups ($p = 0.872$).

Discussion

The anterior capsule opening decreases in area when LECs remaining on the IOL surface proliferate and undergo fibrous metaplasia upon contacting the IOL [24]. The imbalance between the centripetal force

Table 3 Mean Area of the Anterior Capsule Opening and Change after Cataract Surgery at Postoperative Follow Up (mm2)

Follow up	1wk	2 m		6 m	
	CCC size	CCC size	Change from 1 week(percentage)	CCC size	Change from 2 months(percentage)
Precizon (IOL A)	20.69 ± 1.50	17.17 ± 3.23	−3.53 ± 3.31 (17.06 ± 15.99%)	17.01 ± 3.11	− 0.16 ± 1.31 (0.64 ± 6.21%)
Microflex (IOL B)	21.70 ± 0.86	21.07 ± 1.50	− 0.62 ± 1.32 (2.87 ± 6.03%)	20.48 ± 1.09	− 0.60 ± 1.51 (2.47 ± 6.91%)
Asphina (IOL C)	21.43 ± 1.09	20.34 ± 1.60	−1.09 ± 1.53 (4.72 ± 6.10%)	19.86 ± 1.58	−0.48 ± 1.19 (2.12 ± 5.25%)
P-value†	0.068	< 0.001	< 0.001	< 0.001	0.170

†one-way ANOVA

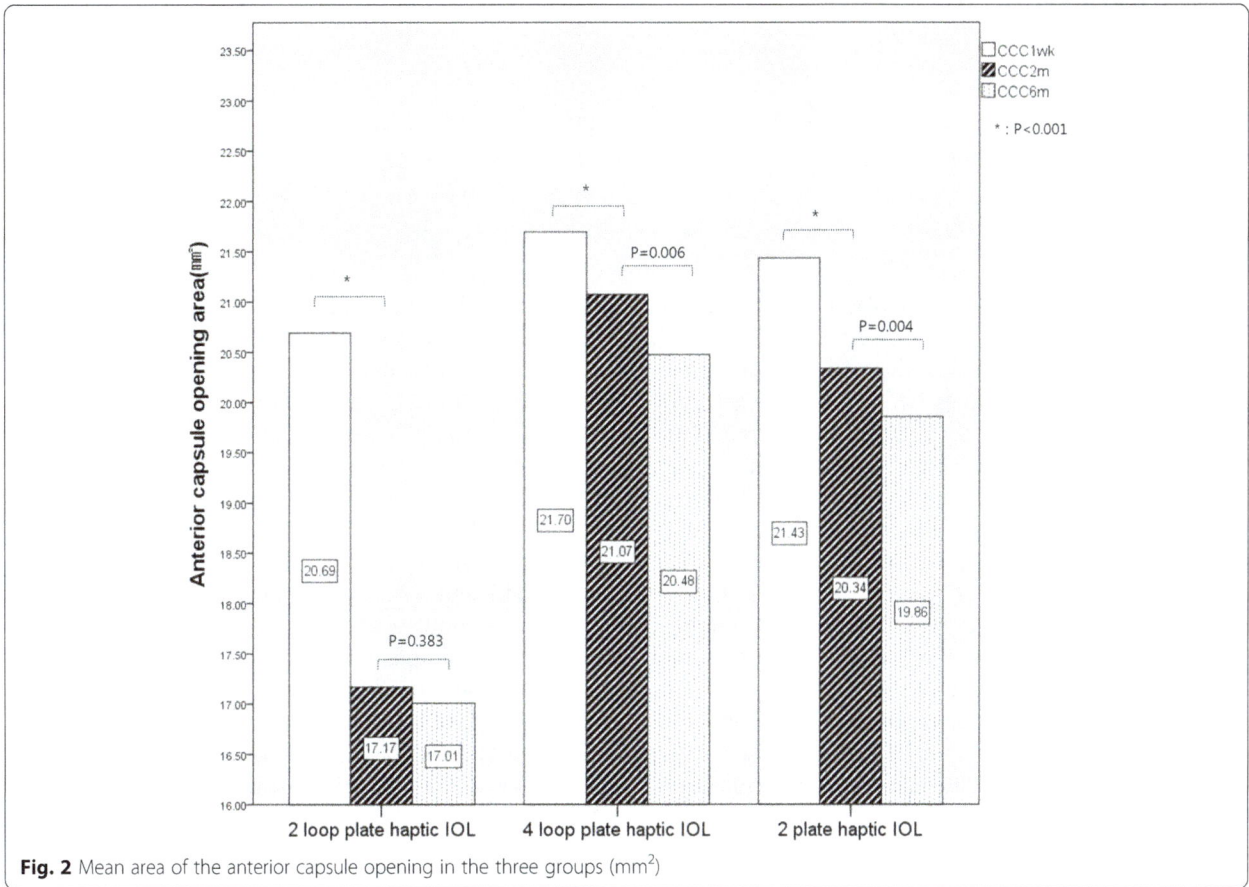

Fig. 2 Mean area of the anterior capsule opening in the three groups (mm²)

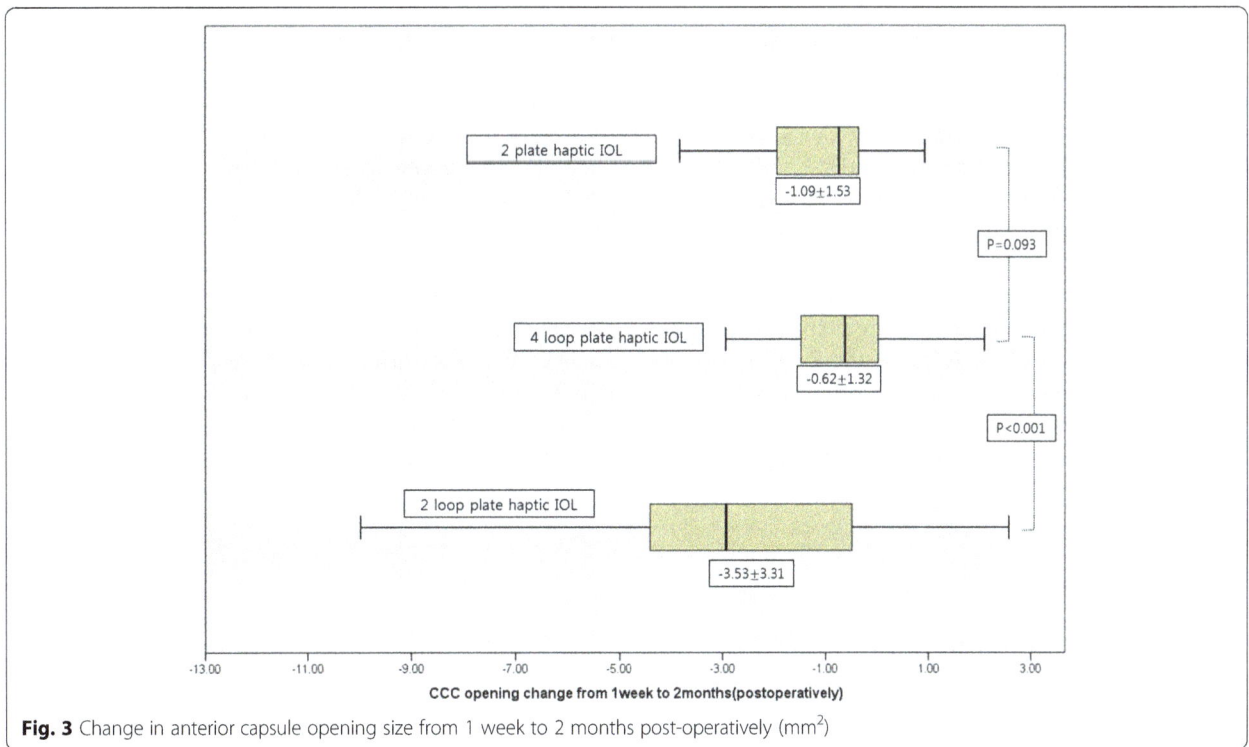

Fig. 3 Change in anterior capsule opening size from 1 week to 2 months post-operatively (mm²)

Table 4 Mean PCO score and grade at Postoperative Follow Up

Follow up	1wk		2 m		6 m	
	Score	Grade	Score	Grade	Score	Grade
Precizon (IOL A)	6.51 ± 3.34	0.06 ± 0.03	11.09 ± 6.81	0.12 ± 0.09	13.75 ± 7.49	0.15 ± 0.10
Microflex (IOL B)	6.16 ± 3.87	0.06 ± 0.04	27.23 ± 14.90	0.36 ± 0.25	43.26 ± 12.79	0.64 ± 0.32
Asphina (IOL C)	6.46 ± 5.69	0.06 ± 0.06	15.56 ± 8.18	0.16 ± 0.10	16.98 ± 5.48	0.19 ± 0.06
P-value	0.409	0.362	< 0.001	< 0.001	< 0.001	< 0.001

exerted by the LECs (fibrous metaplasia) and the centrifugal force exerted by the zonule induces ACC [18, 19]. Several reports have revealed that ACC occurs more frequently when using silicone IOLs or hydrogel optic IOLs, and that plate-haptic IOLs or thin optic IOLs cause less capsule dilation of the centrifugal haptics [3, 11, 12, 17, 25]. The association between silicone or hydrogel optics and ACC may be due to a weaker adhesion of the optic materials to the lens capsule. Weak adhesion may allow space for active proliferation of LECs and synthesis of extracellular matrix. In contrast, because acrylic optics adhere firmly to the capsule, and remnant LECs are only minimally exposed to various cytokines in the aqueous humor, fibrosis and contraction of the anterior capsule would be reduced when using such IOLs [3, 26, 27]. With specific regard to acrylic IOLs, hydrophilic varieties have shown significantly more frequent ACC than hydrophobic varieties [17], perhaps because hydrophobic IOL material prevents attachment of migrating epithelial cells on the optic and haptic surfaces. Other studies have reported that there is no difference between round- and sharp-edge optic design in terms of ACC prevalence [15, 16]. In summary, studies to date have indicated that optic surface contact with the anterior capsule, the convexity of the optic, and the edges of the optic and haptic, may play a role in LEC growth and anterior capsule contracture.

In the present study, we focused on the number and position of the haptics in the circular zonule, because ACO may be caused by LEC growth, whereas ACC is accelerated by the difference between the centripetal force of the anterior capsule opening margin (fibrotic force) and the centrifugal force of the capsular zonule [18, 19]. Some studies have suggested that four-haptic IOLs confer a large surface that contacts the posterior capsule, as well as more accurate IOL fixation within the

capsular bag, leading to constant tension on the zonular fibers [28]. However, later studies reported that the number and design of haptics were not strongly associated with ACC [27]. In the present study, we noticed that it is not only the number of haptics that matters in ACC, but also the range of the zonule that is supported by the haptics and the location of the haptics within the zonule. In other words, there is little difference, in terms of IOL and zonule support, between an IOL with four haptics and one with two haptics if the haptics cannot support the zonule evenly. Since the zonule system has a circular configuration (360°) along the crystalline lens, force imbalances can occur with any number of haptics, unless the haptics are evenly positioned to support the whole zonule. In the case of the previously reported four-haptic IOLs (Akreos MI-60, BAUSCH+LOMB), even though there are four haptics, the interval between the haptics is larger in the long axis of the IOL, and the overall shape of the IOL is a rectangle with a long and short axis [27]. Thus, even if an IOL has four haptics, it may still provide less zonule support than an IOL with two haptics at a 180° interval, because the haptics are not evenly distributed in the zonule but only located on the long axis of the IOL. However, in the present study, IOL B (Microflex)—the four-loop haptic IOL—had four haptics, with an angle of around 90° between them (96° and 84°), suggesting that four haptics can support a circular zonule uniformly in 360°.

This is more pronounced when compared to the IOL A (2-loop plate haptic IOL). The two-loop plate haptic IOL had maintained a good anterior capsule opening 1 week after surgery, but this had decreased by 17.06% ± 15.99% after 2 months. In contrast, the four-loop plate haptic IOL only showed a 2.87% ± 6.03% decrease between 1 week and 2 months after surgery. In the comparison of the retro-illumination images (Fig. 1), the

Table 5 Mean Refractive Outcomes (SE) at Postoperative Follow Up

Follow up	1wk	2 m	6 m	Refractive change (1 week to 6 months)
Precizon (IOL A)	−0.70 ± 1.02	−0.49 ± 1.03	−0.50 ± 1.11	0.18 ± 0.49
Microflex (IOL B)	−0.52 ± 1.01	−0.49 ± 1.06	−0.52 ± 0.98	−0.01 ± 0.84
Asphina (IOL C)	−0.80 ± 1.27	−0.73 ± 1.34	−0.65 ± 1.28	0.12 ± 0.47
P-value				0.046

SE spherical equivalent

four-loop plate haptic IOL (b-1, b-2, b-3) showed a relatively circular anterior capsule opening after surgery, whereas the openings in the two-loop plate haptic IOL (a-1, a-2, a-3) and the two-plate haptic IOL (c-1, c-2, c-3) groups seemed to become elliptical over time. In particular, capsulorhexis margins appeared relatively stable where haptics were located. Where there were no haptics, the opening seemed to change to a narrower elliptical shape. Thus, it may be that the haptic does not support the zonule evenly and induces ACC. Furthermore, the IOL B group with the least ACC showed minimal change in SE value after surgery, suggesting that the haptic support also affects the position of the capsular bag, as well as the effective lens position (ELP).

Most commercially available IOLs are manufactured to be foldable within an injector to allow micro-incision cataract surgery (MICS). For this reason, IOLs are rectangular, and haptics are positioned at both ends of the long axis so that the IOL can be made smaller when folded. However, due to its shape, the four-loop plate haptic IOL used in the present study cannot be inserted into a 2.2-mm injector. Thus, an incision diameter of 2.4 mm was required to allow insertion. Although this may increase astigmatism after surgery, it may also decrease the risk of ACC and should be considered.

The four-loop plate haptic IOL maintained the anterior capsule opening well. However, the PCO generation was much more severe than in the other IOL groups. The Microflex—the four-loop plate haptic IOL used in the study—has a round-edged optic design, while the other IOLs have sharp-edged optic designs; this design is likely the reason for the severe PCO. Furthermore, the four-loop plate haptic of IOL B confers a large contact area with the capsule. This may allow space for active proliferation of LECs.

ACC can induce IOL decentration or tilting, and even IOL dislocation, whereas PCO, which is more common, can easily be treated using Nd:YAG laser posterior capsulotomy. Anterior capsule opening contraction can also be treated with Nd:YAG laser, and, more recently, femtosecond lasers have been used to enlarge a contracted capsule [29, 30]. Nonetheless, in severe cases, IOL tilting may not be improved after enlargement of the anterior capsule opening. Thus, it is important that surgeons prevent ACC as much as possible during surgery. Although many previous investigations have addressed ACC in Asian patients, the present study may be of significance as it is the first published study to focus on the location of IOL haptics and capsular bag stability. Many of the IOLs currently used may not provide an even force to support the zonule, because the haptics are not located at equal intervals around the haptics.

This study had several limitations. Firstly, the IOLs we compared differed in other characteristics besides haptic number and position. In particular, IOL B had a round optic edge that differed from those of the other IOLs. Therefore, it is problematic simply to compare the PCO among the three IOLs. Nonetheless, the present study may open a new line of inquiry based on the observation of previous studies that the optic edge does not affect the ACC [15, 16]. Secondly, although all known additional risk factors for ACC were excluded from the present study, there may be intrinsic factors other than IOL haptics that affect ACC. Thirdly, the ORGC size differed in the IOL A group (5.2 mm—0.2 mm smaller than in the IOL B and IOL C groups); this might have affected ACC. However, a previous paper reported that CCC size did not have a significant effect on capsule contraction. [31] Furthermore, significant ACC difference has been observed between groups with a CCC size of < 4.5 mm and those with a CCC size of 4.6–6.0 mm. [31] Based on previous reports, an ORGC difference of 0.2 mm would not have a significant effect on ACC.

In conclusion, the present study demonstrated that contraction of the anterior capsule opening was much smaller with the four-loop plate haptic IOL than with the two-loop plate haptic and two-plate haptic IOLs. ACC and IOL decentration vary depending on the location of the haptics within the capsular bag. Based on these results, when zonular weakness is detected during surgery, or when a condition that increases zonular instability is detected in the pre-operative examination, clinicians should consider selecting a four-plate haptic IOL that can support the zonule evenly.

Further studies, both clinical and histological, will be necessary to further elucidate the role of haptic position in ACC. It will also be necessary to develop a new IOL design that has evenly distributed haptics positioned within the capsular bag so that the rates of ACC and PCO can be lowered.

Conclusions

The number and position of haptics within the capsular bag may affect ACC. We assume that supporting the zonules evenly plays a role in anterior capsular stability.

Abbreviations

ACC: Anterior capsule contraction; ACO: Anterior capsule opacification; CCC: Continuous curvilinear capsulorhexis; CDVA: Corrected distance visual acuity; I/A: Irrigation/aspiration; IOL: Intraocular lens; LECs: Residual lens epithelial cells; MICS: Micro-incision cataract surgery; Nd:YAG: Neodymium:yttrium-aluminum-garnet; ORGC: Open Ring-shaped Guide for continuous curvilinear capsulorhexis; OVD: Ophthalmic viscoelastic devices; PCO: Posterior capsule opacification

Acknowledgements

We would like to thank all the patients for kindly participating in the study.

Funding

None.

Authors' contributions

Conception and design of the study: MC, CKJ. Acquisition of data: MC, MK, JL. Analysis and interpretation of data: MC, MK, JL. Drafting of the manuscript: MC, MZL. Critically revision of the manuscript: MC, MZL, CKJ. All authors read and approved the final version to be published.

Competing interests

The authors declare that they have no competing interests.

Author details

[1]Department of Ophthalmology, College of Medicine, Seoul St. Mary's Hospital, The Catholic University of Korea, 222, Banpo-daero, Seocho-gu, Seoul 06591, Republic of Korea. [2]Catholic Institute for Visual Science, College of Medicine, Seoul St. Mary's Hospital, The Catholic University of Korea, Seoul, Republic of Korea.

References

1. Nguyen CL, Francis IC. Mechanical anterior lens capsule polishing under viscoelastic during phacoemulsification cataract surgery. Clin Exp Ophthalmol. 2017;45:654–6.
2. Shah SK, Praveen MR, Kaul A, Vasavada AR, Shah GD, Nihalani BR. Impact of anterior capsule polishing on anterior capsule opacification after cataract surgery: a randomized clinical trial. Eye (Lond). 2009;23:1702–6.
3. Hayashi K, Hayashi H. Intraocular lens factors that may affect anterior capsule contraction. Ophthalmology. 2005;112:286–92.
4. Ohmi S. Decentration associated with asymmetric capsular shrinkage and intraocular lens size. J Cataract Refract Surg. 1993;19:640–3.
5. Kim MH, Chung TY, Chung ES. Long-term efficacy and rotational stability of AcrySof toric intraocular lens implantation in cataract surgery. Korean J Ophthalmol. 2010;24:207–12.
6. Swiątek B, Michalska-Małecka K, Dorecka M, Romaniuk D, Romaniuk W. Results of the AcrySof Toric intraocular lenses implantation. Med Sci Monit. 2012;18:PI1–4.
7. Leydolt C, Schartmüller D, Schwarzenbacher L, Schranz M, Schriefl S, Menapace R. Comparison of posterior capsule opacification development with 2 single-piece intraocular lens types. J Cataract Refract Surg. 2017;43: 774–80.
8. Ernest PH. Posterior capsule opacification and neodymium: YAG capsulotomy rates with AcrySof acrylic and PhacoFlex II silicone intraocular lenses. J Cataract Refract Surg. 2003;29:1546–50.
9. Wesolosky JD, Tennant M, Rudnisky CJ. Rate of retinal tear and detachment after neodymium:YAG capsulotomy. J Cataract Refract Surg. 2017;43:923–8.
10. Tognetto D, Toto L, Sanguinetti G, Cecchini P, Vattovani O, Filacorda S, et al. Lens epithelial cell reaction after implantation of different intraocular lens materials: two-year results of a randomized prospective trial. Ophthalmology. 2003;110:1935–41.
11. Kato S, Suzuki T, Hayashi Y, Numaga J, Hattori T, Yuguchi T, et al. Risk factors for contraction of the anterior capsule opening after cataract surgery. J Cataract Refract Surg. 2002;28:109–12.
12. Cochener B, Jacq PL, Colin J. Capsule contraction after continuous curvilinear capsulorhexis: poly(methyl methacrylate) versus silicone intraocular lenses. J Cataract Refract Surg. 1999;25:1362–9.
13. Hirnschall N, Nishi Y, Crnej A, Koshy J, Gangwani V, Maurino V, et al. Capsular bag stability and posterior capsule opacification of a plate-haptic design microincision cataract surgery intraocular lens: 3-year results of a randomised trial. Br J Ophthalmol. 2013;97:1565–8.
14. Hayashi K, Hayashi H, Nakao F, Hayashi F. Reduction in the area of the anterior capsule opening after polymethylmethacrylate, silicone, and soft acrylic intraocular lens implantation. Am J Ophthalmol. 1997;123:441–7.
15. Hayashi K, Hayashi H. Comparison of the stability of 1-piece and 3-piece acrylic intraocular lenses in the lens capsule. J Cataract Refract Surg. 2005;31:337–42.
16. Sacu S, Menapace R, Findl O. Effect of optic material and haptic design on anterior capsule opacification and capsulorrhexis contraction. Am J Ophthalmol. 2006;141:488–93.
17. Tsinopoulos IT, Tsaousis KT, Kymionis GD, Symeonidis C, Grentzelos MA, Diakonis VF, et al. Comparison of anterior capsule contraction between hydrophobic and hydrophilic intraocular lens models. Graefes Arch Clin Exp Ophthalmol. 2010;248:1155–8.
18. Weiblinger RP. Review of the clinical literature on the use of the Nd:YAG laser for posterior capsulotomy. J Cataract Refract Surg. 1986;12:162–70.
19. Spalton DJ. Posterior capsular opacification after cataract surgery. Eye (Lond). 1999;13(Pt 3b):489–92.
20. Chomańska U, Kraśnicki P, Proniewska-Skretek E, Mariak Z. Anterior capsule contraction syndrome after cataract phacoemulsification surgery. Klin Ocz. 2010;112:243–6.
21. Lee YE, Joo CK. Open ring-shaped guider for circular continuous curvilinear capsulorhexis during cataract surgery. J Cataract Refract Surg. 2015;41:1349–52.
22. Gao Y, Dang GF, Wang X, Duan L, Wu XY. Influences of anterior capsule polishing on effective lens position after cataract surgery: a randomized controlled trial. Int J Clin Exp Med. 2015;8:13769–75.
23. Bender L, Spalton DJ, Uyanonvara B, Boyce J, Heatley C, Jose R, et al. POCOman: new system for quantifying posterior capsule opacification. J Cataract Refract Surg. 2004;30:2058–63.
24. Nishi O, Nishi K. Intraocular lens encapsulation by shrinkage of the capsulorhexis opening. J Cataract Refract Surg. 1993;19:544–5.
25. Dahlhauser KF, Wroblewski KJ, Mader TH. Anterior capsule contraction with foldable silicone intraocular lenses. J Cataract Refract Surg. 1998;24:1216–9.
26. Nagata T, Minakata A, Watanabe I. Adhesiveness of AcrySof to a collagen film. J Cataract Refract Surg. 1998;24:367–70.
27. Kim SY, Yang JW, Lee YC, Kim SY. Effect of haptic material and number of intraocular lens on anterior capsule contraction after cataract surgery. Korean J Ophthalmol. 2013;27:7–11.
28. Mingels A, Koch J, Lommatzsch A, Pauleikhoff D, Heiligenhaus A. Comparison of two acrylic intraocular lenses with different haptic designs in patients with combined phacoemulsification and pars plana vitrectomy. Eye (Lond). 2007;21:1379–83.
29. Deokule SP, Mukherjee SS, Chew CK. Neodymium:YAG laser anterior capsulotomy for capsular contraction syndrome. Ophthalmic Surg Lasers Imaging. 2006;37:99–105.
30. Schweitzer C, Tellouck L, Gaboriau T, Leger F. Anterior capsule contraction treated by femtosecond laser capsulotomy. J Refract Surg. 2015;31:202–4.
31. Joo CK, Shin JA, Kim JH. Capsular opening contraction after continuous curvilinear capsulorhexis and intraocular lens implantation. J Cataract Refract Surg. 1996;22:585–90.

Ocular biometric characteristics of cataract patients in western China

Qing Huang, Yongzhi Huang, Qu Luo and Wei Fan[*]

Abstract

Background: We aimed to measure ocular biometric characteristics in older cataract patients from western China.

Methods: Ocular biometry records were retrospectively analyzed for 6933 patients with cataracts (6933 eyes) at least 50 years old who were treated at West China Hospital of Sichuan University.

Results: Partial coherence laser interferometry gave the following population averages: axial length (AL), 24.32 ± 2.42 mm; anterior chamber depth (ACD), 3.08 ± 0.47 mm; keratometric power (K), 44.23 ± 1.66 diopters; and corneal astigmatism (CA), 1.00 ± 0.92 diopters. The percentage of individuals with AL > 26.5 mm was 13.66%, while the percentage with CA > 1.0 diopters was 35.54%. Mean AL and ACD showed a trend of decrease with increasing age ($P < 0.001$). AL correlated positively with ACD (Spearman coefficient, 0.542) and CA (0.111), but negatively with K (-0.411) (all $P < 0.01$). K also correlated negatively with ACD (-0.078, $P < 0.01$).

Conclusions: These results show, for the first time, that older cataract patients from western China have similar ocular biometric characteristics as other populations. The high prevalence of severe axial myopia warrants further investigation.

Keywords: Axial length, Anterior chamber depth, Keratometric power, Corneal astigmatism, Myopia, IOL master

Background

Cataract surgery is the most commonly performed surgical procedure worldwide. Advances in surgical instruments and intraocular lens design have increased the expectations of surgeons and patients for satisfactory postoperative refractive results. To achieve this goal, accurate biometric measurements are crucial. The ocular biometric characteristics of a population, including axial length (AL), anterior chamber depth (ACD), keratometric power (K) and corneal astigmatism (CA), are important to know in order to help engineers design intraocular lenses and to help surgeons select the most appropriate lenses for patients. Partial coherence laser interferometry is used most frequently in the clinic to determine these parameters, and it is routinely used to calculate lens implant power for cataract surgery [1, 2].

Studies have described ocular biometric characteristics of various populations [3–12], including several from China [10–12]. To our knowledge, the values of ocular biometry parameters have never been published for

populations from western China. The present work provides the first hospital-based population study of ocular biometric characteristics of cataract patients 50 yr. and older from western China.

Methods

Medical records were retrospectively reviewed for a consecutive series of patients aged 50 years and older with cataracts treated at West China Hospital of Sichuan University (Chengdu, China) from November, 2011 to August, 2014. Patients who lived outside western China or who underwent photorefractive surgery were excluded, as were patients with retinal detachment, eye trauma, eyeball atrophy, or severe cataracts that could not be analyzed using the IOL Master device. The study was carried out in accordance with the Declaration of Helsinki. The study protocol was approved by the Ethics Committee of the West China Hospital of Sichuan University (2016–324), and procedures were performed in accordance with relevant guidelines and regulations.

Ocular biometry was performed using the IOL Master system (IOL Master 500, Carl Zeiss Meditec AG, Jena,

* Correspondence: fanwei55@yahoo.com
Department of Ophthalmology, West China Hospital of Sichuan University, Sichuan Province, Chengdu, China

Germany), which uses signals from the tear film and retinal pigment epithelium to measure AL. AL measurements were performed a minimum of five times in each eye, the AL was obtained from the composite mean value of five measurements. ACD was defined as the distance from the anterior corneal surface to the anterior lens surface, and it was measured a minimum of five times. Minimal K (K1) and maximal K (K2) were determined at the maximal and minimal radii of curvature, and the two values were averaged to obtain K. Keratometric measurements were also taken three times. CA was calculated as the absolute difference between K values at the two meridians. We classified astigmatism as "with-the-rule" (WTR) when the steep meridian on the corneal surface was 60–120 degrees, or "against-the-rule" (ATR) when the steep meridian was 0–30 degrees or 150–180 degrees [10, 13]. Other cases of astigmatism were classified as oblique. Since biometric characteristics were similar within pairs of eyes [3], the right or left eye of each patient was randomly selected for all analyses. Similar results were obtained when data from only the right eyes of all patients were used (data not shown).

Statistical analyses were performed using SPSS 19.0 (IBM, USA). Only patients with complete data were included in analyses. Normality of data was tested for all variables using the Kolmogorov-Smirnov (K-S) test, which was taken to indicate skewed distribution if $P < 0.05$. Differences between two groups were assessed for significance using the t test if data were normally distributed, and the Mann-Whitney U test otherwise. Differences among more than two groups were assessed using analysis of variance (ANOVA) followed by the least-squares difference post-hoc test when data were normally distributed. When data were skewed, differences were assessed using the Kruskal-Wallis test. Severe axial myopia was defined as AL longer than 26.5 mm in this study. Differences between groups in the percentage of severe axial myopia were assessed using the Pearson chi-squared test. Possible correlations between biometric parameters were assessed using Spearman's correlation coefficient, while possible associations among AL, ACD, K and CA were assessed using polynomial regression. The threshold of significance was defined as $P < 0.05$.

Results
The final study population included 6933 cataract patients from western China (3311 men, 3622 women) ranging in age from 50 to 98 years. The population was divided into four age groups: 50–59 yr., 17.73% of the total population, mean age 55.40 ± 2.98 yr.; 60–69 yr., 35.41%, 64.68 ± 2.92 yr.; 70–79 yr., 34.50%, 74.12 ± 2.78 yr.; and 80+ yr., 12.36%, 83.22 ± 3.84 yr.

Population distribution of ocular biometry characteristics
Figure 1 shows the distribution of ocular biometric characteristics across the entire study population. The AL distribution (mean, 24.32 ± 2.42 mm) was positively skewed (1.914) and peaked, with kurtosis of 3.963 (K-S test, $P < 0.001$). The ACD distribution (mean, 3.08 ± 0.47 mm) was normal (K-S test, $P = 0.097$). The K distribution (mean, 44.23 ± 1.66 diopters [D]) was negatively skewed (– 0.29), with kurtosis of 3.611 (K-S test, $P < 0.001$). The CA distribution (mean, 1.00 ± 0.92 D) was skewed towards the right (5.485) and strongly peaked, with kurtosis of 73.32 (K-S test, $P < 0.001$).

Distribution of ocular biometry characteristics by sex
Table 1 shows ocular biometry characteristics stratified by sex. Mean AL was significantly longer in men (24.79 ± 2.48 mm) than in women (23.88 ± 2.27 mm, $P < 0.001$), and ACD was deeper in men (3.16 ± 0.47 vs 3.01 ± 0.47 mm, $P < 0.001$). Conversely, mean K was significantly greater in women (44.56 ± 1.61 vs 43.87 ± 1.65 D, $P < 0.001$). Mean CA was similar between men and women (0.99 ± 0.84 vs 1.0 ± 0.99 D, $P = 0.398$).

Distribution of ocular biometry characteristics by age
Mean AL and ACD showed a trend of decrease with increasing age (both $P < 0.001$; Table 2, Figs. 2 and 3). While CA varied significantly between some age groups ($P < 0.001$; Table 2, Fig. 4), there were no differences between others (age group 50–59 and 60–69, $P = 0.143$; group 50–59 and 70–79, $P = 0.091$), suggesting there was no trend change with age. The percentage of patients with AL > 26.5 mm also showed a trend of decrease with increasing age ($P < 0.001$, Table 3). The percentage was 13.66% across the entire population (Table 3), and it rose to 21.72% in the youngest patient group (50–59 years). Furthermore, 9.29% of all patients had AL > 28 mm (Table 4). In addition, it was noted that, in the group of patients with AL > 26.5 mm, male accounted for 58.82% (Table 3).

Corneal astigmatism: Severity, type and variation with age
Corneal astigmatism was less than 0.5 D in 26.94% of eyes, 0.5–1.0 D in 37.52%, 1.0–2.0 D in 27.03%, 2.0–3.0 D in 5.76%, and > 3.0 D in 2.75% (Fig. 5). It was WTR in 34.76% of eyes, ATR in 44.09%, and oblique in 21.15%. The distributions of astigmatism axes varied significantly with age ($P < 0.001$, Fig. 6). The percentage of patients with WTR astigmatism decreased with age, while the percentage with ATR astigmatism increased with age.

Correlations between ocular biometric characteristics
AL correlated positively with ACD (Spearman coefficient, 0.542) and with CA (0.111), but negatively with K

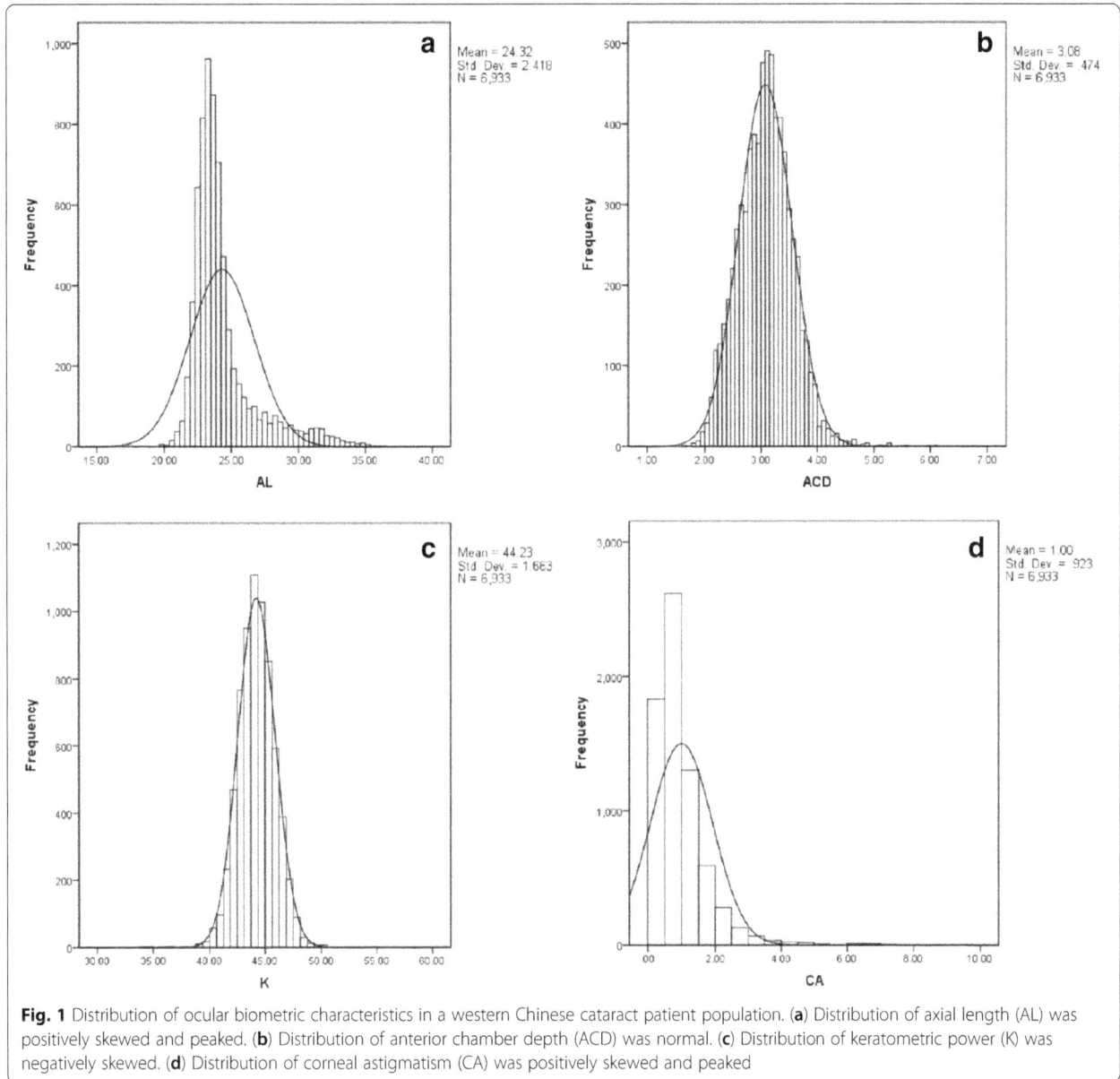

Fig. 1 Distribution of ocular biometric characteristics in a western Chinese cataract patient population. (**a**) Distribution of axial length (AL) was positively skewed and peaked. (**b**) Distribution of anterior chamber depth (ACD) was normal. (**c**) Distribution of keratometric power (K) was negatively skewed. (**d**) Distribution of corneal astigmatism (CA) was positively skewed and peaked

Table 1 Ocular biometric characteristics of western Chinese adult cataract patients, stratified by sex

Gender	AL (mm)	ACD (mm)	K (D)	CA (D)
Male (n = 3311)	24.79 ± 2.48	3.16 ± 0.47	43.87 ± 1.65	0.99 ± 0.84
Female (n = 3622)	23.88 ± 2.27	3.01 ± 0.47	44.56 ± 1.61	1.0 ± 0.99
Total (n = 6933)	24.32 ± 2.42	3.08 ± 0.47	44.23 ± 1.66	1.0 ± 0.92
P[a]	< 0.001[b]	< 0.001[c]	< 0.001[b]	0.398[b]

[a]Difference between males and females
[b]Mann-Whitney U-test
[c]t test

(− 0.411) (all $P < 0.01$; Table 5). K correlated negatively with ACD (− 0.078, $P < 0.01$) and positively with CA (0. 054, $P < 0.01$). ACD correlated negatively with CA (− 0. 003, $P = 0.79$). ACD showed an increasing trend when AL fell below 29.9 mm (Fig. 7a), while K showed a decreasing trend when AL fell below 28.6 mm (Fig. 7b). CA increased with AL (Fig. 7c).

Discussion

Few studies have focused on large populations of Chinese cataract patients, especially from western China. This study aimed to describe a hospital-based distribution of ocular biometric parameters in western Chinese cataract patients. As most patients came from Sichuan which is the most heavily populated province in western China, the

Table 2 Distribution of ocular biometric parameters by age group and sex

Age & sex	N	AL (mm)	ACD (mm)	K (D)	CA (D)
50–59 yr					
Male	535	25.4 ± 3.07	3.33 ± 0.44	43.66 ± 1.76	0.96 ± 0.88
Female	694	24.53 ± 2.98	3.21 ± 0.44	44.37 ± 1.83	1.0 ± 1.18
Total	1229	24.91 ± 3.05	3.26 ± 0.45	44.06 ± 1.83	0.98 ± 1.06
60–69 yr					
Male	1095	25.13 ± 2.68	3.25 ± 0.44	43.96 ± 1.55	0.95 ± 0.85
Female	1360	23.92 ± 2.29	3.06 ± 0.45	44.66 ± 1.53	0.91 ± 0.89
Total	2455	24.46 ± 2.54	3.14 ± 0.46	44.31 ± 1.58	0.93 ± 0.88
70–79 yr					
Male	1183	24.49 ± 2.12	3.09 ± 0.46	44.01 ± 1.5	0.98 ± 0.79
Female	1209	23.62 ± 1.87	2.92 ± 0.45	44.65 ± 1.69	1.04 ± 0.99
Total	2392	24.05 ± 2.04	3.0 ± 0.46	44.28 ± 1.61	1.0 ± 0.9
> 80 yr					
Male	498	24.12 ± 1.76	2.94 ± 0.45	43.87 ± 1.65	1.17 ± 0.88
Female	359	23.36 ± 1.44	2.76 ± 0.43	44.56 ± 1.61	1.2 ± 0.9
Total	857	23.81 ± 1.67	2.86 ± 0.45	44.23 ± 1.61	1.18 ± 0.89
P[a]		< 0.001	< 0.001	0.004	< 0.001

[a]Difference between age groups

results may be representative, to some extent, of the larger population of western China. In addition to providing a rich description of ocular characteristics to serve as a reference for future work, we found a high prevalence of severe axial myopia, particularly in relatively younger patients, which merits further study.

The AL distribution in our population showed positive skew and significant kurtosis, similar to that observed in a healthy Caucasian population [4], but different from that observed in healthy Singaporean Malays [9]. Mean AL was shorter in our population (24.32 ± 2.42 mm) than in cataract patients from eastern China (24.86 ± 2.72 mm) [14]. The possible explanation may be that

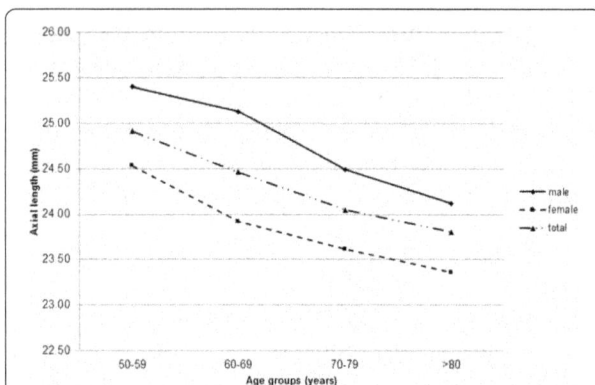

Fig. 3 Distribution of anterior chamber depth across the four age groups of the cataract population. Mean anterior chamber depth showed a decreasing trend with age

the previous study in eastern China [14] included patients aged 18–95 years old; their participants aged 18–49 yr. had longer AL than older participants, making their mean AL longer than ours. At the same time, mean AL was longer in our patients than in cataract patients from southern China (24.07 ± 2.14 mm) [10] and in healthy individuals from southern China (23.48 mm) [15], Europe (23.43 ± 1.51 mm) [5], Latin America (23.38 mm) [6], and other parts of Asia (23.13 ± 1.15 mm [7], 23.13 ± 1.00 mm [8] and 23.55 mm [9]). One likely explanation for these differences between our study and others is ethnicity of Sichuan, which is one of the provinces with most populous ethnic groups of Han Chinese. Another explanation is the relatively high proportion of our cataract patients with severe axial myopia, often defined as AL > 26.5 mm [16, 17]. Our hospital attracts many such patients from Sichuan and other neighbor provinces in western China. Indeed, the proportion of severely axial myopic eyes in our study (13.66%), especially among those aged 50–59 years (21.72%), was higher than in a study of

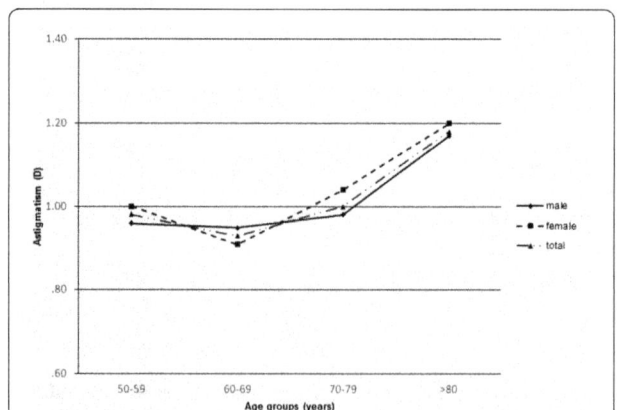

Fig. 2 Distribution of axial length across the four age groups of the cataract population. Mean axial length showed a decreasing trend with age

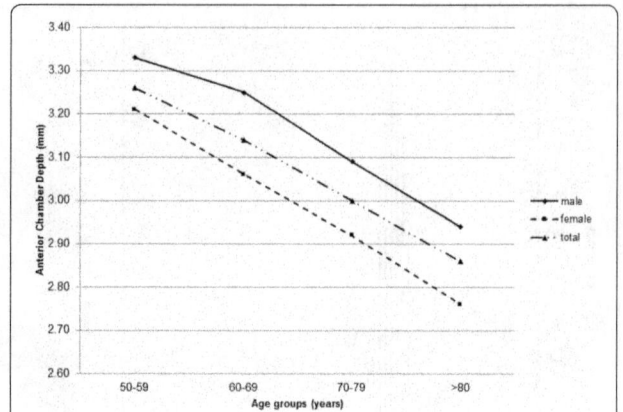

Fig. 4 Distribution of corneal astigmatism across the four age groups of the cataract population. Mean corneal astigmatism did not vary with age

Table 3 Percentages of cataract patients with axial length > 26.5 mm in each age group

Age (yr)	n1[a]	n2[b]	n1/n2 (%)	Nm[d]	Nf[e]	Nm/n1 (%)
50-59	267	1229	21.72	140	127	52.43
60-69	381	2455	15.52	230	151	60.37
70-79	249	2392	10.41	153	96	61.45
> 80	50	857	5.83	34	16	68.0
Total	947	6933	13.66	557	390	58.82
p[c]			< 0.001			

[a]no. with axial length > 26.5 mm in this age group
[b]Total N in this age group
[c]Difference between age groups
[d]No. of male with axial length > 26.5 mm in this age group
[e]No. of female with axial length > 26.5 mm in this age group

cataract patients from southern China (11.9%) [10]. These results may suggest that patients with severe axial myopia tend to develop cataracts at a younger age and therefore require earlier cataract surgery [10, 18]. In any event, our results are consistent with numerous reports of high global prevalence of myopia. In East Asian countries, this prevalence may reach 70–80% [11, 12, 19, 20], with prevalence of severe myopia ranging from 8.4% to 38% [11, 21, 22]. In Western countries, prevalence of myopia ranges from 25% to 40% [23, 24].

AL in our population showed a gender bias: mean AL was longer in men (24.79 ± 2.48 mm) than in women (23.88 ± 2.27 mm). This echoes findings from studies of cataract populations in the US [25], among Singaporean Chinese [26], and among Chinese from the southern part of the mainland [10, 13]. Our result also echoes findings from studies of healthy eyes in Chinese from the southern part of the mainland [15], Latin Americans [6] and Icelanders [27]. The AL difference between men and women in our study (0.91 mm) was longer than that in the previous studies. This may be caused by the relatively high proportion of male patients with severe axial myopia (58.82% in male vs 41.18% in female). In addition, many cross-sectional studies showed body height was positively correlated with AL, men had taller stature than women, and the association between male

Table 4 Distribution of anterior chamber depth (ACD) across patient subgroups with different axial lengths (AL)

AL (mm)	N (%)	ACD (mm)
< 22	348 (5.02)	2.6 ± 0.41
22–25	5069 (73.11)	3.01 ± 0.43
25–28	872 (12.58)	3.38 ± 0.4
> 28	644 (9.29)	3.51 ± 0.41
Total	6933	3.08 ± 0.47
p[a]		< 0.001

[a]Difference between groups

gender and longer AL may reflect the difference in stature between the sexes [3, 28–30].

We found that AL showed a trend of decrease with increasing age, as reported in cross-sectional studies from the UK [31, 32], US [33], and southern China [10]. Studies of Singaporeans suggest that this association may reflect that younger generations are generally taller, so it may be a cohort effect associated with improved nutrition [3, 34]. Other studies have proposed that the reduction of AL in the adult eye may serve as an emmetropizing mechanism, correlating with the increase in refractory power [3, 31]. Another possible explanation, at least in our study, is that younger cataract patients are more likely to have axial myopia. Because of the cross-sectional nature of our study, our comparison of different age groups is confounded with generational effects, so prospective studies are needed to determine why AL decreases with age.

ACD showed normal distribution in our population, with greater depth occurring in male patients and younger patients. This is consistent with findings from other studies [8, 9, 13, 15, 26]. This variation of ACD with sex has been attributed to differences in stature, particularly height, between men and women [4, 26]. The variation of ACD with age has been attributed to age-related lens thickening [10, 33], which may shift the iris forward, making the anterior chamber shallower [6]. Our finding of shallower ACD in older women is consistent with the higher prevalence of angle-closure glaucoma in this population [35]. The reported ability of cataract surgery to significantly deepen the anterior chamber [36] implies that older women with cataracts may benefit from earlier surgery [13]. Unfortunately, we could not verify whether cataract surgery deepened the anterior chamber in our population because the IOL Master system does not measure lens thickness or other relative ocular characteristics. Further study is needed to address this question directly.

The K distribution in our population was skewed. K did not clearly increase with age, in contrast to other studies [37, 38], and K was greater in women than men, similar to other studies [5, 9]. Greater mean K in women indicates higher corneal refractory power, which may be an emmetropizing mechanism to compensate for shorter AL.

CA did not increase or decrease with age as other studies [13, 37, 39, 40]. Consistent with the idea that many cataract patients suffer from corneal astigmatism, 35.54% of eyes in our population had CA > 1.0 D, with similarly high proportions reported in Spain (34.8%) [40] and Japan (36.4%) [41]. These results highlight the importance of astigmatism correction during cataract surgery. Toric intraocular lenses can correct corneal astigmatism of 0.7–8.4 D during cataract surgery [40], and such lenses are now widely used in China. Our

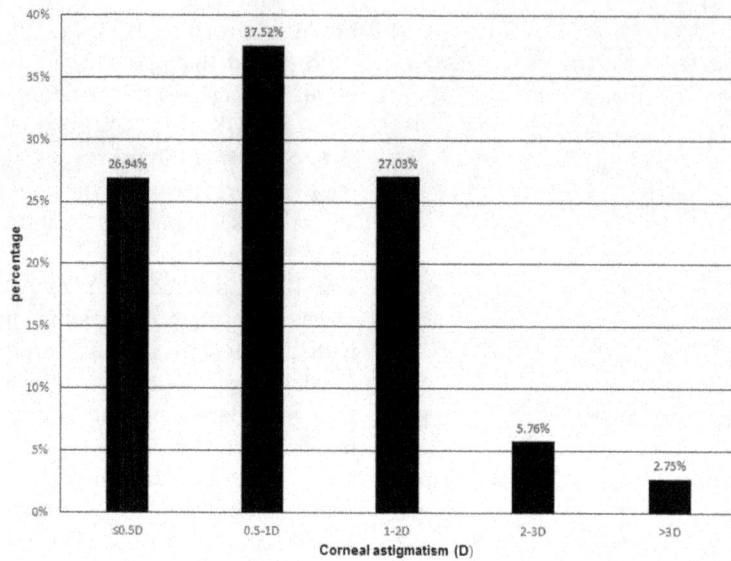

Fig. 5 Distribution of corneal astigmatism (in diopters, D) across the entire cataract population

results, together with those from other populations, may be of interest to hospitals and lens manufacturers.

Prevalence of WTR corneal astigmatism decreased with increasing age, while prevalence of ATR corneal astigmatism rose. Other studies have reported a similar age-related change in astigmatism axis [10, 13, 42]. This change has been attributed to extraocular muscle tension, visual feedback, corneal tissue degeneration, reduction in eyelid pressure and effects of intraocular pressure on corneal curvature [43]. These findings may help ophthalmologists take into account the effects of aging on the age-related change of astigmatism axis when selecting toric lenses.

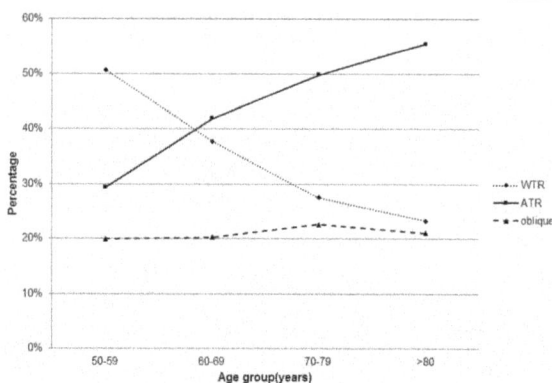

Fig. 6 Distribution of corneal astigmatism axes across the four age groups of the cataract population. Across all age groups, the prevalence of oblique astigmatism was lower than that of with-the-rule (WTR) or against-the-rule (ATR) astigmatism. The prevalence of WTR astigmatism showed a decreasing trend with age, whereas the prevalence of ATR astigmatism showed an increasing trend with age

AL in our population correlated positively with ACD, as reported in other work [10, 15, 44], while it correlated negatively with K, as reported previously [10, 14, 15, 45]. The positive correlation with ACD may reflect a tendency of shorter eyes to have smaller anterior chambers. The negative correlation with K may reflect a tendency of shorter eyes to have steeper corneas and longer eyes to have flatter corneas [45], suggesting an emmetropic mechanism.

While the present study appears to be the first description of ocular biometric characteristics in such a large population of cataract surgery candidates from western China, we cannot exclude selection bias because ours is a hospital-based population from a single medical center. This is particularly important to keep in mind when speculating about the reasons for the high prevalence of severe axial myopia in our patients, particularly younger ones. The fact that we examined 6933 patients suggests that our findings may be relevant to the broader population of individuals with cataracts in western China, although the IOL Master system can fail in 36–38% of patients with dense or posterior

Table 5 Pairwise correlations among axial length (AL), anterior chamber depth (ACD), keratometric power (K) and corneal astigmatism (CA)

	ACD (mm)	K (D)	CA (D)
AL (mm)	0.542[a]	− 0.411[a]	0.111[a]
ACD (mm)	–	− 0.078[a]	− 0.003[b]
K (D)	–	–	0.054[a]

[a]a < 0.01
[b]P = 0.79

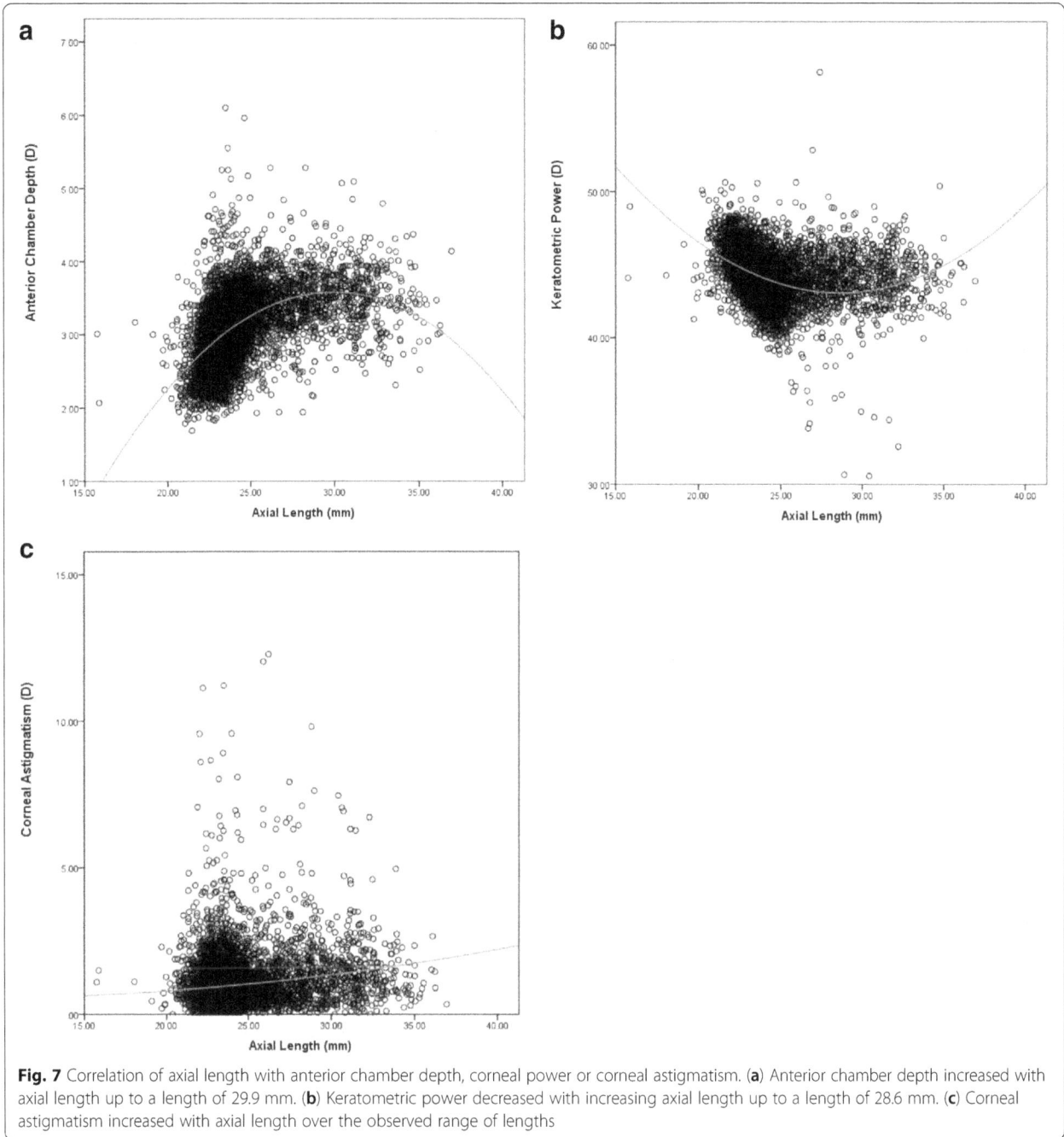

Fig. 7 Correlation of axial length with anterior chamber depth, corneal power or corneal astigmatism. (**a**) Anterior chamber depth increased with axial length up to a length of 29.9 mm. (**b**) Keratometric power decreased with increasing axial length up to a length of 28.6 mm. (**c**) Corneal astigmatism increased with axial length over the observed range of lengths

subcapsular cataracts [46, 47], and we excluded patients with severe cataracts. In addition, the retrospective nature of our study means that some relevant biometric parameters were not measured, limiting the analyses that we could perform. For example, cataract grading scale was unavailable for many patients in this retrospective study, and this parameter can influence ocular biometric characteristics [6, 48].

Conclusion
This study provides data on ocular biometric parameters and their relationships in a large, representative population of cataract patients at least 50 years old from western China. The present work helps expand the reference database on ocular biometric characteristics of Asian cataract populations. It also highlights the need for further studies into the factors that may contribute to the high prevalence of severe axial myopia.

Abbreviations

ACD: Anterior chamber depth; AL: Axial length; ATR: Against-the-rule; CA: Corneal astigmatism; K: Keratometric power; K1: Minimal keratometric power; K2: Maximal keratometric power; WTR: With-the-rule

Acknowledgments

The authors thank ophthalmology technicians at West China Hospital for providing ocular biometric data, as well as Professor Jan Dietrich Reinhardt (Sichuan University) for helping revise the manuscript.

Authors' contributions

WF conceived, designed and coordinated the study. QH analyzed and interpreted the data, and drafted the manuscript. YH helped prepare the data. QL participated in statistical analysis. All authors read and approved the final manuscript.

Competing interests

The authors declare that they have no competing interests.

References

1. Hill W, Angeles R, Otani T. Evaluation of a new IOLMaster algorithm to measure axial length. J Cataract Refract Surg. 2008;34:920–4.
2. Suto C, Sato C, Shimamura E, Toshida H, Ichikawa K, Hori S. Influence of the signal-to-noise ratio on the accuracy of IOLMaster measurements. J Cataract Refract Surg. 2007;33:2062–6.
3. Wong TY, Foster PJ, Johnson GJ, Klein BE, Seah SK. The relationship between ocular dimensions and refraction with adult stature: the Tanjong Pagar survey. Invest Ophthalmol Vis Sci. 2001;42:1237–42.
4. Fotedar R, Wang JJ, Burlutsky G, Morgan IG, Rose K, Wong TY, Mitchell P. Distribution of axial length and ocular biometry measured using partial coherence laser interferometry (IOL master) in an older white population. Ophthalmology. 2010;117:417–23.
5. Hoffmann PC, Hutz WW. Analysis of biometry and prevalence data for corneal astigmatism in 23,239 eyes. J Cataract Refract Surg. 2010;36:1479^{-85}.
6. Shufelt C, Fraser-Bell S, Ying-Lai M, Torres M, Varma R. Refractive error, ocular biometry, and lens opalescence in an adult population: the Los Angeles Latino eye study. Invest Ophthalmol Vis Sci. 2005;46:4450–60.
7. Wickremasinghe S, Foster PJ, Uranchimeg D, Lee PS, Devereux JG, Alsbirk PH, Machin D, Johnson GJ, Baasanhu J. Ocular biometry and refraction in Mongolian adults. Invest Ophthalmol Vis Sci. 2004;45:776–83.
8. Mallen EA, Gammoh Y, Al-Bdour M, Sayegh FN. Refractive error and ocular biometry in Jordanian adults. Ophthalmic Physiol Opt. 2005;25:302–9.
9. Lim LS, Saw SM, Jeganathan VS, Tay WT, Aung T, Tong L, Mitchell P, Wong TY. Distribution and determinants of ocular biometric parameters in an Asian population: the Singapore Malay eye study. Invest Ophthalmol Vis Sci. 2010;51:103–9.
10. Cui Y, Meng Q, Guo H, Zeng J, Zhang H, Zhang G, Huang Y, Lan J. Biometry and corneal astigmatism in cataract surgery candidates from southern China. J Cataract Refract Surg. 2014;40:1661–9.
11. Sun J, Zhou J, Zhao P, Lian J, Zhu H, Zhou Y, Sun Y, Wang Y, Zhao L, Wei Y, et al. High prevalence of myopia and high myopia in 5060 Chinese university students in shanghai. Invest Ophthalmol Vis Sci. 2012;53:7504^{-9}.
12. He M, Zeng J, Liu Y, Xu J, Pokharel GP, Ellwein LB. Refractive error and visual impairment in urban children in southern China. Invest Ophthalmol Vis Sci. 2004;45:793–9.
13. Chen W, Zuo C, Chen C, Su J, Luo L, Congdon N, Liu Y. Prevalence of corneal astigmatism before cataract surgery in Chinese patients. J Cataract Refract Surg. 2013;39:188–92.
14. Feng CL, Yuan YZ, Yuan F, Ma XP, Zhang CH. Biometric analysis of adult cataract surgery candidates in shanghai, China. West Indian Med J. 2015;
15. Chen H, Lin H, Lin Z, Chen J, Chen W. Distribution of axial length, anterior chamber depth, and corneal curvature in an aged population in South China. BMC Ophthalmol. 2016;16:47.
16. Hayashi M, Ito Y, Takahashi A, Kawano K, Terasaki H. Scleral thickness in highly myopic eyes measured by enhanced depth imaging optical coherence tomography. Eye (Lond). 2013;27:410–7.
17. Liang IC, Shimada N, Tanaka Y, Nagaoka N, Moriyama M, Yoshida T, Ohno-Matsui K. Comparison of clinical features in highly myopic eyes with and without a dome-shaped macula. Ophthalmology. 2015;122:1591–600.
18. Hoffer KJ. Axial dimension of the human cataractous lens. Arch Ophthalmol. 1993;111:914–8.
19. Lin LL, Shih YF, Hsiao CK, Chen CJ. Prevalence of myopia in Taiwanese schoolchildren: 1983 to 2000. Ann Acad Med Singap. 2004;33:27–33.
20. Lee JH, Jee D, Kwon JW, Lee WK. Prevalence and risk factors for myopia in a rural Korean population. Invest Ophthalmol Vis Sci. 2013;54:5466–71.
21. Pan CW, Zheng YF, Anuar AR, Chew M, Gazzard G, Aung T, Cheng CY, Wong TY, Saw SM. Prevalence of refractive errors in a multiethnic Asian population: the Singapore epidemiology of eye disease study. Invest Ophthalmol Vis Sci. 2013;54:2590–8.
22. Wang TJ, Chiang TH, Wang TH, Lin LL, Shih YF. Changes of the ocular refraction among freshmen in National Taiwan University between 1988 and 2005. Eye (Lond). 2009;23:1168–9.
23. Kempen JH, Mitchell P, Lee KE, Tielsch JM, Broman AT, Taylor HR, Ikram MK, Congdon NG, O'Colmain BJ. The prevalence of refractive errors among adults in the United States, Western Europe, and Australia. Arch Ophthalmol. 2004;122:495–505.
24. Vitale S, Sperduto RD, Ferris FL, 3rd. Increased prevalence of myopia in the United States between 1971-1972 and 1999-2004. Arch Ophthalmol 2009; 127:1632–1639.
25. Jivrajka R, Shammas MC, Boenzi T, Swearingen M, Shammas HJ. Variability of axial length, anterior chamber depth, and lens thickness in the cataractous eye. J Cataract Refract Surg. 2008;34:289–94.
26. Wong TY, Foster PJ, Ng TP, Tielsch JM, Johnson GJ, Seah SK. Variations in ocular biometry in an adult Chinese population in Singapore: the Tanjong Pagar survey. Invest Ophthalmol Vis Sci. 2001;42:73–80.
27. Olsen T, Arnarsson A, Sasaki H, Sasaki K, Jonasson F. On the ocular refractive components: the Reykjavik eye study. Acta Ophthalmol Scand. 2007;85:361–6.
28. Nangia V, Jonas JB, Matin A, Kulkarni M, Sinha A, Gupta R. Body height and ocular dimensions in the adult population in rural Central India. The Central India eye and medical study. Graefes Arch Clin Exp Ophthalmol. 2010;248: 1657–66.
29. Nangia V, Jonas JB, Sinha A, Matin A, Kulkarni M, Panda-Jonas S. Ocular axial length and its associations in an adult population of central rural India: the Central India eye and medical study. Ophthalmology. 2010;117:1360–6.
30. Yin G, Wang YX, Zheng ZY, Yang H, Xu L, Jonas JB, Beijing Eye Study G. Ocular axial length and its associations in Chinese: the Beijing eye study. PLoS One. 2012;7:e43172.
31. Grosvenor T. Reduction in axial length with age: an emmetropizing mechanism for the adult eye? Am J Optom Physiol Optic. 1987;64:657–63.
32. Leighton DA, Tomlinson A. Changes in axial length and other dimensions of the eyeball with increasing age. Acta Ophthalmol. 1972;50:815–26.
33. Brown NP, Koretz JF, Bron AJ. The development and maintenance of emmetropia. Eye (Lond). 1999;13(Pt 1):83–92.
34. Saw SM, Chua WH, Hong CY. Wu HM, chia KS, stone RA, tan D. Height and its relationship to refraction and biometry parameters in Singapore Chinese children. Invest Ophthalmol Vis Sci. 2002;43:1408–13.
35. Salmon JF. Predisposing factors for chronic angle-closure glaucoma. Prog Retin Eye Res. 1999;18:121–32.
36. Lee RY, Kasuga T, Cui QN, Huang G, Wang SY, Lin SC. Ethnic differences in intraocular pressure reduction and changes in anterior segment biometric parameters following cataract surgery by phacoemulsification. Clin Exp Ophthalmol. 2013;41:442–9.
37. KhabazKhoob M, Hashemi H, Yazdani K, Mehravaran S, Yekta A, Fotouhi A. Keratometry measurements, corneal astigmatism and irregularity in a normal population: the Tehran eye study. Ophthalmic Physiol Opt. 2010;30:800–5.
38. Eysteinsson T, Jonasson F, Sasaki H, Arnarsson A, Sverrisson T, Sasaki K, Stefansson E. Central corneal thickness, radius of the corneal curvature and intraocular pressure in normal subjects using non-contact techniques: Reykjavik eye study. Acta Ophthalmol Scand. 2002;80:11–5.
39. Khan MI, Muhtaseb M. Prevalence of corneal astigmatism in patients having routine cataract surgery at a teaching hospital in the United Kingdom. J Cataract Refract Surg. 2011;37:1751–5.
40. Ferrer-Blasco T, Montes-Mico R, Peixoto-de-Matos SC, Gonzalez-Meijome JM, Cervino A. Prevalence of corneal astigmatism before cataract surgery. J Cataract Refract Surg. 2009;35:70–5.

41. Miyake T, Kamiya K, Amano R, Shimizu K. Corneal astigmatism before cataract surgery. Nihon Ganka Gakkai Zasshi. 2011;115:447–53.
42. Yuan X, Song H, Peng G, Hua X, Tang X. Prevalence of corneal astigmatism in patients before cataract surgery in northern China. J Ophthalmol 2014; 2014:536412.
43. Read SA, Collins MJ, Carney LG. A review of astigmatism and its possible genesis. Clin Exp Optom. 2007;90:5–19.
44. Hosny M, Alio JL, Claramonte P, Attia WH, Perez-Santonja JJ. Relationship between anterior chamber depth, refractive state, corneal diameter, and axial length. J Refract Surg. 2000;16:336–40.
45. Jonas JB, Nangia V, Sinha A, Gupta R. Corneal refractive power and its associations with ocular and general parameters: the Central India eye and medical study. Ophthalmology. 2011;118:1805–11.
46. McAlinden C, Wang Q, Pesudovs K, Yang X, Bao F, Yu A, Lin S, Feng Y, Huang J. Axial length measurement failure rates with the IOLMaster and Lenstar LS 900 in eyes with cataract. PLoS One. 2015;10:e0128929.
47. McAlinden C, Wang Q, Gao R, Zhao W, Yu A, Li Y, Guo Y, Huang J. Axial length measurement failure rates with biometers using swept-source optical coherence tomography compared to partial-coherence interferometry and optical low-coherence interferometry. Am J Ophthalmol. 2017;173:64–9.
48. Kubo E, Kumamoto Y, Tsuzuki S, Akagi Y. Axial length, myopia, and the severity of lens opacity at the time of cataract surgery. Arch Ophthalmol. 2006;124:1586–90.

Combined 23-gauge transconjunctival vitrectomy and scleral fixation of intraocular lens without conjunctival dissection in managing lens complications

Ling Yeung[1,2], Nan-Kai Wang[2,3], Wei-Chi Wu[2,3] and Kuan-Jen Chen[2,3*]

Abstract

Background: To evaluate the safety and efficacy of combined 23-gauge transconjunctival pars plana vitrectomy and scleral fixation of intraocular lens (IOL) without conjunctival dissection.

Methods: A retrospective study in Chang Gung Memorial Hospital, Keelung and Taoyuan, Taiwan. Patients receiving combined 23-gauge transconjunctival pars plana vitrectomy and scleral fixation of IOL without conjunctival dissection were enrolled. The ocular findings, causes of lens complication, surgical procedures, type of IOL used, and complications were documented.

Results: We included 40 eyes from 39 patients (27 male, 12 female) with a mean age of 59.5 [standard deviation (±) 14.8] years old. The mean follow-up duration was 6.8 ± 5.4 months. The cause of lens complications was ocular trauma in 24 (60%) eyes, cataract surgery complications in 11 (28%) eyes, and spontaneous subluxation of crystalline lens in 5 (13%) eyes. The overall best corrected visual acuity (BCVA) (logMAR) improved from 1.359 ± 0.735 to 0.514 ± 0.582 ($p < 0.001$). The BCVA also improved significantly in each group with different causes of lens complications. Preoperative BCVA was the only factor associated with the postoperative visual outcome ($p = 0.008$). Most surgery-related complications were self-limited, including mild vitreous hemorrhage (5%), microhyphema (5%), transient elevated intraocular pressure (3%), and transient hypotony (3%). Cystoid macular edema and IOL decentration was found in 3 (8%) eyes and 1 (3%) eye respectively.

Conclusions: Combined 23-gauge transconjunctival vitrectomy and scleral fixation of IOL without conjunctival dissection is effective and safe in managing a wide variety of lens complications, with good postoperative comfort and visual recovery.

Keywords: Cataract surgery, Intraocular lens, Lens dislocation, Lens subluxation, Scleral fixation

Background

Lens-related complications are common in clinical practice. These include crystalline lens subluxation or dislocation due to ocular trauma or systemic diseases (such as Marfan syndrome), complicated cataract surgeries with retained lens materials or inadequate capsular support for intraocular lens (IOL), and spontaneous IOL dislocation. More devastating and serious complications such as persistent corneal edema, secondary glaucoma, uveitis, vitreous hemorrhage, cystoid macular edema and retinal detachment may occur if untreated [1]. Vitrectomy with or without lensectomy are the standard procedures to clean up the vitreous incarceration and lens materials, followed by IOL implantation, reposition or exchange [1, 2]. Nowadays, small gauge (23-gauge or 25-gauge) transconjunctival pars plana vitrectomies have the advantages of avoiding conjunctival dissection, smaller

* Correspondence: cgr999@gmail.com
[2]College of Medicine, Chang Gung University, Taoyuan, Taiwan
[3]Department of Ophthalmology, Chang Gung Memorial Hospital, No 5, Fu Hsing Street, Kuei Shan, Taoyuan, Taiwan
Full list of author information is available at the end of the article

sclerotomies, and omitting sutures required for sclerotomy and conjunctival wounds when compared with 20-gauge vitrectomies. This improves the postoperative comfort in patients.

After vitrectomy, IOL can be implanted either into the anterior chamber (AC) or the posterior chamber (PC). Although it involves a more complicated surgical process, PC IOL in ciliary sulcus is more compatible with the physiological location of the lens and less likely to damage the angle structure and corneal endothelial cell. Hoffmann et al. proposed a method to fixate the in-the-bag IOL dislocation by creating a "reverse" scleral pocket [3]. The "reverse" scleral pocket was dissected outward from a clear cornea incision and conjunctival dissection was not required. This method was also reported in the handling of other IOL complications [4, 5]. By combining this technique with the small gauge transconjunctival pars plana vitrectomy, a wide variety of lens complications can theoretically be managed by a single surgery with a more comfortable postoperative condition and faster visual recovery. However, the efficacy and safety of these concurrent surgeries are unknown.

The purpose of the current study is to evaluate the safety and efficacy of concurrent 23-gauge transconjunctival pars plana vitrectomy and scleral fixation of IOL by a modified version of Hoffmann's technique. No conjunctival dissection was needed throughout the whole surgery. The postoperative complications, choice of IOLs, and the surgical tips are also discussed.

Methods

This was a retrospective study conducted at Chang Gung Memorial Hospital, Keelung and Taoyuan, Taiwan. The study was approved by the Institutional Review Board of Chang Gung Memorial Hospital and adhered to the tenets and guidelines of the Declaration of Helsinki. Patients receiving concurrent 23-gauge transconjunctival pars plana vitrectomy and scleral fixation of IOL without conjunctival dissection between October 2014 and December 2015 were included. The major exclusion criteria were: (1) using 20-gauge pars plana vitrectomy; (2) performing scleral fixation of IOL without simultaneous pars plana vitrectomy; (3) performing scleral fixation with other surgical techniques different from this study; (4) postoperative follow up of less than 1 month. Medical records, including clinical history, cause of lens complication, findings in ocular examinations, surgical procedures, type of IOL and postoperative complications were reviewed. The postoperative best corrected visual acuity (BCVA) was defined as the best visual acuity measurement between 1 to 3 months after surgery. The BCVA was measured using the Snellen chart and was converted to a logarithm of the minimum angle of resolution (logMAR) visual acuity for calculation. Counting fingers, hand movement, and light

perception vision were allocated to 1/200, 1/400 and 1/800 respectively [6].

Surgical techniques

(Also see Additional file 1: Video S1 which demonstrates the surgical techniques)

Step 1: Creating Hoffmann scleral pockets. This technique is modified from that described by Hoffmann et al. [3]. A #11 beaver blade was used to create 2 corneal incisions just anterior to the conjunctival insertion at 180 degrees apart from the desired meridian (Fig. 1a). The incisions were about 1 clock hour in width and one-third of the corneal thickness in depth. Some surgeons may omit this procedure to avoid surgically induced astigmatism (Additional file 1: Video S1). A metal crescent blade (Crescent Knife, Satin Cresecent™ Angled Bevel Up, Alcon) was used to make 2 scleral pockets by posterior lamellar dissection from the corneal incisions to about 3 mm posterior to the incisions (Fig. 1b). A spatula was used to check the width and depth of the scleral pockets (Fig. 1c).

Step 2: Setting 23-gauge transconjunctival pars plana vitrectomy system. Standard 3-port 23-gauge transconjunctival pars plana vitrectomy trocars were inserted at 3.5 - 4 mm from the limbus with infusion at the inferotemporal quadrant (Fig. 1d). Pars plana vitrectomy, pars plana lensectomy or other vitreoretinal surgical procedures can be done at this stage; or alternatively, at a later stage after scleral fixation of IOL. A clear corneal incision was done at the superior quadrant by a

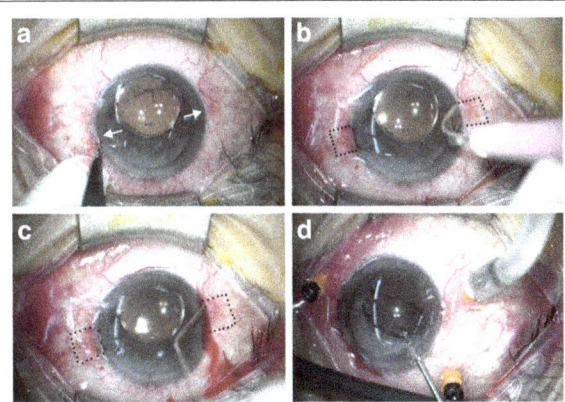

Fig. 1 a A #11 beaver blade was used to create 2 corneal incisions (white arrows) just anterior to the conjunctival insertion at 180 degrees apart on the desired meridian. **b** A metal crescent blade was used to make 2 scleral pockets by posterior lamellar dissection from the corneal incisions to about 3 mm posterior to the incisions. **c** A spatula was used to check the width and depth of the scleral pockets. The margins of the scleral pockets were indicated by the black dots in (**b**) and (**c**). **d** Standard 3-port 23-gauge transconjunctival pars plana vitrectomy trocars were set up with infusion at the temporal inferior quadrant. 23-gauge micro forceps were used to grasp the intraocular lens from ciliary sulcus into the anterior chamber

2.65 mm blade (EdgeAhead® Slit Knife 2.65 mm(40°), Beaver-Visitec International Ltd., Warwickshire, UK) The anterior chamber was filled with viscoelastic materials. In patients who required IOL reposition, the original IOL was moved to the anterior chamber by a 23-gauge micro forceps (Fig. 1d). In crystalline lens subluxation patients with some residue zonules and intact capsular bags, we could hold the capsular bag by iris retractors, and performed phacoemulsification to remove the cataract as much as possible if there was no vitreous prolapsed.

Step 3: Fixating the IOL haptics with 10-0 polypropylene sutures. A single-armed 10-0 polypropylene suture on a long straight needle (AUM-5 & SC-5, Alcon) was inserted into the eye at one side by passing through the conjunctiva and the full thickness of the scleral pocket at 1.5 mm posterior to the surgical limbus (Fig. 2a). A 27-gauge needle was passed through the conjunctiva and scleral pocket at 1.5 mm posterior to the surgical limbus in the opposite side. The long straight needle was docked with the 27-gauge needle and externalized (Fig. 2a). The above procedures were repeated in the opposite direction. The long straight needle was inserted again into the eye at the location just beside the exit. It was docked with a 27-gauge needle again and passed out beside the initial entry site. The 10-0 polypropylene sutures were pulled out from the superior corneal incision by a Jaffe-Knolle Iris Hook (Fig. 2b). Each 10-0 polypropylene suture was cut at the center. In patients who required IOL implantation, a foldable IOL was inserted into the anterior chamber at the current stage. One haptic of the IOL will be pulled out from the superior corneal incision and tightened with the two 10-0 polypropylene sutures from one of the scleral pockets (Fig. 2c). The haptic was then pushed back into the anterior chamber; and the process repeated with another haptic and the two 10-0 polypropylene sutures from another scleral pocket. Alternatively, for those IOLs with haptics that are difficult to externalize, we can pass the 10-0 Polypropylene suture first beneath the haptic and then above the haptic to form a loop to fix the haptic to ciliary sulcus (Fig. 2d).

Step 4: Retrieved the 10-0 polypropylene sutures from scleral pockets and tightened the knots. The sutures were retrieved from the scleral pockets by a Sinskey hook (Fig. 3a). The IOL was moved to the posterior chamber and the centration was ensured by adjusting the tightness of sutures in both scleral pockets (Fig. 3b). The knots buried themselves inside the scleral pocket spontaneously when they were tightened.

Step 5: Cleaning up and concluding the surgery. Residue vitreous, lens materials, or viscoelastic materials were all removed by vitrectomy or simcoe cannula (Fig. 3c). The 23-gauge vitrectomy trocars were then removed. The corneal wound was hydrated by balanced salt solution or sutured with 10-0 nylon if necessary (Fig. 3d).

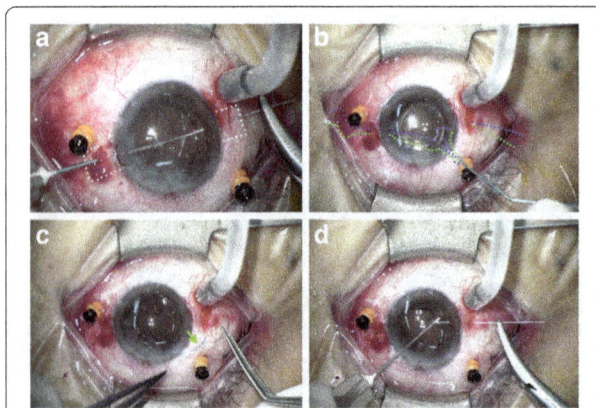

Fig. 2 a A single-armed 10-0 Polypropylene suture on a long straight needle was inserted into eye at one side at 1.5 mm posterior to the surgical limbus (right side). A 27-gauge needle was also inserted into the eye at the scleral pocket at 1.5 mm posterior to the surgical limbus in the opposite side (left side). The long straight needle was docked with the 27-gauge needle and externalized. Then this procedure was repeated in the opposite direction. The margins of the scleral pockets were indicated by white dots. **b** The two 10-0 polypropylene sutures (indicated by blue dots and green dots) were pulled out from the superior corneal incision by a Jaffe-Knolle Iris Hook. **c** One haptic of the IOL was pulled out from the superior corneal incision and was tightened with the 10-0 polypropylene sutures (green arrow). The haptic was then pushed back into the anterior chamber and the process repeated with another haptic. **d** Alternatively, we can also pass the 10-0 polypropylene suture first beneath the haptic and then above the haptic to form a loop to fix the haptic to ciliary sulcus

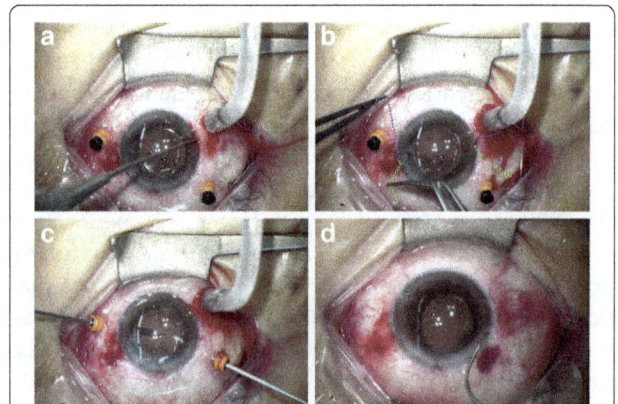

Fig. 3 a The 10-0 polypropylene sutures were retrieved out from scleral pockets by a Sinskey hook. The IOL centricity was ensured by adjusting the tightness of sutures in both scleral pockets. **b** The sutures buried themselves inside the scleral pocket spontaneously when they were tightened. **c** The residue vitreous, lens materials, or viscoelastic materials were then removed. **d** The 23-gauge vitrectomy trocars were removed. The corneal wound was hydrated by balanced salt solution or sutured with 10-0 nylon if necessary

Statistical analysis

Statistical analysis was performed using SPSS 17.0 (SPSS Inc., Chicago, IL). Continuous data were reported as the mean ± standard deviation, and categorical data were reported as n (%).Paired sample *t*-test and chi-square test were used for comparing the preoperative BCVA to the postoperative BCVA. One way ANOVA was used to determine the difference in the preoperative BCVA and the postoperative BCVA among eyes with different causes of lens complications. Linear regression model was used to evaluate the factors associated with the postoperative BCVA. A *p* value < 0.05 was considered statistically significant in this study.

Results

A total of 40 eyes from 39 patients (male: female = 27:12) were enrolled in this study. The mean age was 59.5 [range 22 - 90, standard deviation (±) 14.8] years old and the mean postoperative follow-up duration was 6.8 (± 5.4) months. Table 1 shows the cause of lens complications, prior surgeries and the preoperative lens status. The most common cause of lens complications was ocular trauma (24 eyes, 60%), which included open globe injury in 6 eyes (15%) and closed globe injury in 18 eyes (45%), followed by cataract surgery complications (11 eyes, 28%) and spontaneous subluxation of crystalline lens (5 eyes, 13%). The surgical procedures and type of IOL used in the current surgery are summarized in Table 2. All patients received 23-gauge vitrectomy and scleral fixation of IOL.

Table 1 Clinical characteristics of patients

Total number of eyes	40
Total number of patients	39
Male: Female	27: 12
Age, mean ± standard deviation	59.5 ± 14.8
Cause of lens complications, *n* (%)	
Ocular trauma	24 (60)
Cataract surgery complications	11 (28)
Spontaneous subluxation of crystalline lens	5 (13)
Prior surgeries, *n* (%)	
Cataract surgery	19 (48)
Vitrectomy	4 (10)
Primary repair of open globe injury	2 (5)
Scleral buckle	1 (3)
Scleral fixation	1 (3)
Preoperative lens status, *n* (%)	
Crystalline lens subluxation / dislocation	19 (48)
IOL dislocation	13 (33)
Aphakia	6 (15)
Retained lens fragments	2 (5)

Abbreviation: IOL intraocular lens

Table 2 Surgical procedures and type of intraocular lens used in the study

	Number of eyes (%)
Procedures performed	
23-gauge pars plana vitrectomy	40 (100)
Phacoemulsification / pars plana lensectomy	19 (48)
Epiretinal membrane peeling	1 (3)
IOL related procedures	
IOL implantation	28 (70)
IOL reposition	10 (25)
IOL exchange	2 (5)
Type of IOL used	
Rayner 570C / 620H / 920H / 970C	20 (50)
Alcon SA60AT / SN60WF	6 (15)
AMO Sensar AR40e	3 (8)
AMO AAB00	1 (3)
Bausch & Lomb MX60	1 (3)
Alcon CZ70BD	4 (10)
Using original IOL which type unknown	5 (13)

Abbreviation: IOL intraocular lens

Phacoemulsification or pars plana lensectomy was performed in 17 (43%) eyes. Foldable (soft) IOLs were implanted in 31 (78%) eyes and PMMA IOLs were used in 4 (10%) eyes.

Table 3 shows the changes in BCVA. None of the patients showed decreased BCVA after the surgery. The BCVA improved significantly from 1.359 (Snellen equivalent 20/457)

Table 3 Change in the best corrected visual acuity

	Preoperative	Postoperative	*p* value
BCVA level, *n* (%)			0.001*
< 20/200	19 (48)	3 (8)	
20/200 - 20/40	21 (53)	22 (55)	
> 20/40	–	15 (38)	
BCVA in logMAR (Mean ± SD)			
Overall (*n* = 40)	1.359 ± 0.735	0.514 ± 0.582	< 0.001 †
Ocular trauma (*n* = 24)	1.265 ± 0.669	0.477 ± 0.603	< 0.001 †
Cataract surgery complications (*n* = 11)	1.675 ± 0.866	0.711 ± 0.609	0.006 †
Spontaneous subluxation of crystalline lens (*n* = 5)	1.114 ± 0.645	0.264 ± 0.295	0.036 †
p value	0.230‡	0.328‡	

Abbreviation: BCVA best corrected visual acuity, *logMAR* logarithm of the minimum angle of resolution, *SD* standard deviation
*Comparing the postoperative BCVA level to the preoperative BCVA level, *p* value was calculated by chi-square test
† Comparing the postoperative BCVA (logMAR) to the preoperative BCVA (logMAR), *p* values were calculated by paired sample t-test
‡ Comparing the BCVA among 3 different causes of lens complications (i.e. ocular trauma, cataract surgery complications, and spontaneous subluxation of crystalline lens), *p* values were calculated by one way ANOVA

preoperatively to 0.514 (Snellen equivalent 20/65) postoperatively ($p < 0.001$) in study patients as a whole. The BCVA improved by 3 lines or more in 32 (80%) eyes. When the patients were divided into three groups according to different causes of lens complications (i.e. ocular trauma, cataract surgery complications, and spontaneous subluxation of crystalline lens), there were no intergroup differences in the preoperative BCVA and the postoperative BCVA. All three groups of patients showed significant improvement in BCVA after the surgery. (Table 3) The linear regression model showed that only the preoperative BCVA ($p = 0.008$) was correlated with the postoperative BCVA. Other factors including age, gender, cause of lens complication, prior cataract surgery, prior vitrectomy, concurrent phacoemulsification / lensectomy, type of IOL procedure, and type of IOL used were not correlated with the postoperative BCVA.

No major intraoperative complications such as retinal tear, retinal detachment, or suprachoroidal hemorrhage were noted. The postoperative complications are summarized in Table 4. The majority of surgery-related complications were self-limited, such as mild vitreous hemorrhage, microhyphema, transient elevated intraocular pressure, and transient ocular hypotony. All of these self-limited complications resolved within 1 to 2 weeks after surgery. Three (8%) eyes with cystoids macular edema required topical nonsteroidal anti-inflammatory (NSAID) drugs or intravitreal injection of steroid. One (3%) eye receiving IOL reposition had IOL decentration at 2 months after surgery due to vigorous eye rubbing.

Discussion

Our results show that combined 23-gauge transconjunctival vitrectomy and scleral fixation of IOL without conjunctival dissection is an effective and safe method in handling a wide variety of lens complications within a single surgery. Preoperative BCVA is the only factor correlated with postoperative visual outcome. Concurrent phacoemulsification / lensectomy, type of IOL procedure (implantation / reposition / exchange), and type of IOL used were not associated with visual outcome. Most complications related to the current surgical procedure were self-limited.

In patients without adequate capsular support, many surgical methods were introduced to fixate the PC IOL into the ciliary sulcus. However, most of them involve conjunctival peritomy and creating a scleral flap or glove to embed the stitches or haptics of IOL [2]. In this study, by combining a modified form of Hoffmann's "reverse" scleral pocket technique and 23-gauge transconjunctival vitrectomy, a wide variety of lens complications were treated without conjunctival periotomy. These provided rapid surgical wounds recovery and less postoperative discomfort in patients (Fig. 4).

No major intraoperative complications were noted. Most of the vision-threatening complications were related to prior underlying ocular diseases (Table 3). Most complications related to current surgical procedures were self-limited, including mild vitreous hemorrhage, microhyphema, transient elevated intraocular pressure, and transient hypotony. All of these complications resolved within 1 to 2 weeks. Cystoid macular edema occurred in 8% of patients. This is comparable to previous studies [7]. Pseudophakic cystoid macular edema was observed on optical coherence tomography in 4-11% of patients, and may be further increased in

Table 4 Postoperative complications

	Number of eyes (%)
Complications related to prior underlying ocular disorders	
Traumatic optic neuropathy	2 (5)
Recurrent retinal detachment	1 (3)
Corneal irregular astigmatism	1 (3)
Progression of epiretinal membrane	1 (3)
Complications related to current surgical procedures	
Cystoid macular edema	3 (8)
Mild vitreous hemorrhage	2 (5)
Mild hyphema	2 (5)
Transient elevated intraocular pressure	1 (3)
Transient hypotony	1 (3)
Intraocular lens decentration	1 (3)
Intraocular lens dislocation	0 (0)

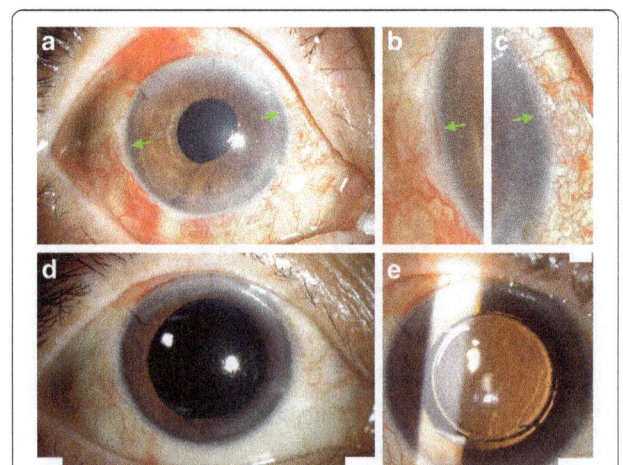

Fig. 4 External photos of the same patient in Figs. 1, 2 and 3. **a** Minimal residual corneal edema and conjunctival hemorrhage at 3 days after surgery. Incison wounds (indicated by green arrows) of both scleral pockets were healing well. **b-c** The manified image of temporal and nasal scleral pocket incision wounds (green arrows). **d** No more corneal edema and conjunctival hemorrhage could be found at 10 days after surgery. **e** Intraocular lens centration was good

complicated cataract surgeries [7]. In considering the complexity of the surgeries in this study, it is reasonable that 8% of eyes developed cystoid macular edema. Nowadays, most cystoid macular edema can be successfully treated by topical NSAID or local (intravitreal or sub-Tenon) injection of corticosteroid [7]. In this study, IOL decentration was noted in an 86 years old male patient after vigorous eye rubbing. None of the patients had IOL dislocation to vitreous cavity after surgery.

In our study, a soft foldable IOL was used in 31 (78%) eyes. Recent reports showed that different types of foldable IOLs can be used safely for scleral fixation in aphakic eyes [8–12]. The advantages include small incision, short surgical time, less likelihood of intraoperative hypotony-related complications, and faster recovery [8–12]. For patients with IOL subluxation / dislocation, we prefer to use the original IOLs for reposition whenever possible. The advantage of this is that only a small corneal incision (2.2 mm - 2.65 mm) is required for externalization and fixation of the haptics of the IOL. The small corneal incision can be easily sealed by balanced salt solution hydration or a 10-0 nylon suture at the end of surgery. For patients with crystalline lens subluxation / dislocation or in aphakic status, we prefer to use closed-loop foldable IOLs (e.g. Rayner 570C / 620H / 920H / 970C). In fact, this is the most common type of IOL used in this study. It is easy for the suture to pass through the closed-loop and we do not need to worry about the suture slipping out of the haptic after surgery. A 2.65 mm – 2.8 mm corneal incision is adequate for the implantation of a foldable IOL. Other factors that we may consider include the presence of corneal astigmatism, the size of iris defect, and the availability of specific types of IOL among the participating hospitals. However, our study showed that the current surgical technique is feasible for a wide variety of IOLs. The suture technique is quite similar for different type of IOLs. The type of IOL used was not correlated with postoperative visual outcome.

The surgical technique in this study is moderately difficult in its learning curve. The most difficult part of the surgery is in creating the scleral pockets. There are some tips in this procedure. Firstly, it is better to create the scleral pockets at the beginning of the surgery, before inserting 23-gauge vitrectomy trocars and performing anterior chamber paracentesis. This maintains adequate intraocular pressure and firmness of eyeball for easier dissection of the scleral pocket. Secondly, the dissection of the scleral pockets may be difficult at some surgical angles. This can be facilitated by rotating the eyeball to the opposite direction, so the scleral pocket dissection can be done at the horizontal plane in an easier manner. Thirdly, we recommend checking the width and depth of the scleral pocket with a spatula after dissection (Fig. 1c). The depth of the scleral pocket can be easily

estimated by measuring the bloodstain or water mark on the spatula. Inadequate width and depth of the scleral pockets may lead to difficulty in retrieving the sutures in Step 3.

Our study was limited by its retrospective nature and a short follow up duration. The follow up duration is relative short in this study because most referred patients will be referred back to primary care general ophthalmologists once their postoperative conditions have stabilized. However, our short-term results are promising. Our study also limited by lacking a comparative group. It requires further studies to evaluate the success rate, the visual outcome, and the complications when compare to other surgical methods.

Conclusions
Combined 23-gauge transconjunctival vitrectomy and scleral fixation of intraocular lens without conjunctival dissection is an effective and safe surgical technique in handling a wide variety of lens complications within a single surgery. Visual acuity improved significantly in all groups with different causes of lens complications. Most complications related to the current surgical technique are self-limited.

Abbreviations
AC: Anterior chamber; BCVA: Best corrected visual acuity; IOL: Intraocular lens; LogMAR: Logarithm of the minimum angle of resolution; NSAID: Nonsteroidal anti-inflammatory; PC: Posterior chamber

Authors' contributions
LY, NKW, and WCW analyzed and interpreted the patient data regarding this surgical techinque. LY and KJC were major contributors in writing the manuscript. All authors read and approved the final manuscript.

Competing interests
The authors declare that they have no competing interests.

Author details
[1]Department of Ophthalmology, Chang Gung Memorial Hospital, Keelung, Taiwan. [2]College of Medicine, Chang Gung University, Taoyuan, Taiwan. [3]Department of Ophthalmology, Chang Gung Memorial Hospital, No 5, Fu Hsing Street, Kuei Shan, Taoyuan, Taiwan.

References
1. Nagpal M, Jain P. Dropped lens fragment, dislocated intraocular lens. Dev Ophthalmol. 2014;54:234–42.
2. Holt DG, Young J, Stagg B, Ambati BK. Anterior chamber intraocular lens, sutured posterior chamber intraocular lens, or glued intraocular lens: where do we stand? Curr Opin Ophthalmol. 2012;23:62–7.
3. Hoffman RS, Fine IH, Packer M. Scleral fixation without conjunctival dissection. J Cataract Refract Surg. 2006;32:1907–12.
4. Das S, Nicholson M, Deshpande K, Kummelil MK, Nagappa S, Shetty BK. Scleral fixation of a foldable intraocular lens with polytetrafluoroethylene sutures through a Hoffman pocket. J Cataract Refract Surg. 2016;42:955–60.
5. Long C, Wei Y, Yuan Z, Zhang Z, Lin X, Liu B. Modified technique for transscleral fixation of posterior chamber intraocular lenses. BMC Ophthalmol. 2015;15:127.

6. Scott IU, Schein OD, West S, Bandeen-Roche K, Enger C, Folstein MF.
    Functional status and quality of life measurement among ophthalmic
    patients. Arch Ophthalmol. 1994;112:329–35.
7. Guo S, Patel S, Baumrind B, Johnson K, Levinsohn D, Marcus E, et al.
8. Takayama K, Akimoto M, Taguchi H, Nakagawa S, Hiroi K. Transconjunctival
    sutureless intrascleral intraocular lens fixation using intrascleral tunnels guided
    with catheter and 30-gauge needles. Br J Ophthalmol. 2015;99:1457–9.
9. Wallmann AC, Monson BK, Adelberg DA. Transscleral fixation of a foldable
    posterior chamber intraocular lens. J Cataract Refract Surg. 2015;41:1804–9.
10. Wilgucki JD, Wheatley HM, Feiner L, Ferrone MV, Prenner JL. One-year
    outcomes of eyes treated with a sutureless scleral fixation technique for
    intraocular lens placement or rescue. Retina. 2015;35:1036–40.
11. Terveen DC, Fram NR, Ayres B, Berdahl JP. Small-incision 4-point scleral
    suture fixation of a foldable hydrophilic acrylic intraocular lens in the
    absence of capsule support. J Cataract Refract Surg. 2016;42:211–6.
12. Kim SJ, Lee SJ, Park CH, et al. Long-term stability and visual outcomes
    of a single-piece, foldable, acrylic intraocular lens for scleral fixation.
    Retina. 2009;29:91–7.

6

Metabolic characterization of human aqueous humor in the cataract progression after pars plana vitrectomy

Yinghong Ji, Xianfang Rong and Yi Lu*

Abstract

Background: While pars plana vitrectomy (PPV) has become the third most commonly performed surgery in the world, it can also induce multiple post complications easily. Among them, cataract progression is the most frequent one that can lead to blindness eventually.

Methods: To understand the underlying mechanisms of post PPV cataract progression, we performed comprehensive metabolic characterization of aqueous humor (AH) samples from 20 cataract patients (10 post PPV complication and 10 none PPV cataract) by a non-targeted metabolomic analysis using gas chromatography combined with time-of-flight mass spectrometer (GC/TOF MS).

Results: A total of 263 metabolites were identified and eight of them are determined to be significantly different (VIP ≥ 1 and $p \leq 0.05$) between post PPV group and none PPV control group. The significantly changed metabolites included glutaric acid and pelargonic acid that play key roles in the regulation of oxidative stress and inflammatory responses. Furthermore, we constructed a metabolic regulatory network in each group based on metabolite-metabolite correlations, which reveals key metabolic pathways and regulatory elements including amino acids and lipids metabolisms that are related to cataract progression.

Conclusions: Altogether, this work discovered some potential metabolite biomarkers for post PPV cataract diagnostics, as well as casted some novel insights into the underlying mechanisms of cataract progression after PPV.

Keywords: Aqueous humor (AH), Metabolite-metabolite correlation, Metabolomics, Pars plana vitrectomy (PPV)

Background

Pars plana vitrectomy (PPV) was first introduced about 35 years ago. The procedure is relatively safe, but unintended long-term complications may still occur that endangers complete visual rehabilitation of patients [1–3]. For example, cataract formation is known to be the most frequently happened complication of PPV, and more than 80% of patients develop cataract within 2 years after surgery [4]. Two types of cataract are most common after vitrectomy: posterior subcapsular cataract and nuclear sclerotic cataract. Nuclear sclerotic cataract progression after PPV has been known for many years,

which may be caused by the deficiency of ascorbate, a powerful antioxidant [5].

Metabolomics analysis can provide comparative, semi-quantitative information of a large number of metabolites in biological samples from different groups at a specific time [6]. In recent years, this powerful –omics technology has been applied in ophthalmology researches such as diabetic retinopathy, glaucoma, and cataract progression, aiming to identify metabolic biomarkers and pathways that are important for understanding disease mechanisms and developing novel diagnosis and therapies [6–8]. Pushpot et al. performed metabolic profiling of serum and urine samples collected from patients with atrophic age-related macular degeneration (AMD) and neovascular AMD. They found that while arginine increases in neovascular AMD samples, glucose, lactate, glutamine and reduced glutathione decrease [9]. Mayordomo-Febrer et al.

* Correspondence: luyieent@126.com
Department of Ophthalmology and Eye Institute, Eye and ENT Hospital of Fudan University, Key Laboratory of Myopia of State Health Ministry, and Key Laboratory of Visual Impairment and Restoration of Shanghai, No. 83 Fenyang Road, Shanghai 200031, China

used high-resolution 1H NMR to analyze aqueous humor (AH) samples from control and glaucoma patients, and showed that levels of amino acids, carbohydrates, and lipids are all significantly altered after sodium hyaluronate injection series [7]. It was believed that these metabolic changes may play important roles in the pathogenesis of glaucoma.

AH is a very important intraocular fluid which is necessary for normal eye functions [10]. Knowledge gained from metabolic characterization of AH samples can be very helpful in advancing researches of many eye diseases. AH samples have been studied using nuclear magnetic resonance (NMR), liquid chromatography combined with mass spectrometry (LC-MS), and capillary electrophoresis combined with mass spectrometry (CE-MS), but to our knowledge, the metabolome for patients after PPV has never been determined using GC-MS technology [7, 10–12].

In this study, we analyzed AH samples from 20 patients using GC/TOF MS technology. Ten of the patients had received PPV and the other 10 did not. Significant metabolic variations were discovered between the two groups. Metabolite-metabolite correlation network in each group was also constructed, which reveals key regulatory pathways including amino acid and lipid metabolism pathways that are related to post PPV cataract progression. Altogether, the identified metabolites and regulatory metabolic pathways that changed significantly in the AH of

patients after PPV may play important roles in the development of post PPV cataract.

Methods
Subjects
Totally 20 subjects were recruited for the present study: 10 post PPV complication and 10 none PPV cataract (Table 1). In the former group, a standard 23-gauge 3-port PPV was employed as the previous study, and the PPV surgery has been performed for more than half a year [13]. The intraoperative lens injuries during PPV were excluded. The other 10 controls had age-related cataract. Besides, all collected subjects met inclusion criteria, which had no history or slit-lamp evidence of ocular trauma, no use of systemic antimetabolites, corticosteroids, or immunosuppressants, and no unrelated ocular disease other than cataract. Furthermore, all patients signed the consent form, which was approved by the Ethics Committee of Eye & ENT Hospital of Fudan University, Shanghai, China.

Sample extraction and preparation
Samples of AH were collected from Eye &ENT Hospital of Fudan University and extracted as the same with our previous study [14, 15]. After final centrifuging, all the samples were rapidly stored at − 80 °C until further analysis.

Table 1 Summary of human aqueous humor samples

Group	Patient ID	Gender	Age range (Years old)	Axial length	LOCSIII
Controls	A36_1	Female	50–55	24.32	C3N3P3
	A37_1	Female	50–55	24.75	C2N2P5
	A38_1	Female	50–55	24.63	C3N4P2
	A39_1	Female	55–60	22.59	C3N3P2
	A40_1	Male	60–65	24.65	C2N3P2
	A41_1	Male	60–65	23.2	C3N2P4
	A42_1	Male	65–70	23.8	C3N3P3
	A43_1	Male	65–70	24.01	C4N5
	A44_1	Female	65–70	22.96	C4N5
	A45_1	Male	70–75	23.63	C5N4P2
Patients after pars plana vitrectomy	P1_1	Male	50–55	26.92	C2N5P3
	P2_1	Male	50–55	25.76	C2N4P2
	P3_1	Male	50–55	29.63	C3N5P4
	P4_1	Female	55–60	27.79	C2N3P3
	P5_1	Female	55–60	25.63	C3N3P2
	P6_1	Female	60–65	26.53	C3N4P3
	P7_1	Female	60–65	23.94	C3N4P3
	P8_1	Female	60–65	24.91	C2N3P2
	P9_1	Male	60–65	25.45	C2N3P2
	P10_1	Male	70–75	25.78	C3N4P3

GC/TOF MS analysis

The metabolic profiling for all 20 samples was performed as the same with our previous study [15]. After derivatization, the samples were analyzed by gas chromatograph (Agilent 7890A, Agilent, USA) combined with a Pegasus 4D time-of- flight mass spectrometer (LECO ChromaTOF PEGASUS 4D, LECO, USA). Meanwhile, mass spectrometry data were acquired with the m/z range of 20–600 and then mapped to spectra in the National Institute of Standards and Technology (NIST, http://www.nist.gov/index.html) and Fiehn databases as our previous report [15].

Data analysis

Data normalization was firstly performed as previous studies [15–17]. Briefly, raw area counts of each compound were divided by its median value, while missing values (if any) were assumed to be below the limits of detection and were imputed with the observed minimum. The data after normalization step followed normal distribution, which was confirmed by SPSS 17.0 software. Mev (MultiExperiment Viewer) 4.8 was employed for K-Medians clustering analysis. Significant changed metabolites were determined in partial least squares discriminant analysis (PLS-DA) model, followed by independent t tests (SPSS 17.0 software) as other studies and our previous study [15–19]. Metabolites with both VIP (variable importance in the projection) values in PLS-DA model more than 1 and p values (in t tests) less than 0.05 were considered to be significant. The metabolite-metabolite correlation analysis was performed by using the R statistical software.

Results

AH samples collection

In the present study, these 20 samples were patients with moderate or even severe cataract, preparing for cataract surgery. They included 10 from controls of age-related cataract (ARC), and 10 from patients after PPV. The details for the 20 subjects including sex, age, and axial length were listed in Table 1. The average age of the patients after PPV was nearly 59, while the average age for the controls was about 60. Obviously, there was no statistical significance between those two groups for both sex and age. Furthermore, further binary logistic regression analysis based on the ratio $C/(C + N + P)$ indicated the type between the two groups was significantly different ($p \leq 0.05$). As a result, the present study emphasized on uncovering the underlying mechanism that patients after PPV easily develop nuclear and posterior capsular cataract instead of cortical cataract.

Metabolic profiling of human AH

Taking advantage of a non-targeted metabolomic technology, we here employed GC/TOF MS to fully uncover AH metabolome. 263 metabolites in total were identified in those 20 AH samples including 10 patients after PPV and 10 patients for controls (Additional file 1: Table S1). The identified 263 metabolites contained 32 amino acids, 13 lipids, 44 carbohydrates, 6 nucleotides and other 168 biochemicals. Among those 168 metabolites, there were 39 named metabolites and 68 metabolites identified as analytes, and 61 metabolites determined to be unknown. Hence, the result here revealed 134 named biochemicals of the identified 263 metabolites, which involves in major metabolism pathways such as super pathway of amino acid, lipid, carbohydrate, nucleotide, etc. Importantly, as compared to previous studies, the result uncovered the broadest AH metabolome for human to date [7, 10–12, 15].

Metabolomic study with patients after PPV and the controls

To review metabolic variation between the controls and patients after PPV, we performed clustering analysis by MEV 4.8, showing a plot of all the 263 biochemicals vs 20 samples, which were finally grouped into 6 classes (Fig. 1a). Obviously, the abundances of those 263 metabolites showed significant diversity across the 20 AH samples and more importantly, certain enriched metabolites seemed to be group-specific or individual-specific. For example in class 1, 60 of 67 metabolites appeared to be very high levels only in P8_1, while certain metabolites were enriched in patients after PPV including P1_1 (class 5), P9_1 (class 1), and P9_1 (class 4). Conversely, in class 3, 34 of 40 metabolites were abundant only in A36_1. Furthermore, several metabolites were specifically enriched in both two groups. For instance, certain metabolites in class 2 were enriched in P6_1, P7_1, P8_1, P9_1, A41_1, and A42_1.

The widely used supervised method, PLS-DA, was then employed for determining metabolic changes between the controls and patients after PPV. As shown in Fig. 1b, ten samples from patients after PPV were completely apart from those from the controls. Further statistical analysis including independent t tests showed that eight metabolites (Table 2 and Fig. 1c) were significantly different ($p \leq 0.05$), responsible for the separation for those two group. These eight metabolites including 2 increased and 6 decreased biochemicals referred to 3 super pathways such as amino acid super pathway, lipid super pathway, and others. The only two increased metabolites were 3-(2-Hydroxyphenyl)propionic acid and unknown 029, whose ratio between patients after PPV and the controls were respectively 2.04 and 1.55. On the other hand, the left six decreased metabolites ranged from 0.34 to 0.70 folds including 4-acetamidobutyric acid 1, glutaric acid, and pelargonic acid.

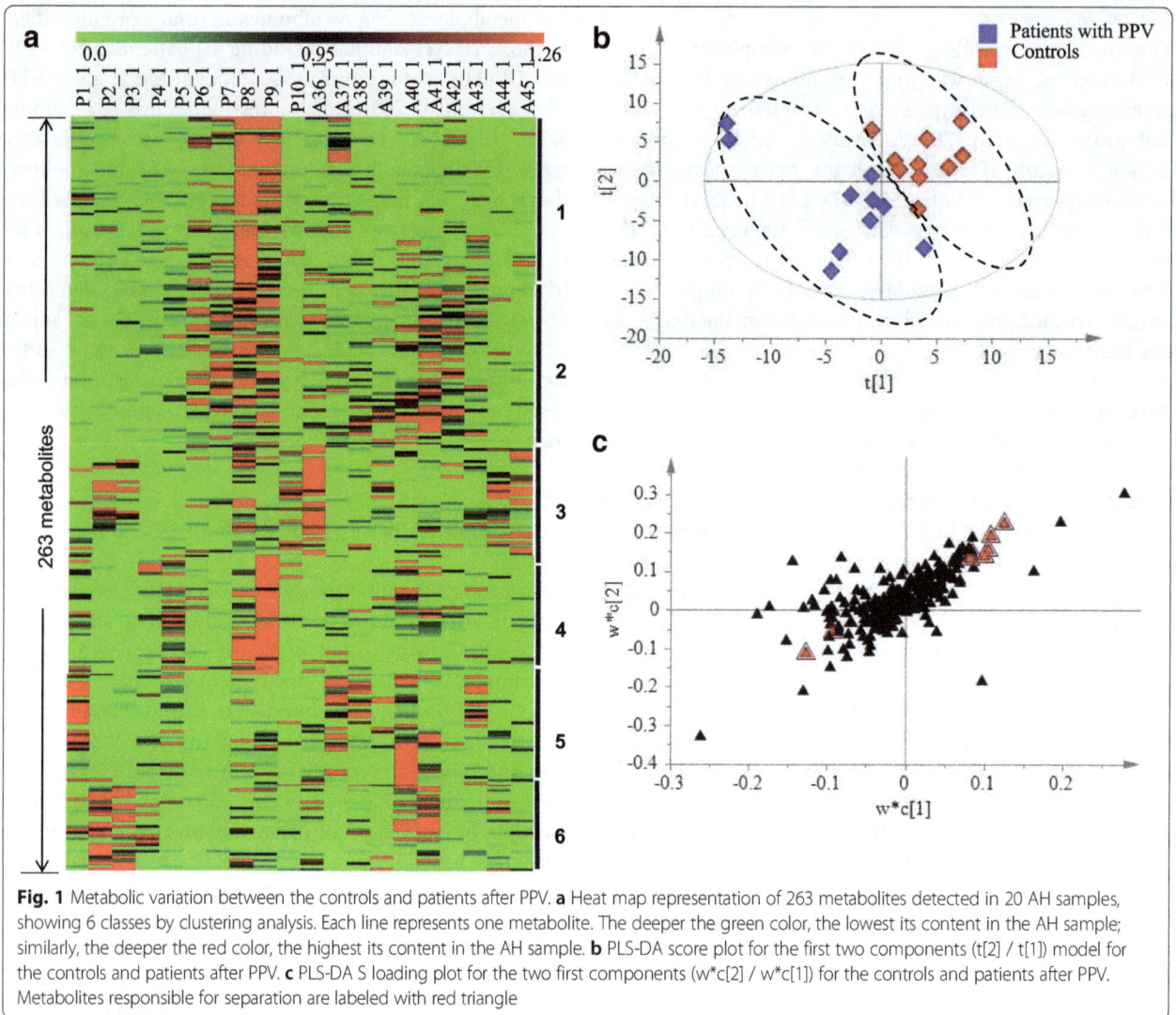

Fig. 1 Metabolic variation between the controls and patients after PPV. **a** Heat map representation of 263 metabolites detected in 20 AH samples, showing 6 classes by clustering analysis. Each line represents one metabolite. The deeper the green color, the lowest its content in the AH sample; similarly, the deeper the red color, the highest its content in the AH sample. **b** PLS-DA score plot for the first two components (t[2] / t[1]) model for the controls and patients after PPV. **c** PLS-DA S loading plot for the two first components (w*c[2] / w*c[1]) for the controls and patients after PPV. Metabolites responsible for separation are labeled with red triangle

Metabolic network variation based on metabolite-metabolite correlation

In order to uncover the regulatory of metabolic network in AH, we conducted metabolite-metabolite correlation analysis for both groups. As in the control group, there were a total of 31,626 associations, ranging from − 0.9769 for lysine and analyte 381 to 0.9988 for analyte 30 and analyte 32 (Fig. 2). Moreover, 1666 significant associations were then determined ($r \geq 0.7$ & $r \leq - 0.7$ and $p \leq 0.05$), among which 1415 were positive associations while 251 were negative ones. Notably similar with our previous study in relation to high myopia, here amino acids also

Table 2 List of different metabolites between patients after PPV and the controls, responsible for the separation

Super Pathway	Biochemical Name	Retention time (minutes)	Ratio(PPV/ARC)[*]	p value
Amino acid	4-Acetamidobutyric acid 1	9.96	0.34	0.0347
Lipids	Glutaric Acid	9.31	0.43	0.0371
	Pelargonic acid	9.05	0.67	0.0173
Others	3-(2-Hydroxyphenyl)propionic acid	11.16	2.04	0.0019
	Analyte 389	14.16	0.59	0.0457
	unknown 029	9.64	1.55	0.0183
	unknown 037	10.39	0.70	0.0198
	unknown 056	13.85	0.60	0.0142

[*]ARC represented the controls

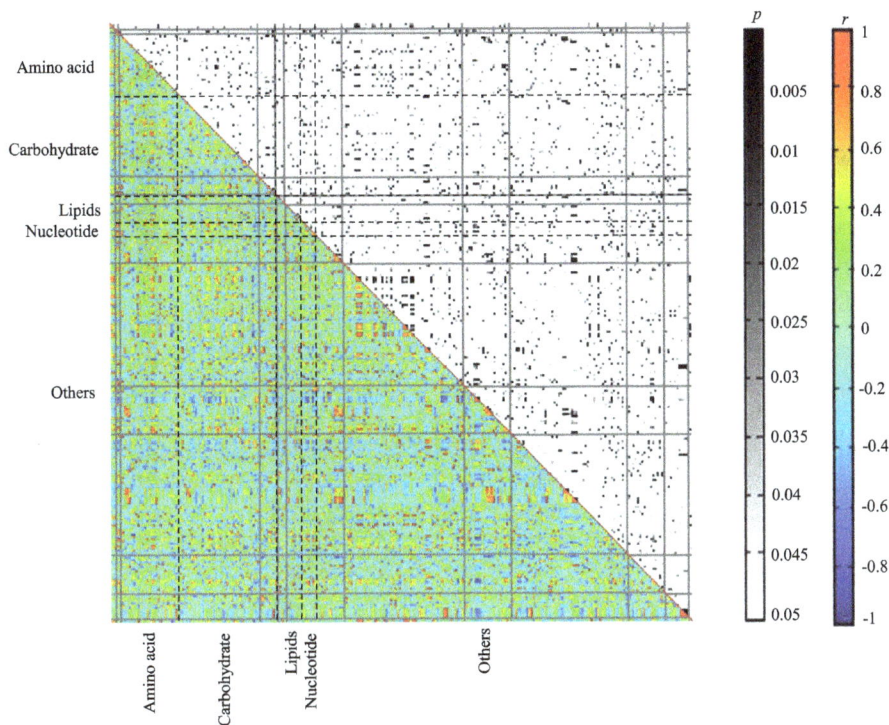

Fig. 2 Metabolite-metabolite correlation analysis in the controls (The control group). Metabolites were shown in X and Y-axes, grouped by pathway information. Both *p* and *r* values of the correlations between every two metabolites were displayed in distinct colors

dominated the significant metabolite-metabolite associations (395 associations) including 54 negative ones [20]. All 20 standard amino acids except cysteine, arginine, glutamic acid, aspartic acid, histidine, threonine, and leucine had 150 significant associations, including 25 negative ones. Asparagine had 20 significant associations with only one negative correlation. Likewise, lysine had 20 significant associations but including 18 negative ones. Moreover, 43 carbohydrates had 402 significant associations including 69 negative ones. Among them, fructose had 8 positive associations and 3 negative ones. Similarly, 12 of 13 lipids had 103 significant associations with six negative ones. Especially, 19 associations were connected with linoleic acid methyl ester, which were all positive.

Likewise based on the identified 263 metabolites in patients after PPV, metabolic network was also constructed to analyze the regulatory. As shown in Fig. 3, a total of 32,640 associations were identified, ranging from − 0.92452 for purine riboside and analyte 48 to 0.99997 for analyte 363 and analyte 402.Moreover, there were 3575 significant associations (r ≥ 0.7 & r ≤ − 0.7 and $p \leq 0.05$): 3482 positive associations and 93 negative ones. Likewise in patients after PPV, amino acids still dominated the significant associations as the same with control group. A total of 1044 significant associations (including 22 negative associations) were determined for amino acids. Among them, all 20 standard amino acids except

glutamic acid, cysteine, arginine, leucine, aspartic acid, histidine, and threonine had 493 significant associations including three negative associations. All the negative associations were associated with proline. Notably, 71, 67, and 64 associations were respectively associated with serine 1, asparagine 4, and lysine. Moreover, 42 carbohydrates had 634 significant associations including 40 negative associations. Among them, there were 23 positive associations for fructose. 11 of 13 lipids had 208 significant associations including four negative ones, and 17 associations were positively associated with linoleic acid methyl ester.

Discussion
Cataract is one of the highest frequently eye diseases, which can eventually lead to blindness. It's possible now to cure cataract through surgery for removing the diseased lens and replacing by a clear one, but it is difficult to efficiently control cataract in the nearby future. Hence, it is very important for us to reveal the underlying mechanism of the formation of cataract. We previously reported the metabolic characterization of human aqueous humor associated with high myopia [15]. The results showed considerable metabolic variations including both metabolite abundances and the metabolite-metabolite associations in the development of nuclear and posterior capsular cataract due to high myopia.

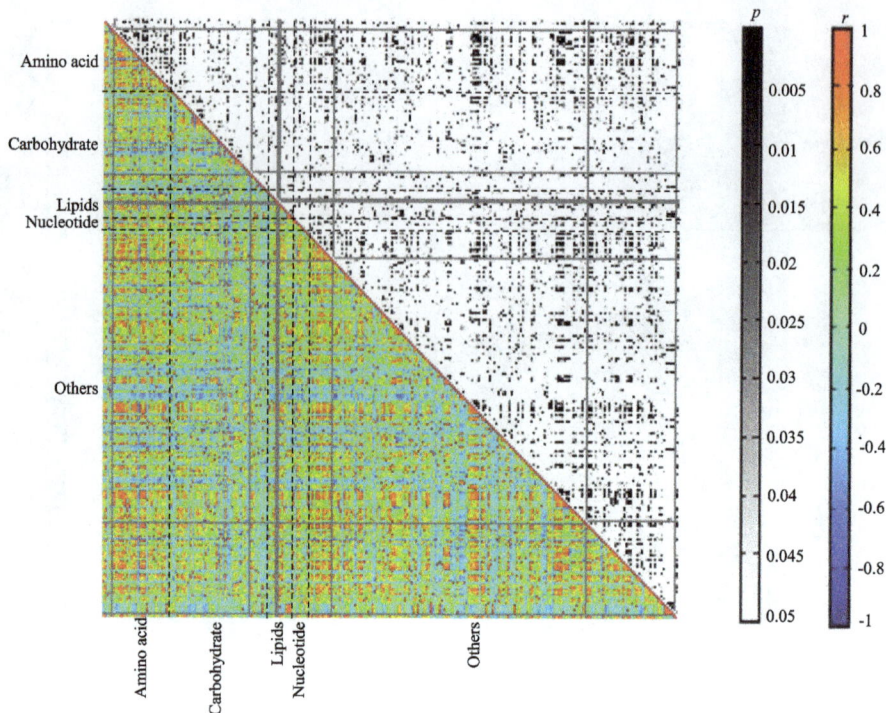

Fig. 3 Metabolite-metabolite correlation analysis in patients after PPV (The experiment group). Metabolites were shown in X and Y-axes, grouped by pathway information. Both *p* and *r* values of the correlations between every two metabolites were displayed in distinct colors

Similarly, PPV have long been reported to be associated with the development of nuclear and posterior capsular cataract. However, we believed patients after PPV may easier develop cataract than those with high myopia, since full of the vitreous cavity in patients after PPV is aqueous humor without normal function acting as a gel and interconnected meshwork. In order to reveal the underlying mechanism in the cataract progression after PPV, in the present study by using the same technology, we collected 20 aqueous humor samples from 20 cataract patients (10 post PPV complication and 10 none PPV cataract for metabolomics analysis. It should be pointed that both two groups of patients were with cataract, while patients in the control group had age-related cataract. As a result, the study here might emphasis on revealing metabolic changes at progressive stage of cataract development for patients after PPV other than pathogenesis of cataract at early time.

Obviously, significant different metabolic characterization could be observed in patients after PPV when compared with those in patients with high myopia, which demonstrated that there is a different underlying mechanism in the cataract progression after PPV. Firstly based on the same metabolomics technology and data analysis methods, totally 263 metabolites were identified in this study, which was larger than that in our previous study on high myopia. Secondly, very few significantly changed metabolites were determined between patients after PPV and the controls.

Here eight metabolites were significantly different ($p \leq 0.05$), responsible for the separation for these two groups, while 29 metabolites were determined to be significantly different in patients with high myopia. Finally, more (significant) correlation analyses were identified in the present study. Especially, there were a total of 1044 significant associations (including 22 negative associations) between amino acids and metabolites in other super pathways or among amino acids in patients after PPV, while only 703 significant associations for amino acids in patients with high myopia.

As a matter of fact, there has been already a nutrient theory of cataractogenesis as a function of altered aqueous fluid dynamics [5]. For example, Chung et al. (2001) observed that after removal of part of the vitreous, nuclear cataract may be resulted from altered lens metabolism [20]. It is believed that powerful antioxidant ascorbate is deficient in the vitreous cavity after vitrectomy, which may be one of the factors to trigger the development of cataract. Moreover, another a major mechanism resulting in senile nuclear cataract is posttranslational modification of lens crystallins through glycation, which includes glucose and the oxidative products of ascorbic acid: dehydroascorbate, 2,3 diketogulonic acid, xylosone, and threose [5]. In the present study, eight metabolites of 263 detected metabolites were found to be significantly changed in patients after PPV, including one amino acid and two lipids. These significantly changed metabolites may play very important roles in cataract development, which are likely to be potential biomarkers for cataract diagnostics. For example, glutaric acid was reported to be involved in the regulation of oxidative stress, which is an initiating factor for the progression of maturity onset cataract [21]. So the change of the level of glutaric acid in patients after PPV may help explain the progression of cataract after PPV [22]. Meanwhile, inflammation has also been reported to induce cataract (especially for PSC) after vitrectomy [5]. Here we found a lower level of pelargonic acid in patients after PPV, which was reported to have antifungal property [23]. Thus the change of this metabolite may involve in inflammatory response that contributes to cataract progression.

The metabolite-metabolite correlation analysis is supposed to dissect putative key regulatory elements or pathways for metabolism regulation, and proved to be helpful for discovering novel pathways [15, 17]. Correlation analysis of metabolomics data in our study indicated much more (significant) correlation analyses for amino acids and lipids in patients after PPV than those in the control group. The results here suggested both the metabolism of amino acids and lipids may play significant roles in the progression of cataract after PPV [5]. Usually, more active of amino acids or proteins could be observed in the development of cataract, which has been reported by other studies and our previous studies [14, 15]. And especially in the present study among the standard amino acids, serine 1 accounted for the most associations in patient after PPV, which was reported to be associated with the formation of human age-related conditions such as cataract [24].

Conclusions

In conclusion, taking advantage of an unbiased technology GC-TOF-MS, we fully showed the metabolic characterization of AH in patients after PPV. More importantly, the significant metabolic variation including metabolite abundances and metabolic networks in PPV revealed key regulatory elements or pathways especially referred to amino acids and lipids metabolism in relation to cataract progression. The results here would extend our understanding on the underlying mechanism and may provide potential biomarkers for cataract diagnostics. However in the present study, there were still some deficiencies including the small number of samples and proper samples for control group due to ethical issues. At the same time, further studies with a great number of samples and much more effort are supposed to be done for validating the potential biomarkers for cataract diagnostics. Additionally in combination with other data/technologies including genomics and proteomics, these findings on metabolic changes need further explore to fully reveal the underlying mechanism in the cataract progression after PPV.

Abbreviations
AH: Aqueous humor; AMD: Age-related macular degeneration; ARC: Age-related cataract; BSS: Balanced salt solution; CE-MS: Capillary electrophoresis–mass spectrometry; CME: Cystoid macular edema; ERM: Epiretinal membrane; GC/TOF MS: Gas chromatography coupled to time-of-flight mass spectrometer; GC-MS: Gas chromatography-mass spectrometry; LC-MS: Liquid chromatography-mass spectrometry; LOCSIII: Lens opacities classification system III; NMR: Nuclear magnetic resonance; PCED: Persistent corneal epithelial defects; PLS-DA: Partial least squares discriminant analysis; PPV: Pars plana vitrectomy; RRD: Rhegmatogenous retinal detachment; VIP: Variable importance in the projection

Acknowledgements
Not applicable.

Funding
This study was supported by Grant No.81300745 and No. 81670835 from National Natural Science Foundation of China. The funders had no role in the design of the study and collection, analysis, and interpretation of data and in writing the manuscript.

Authors' contributions
Authors YHJ, XFR, and YL designed the study. YHJ, and XFR conducted the entired experiment. XFR participated in the data collection, analysis and interpretation. YHJ, XFR, YL participated in writing and revising of the manuscript. All authors read and approved the final manuscript.

Competing interests
The authors declare that they have no competing interests.

References
1. Machemer R, Buettner H, Norton EW, Parel JM. Vitrectomy: a pars plana approach. Trans Am Acad Ophthalmol Otolaryngol. 1971;75:813–20.
2. Mahdavi P, Tornambe PE. Pars Plana Vitrectomy. In: Rosenberg ED, Nattis AS, Nattis, RJ, editors. Operative Dictations in Ophthalmology. Switzerland: Springer International Publishing; 2017. p. 297–9.
3. Lalezary M, Kim SJ, Jiramongkolchai K, Recchia FM, Agarwal A, Sternberg P. Long-term trends in intraocular pressure after pars plana vitrectomy. Retina. 2011;31:679–85.
4. Shousha MA, Yoo SH. Cataract surgery after pars plana vitrectomy. Curr Opin Ophthalmol. 2010;21:45–9.
5. Ling CA, Weiter JJ, Buzney SM, Lashkari K. Competing theories of cataractogenesis after pars plana vitrectomy and the nutrient theory of cataractogenesis: a function of altered aqueous fluid dynamics. Int Ophthalmol Clin. 2005;45:173–98.
6. Chen L, Zhou L, Chan EC, Neo J, Beuerman RW. Characterization of the human tear metabolome by LC-MS/MS. J Proteome Res. 2011;10:4876–82.
7. Mayordomo-Febrer A, Lopez-Murcia M, Morales-Tatay JM, Monleon-Salvado D, Pinazo-Duran MD. Metabolomics of the aqueous humor in the rat glaucoma model induced by a series of intracamerular sodium hyaluronate injection. Exp Eye Res. 2015;131:84–92.
8. Tsentalovich YP, Verkhovod TD, Yanshole VV, Kiryutin AS, Yanshole LV, Fursova AZH, et al. Metabolomic composition of normal aged and cataractous human lenses. Exp Eye Res. 2015;134:15–23.
9. Pushpot S, Fitzpatrick M, Young S, Yang Y, Talks J, Wallace G. Metabolomic analysis in patients with age related macular degeneration. Invest Ophthalmol Vis Sci. 2013;54:3662.
10. Barbas-Bernardos C, Armitage EG, García A, Mérida S, Navea A, Bosch-Morell F, et al. Looking into aqueous humor through metabolomics spectacles-exploring its metabolic characteristics in relation to myopia. J Pharm Biomed Anal. 2016;127:18–25.
11. Brown JC, Sadler PJ, Spalton DJ, Juul SM, Macleod AF, Sšnksen PH. Analysis of human aqueous humour by high resolution ^{1}H NMR spectroscopy. Exp Eye Res. 1986;42:357–62.
12. Midelfart A, Gribbestad IS, Knutsen BH, Jørgensen L. Detection of metabolites in aqueous humour from cod eye by high resolution ^{1}H NMR spectroscopy. Comp Biochem Phys B. 1996;113:445–50.

13. Rossi T, Querzoli G, Angelini G, Rossi A, Malvasi C, Iossa M, et al. Ocular perfusion pressure during pars plana vitrectomy: a pilot study. Invest Ophthalmol Vis Sci. 2014;55:8497–505.

14. Ji Y, Rong X, Ye H, Zhang K, Lu Y. Proteomic analysis of aqueous humor proteins associated with cataract development. Clin Biochem. 2015;48:1304–9.

15. Ji Y, Rao J, Rong X, Lou S, Zheng Z, Lu Y. Metabolic characterization of human aqueous humor in relation to high myopia. Exp Eye Res. 2017;159: 147–55.

16. Liu B, Gu Y, Xiao H, Lei X, Liang W, Zhang J. Altered metabolomic profiles may be associated with sevoflurane-induced neurotoxicity in neonatal rats. Neurochem Res. 2015;40:788–99.

17. Rao J, Cheng F, Hu CY, Quan S, Lin H, Wang J, et al. Metabolic map of mature maize kernels. Metabolomics. 2014;10:775–87.

18. Luo D, Deng T, Yuan W, Deng H, Jin M. Plasma metabolomic study in Chinese patients with wet age-related macular degeneration. BMC Ophthalmol. 2017;17:165.

19. Rao J, Yang L, Guo J, Quan S, Chen G, Zhao X, et al. Metabolic changes in transgenic maize mature seeds over-expressing the *Aspergillus niger* phyA2. Plant Cell Rep. 2016;35:429–37.

20. Chung CP, Hsu SY, Wu WC. Cataract formation after pars plan vitrectomy. Kaoshiung J Med Sci. 2001;17:84–9.

21. Groves N. IOP elevations induce oxidative stress. Ophthalmol Times. 2007; 32:38.

22. de Oliveira MF, Hagen MEK, Pederzolli CD, Sgaravatti AM, Durigon K, Testa CG, et al. Glutaric acid induces oxidative stress in brain of young rats. Brain Res. 2003;964:153–8.

23. Pohl CH, Kock JLF, Thibane VS. Antifungal free fatty acids: a review. Sci microb pathog. 2011;1:61–71.

24. Hooi M, Raftery MJ, Truscott RJW. Age-dependent racemization of serine residues in a human chaperone protein. Protein Sci. 2013;22:93–100.

7

Analysis of intraocular positions of posterior implantable collamer lens by full-scale ultrasound biomicroscopy

Xi Zhang[1,2,3], Xun Chen[2,3], Xiaoying Wang[2,3*], Fei Yuan[1] and Xingtao Zhou[2,3]

Abstract

Background: To analyze the positions of intraocular posterior Implantable Collamer Lens (ICL) and its possible relationship with vault.

Methods: This cross-sectional study included 72 patients with high myopia (134 eyes) who were followed up after phakic intraocular lens implantation. The postoperative time ranged from 1 week to 7 years. We obtained the images of ICL by using Compact Touch STS UBM and observed the position of ICL in posterior chamber and ciliary sulcus. The horizontal lines vault was measured and recorded.

Results: There were various positions in the posterior chamber as observed by full-scale ultrasound biomicroscopy and the haptics were inserted at different positions. -Eight seven eyes (64.9%) that obtained ideal vault, 29 eyes (21.6%) had insufficient vaults and 18 eyes (13.4%) had excessive vault. The vault with various positions of haptics was in ideal range (250 μm–750 μm) almost in each group. Three eyes in this study with haptics on the top of ciliary sulcus obtained excessive vault (mean vault, 850.00 ± 70.71 μm) and one eye appeared one side haptics pushing forward the iris. Among five eyes (3.7%) with iridociliary body cysts, three eyes (60%) obtained ideal vault. One eye (0.7%) with ICL decentralization after implantation surgery had an ideal vault, but the patient had serious glare.

Conclusions: Though ICL in the posterior chamber had different positions and the haptics in most cases were not in the ciliary sulcus, the postoperative vault was almost in the ideal range.

Keywords: High myopia, Phakic intraocular Lens, Implantable Collamer Lens, Ultrasound biomicroscopy, Vault

Background

Phakic intraocular lens (PIOL) implantation is a technique to correct high ametropia as the condition cannot be corrected by laser in situ keratomileusis (LASIK). The implantable collamer lens (Visian ICL; STAAR Surgical, Nidau, Switzerland) is a posterior chamber phakic IOL and was approved by FDA in December 2005 for commercial use in the United States for myopia -3D to -20D [1]. It is made of a porcine collagen/hema copolymer material which is thin, flexible, and hydrophilic. It is 7.0 mm wide and the length of myopia model varies from 11.5 to 13. 0 mm. The diameter of the optic zone varies from 4. 5 to 5.5 mm according to the diopter power of the lens. The Toric implantable collamer lens (TICL) correct – 3.00 to – 6.00D astigmatism [2]. ICL/TICL is most widely adopted for correction of high myopia in the world due to their safe and effective strategies than laser corneal surgery [3–7].

Ultrasound biomicroscopy is a high-frequency ultrasound technology that provides information of posterior iris, which cannot be evaluated through slit-lamp microscopy or Pentacam anterior segment analyzer before and after ICL/TICL implantation. Preoperatively, ultrasound biomicroscopy is helpful in discovering the existence of post-iris anomalies [8–10]. Postoperatively, ultrasound biomicroscopy evaluates the appropriate

* Correspondence: doctxiaoyingwang@163.com
[2]Department of Ophthalmology, Eye and ENT Hospital of Fudan University, Shanghai, People's Republic of China
[3]Department of Ophthalmology, Myopia Key Laboratory of the Health Ministry, Shanghai, People's Republic of China
Full list of author information is available at the end of the article

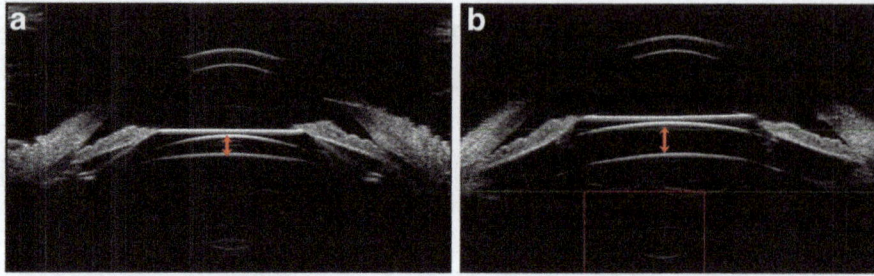

Fig. 1 Images of normal anterior segment on horizontal (**a**) and vertical (**b**) meridians as measured by Compact Touch STS UBM. Arrows showed the vault of horizontal and vertical meridian, respectively

position of phakic IOL of posterior chamber, including the optical zone, bilateral haptics and relation to iris, crystalline lens, zonules and ciliary body [11, 12].

As we know, the ideal phakic IOL position show the optical zone located on the center of the pupil, and both haptics on the sulcus with an appropriate vault (250 μm -750 μm). Because excessive (> 750 μm) or insufficient (< 250 μm) vault lead to complications such as pigmentary loss, glaucoma or cataract, and the stability of vault becomes the major concern after ICL implantation [13]. The ICL dislocation usually results in an inappropriate vault [14]. To our knowledge, the relationship between different kinds of dislocation of ICL haptics and vault has not been reported till date. The purpose of this study is to evaluate the various positions of ICL haptics after implantation in high myopic eyes by capturing the images using full-scan ultrasound biomicroscopy and its effect on the vault.

Methods
Subjects
This cross-sectional study included 72 patients with high myopia (134 eyes) who were followed up after phakic intraocular lens implantation in the Eye and ENT Hospital of Fudan University from May to July

in 2014. The mean age was 29.78 ± 7.61 years old (range 19–48 years old). The preoperative spherical diopter ranged from − 22.50D to − 5.50D and the mean spherical equivalent was − 13.32 ± 5.10D. The postoperative time ranged from 1 week to 7 years. Before surgery, all patients had a complete ophthalmic examination, such as uncorrected visual acuity (UCVA), best corrected visual acuity (BCVA), manifest and cycloplegic refraction, anterior chamber depth (ACD), corneal keratometry, intraocular pressure, retinal examination through a dilated pupil and ultrasound biomicroscopic examination. The inclusion criteria were as follows: spectacles and/or contact lens intolerance, stable refraction for at least 1 year before preoperative examination, the endothelial cell density (ECD) ≥2100 cell/mm, anterior chamber depth ≥ 2.8 mm, no history of cataract, glaucoma, uveitis, uncontrolled diabetes, collagen vascular disease, or previous intraocular surgery.

ICL size calculation
Size of the myopic lens was determined by the horizontal white-to-white (WTW) and the anterior chamber depth (ACD) measurements. The lens size was calculated by adding 0.5 mm to the white-to-white

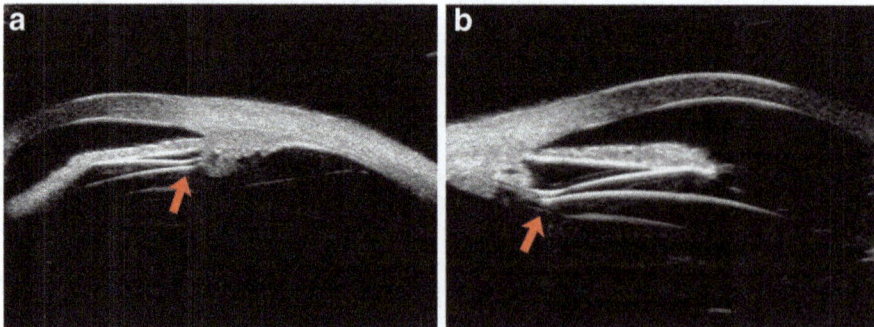

Fig. 2 Images of ICL haptics position on temporal (**a**) and nasal (**b**) as measured by Compact Touch STS UBM. Arrows showed the haptics position

measurement when eyes exhibited an ACD between 2.8 and 3.5 mm and 1.0 mm to the white-to-white measurement when the ACD was greater than 3.5 mm. All lens power calculations were performed by STAAR Surgical Company.

Surgical procedure

At least 1 week before ICL implantation, patients received two peripheral laser Nd:YAG iridotomies at 10:30 and 1: 30 clock positions. On the day of surgery, 2.5% phenylephrine for mydriasis and 0.4% oxybuprocain hydrochloride eye drops were applied to the operative eye before surgery. All ICL/TICL implantations into the posterior chamber were performed with an injector cartridge designed by STAAR Surgical through a 3.2 mm corneal tunnel incision in the horizontal meridian using peribulbar anesthesia. The anterior chamber was filled with sodium hyaluronate 1% (Provisc), which was completely removed at the end of surgery. During TICL implantation, the surgeon marked the zero horizontal axis at the 3- and 9-o'clock limbus using a marking pen with the patient sitting upright at a slit lamp. The surgeon also used a Mendez ring to measure the required rotation from horizontal during the surgical procedure and the lens was rotated to the required axis using a modified intraocular spatula. Tobramycin eye drops were used four times a day for 7 days, 0.1% fluorometholone eye drops were instilled six times a day from the second day after surgery and minus one time every three days for one month.

Postoperative full-scale ultrasound biomicroscopy examination

During the follow-up period, all subjects underwent postoperative Compact Touch STS UBM (Quantel Medical, France) examination whose linear scanning frequency is 50 MHz; scanning depth and width is 9 *16 mm; the resolution of axial and vertical is 35 μm, 60 μm, respectively. Its reliability has been reported in the previous study [15]. Examinations were performed using an eyecup filled with methylcellulose solution after topical oxybuprocaine hydrochloride was instilled to anesthetize the cornea, while the subjects were asked to fixate on a ceiling target and keep head still in the spine position. The examiner adjusts the probe perpendicular to the eyes, choose the UBM/STS pattern and acquires vertical (6 o'clock – 12 o'clock) and horizontal (3 o'clock - 9 o'clock) lines images. The patients were then asked to gaze at the nasal and temporal angles for acquiring images of ICL haptics in ciliary sulcus, and record the horizontal vault. Figs 1 and 2 showed the images of normal anterior segment taken by UBM after phakic IOL implantation as measured by Compact Touch STS UBM. All image acquisitions were completed by the same physician.

Results

In this study, ICL implantation in the posterior chamber was observed at various positions and 74. 1% eyes had ICL or ICL haptics dislocation such as

Table 1 ICL/TICL and haptics posterior chamber position in 72 patients (134 eyes)

Position	Eyes(%)	Vault(μm, mean ± SD)	Ideal vault eyes (250 μm–750 μm)	Insufficient vault eyes(<250 μm)	Excessive vault eyes(>750 μm)
In ciliary sulcus	29(21.6%)	573.10 ± 253.94	23(79.3%)	4(13.8%)	2(6.9%)
On the top of ciliary sulcus	3(2.2%)	850.00 ± 70.71	0	0	3(100%)
In ciliary process	17(12.7%)	453.53 ± 215.09	13(76.5%)	3(17.6%)	1(5.9%)
Under ciliary sulcus	14(10.4%)	498.57 ± 200.92	11(78.6%)	2(14.3%)	1(7.1%)
Inserted in the ciliary body	43(32.1%)	520.73 ± 329.40	22(51.2%)	13(30.2%)	8(18.6%)
One haptics under the ciliary sulcus	6(4.5%)	725.00 ± 249.78	5(83.3%)	0	1(16.7%)
One haptics on the ciliary process, another haptics inserted the ciliary body	10(7.5%)	300.00 ± 208.91	4(40%)	6(60%)	0
One haptics on the ciliary process, another haptics under the ciliary body	4(3.0%)	533.33 ± 190.35	4(100%)	0	0
One haptics under the ciliary sulcus, another haptics inserted the ciliary body	2(1.5%)	375.00 ± 388.91	1(50%)	1(50%)	0
With iris ciliary body cysts	5(3.7%)	656.00 ± 283.69	3(60%)	0	2(40%)
ICL decentralization	1(0.7%)	550	1(100%)	0	0
Total	134		87(64.9%)	29(21.6%)	18(13.4%)

in the ciliary process; on the top of ciliary sulcus; under ciliary sulcus; the haptics inserted in the ciliary body; one haptics under the ciliary sulcus; One haptics on the ciliary process, another haptics inserted the ciliary body; one haptics on the ciliary process, another haptics under the ciliary body; one haptics under the ciliary sulcus, another haptics inserted in the ciliary body; ICL decentralization through the UBM images of the subjects having ICL/TICL implantation. Even though, the mean vault of each kind of position observed in this study was in ideal range (250 μm -750 μm) except in three eyes with haptics on the top of ciliary sulcus (850.00 ± 70.71 μm). Among the three eyes, one eye appeared with haptics pushing forward the iris. More than half eyes (64.9%) in 134 eyes acquired ideal vault. Five eyes were with iridociliary cysts preoperatively and three eyes (60%) had ideal vault. Information regarding the population of the position of phakic IOL and the vault was seen in Table 1.

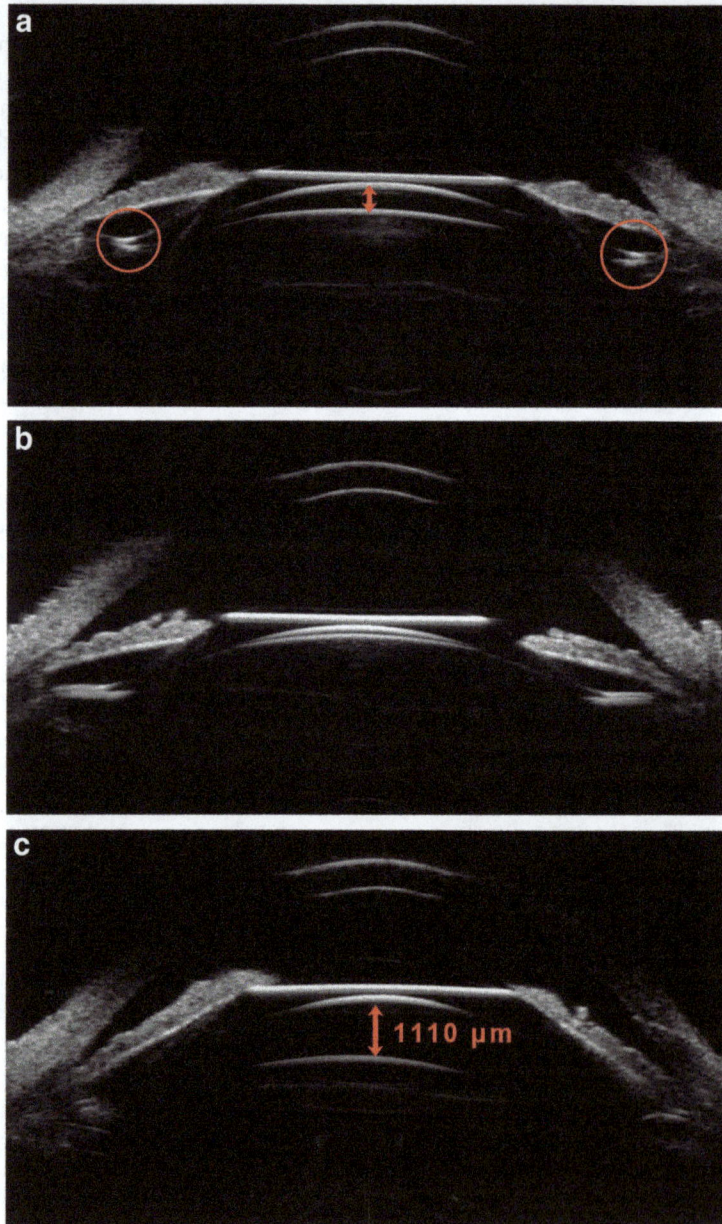

Fig. 3 UBM images of ideal ICL posterior chamber position after implantation. **a** UBM images of one patient with ideal vault; **b** UBM images of one patient with the vault barely disappeared, while the ICL was at normal position; **c** UBM images of one patient with excessive vault, while the ICL was at normal position. The arrowes showed the vault; the red circles showed haptics position

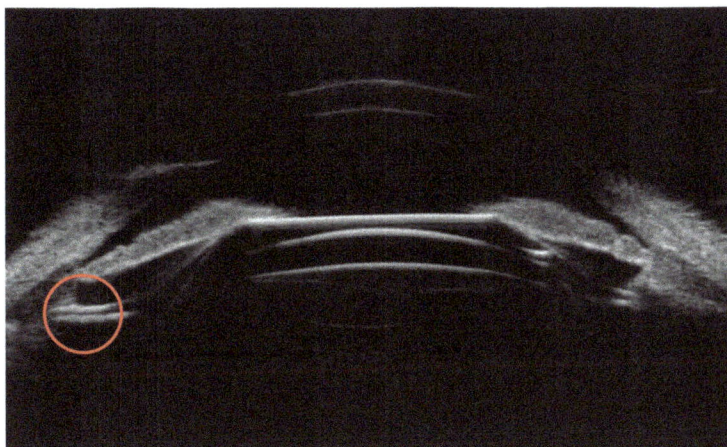

Fig. 4 UBM images of one patient with an ideal vault, while one haptic was inserted into the ciliary body. The red circles showed the haptics position

Figure 3 shows the different vault when ICL had an ideal position -optical zone in the center of the pupil and the haptics located in the ciliary sulcus.

Figures 4, 5, 6 shows the different vault when ICL haptics inserted in the ciliary body.

Figures 7, 8, 9 shows the different vault when ICL haptics dislocation including on the top of sulcus, in the ciliary process and under the sulcus. In this study, all eyes with haptics on the top of sulcus obtained excessive vault, while another showed dislocation of haptics with no eyes exhibiting excessive vault.

In our study, some patients underwent ICL implantation surgery with preoperative iris ciliary cysts. The incidence of iridociliary cysts ranged from 4.9% (1157 patients) to 54.3% (116 patients), which showed no consensus and the large iridociliary cysts caused anterior chamber angle closure and increased the risk of secondary glaucoma [10, 16, 17]. Most of the diameter of the cysts are less than 1 mm and have no effect on phakic IOL implantation. However, huge (diameter > 2 mm) or multiple cysts could increase the risk of ICL dislocation, the operator preoperatively should carefully estimate and avoid the cysts intra-operatively. Figure 10 showed the UBM image of preoperative iris ciliary cysts. Figure 11 showed the UBM image after implantation surgery in patients with preoperative iris ciliary cysts.

One case in our study demonstrated the optical zone of ICL departure from the center of the pupil and complained with severe glare. Figure 12 showed the UBM images of this patient.

Discussion

The central vault concept is defined as the distance between the back of the surface of the ICL and the

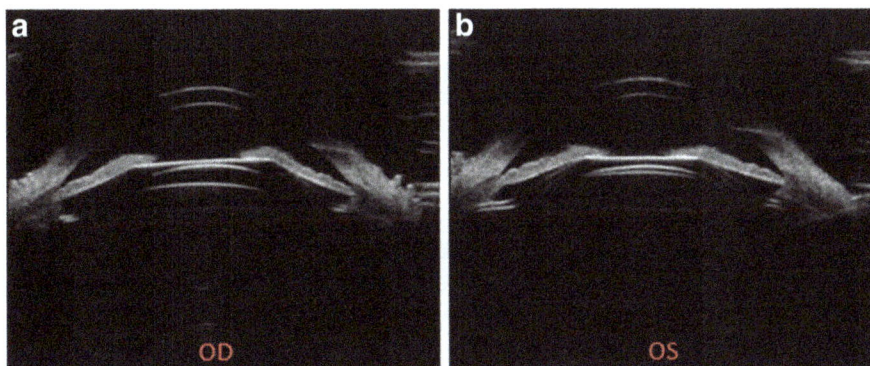

Fig. 5 UBM images of one patient (2 eyes) with different vaults –the right eye obtained an ideal vault (**a**), while the left vault barely disappeared when the one haptic was inserted into the ciliary body (**b**)

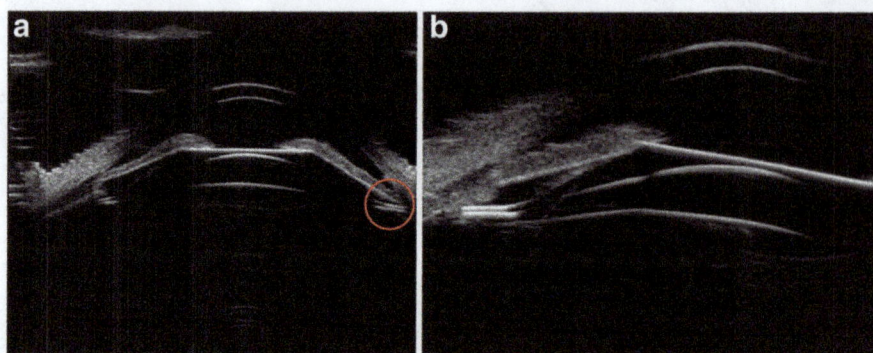

Fig. 6 UBM images of one patient with an excessive vault, while one haptic was inserted into the ciliary body. (**a**) Full-scale images of the ICL in the posterior chamber position; (**b**) the haptics position on the nasal. The red circles showed the haptics position

anterior crystalline lens pole. The vault is considered as an important index to evaluate the security after ICL implantation. Although most of the postoperative patients can obtain ideal vault, excessive or insufficient vaults cannot be avoided. The vault is a dynamic range but a fixed value and is influenced by many factors such as ICL size, ICL posterior chamber position, ages, pupil size [18]. The inappropriate ICL size, especially too large ICL size, caused by the preoperative white to white inaccurate measurement usually leads to shallow anterior chamber, pigmentary loss, glaucoma and corneal endothelial loss because of the excessive vault. Besides the size, the thickness of ICL was increased with refractive diopter. However, the thickness of ICL ranged from 1.19 mm to 1.09 mm according to the refractive diopter, and a difference of 0.9 mm could be ignored. Lege, B. A. [19] had reported that the vault tended to decrease with age. It was possibly related with anterior lens capsule thickening with age and decreased the distance between lens anterior capsule and back of the surface of the ICL.

According to a previous study on pupil size, miosis caused by natural light could decrease the vault as compared with the drug-induced miosis [20]. The ICL in the posterior chamber position was closely associated with some complications postoperatively, but it is fully observed only by full-scale ultrasound biomicroscopy after implantation surgery and hence we implanted the ICL into the posterior chamber intra-operatively without a thorough view. In another word, the implant surgery was performed in blind, thus lead to the ICL placement does not always obtain an ideal position, especially the ICL haptics. Though UBM could be used during operation to provide a straight view, the operators always performed the implantation based on the experience due to the inconvenience of UBM and helpless for the postoperative safety and efficacy. We expect a more excellent technique to be used and prevent the dislocation of ICL and haptics.

In this study, firstly, we found that the haptics position after implantation was inserted into the ciliary body (32.1%) and 21.6% eyes with haptics in the

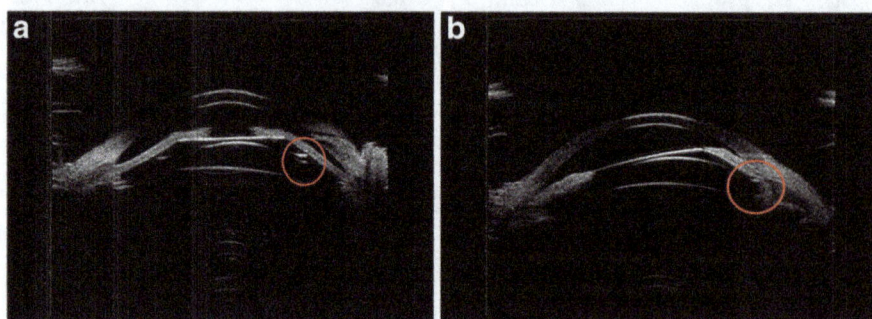

Fig. 7 UBM images of ICL, one side haptic on the top of the ciliary sulcus and iris losing the normal arc shape because of being pushed by haptics. The vault exhibited more than 750 μm in (**a**) and (**b**). The red circles showed the haptics position

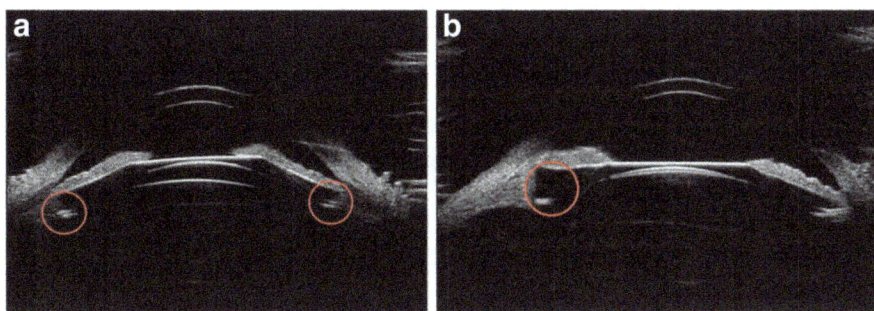

Fig. 8 UBM images of ICL, one side haptic in the ciliary process with an ideal vault (**a**) and ciliary sulcus distortion with the vault disappearing because of the process being pushed by haptics (**b**). The red circles showed the haptics position

ciliary sulcus, which was probably due to the ICL size choice preoperatively and invisible intraoperatively. Secondly, though the haptics located on various positions postoperatively, almost each group vault with different positions of the haptics was in normal range. There were 64.9% eyes obtained normal vault in total, while 21.6% eyes (29/134) with insufficient vault and only 13.4% eyes (18/134) with excessive vault. Of these, all three eyes with haptics on the top of ciliary body obtained excessive vault and one eye with haptics pushing forward the iris. This meant that the vault after surgery overall tended to be normal and were less susceptible to be excessive in various positions of haptics. This could be due to the excessive vault, which always appears after implanting too large ICL, would be adjusted during postoperative in early stage and the vault tend to decrease with time after implantation of appropriate ICL size. Thirdly, to find the relationship between follow-up time period and vault, we analyzed the vault of patients after implantation surgery who were followed-up less and more than 1 year, respectively. In 107 eyes of 58 patients were followed-up in less than a year, there were 31 eyes (29.0%) with vault less than 250 μm, and in 14 patients (27 eyes) with follow-up longer than 1 year, 16 eyes (59.3%) with insufficient vault compared to the rest of the 11 eyes with normal vault. We speculate that the vault tend to decrease with postoperative time increasing, which was in accordance with previous research [21, 22]. Among 8 patients (15 eyes) who were more than 40 years old in our study, only 5 eyes (33.3%) obtained insufficient vault and was far less than the results that were reported previously [19]. It might be due to the small sample size and we need to expand the sample size for further analysis.

How to deal with the various haptics position in different vaults is also our major concern and finding a reasonable solution would be more helpful for preoperative and postoperative estimation. In this study, we obtained the following conclusions by observing various haptics positions and took different relevant treatment depending on different situations: (a) the haptics inserting into the ciliary body (32.1%) and in ciliary sulcus (21.6%) were relatively common

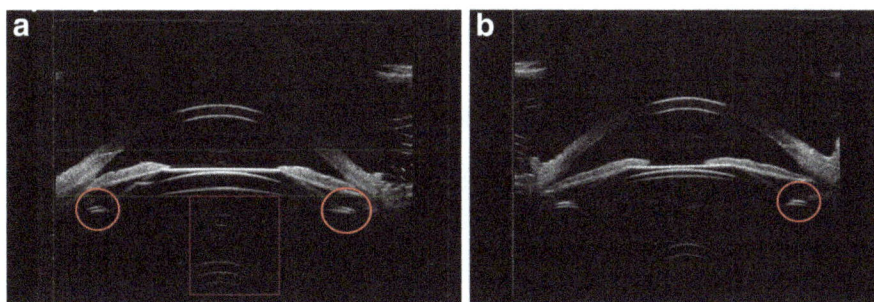

Fig. 9 UBM images of ICL haptics under the ciliary sulcus. (**a**) bilateral haptics under the ciliary sulcus with an ideal vault. (**b**) one side of the haptics under the ciliary sulcus with insufficient vault. The red circles showed the haptics position

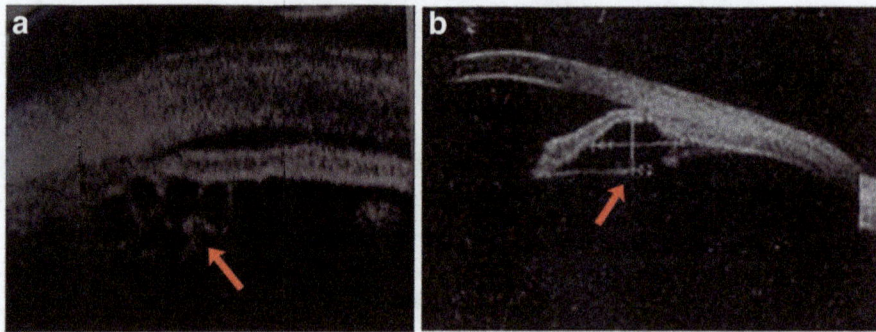

Fig. 10 UBM images of multiple cysts (**a**) and huge cysts (diameter > 2 mm, (**b**)). Arrows showed the cysts

after the implantation surgery (b) most eyes (79.3%) with haptics in ciliary sulcus obtained ideal vault, except 4 eyes with insufficient vault and 2 eyes with an excessive vault. Among them, 2 eyes with insufficient vault were speculated to have implanted with smaller ICL due to shallow anterior chamber diameter preoperatively. No treatment was provided to the eye with excessive vault, which showed no complications of IOP rising or angle closure postoperatively. So, we could followed-up the cases with haptics in ciliary sulcus (c) the cases with ICL haptics inserted into the ciliary body were inclined to have insufficient vault, which might be due to the haptics position which reduced the distance between ICL and crystalline lens. Beyond this, some patients with vault less than 250 μm might be due to the implantation of smaller ICL size. The cases in this situation could receive follow-up observation (d) the haptics dislocation included on the top of ciliary sulcus, in the ciliary process and under ciliary sulcus. One eye in this study with haptics on the top of ciliary sulcus had iris pushed by haptics and lost the normal arc shape, so that the vault appeared far more than 750 μm. It was probably because the operator could not see the back of the iris straightly and the haptics were not incorrectly placed, which induced the ICL abnormal arching. In the case of those patients with implantation of inappropriate ICL size, we should topically instill pilocarpine to contract the pupil and observe for one week. If the vault still remains excessive and have risk of angle closure after one week, the haptics or the ICL should be adjusted through the operation. If the haptics in the ciliary process lead to the abnormal structure of ciliary sulcus, the ICL might shift downwards and the vault might usually be less than 250 μm. The haptics under the ciliary sulcus had less impact on the distance between ICL and crystalline and need follow-up observation. (e) Compared

with the incidence of iridociliary cysts in the previous report (4.9–54.3%), the incidence in our study was significantly lower (3.7%). This probably might be due to small sample size. The iridociliary cysts probably effected the haptics position and induced some patients obtaining abnormal vault. For these cases, special treatment was unnecessary if the IOP was not increased. (f) One patient with the ICL optical zone decentralization in our study complained of having sever glare and the UBM images showed the vault to be in ideal range. We speculated that the postoperative visual quality was closely related with ICL position. Further research on larger sample size is warranted to conclude the results of glare or poor visual quality and explore the inner relationship between visual quality and ICL or ICL haptics position.

In this cross-sectional study, we recruited the patients who were performed with ICL V4 implantation surgery and the postoperative period ranged from 1 week to 7 years. We obtained the UBM images of every patient and mainly investigated the relationship between various haptic positions and the vault in different postoperative period. Though the changes of the haptics and ICL positions in different follow-up period of one patient were not observed in our study, the comprehensive analysis and numerous of UBM images were considered to being helpful for surgeons to deal with various ICL positions and vault. In the future, a prospective study should be performed to investigate the changes of haptics and ICL positions as the postoperative time prolonging.

Conclusion

In conclusion, full-scale ultrasound biomicroscopy provides a straight view regarding various positions of ICL or haptics in posterior chamber after implantation. And in this study, we noticed that the location of haptics placed inappropriately (not in ciliary

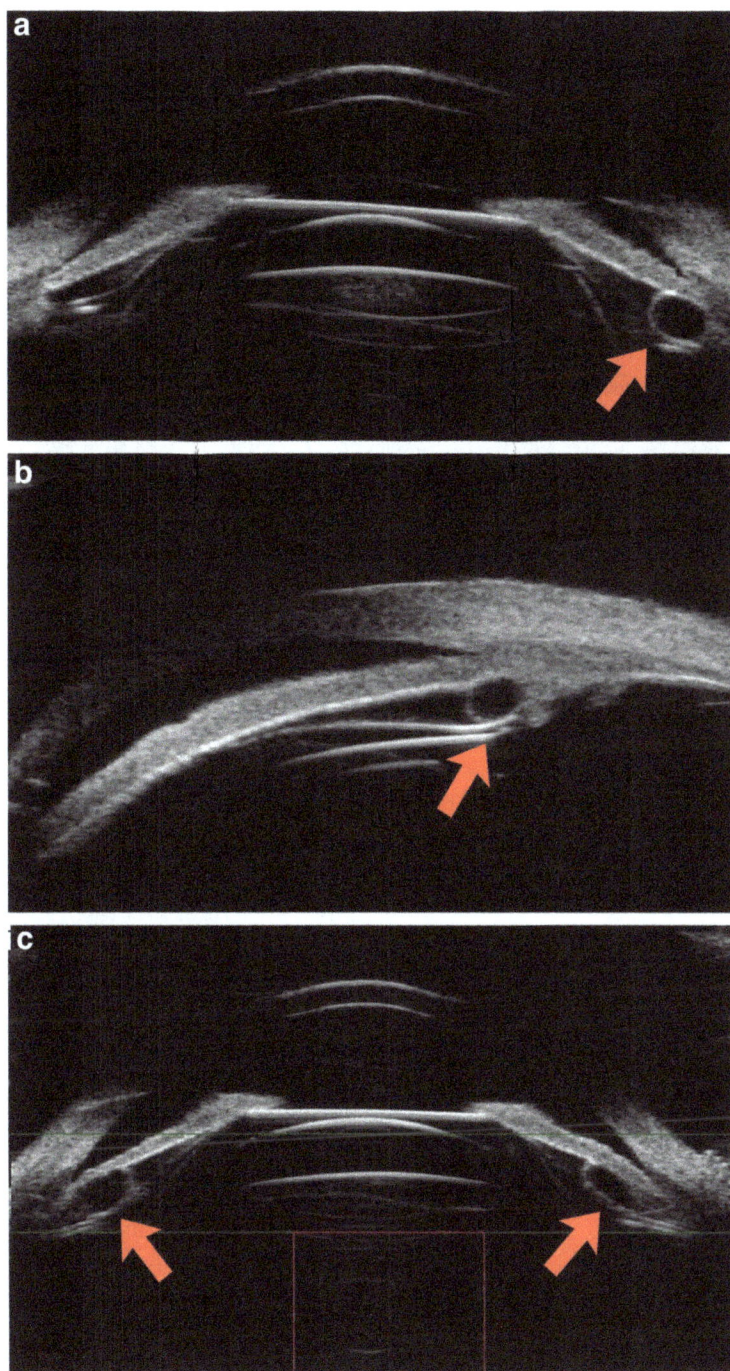

Fig. 11 UBM images after implantation in patients with iris ciliary cysts. (**a**, **b**, **c**) listed various position of haptics. Arrows showed the haptics

sulcus) might be one of the factors influencing the vault through observing positions of ICL and haptics in the posterior chamber after implantation by recording UBM images and the incidences of different vault (less than 250 μm; 250~750 μm; and more than 750 μm) in various situations. Though we had not abstract the exact relationship between the haptics position and vault due to the small sample size in this study, our research on ICL or ICL haptics position in posterior chamber was undoubtedly helpful for the surgeons to directly estimate the appropriateness of ICL size, the ICL implanted position and find out the possible reasons of less-than-ideal vault. Follow-up observation is usually recommended

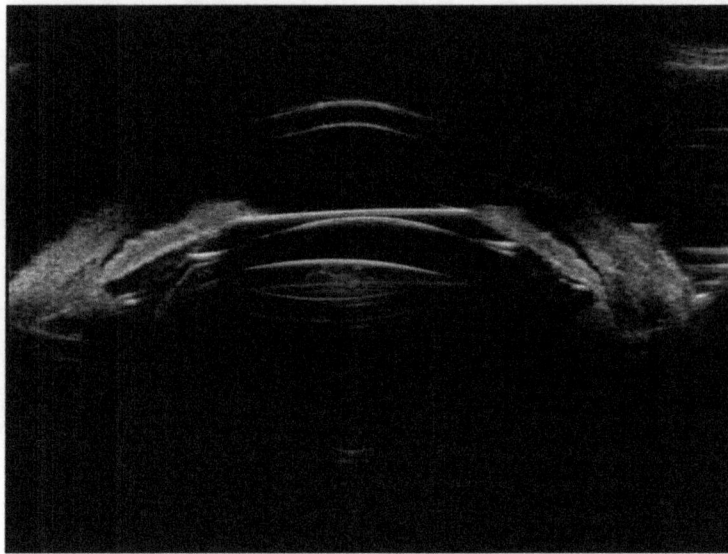

Fig. 12 UBM images of the eye with ICL optical zone departure from the center of the pupil and an ideal vault

in patients with insufficient vault; but if the positions of ICL or haptics resulted in excessive vault, topical pilocarpine is applied to contract the pupil followed by observation for one week and if the excessive vault is due to a large ICL size, then the best course of action is to exchange the ICL. The accurate assessment of these cases is undoubtedly beneficial for the surgeons to accumulate more experience on evaluating the safety of the surgical outcome and dealing with the dislocation and less-than-ideal vault caused by various reasons.

Abbreviations
ACD: Anterior chamber depth; BCVA: Best corrected visual acuity; ICL: Implantable Collamer Lens; LASIK: Laser in situ keratomileusis; PIOL: Phakic intraocular lens; TICL: Toric implantable collamer lens; UCVA: Uncorrected visual acuity

Funding
The project from the Shanghai Shenkang Hospital Development Center (Grant No. SHDC12016207): design of the study and collection, analysis, and interpretation of data. The project from the Health and Family Planning Committee of Pudong New District of Shanghai, China (Grant No. PW2014D-1): write the manuscript and pay for a professional language editing service.

Authors' contributions
XZ and XC carried out the studies, participated in collecting data and performed the statistical analysis. XZ drafted the manuscript. XZ and FY prepare and review of the manuscript. XYW and FY participated in the design of the study. XYW and XTZ have revised it critically for important intellectual content and given final approval of the version to be published. All authors read and approved the final manuscript.

Competing interests
The authors declare that they have no competing interests.

Author details
[1]Department of Ophthalmology, Zhongshan Hospital of Fudan University, Shanghai, People's Republic of China. [2]Department of Ophthalmology, Eye and ENT Hospital of Fudan University, Shanghai, People's Republic of China. [3]Department of Ophthalmology, Myopia Key Laboratory of the Health Ministry, Shanghai, People's Republic of China.

References
1. Sanders DR, Doney K, Poco M. United States Food and Drug Administration clinical trial of the implantable Collamer Lens (ICL) for moderate to high myopia: three-year follow-up. Ophthalmology. 2004;111(9):1683–92.
2. Sanders DR, Schneider D, Martin R, Brown D, Dulaney D, Vukich J, et al. Toric implantable Collamer Lens for moderate to high myopic astigmatism. Ophthalmology. 2007;114(1):54–61.
3. Sanders DR, Vukich JA. Comparison of implantable contact lens and laser assisted in situ keratomileusis for moderate to high myopia. Cornea. 2003; 22(4):324–31.
4. Sanders DR, Sanders ML. Comparison of the toric implantable collamer lens and custom ablation LASIK for myopic astigmatism. J Refract Surg. 2008; 24(8):773–8.
5. Alfonso JF, Lisa C, Fernandez-Vega Cueto L, Fernandes P, Gonzalez-Meijome JM, Montes Mico R. Comparison of visual and refractive results of Toric implantable Collamer Lens with bioptics for myopic astigmatism. Graefes Arch Clin Exp Ophthalmol. 2013;251(3):967–75.
6. Kamiya K, Shimizu K, Kobashi H, Igarashi A, Komatsu M, Nakamura A, et al. Three-year follow-up of posterior chamber toric phakic intraocular lens implantation for the correction of high myopic astigmatism in eyes with keratoconus. Br J Ophthalmol. 2015;99(2):177–83.
7. Sayman Muslubas IB, Kandemir B, Aydin Oral AY, Kugu S, Dastan M. Long-term vision-threatening complications of phakic intraocular lens implantation for high myopia. Int J Ophthalmol. 2014;7(2):376–80.
8. Oh J, Shin HH, Kim JH, Kim HM, Song JS. Direct measurement of the ciliary sulcus diameter by 35-megahertz ultrasound biomicroscopy. Ophthalmology. 2007;114(9):1685–8.

9.   Kim KH, Shin HH, Kim HM, Song JS. Correlation between ciliary sulcus diameter measured by 35 MHz ultrasound biomicroscopy and other ocular measurements. J Cataract Refract Surg. 2008;34(4):632–7.

10. Kunimatsu S, Araie M, Ohara K, Hamada C. Ultrasound biomicroscopy of ciliary body cysts. Am J Ophthalmol. 1999;127(1):48–55.

11. Choi KH, Chung SE, Chung TY, Chung ES. Ultrasound biomicroscopy for determining visian implantable contact lens length in phakic IOL implantation. J Refract Surg. 2007;23(4):362–7.

12. Pitault G, Leboeuf C, Leroux Les Jardins S, Auclin F, Chong-Sit D, Baudouin C. Ultrasound biomicroscopy of posterior chamber phakic intraocular lenses: a comparative study between ICL and PRL models. J Fr Ophtalmol. 2005; 28(9):914–23.

13. Du GP, Huang YF, Wang LQ, Wang DJ, Guo HL, Yu JF, et al. Changes in objective vault and effect on vision outcomes after implantable Collamer lens implantation: 1-year follow-up. Eur J Ophthalmol. 2012;22(2):153–60.

14. Shi M, Kong J, Li X, Yan Q, Zhang J. Observing implantable collamer lens dislocation by panoramic ultrasound biomicroscopy. Eye (Lond). 2015;29(4): 499–504.

15. Li DJ, Wang NL, Chen S, Li SN, Mu DP, Wang T. Accuracy and repeatability of direct ciliary sulcus diameter measurements by full-scale 50-megahertz ultrasound biomicroscopy. Chin Med J. 2009;122(8):955–9.

16. Aman-Ullah M, Gimbel HV, Camoriano GD. Toric implantable collamer lens implantation in a case with bilateral primary peripheral iris cysts. Ophthalmic Surg Lasers Imaging. 2012;43(Online):e18–21.

17. Cronemberger S, Ferreira DM, Diniz Filho A, Merula RV, Calixto N. Iridociliary cysts on ultrasound biomicroscopic examinations. Arq Bras Oftalmol. 2006; 69(4):471–5.

18. Mori T, Yokoyama S, Kojima T, Isogai N, Ito M, Horai R, et al. Factors affecting rotation of a posterior chamber collagen copolymer toric phakic intraocular lens. J Cataract Refract Surg. 2012;38(4):568–73.

19. Lege BA, Haigis W, Neuhann TF, Bauer MH. Age-related behavior of posterior chamber lenses in myopic phakic eyes during accommodation measured by anterior segment partial coherence interferometry. J Cataract Refract Surg. 2006;32(6):999–1006.

20. Petternel V, Koppl CM, Dejaco-Ruhswurm I, Findl O, Skorpik C, Drexler W. Effect of accommodation and pupil size on the movement of a posterior chamber lens in the phakic eye. Ophthalmology. 2004;111(2):325–31.

21. Alfonso JF, Fernandez-Vega L, Lisa C, Fernandes P, Jorge J, Montes Mico R. Central vault after phakic intraocular lens implantation: correlation with anterior chamber depth, white-to-white distance, spherical equivalent, and patient age. J Cataract Refract Surg. 2012;38(1):46–53.

22. Kamiya K, Shimizu K, Komatsu M. Factors affecting vaulting after implantable collamer lens implantation. J Refract Surg. 2009;25(3):259–64.

8

Surgical factors affecting oculocardiac reflex during strabismus surgery

Suk-Gyu Ha[1,2], Jungah Huh[1,2], Bo-Ram Lee[1,2] and Seung-Hyun Kim[1,2]*

Abstract

Background: To investigate surgical factors associated with the occurrence of oculocardiac reflex (OCR) and changes in heart rate (HR) during strabismus surgery.

Methods: Patients who underwent strabismus surgery under general anesthesia were enrolled in this study. The HR during surgery was measured at baseline, and at the following points during surgery: traction of the muscle, maximal increase after traction (adrenergic phase), and the cutting of the muscle. OCR was defined as an HR reduction of more than 20% at traction of the muscle, when compared to baseline HR. The HR at each stage during the surgery was compared between patients with and without OCR.

Results: A total of 162 operated muscles from 99 patients were enrolled. The incidence of OCR was 65% in patients. In patients with two muscle surgeries, there were significantly more OCRs in the first operated muscle than in the second operated muscle ($p < 0.01$). The difference in the decrease in HR in patients with OCR was significantly lower than that in patients without OCR at traction of the muscle, the adrenergic phase, and the cutting of the muscle (all, $p < 0.01$). The first operated muscle was a significant risk factor associated with the occurrence of OCR ($OR = 3.95$, $p < 0.01$).

Conclusion: The first operated muscle in patients with two muscle surgeries was a significant risk factor for OCR. Decreased HR at the traction of the muscle during surgery did not fully recover in patients with OCR.

Keywords: Oculocardiac reflex, Strabismus, Surgery

Background

Oculocardiac reflex (OCR) is a phenomenon defined by bradycardia or dysrhythmia during strabismus surgery [1]. Although the definition of OCR has not yet been formally established, prevalence of OCR ranges from 14% to 90%, based on varying published definitions [2, 3]. Oculocardiac reflex is commonly caused by the traction on the extraocular muscle (EOM), which, through the ophthalmic branch of trigeminal nerve, stimulates the vagal center. The afferent arm of the reflex is the ophthalmic branch of the trigeminal nerve, and the efferent arm is the vagus nerve, which diminishes sinoatrial node impulses and leads to bradycardia [1, 4]. Transient cardiac arrest has been reported to occur in about 1/2200 cases during strabismus surgery [5]. Sino-atrial arrests and ventricular fibrillation have been reported [6, 7].

Previous studies have investigated the effect of anesthetic medication on the occurrence of OCR. To reduce OCR, retrobulbar block and premedication with anticholinergics have been applied. [3, 8–10] In spite of these attempts, methods of preventing OCR have not yet been found to be consistently effective. In addition, there are only a few studies that evaluate the relationship between strabismus surgery and OCR [11, 12].

The OCR commonly occurs following the traction of the EOM. Routine strabismus surgery requires 100–200 g tension on rectus muscles. Deliberately gentle surgery may take 50 g tension [13]. Braun et al. showed that sustained traction of 600 g of the EOM induced a counter-regulatory effect against OCR and increased the heart rate (HR) following the occurrence of OCR [14]. This phenomenon was referred to as the adrenergic phase of OCR. During strabismus surgery, several manipulations of the EOM, such as traction, re-traction, and cutting, are performed on the same muscle. Thus, stimulation of the EOM may be repeated and may vary, depending

* Correspondence: ansaneye@hanmail.net

[1]Department of Ophthalmology, Korea University College of Medicine, Seoul, Korea

[2]Department of Ophthalmology, Korea University Anam Hospital, 73, Inchon-ro, Seongbuk-gu, Seoul 02841, South Korea

on the surgical method and other surgical factors, during the strabismus surgery.

The aim of this study is to investigate surgical factors associated with the occurrence of OCR and changes of HR in patients with OCR during strabismus surgery.

Methods

The study protocol was approved by the Korea University Anam Hospital Institutional Review Board and adhered to the tenets of the Declaration of Helsinki. The medical charts of the patients who had undergone strabismus surgery under general anesthesia, at Korea University Anam Hospital, Seoul, Korea, between October 2015 and January 2016, were reviewed retrospectively. Patients classified as American Society of Anesthesiologists class I or II were selected. Patients were excluded if they had a history of bronchial asthma, congenital heart disease, central nervous disease, or other organic dysfunction. In pediatric patients under 18 years of age, intravenous atropine (0.01 mg/kg) was administered as a premedication and all patients were instructed not to eat or drink for 8 h prior to surgery. During the operation, thiopentone (5 mg/kg) and rocuronium (0.6 mg/kg) were administered to facilitate endotracheal intubation. Anesthesia was maintained with sevoflurane, an inhalational anesthetic. The HR was monitored every 5 s during anesthesia.

Recession or resection surgery of the EOM were performed based on their diagnosis. One single surgeon (SHK) performed all of the surgeries. Under general anesthesia, a fornix incision of conjunctiva was made. The EOM was engaged with a muscle hook and completely exposed with traction. The intramuscular septum was incised. In recession surgery, a suture was passed 1 mm from the insertion on the tendon and a locking bite suture was done in the superior and inferior margin of the muscle. The tendon was cut from the sclera. The EOM was reattached to the sclera according to the surgical amount. In resection surgeries, a suture was made at the superior and inferior margin of the muscle apart from the insertion according to the surgical amount. Though a tension gauge was not employed, the surgeon manipulated the extraocular muscle gently with uniformed tension in each of procedures. For recession of the inferior oblique muscle, following the isolation of the muscle, posterior fibers of the inferior oblique muscle were bunched using a single suture, toward the main muscle belly. The isolated inferior oblique muscle was placed next to vortex vein, behind the inferior rectus muscle. Based on the preoperative angle of deviation in patients, recession of the ipsilateral superior rectus muscles was performed in combination. The procedure of inferior oblique recession was similar to that for recession rectus muscle surgery. The surgical amount was determined by the patient's angle of deviation, according to

standardized values. The conjunctiva were closed with interrupted sutures at two points.

The data, collected preoperatively, included information regarding age at surgery, gender, and type of strabismus. During strabismus surgery, the number and sequence of the operated muscles, HR before traction of the EOM (baseline HR), maximum decreased HR after traction of the EOM, HR at maximum recovery from decreased HR and maintained during traction of the EOM (adrenergic HR), and HR at the cutting of the muscle, were collected. Oculocardiac reflex was defined as a decrease in HR greater than or equal to 20% rather than maximum at first traction of the muscle.

If a decrease of HR was noted during traction, we monitored the HR until a maximized increase was reached that was close to the baseline HR. Once the HR had been maintained for 10 s without a decrease, we defined the HR as adrenergic HR.

Prevalence of OCR was investigated and patients were divided into two subgroups according to the occurrence of OCR. In addition, prevalence of OCR was compared according to the patient's diagnosis, and, in patients who underwent two muscle surgeries, also the number and sequence of the operated muscles (first and second operated muscle). Additionally, the prevalence of OCR between the specific operated muscle groups were compared. The surgical factors associated with the occurrence of OCR were analyzed. The changes in HR each stage during the surgery were evaluated and compared between patients with and without OCR.

The data were analyzed using SPSS software version 21.0 (SPSS Inc., Chicago, IL, USA), and the clinical values were compared and analyzed using the Mann-Whitney test and Chi-square test. Multivariate logistic regression was used to analyze the risk factors associated with the occurrence of OCR. A p-value ≤ 0.05 was considered statistically significant.

Results

A total of 99 patients, with 162 operated muscles, who underwent strabismus surgery, were included in this study. During surgery, OCR occurred in 64 (65%) patients. The mean age was 11.1 ± 8.9 years in patients with OCR, and 7.9 ± 6.8 years in patients without OCR. Male patients accounted for 36 (56%) and 14 (40%) patients in each group, respectively. There were no significant differences in age and gender between patients with and without OCR. In total, 79 patients (80%) were diagnosed with exotropia, 9 patients (9%) with esotropia, and 13 patients (11%) with superior oblique palsy. There were no significant differences of strabismus diagnosis in patients with and without OCR ($p = 0.28$). Basic demographics are presented in Table 1.

Table 1 Preoperative demographics of the patients

	OCR ($n = 64$)	without OCR ($n = 35$)	p
Age, years (range)	$11.1 \pm 8.9(2-52)$	$7.9 \pm 6.8(1-42)$	0.07[a]
Male (%)	36(56)	14(40)	0.12[b]
Diagnosis (%)			0.28[b]
Exotropia	54(84)	25(72)	
Esotropia	5(8)	4(11)	
Superior oblique palsy	5(8)	6(17)	

OCR, oculocardiac reflex
[a]Mann-Whitney test
[b]Chi-square test

The mean number of operated muscles was 1.6 ± 0.5 in patients with OCR and 1.7 ± 0.5 in patients without OCR. There was no difference between the groups ($p = 0.56$). Baseline HR was higher in patients without OCR (131.1 ± 16.3 beat/min) than in patients with OCR (122.2 ± 17.5 beat/min) however, there was no statistical difference of HR between 2 groups. Thirty-eight (59%) patients with OCR underwent two muscle surgeries, compared to 22 (63%) patients without OCR. However, there was no significant difference between the groups ($p = 0.39$). The incidence of OCR in muscles undergoing recession, resection and oblique surgery was 70 (41%), 12 (7%) and 4 (3%), respectively ($p = 0.02$). In the surgical techniques, resection surgeries were significantly prevalent in patients with OCR than in patients without OCR ($p = 0.03$).

In the 162 muscles that were operated on, 122 (76%) were lateral rectus; 26 (16%), medial rectus; 2 (1%), superior rectus; and 12 (7%), inferior rectus. There was no significant difference in the occurrence of OCR according to the operated muscle ($p = 0.36$). Table 2 details the surgical information.

Sixty (60%) patients underwent two muscle surgeries. In the analysis based on the sequence of the operated muscles, incidence of OCR were significantly higher in the first ($n = 48$, 80%) than the second operated muscle ($n = 18$, 30%) ($p = 0.01$). Additionally, there were 46 (46%) patients with bilateral rectus muscle recession muscle surgery in this study. According to the sequence of operated muscle, the prevalence of OCR was higher in first operated lateral rectus muscle than second lateral rectus muscle ($p < 0.01$) (Table 3 and Table 4).

In multivariate logistic regression analysis, age, gender, and single muscle surgery were not associated with the occurrence of OCR ($p = 0.08$, 0.12 and 0.82). Resection and medial rectus muscle surgeries were highly associated with a greater occurrence of OCR (OR = 3.57 and 3.31, respectively); however, they were not significantly correlated ($p = 0.06$ and 0.11, Table 5). Additionally, the first operated EOM at surgery was significantly associated with the occurrence of OCR (OR = 3.95, $p < 0.01$, Table 5).

Table 2 Surgical measurements stratified by the occurrence of oculocardiac reflex

	OCR (n = 64)	without OCR (n = 35)	p
Number of operated muscle (range)	$1.6 \pm 0.5(1-2)$	$1.7 \pm 0.5(1-2)$	0.56[a]
Operated muscle (%)			0.36[b]
Lateral rectus muscle	59(72)	63(79)	
Medial rectus muscle	17(21)	9(11)	
Superior rectus muscle	2(2)	1(1)	
Inferior oblique muscle	4(5)	7(9)	
Baseline HR, beat/min	122.2 ± 17.5 (78–162)	131.1 ± 16.3 (89–166)	0.06[a]
Two muscle surgery (%)	38(59)	22(63)	0.39[a]
Surgery (%)			
Recession	70(41)	76(43)	0.02[b]
Resection	12(7)	3(2)	
Oblique surgery	4(3)	7(4)	

Recession surgery included the rectus muscle and inferior oblique muscle recession, OCR, oculocardiac reflex; HR, heartrate
[a]Mann-Whitney test
[b]Chi-square test

Discussion

The OCR is a common occurrence in strabismus surgery. The incidence of OCR reported in previous studies is greatly varied and depends on the method of evaluation and definition of OCR. In this study, the incidence of OCR, which was defined as the maximum decrease in HR at the first traction of the muscle ($\geq$ 20% reduction from baseline HR) was 65%. This is similar to incidences reported in other studies [11, 12, 15].

Several risk factors, such as the patient's age and gender, use of premedication, anesthetic technique, type of surgery, and the sequence of the operated muscle, have been shown to influence the occurrence of OCR. A number of studies have shown that the occurrence of OCR was higher in female patients, however, there are studies that have reported no difference between the gender of patients with OCR [11, 12]. There was no

Table 3 The occurrence of oculocardiac reflex according to the sequence of operated muscle in two muscle surgery and bilateral lateral rectus recession surgery

	OCR	without OCR	p[a]
Sequence of operated muscle (%)			< 0.01
First muscle	38(63)	22(37)	
Second muscle	18(30)	42(70)	
Sequence of operated muscle in BLR recession (%)			< 0.01
First lateral rectus muscle	33(72)	13(28)	
Second lateral rectus muscle	16(35)	30(65)	

OCR, oculocardiac reflex; BLR, bilateral lateral rectus muscle
[a]Chi-square test

Table 4 The occurrence of oculocardiac reflex and heart rate at each phase in one and two muscle surgery

	One muscle surgery	Two muscle surgery	
		first muscle	second muscle
Patients	39	60	60
OCR (%)	26(67)	38(63)	18(30)
Heart rate, beat/min			
Baseline	125.1 ± 15.9	128.8 ± 17.8	125.1 ± 18.3
Calculated percentage (median, range), %	100	100	100
Traction	89.9 ± 24.4	97.6 ± 24.5	105.7 ± 25.8
Calculated percentage (median, range), %	67.5 ± 12.1 (63.2, 45.1–84.4)	75.1 ± 9.8 (70.4, 38.4–87.6)	83.5 ± 12.2 (83.1,67.7–92.2)
Adrenergic	110.1 ± 19.8	113.1 ± 19.6	117.5 ± 22.1
Calculated percentage (median, range), %	84.1 ± 11.8 (80.2, 68.3–90.2)	89.3 ± 12.4 (85.9,73.2–93.2)	93.4 ± 4.6 (90.3,72.3–98.2)
Cut muscle	114.9 ± 18.9	118.2 ± 19.0	119.8 ± 20.9
Calculated percentage (median, range), %	91.3 ± 9.6 (87.9, 76.4–96.8)	90.7 ± 5.6 (89.4,77.9–98.7)	93.7 ± 3.4 (91.2,78.5–98.2)

OCR, oculocardiac reflex

gender difference between patients with and without OCR in this study. An intravenous anticholinergic agent was used as a premedication in pediatric surgeries, therefore, we could not conclude on a possible preventive effect of premedication on OCR. Additionally, the surgical method and number of operated muscles were not associated with the occurrence of OCR in this study.

The results of this study show that OCR was more prevalent in the resection of EOM; however, no significant association between specific muscles and OCR was found. Previous studies have reported that medial rectus surgery is strongly associated with OCR [11, 12, 15]. However, medial rectus muscle surgery was not significant risk factor for OCR in this study. In this study, most of the operated muscles were lateral rectus muscles unilaterally or bilaterally rather than other muscles, due to the high prevalence of exotropia in Korea, when compared to Western countries. Additionally, most of resection surgeries were performed to medial rectus muscle with exotropia. Clinically, it speculated that the traction of the medial rectus muscle might trigger OCR in resection surgery,

Table 5 Multivariate logistic regression analysis for the occurrence of oculocardiac reflex

Variable	OR	95% CI		p
Age	1.07	0.99	1.15	0.08
Male	0.52	0.22	1.19	0.12
Baseline HR	0.97	0.95	0.99	0.09
Resection	3.57	0.94	13.47	0.06
Medial rectus muscle	3.31	0.76	14.38	0.11
Single muscle surgery	0.91	0.39	2.12	0.82
First operated EOM	3.95	1.85	8.41	< 0.01

HR, heartrate; EOM, extraocular muscle; OR, odds ratio; CI, confidential interval

however, our study did not show support that the surgery on the medial rectus muscle is a risk factor for oculocardiac reflex.

Also, we did not find a statistical difference in the occurrence of OCR between patients with one or two muscle surgeries. However, there was a higher prevalence of OCR in first operated muscle among patients having two muscle surgeries. The first operated muscle was significantly associated with the occurrence of OCR in this study. This is in agreement with Lai et al., who reported that the occurrence of OCR was significantly higher during traction of the first operated muscle [12]. We speculated that the first operated muscle might be more likely to trigger OCR regardless of specific type of EOM. Additionally, we demonstrate that the prevalence of OCR was high in first operated muscle, even though same muscles in both eye although we could not explain this phenomenon exactly.

When OCR occurred after first mechanical stimulation of the EOM, the counter-regulatory process could lead to the adaption of a subsequent stimulus, due to the occurrence of OCR. We speculated that this process could affect the infrequency of OCR in the second operated muscle. Thus, the first operated muscle, with multiple surgeries, might be vulnerable to OCR, regardless of the specific muscle or surgical technique. Machida et al. reported that uniformed and objective EOM tension without atropine as premedication and recovery for OCR were evaluated at the strabismus surgery [13].

Braun et al. first reported the adrenergic phase of OCR in 1992 [14]. It described the counter-regulatory effect that outlasted the period of mechanical stimulation. This phenomenon occurred through the spontaneous recovery of HR after traction of the EOM and is referred to as the 'adrenergic phase' or 'vagal escape' of the OCR [6, 14]. In this study, the maximum recovered HR after traction of the EOM was measured, and interestingly, it did not fully recover until the cutting of the EOM, during surgery in patients with OCR. The mean percentage of the decreased HR, when compared to baseline HR, was 10% at the cutting of the EOM in patients with OCR. We speculated that when the OCR first occurred, it would be relatively difficult for the HR to fully recover to the baseline HR at any point in the surgery. Therefore, it might be important for the surgeon to monitor the occurrence of OCR at the first traction of the EOM.

This study has some limitations. Firstly, the design of this study was retrospective. Secondly, the patients in this study underwent surgery using an anticholinergic agent as a premedication. Thus, the occurrence of OCR could be affected by this pharmacologic agent. However, the use of an anticholinergic agent is still controversial in the prevention of OCR. Secondly, the majority of patients underwent lateral rectus muscles for exotropia. Therefore, there was an unbalanced distribution of operated muscles. As exotropia, such as intermittent exotropia, is common in East Asia, recession of the lateral rectus muscle is a more common procedure, when compared to other EOMs. Lastly, we did not measure objective information of traction muscles such as duration, amount of force. In this study, we hooked the muscle persistently until observing maximal recovery of decreased heart rate comparing with baseline heart rate. Thus, the duration of tension was variable at each surgical cases. These variability of traction could affect incidence of OCR during surgery. We performed the surgery, routinely without the manipulation of traction force.

Conclusions

A reduction in HR at the traction of the muscle during surgery did not fully recover in patients with OCR. The first operated muscle in patients with two muscle surgeries was a significant risk factor for OCR occurrence. Surgeon needs to be more careful while operating first extraocular muscle in strabismus surgery. The occurrence of OCR may be an important surgical consideration for patients with strabismus.

Abbreviations
EOM: Extraocular muscle; HR: Heart rate; OCR: Oculocardiac reflex

Acknowledgements
The authors thank Kyung-Sook Yang, PhD, a biostatistician at the Department of Biostatistics, Korea University College of Medicine, for help with statistical analysis and technical edition of this study.

Authors' contributions
SHK suggested concept of study. SGH and JAH performed to conduct study. BRL and SGH measured and collected data in this study. The measurements were confirmed by SGH and JAH. Analysis data and interpretation of data were performed by SGH and SHK. SGH wrote the manuscript. SHK provided a critical review of the manuscript. All authors approved the manuscript for submission.

Competing interests
The authors declare that they have no competing interests.

References
1. Alexander JP. Reflex disturbances of cardiac rhythm during ophthalmic surgery. Br J Ophthalmol. 1975;59:518–24.
2. Hahnenkamp K, Honemann CW, Fischer LG, Durieux ME, Muehlendyck H, Braun U. Effect of different anaesthetic regimes on the oculocardiac reflex during paediatric strabismus surgery. Paediatr Anaesth. 2000;10:601–8.
3. Gilani MT, Sharifi M, Najafi MN, Etemadi Mashhadi MG. Oculocardiac reflex during strabismus surgery. Reviews in. Clinical Medicine. 2016;3:4–7.
4. Allen LE, Sudesh S, Sandramouli S, Cooper G, McFarlane D, Willshaw HE. The association between the oculocardiac reflex and post-operative vomiting in children undergoing strabismus surgery. Eye (Lond). 1998;12(Pt 2):193–6.
5. Bietti OB. Problems of anesthesia in strabismus surgery. Int Ophthalmol Clin. 1966;6:727–37.
6. Blanc VF, Hardy JF, Milot J, Jacob JL. The oculocardiac reflex: a graphic and statistical analysis in infants and children. Can Anaesth Soc J. 1983;30:360–
7. Smith RB, Douglas H, Petruscak J. The oculocardiac reflex and sino-atrial arrest. Can Anaesth Soc J. 1972;19:138–42.
8. Defalque RJ. Retrobulbar block for oculocardiac reflex: duration of protection by common local anesthetics. Acta Ophthalmol. 1969;47:998–1003.
9. Klockgether-Radke A, Demmel C, Braun U, Mühlendyck H. Emesis and the oculocardiac reflex. Drug prophylaxis with droperidol and atropine in children undergoing strabismus surgery. Anaesthesist. 1993;42:356–60.
10. Tramèr MR, Sansonetti A, Fuchs-Buder T, Rifat K. Oculocardiac reflex and postoperative vomiting in paediatric strabismus surgery. A randomised controlled trial comparing four anaesthetic techniques. Acta Anaesthesiol Scand. 1998;42:117–23.
11. Apt L, Isenberg S, Gaffney WL. The oculocardiac reflex in strabismus surgery. Am J Ophthalmol. 1973;76:533–6.
12. Lai YH, Hsu HT, Wang HZ, Cheng KI, Wu KY. The oculocardiac reflex during strabismus surgery: its relationship to preoperative clinical eye findings and subsequent postoperative emesis. J AAPOS. 2014;18:151–5.
13. Machida CJ, Arnold RW. The effect of induced muscle tension and fatigue on the oculocardiac reflex. Binocul Vis Strabismus Q. 2003;18:81–6.
14. Braun U, Feise J, Muhlendyck H. Is there a cholinergic and an adrenergic phase of the oculocardiac reflex during strabismus surgery? Acta Anaesthesiol Scand. 1993;37:390–5.
15. Welhaf WR, Johnson DC. The Oculocardiac reflex during extraocular muscle surgery. Arch Ophthalmol. 1965;73:43–5.

9

Correlation of subfoveal choroidal thickness with axial length, refractive error, and age in adult highly myopic eyes

Bingqian Liu[1†], Yan Wang[2†], Tao Li[1], Ying Lin[1], Wei Ma[1], Xiaohong Chen[1], Cancan Lyu[1], Yonghao Li[1] and Lin Lu[1*]

Abstract

Background: Subfoveal choroidal thickness (SFCT) in highly myopic eyes was found to be correlated with increasing age, refractive error (spherical equivalent), and axial length. Which factor is the most significant predictor of SFCT remains controversial.

Methods: A hospital-based cohort of highly myopic eyes (with spherical equivalent equal to or over 6.00 diopter) were retrospectively screened. Data from only right eye in those bilateral high myopia, and unilateral high myopia in any eye, were used for analysis. Correlations among the four biometric factors were analyzed. Linear correlation was performed to analyze the predictors of SFCT.

Results: A cohort of 312 eyes from 312 adults (98 men) was enrolled. Statistical analysis showed that axial length ($R = -0.592$), spherical equivalent ($R = -0.471$), and age ($R = -0.296$) were significantly correlated with SFCT ($P < 0.001$). No significant correlation was found between age and axial length, or age and spherical equivalent. Partial correlation with controlled age confirmed that axial length ($R = -0.628$) was a more significant predictor of SFCT than spherical equivalent ($R = -0.507$).

Conclusions: SFCT was inversely correlated with increasing age, spherical equivalent and axial length, with axial length as the most significant predictor of SFCT, in adult highly myopic eyes.

Keywords: High myopia, Subfoveal choroidal thickness, Axial length, Age, Refractive error, Correlation analysis

Background

Myopia is a significant public health concern worldwide [1]. The prevalence of myopia in teenagers and young adults has reached up to 90% in East Asia, up to 50% in United States and Europe, and the overall prevalence of myopia is still increasing [1–11]. High myopia, featured by progressive elongation of the eyeball, is associated with potentially blinding complications such as retinal detachment, macular schisis, macular hole, chorioretinal atrophy, choroidal neovascularization, and peripapillary cavity [7, 8, 12–15]. It is estimated that 1–2% of the population in western countries exhibits high myopia, with a much higher prevalence in East Asian. Population-based studies showed high myopia to be the 1st to 3rd most frequent cause of blindness, and the prevalence of visual impairment attributable to high myopia ranged from 0.1 to 0.5% in European studies and from 0.2 to 1.4% in Asian studies [16].

The severity of myopic macular degeneration was found strongly associated with subfoveal choroidal thicknesses (SFCT) in a recent study [17]. Accurate measurement of choroidal thickness may provide some information about myopic pathologic conditions. The development of enhanced depth imaging (EDI) of spectral-domain optical coherence tomography (SD-OCT) allows for the evaluation of choroidal thickness in vivo [18–20].

Choroidal thickness in highly myopic eyes was reported to be correlated with increasing age, spherical equivalent, and axial length, and SFCT could be considered as a useful predictor of visual function [21–25], but which factor is the most significant predictor remains

* Correspondence: lulin888@126.com
†Bingqian Liu and Yan Wang contributed equally to this work.
[1]State Key Laboratory of Ophthalmology, Zhongshan Ophthalmic Center, Sun Yat-sen University, 54 South Xianlie Road, Guangzhou 510060, Guangdong, China
Full list of author information is available at the end of the article

controversial in previous studies, and the data from different population might be variable according to literatures [21, 25]. The goal of this study was to estimate the correlation of SFCT with age, axial length and spherical equivalent in a hospital-based cohort of highly myopic eyes, and to find which factor was the most significant predictor of SFCT.

Methods

This is a retrospective cross-sectional study, by re-analysis of the project data of "high myopia cohort study in a tertiary eye center". An informed consent was obtained from all of the included subjects for the project but not specifically for this study. Adult patients (age ≥ 18 years) with high myopia from December 2013 to April 2016 collected by high myopia research group at Fundus Disease Center of Zhongshan Ophthalmic Center were screened. The study followed the tenets of the Declaration of Helsinki and was approved by the Zhongshan Ophthalmic Center Institutional Review Board.

Inclusion criteria was spherical equivalent equal to or over 6.00 diopter (D); Exclusion criteria included poor OCT image quality and those choroid borderlines could not be clearly visualized; history of vitrectomy, sclera buckling, glaucoma, or retinal detachment. Data from only right eye were used for analysis in those with bilateral high myopia. Unilateral high myopia in any eye was also included.

Measurements

All the participants underwent ophthalmic examinations including assessment of BCVA, intraocular pressure measurement, slit lamp examination, spherical equivalent, axial length, indirect dilated fundus ophthalmoscopy, fundus photography, and OCT for the mentioned project. Axial length was measured using IOL Master (Carl Zeiss Meditec, Jena, Germany). Spherical equivalent was measured by autorefractometry (Canon, Tokyo, Japan). Horizontal and vertical cross hair scans through central fovea were captured by an SD-OCT machine (Heidelberg, Germany) with EDI modality. Choroidal thickness was defined from the outer edge of the hyperreflective line corresponding to the retinal pigment epithelium to the inner surface of sclera [18, 25, 26]. The SFCT was manually measured and averaged by two independent observers from horizontal and vertical scans. Repeatability of SFCT measurements between the scans and observers were analyzed.

Statistics

Statistical analyses were performed using SPSS 17.0 software. Pearson's correlation was used to analyze the correlation between any two biometric factors. Analysis of multi-predictors (axial length/spherical equivalent and

Table 1 Epidemiological data of included eyes

Variable	Minimum	maximum	mean	SD
age (years)	18	88	47.47	14.11
[a]Refractive error (D)	−6.00	−32.00	−14.58	5.52
Axial length (mm)	24.31	36.23	29.45	2.31
SFCT (um)	10.00	337.00	83.77	54.64

SFCT subfoveal choroidal thickness
[a] Eyes underwent refractive or cataract surgery (n = 31) were not included

age) of SFCT were analyzed using stepwise method. Partial correlations with controlled factor were studied. Analysis of linear regression of SFCT with its predictors of axial length, spherical equivalent, and age was performed. $P < 0.05$ was considered statistically significant.

Results

Correlations among biometric factors in high myopia

Our cohort comprised 312 eyes from 312 patients (98 men). Table 1 shows the demographic and clinical characteristics. The correlation between the measurements of SFCT performed by two independent observers was highly significant ($r = 0.96$; $p < 0.001$). The correlation between SFCT measurements from vertical scan and horizontal scan was also highly significant ($r = 0.89$, $p < 0.001$).

Correlation analysis among the four biometric factors showed that SFCT was significantly negative correlated with axial length ($r = -0.592$, $p < 0.001$), negative correlated with spherical equivalent ($r = -0.471$, $p < 0.001$), and negative correlated with age ($r = -0.296$, $p < 0.001$), respectively, as shown in Table 2. With the increasing of axial length, spherical equivalence and age, the SFCT became gradually thinning. Among these three biometric factors, axial length showed the largest coefficient correlated to SFCT. Axial length and spherical equivalent was highly correlated, as commonly expected ($r = 0.773$, $p < 0.001$). There was no significant correlation between age and axial length. No significant correlation between age and spherical equivalent was found, either.

Table 2 Correlations among biometric factors in high myopia

		SFCT	Age	SE
Correlation Coefficients	Age	−0.296		
	SE	−0.471	0.050	
	AL	−0.592	−0.018	0.773
P values (2-tailed)	Age	< 0.001		
	RE	< 0.001	0.1798	
	AL	< 0.001	0.3855	< 0.001

AL axial length, SE spherical equivalent, SFCT subfoveal choroidal thickness

Table 3 Analysis of multi-predictors (axial length/ spherical equivalent and age) of subfoveal choroidal thickness

Model		B	SE	Hypothesis test		95% Confidence Interval for B		Partial correlations
				t	Sig.	Lower bound	Upper bound	
1	Constant	646.854	34.159	18.936	< 0.001	579.673	714.035	–
	Axial length	−16.804	1.109	−15.153	< 0.001	−18.985	−14.623	−0.628
	Age	−1.422	0.182	−7.832	< 0.001	−1.779	−1.065	−0.385
2	Constant	234.984	12.824	18.324	< 0.001	209.763	260.205	–
	Spherical equivalent	−5.627	0.509	−11.060	< 0.001	−4.626	−6.627	−0.507
	Age	−1.482	0.201	−7.366	< 0.001	−1.878	−1.086	−0.365

Axial length and age, or spherical equivalent and age were predictors for the dependent variable, subfoveal choroidal thickness

Predictors of subfoveal choroidal thickness

Given that axial length, spherical equivalent, and age were all correlated significantly with SFCT. Multi-predictors of subfoveal choroidal thickness were analyzed. Adding all the three factors resulted in confounding results using stepwise method. The models of axial length plus age and spherical equivalent plus age were similar in the statistical fitness (Table 3). Partial correlation with controlled age further confirmed that axial length ($R = − 0.628, p < 0.001$) was a more significant predictor of SFCT than spherical equivalent ($R = − 0.507, p < 0.001$).

Linear regression of SFCT with predictors

The predictors of SFCT were analyzed using linear regression (Table 4). The distribution of SFCT values in eyes with different levels of predictors was shown in box plot, Fig. 1. The SFCT cohort was grouped by sectioned range of axial length (1 mm), age (1 decade), and spherical equivalent (3D). According to the distribution of data (Fig. 1), the speed of SFCT decrease seemed slowing down with the increasing axial length, age, and spherical equivalent, especially with axial length over 30 mm, age older than 50 years, and spherical equivalent over 15 D.

Discussion

In this study, we found that axial length, rather than spherical equivalent, was the more important predictor of SFCT, different to previous reports from another cohort [21]. In a recent study, by comparing eyes with different degree of myopia and healthy eyes, axial length was found to be determining factor of choroidal thickness in some locations including subfoveal [25]. We suggest that axial length may be more accurate in predicting SFCT in high myopia due to the following reasons: 1) the sample size of our cohort was much larger; 2) the axial length may represent more accurately and directly the extent of choroidal stretch in the posterior pole of highly myopic eyes; 3) the refraction might be confused by development of nuclear cataract, which is very common in adult myopes and could result in further myopic shift; 4) for the eyes with cataract removed, spherical equivalent is not applicable to understanding the myopic status.

The choroidal thickness become gradually thinning with the extension of axial length. However, the SFCT seemed decrease faster in eyes with axial length in the range of 24 to 30 mm compared with those axial length over 30 mm (Fig. 1, left).

The second predictor of SFCT is spherical equivalent. The choroidal thickness become gradually thinning with the increasing of refraction. The speed of SFCT decrease looked much faster in eyes with a spherical equivalent from 6 D to 15 D, compared with those spherical equivalent greater than 15 D (Fig. 1, middle).

Our cohort was from a tertiary eye-care center based population, the myopic degree was probably much higher than other cohorts. The SFCT of our high myopia cohort was 83.77 ± 54.64 µm, much thinner than

Table 4 Linear regression of SFCT with its predictors of axial length, spherical equivalent, and age

Parameters	B	SE	Hypothesis Test		95% Confidence Interval for B	
			t	Sig.	Lower Bound	Upper Bound
Constant	573.253	35.530	16.134	< 0.001	503.38	643.13
Axial length (mm, n = 312)	−16.646	1.200	−13.876	< 0.001	− 19.00	− 14.29
Constant	160.458	8.452	18.985	< 0.001	143.84	177.08
[a]Spherical equivalent (D, n = 285)	−5.441	0.545	−9.984	< 0.001	−4.37	−6.51
Constant	148.216	11.755	12.61	< 0.001	125.10	171.34
Age (years, n = 312)	−1.372	0.233	−5.89	< 0.001	−1.83	−0.91

SFCT subfoveal choroidal thickness (µm), was a dependent variable, SE standard error
[a]Eyes underwent refractive or cataract surgery (n = 27) were not included

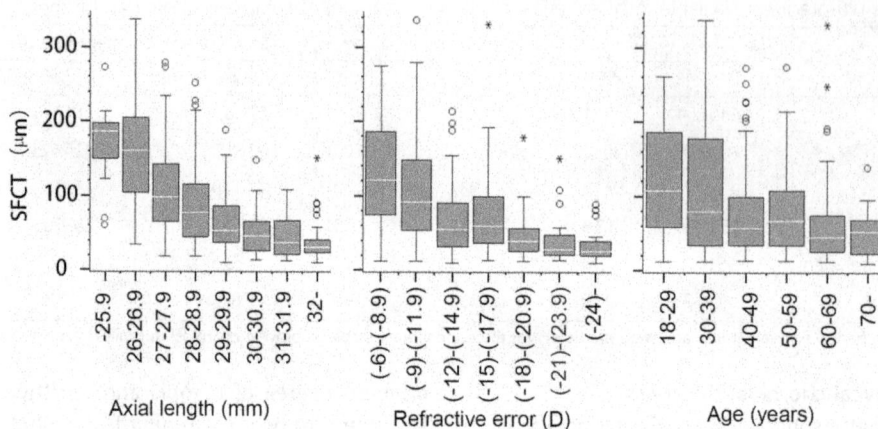

Fig. 1 Distribution of SFCT data associated with predictors. Left: SFCT data associated with axial length; Middle: SFCT data associated with refractive error; Right: SFCT data associated with age; o: Outlier values which were between 1.5 and 3 box lengths from either end of the box. *: Extreme values which are more than 3 box lengths from either end of the box

that in healthy subjects from literatures [27–30]. Our mean SFCT was even thinner than a similar study showing a SFCT of 113.8 ± 53.9 μm in a New York cohort (*n* = 35 eyes), 172.9 ± 72.8 μm in a Japanese cohort (*n* = 110 eyes) [21], 166 ± 88.7 μm in a Spain cohort [22] and 225.87 ± 5.51 μm from a case-control study of young Chinese men in Singapore [31].

Age is associated with SFCT in both high myopic and healthy eyes. In eyes without high myopia, age was found critical for evaluation of SFCT in two healthy Chinese cohorts, one from Guangzhou in southern China, and another from Beijing in northern China [28, 32]. SFCT in subjects older than 60 years of age was much thinner than that in younger subjects, and the SFCT after 60 years of age seemed to keep relatively stable in healthy cohorts [28, 29, 32]. The age of the patients in our cohort was from 18 to 88, but most of the cases were older than 30 years. The speed of SFCT decrease after 50 years of age looked much slower than that from 18 to 49 years of age (Fig. 1, right). Our study did not focus on young myopes. Choroidal thickness in young population [33, 34] might be quite different compared with in older ones.

Our study has several limitations: 1) it is a retrospective cross-sectional study, the data from a hospital-based cohort might represent more severe degree of myopia. 2) some eyes were excluded because of low image quality due to poor focus fixation, or the posterior scleral border was not clear; 3) the correlation of SFCT with other factors, such as gender, visual acuity, retinal thickness, intraocular pressure, ocular biometric parameters, or various maculopathy, was not analyzed, which might be worthy of further investigation; 4) Our cohort does not include patients younger than 18 years. 5) The SFCT may be also affected by other factors including the severity of posterior staphyloma, which was not included in this study.

We included only one eye from each patient to meet statistical requirement. From a recent study, there was larger absolute interocular differences in choroidal thickness of high myopic eyes compared with healthy control eyes [35]. Further study comparing the interocular difference in severity of pathological change and corresponding choroidal thickness and visual function might provide more information for understanding high myopia related changes.

Conclusion

In summary, SFCT in adult highly myopic eyes was inversely correlated with increasing age, spherical equivalent and axial length. Axial length was a more significant predictor of SFCT than spherical equivalent, or age.

Abbreviations
D: Diopter; EDI: Enhanced depth imaging; SD-OCT: Spectral-domain optical coherence tomography; SFCT: Subfoveal choroidal thickness

Acknowledgements
The authors thank Mr. Jun Chen from Guangzhou Women and Children's Medical Center for statistical assistant, Mrs. Xiaofang Li, Shaofen Lin, and Qiufen Yang from Zhongshan Ophthalmic Center for OCT imaging support.

Funding
This study was supported by National Natural Science Foundation of China (81570862), Natural Science Foundation of Guangdong Province (2014A030313197), Guangzhou Science and Technology Project (2014Y2–00064), and Young Teacher Training Program of Sun Yat-sen University (15ykpy32).

Authors' contributions
BL participated in the design of the study and drafted the manuscript; YW, XC and CL collected and analyzed the data; TL and YLin carried out critical review and revised the manuscript; LL and YLi conceived of the study and revised the manuscript, and contributed as co-corresponding authors. All authors read and approved the final manuscript.

Competing interests

The authors declare that they have no competing interests.

Author details

[1]State Key Laboratory of Ophthalmology, Zhongshan Ophthalmic Center, Sun Yat-sen University, 54 South Xianlie Road, Guangzhou 510060, Guangdong, China. [2]Department of Ophthalmology, Shenzhen Hospital of Southern Medical University, Shenzhen, China.

References

1. Dolgin E. The myopia boom. Nature. 2015;519(7543):276–8.
2. Lyu Y, Zhang H, Gong Y, Wang D, Chen T, Guo X, Yang S, Liu D, Kang M. Prevalence of and factors associated with myopia in primary school students in the Chaoyang District of Beijing, China. Jpn J Ophthalmol. 2015;59(6):421–9.
3. Wu LJ, You QS, Duan JL, Luo YX, Liu LJ, Li X, Gao Q, Zhu HP, He Y, Xu L, et al. Prevalence and associated factors of myopia in high-school students in Beijing. PLoS One. 2015;10(3):e0120764.
4. Williams KM, Bertelsen G, Cumberland P, Wolfram C, Verhoeven VJ, Anastasopoulos E, Buitendijk GH, Cougnard-Gregoire A, Creuzot-Garcher C, Erke MG, et al. Increasing prevalence of myopia in Europe and the impact of education. Ophthalmology. 2015;122(7):1489–97.
5. Saxena R, Vashist P, Tandon R, Pandey RM, Bhardawaj A, Menon V, Mani K. Prevalence of myopia and its risk factors in urban school children in Delhi: the North India myopia study (NIM study). PLoS One. 2015;10(2):e0117349.
6. Jones D, Luensmann D. The prevalence and impact of high myopia. Eye Contact Lens. 2012;38(3):188–96.
7. Henaine-Berra A, Zand-Hadas IM, Fromow-Guerra J, Garcia-Aguirre G. Prevalence of macular anatomic abnormalities in high myopia. Ophthalmic Surg Lasers Imaging Retina. 2013;44(2):140–4.
8. Chang L, Pan CW, Ohno-Matsui K, Lin X, Cheung GC, Gazzard G, Koh V, Hamzah H, Tai ES, Lim SC, et al. Myopia-related fundus changes in Singapore adults with high myopia. Am J Ophthalmol. 2013;155(6):991–9. e991
9. Cheng SC, Lam CS, Yap MK. Prevalence of myopia-related retinal changes among 12-18 year old Hong Kong Chinese high myopes. Ophthalmic Physiolog Opt. 2013;33(6):652–60.
10. Morgan IG. What public policies should be developed to deal with the epidemic of myopia? Optom Vis Sci. 2016;93(9):1058–60.
11. Warner N. Update on myopia. Curr Opin Ophthalmol. 2016;27(5):402–6.
12. Lichtwitz O, Boissonnot M, Mercie M, Ingrand P, Leveziel N. Prevalence of macular complications associated with high myopia by multimodal imaging. J Fr Ophtalmol. 2016;39(4):355–63.
13. Rey A, Jurgens I, Maseras X, Carbajal M. Natural course and surgical management of high myopic foveoschisis. Ophthalmologica. 2014;231(1):45–50.
14. Ripandelli G, Parisi V, Friberg TR, Coppe AM, Scassa C, Stirpe M. Retinal detachment associated with macular hole in high myopia: using the vitreous anatomy to optimize the surgical approach. Ophthalmology. 2004;111(4):726–31.
15. Shimada N, Ohno-Matsui K, Nishimuta A, Tokoro T, Mochizuki M. Peripapillary changes detected by optical coherence tomography in eyes with high myopia. Ophthalmology. 2007;114(11):2070–6.
16. Wong TY, Ferreira A, Hughes R, Carter G, Mitchell P. Epidemiology and disease burden of pathologic myopia and myopic choroidal neovascularization: an evidence-based systematic review. Am J Ophthalmol. 2014;157(1):9–25. e12
17. Wong CW, Phua V, Lee SY, Wong TY, Cheung CM. Is choroidal or scleral thickness related to myopic macular degeneration? Invest Ophthalmol Vis Sci. 2017;58(2):907–13.
18. Fujiwara A, Shiragami C, Shirakata Y, Manabe S, Izumibata S, Shiraga F. Enhanced depth imaging spectral-domain optical coherence tomography of subfoveal choroidal thickness in normal Japanese eyes. Jpn J Ophthalmol. 2012;56(3):230–5.
19. Shao L, Xu L, Chen CX, Yang LH, Du KF, Wang S, Zhou JQ, Wang YX, You QS, Jonas JB, et al. Reproducibility of subfoveal choroidal thickness measurements with enhanced depth imaging by spectral-domain optical coherence tomography. Invest Ophthalmol Vis Sci. 2013;54(1):230–3.
20. Spaide RF, Koizumi H, Pozzoni MC. Enhanced depth imaging spectral-domain optical coherence tomography. Am J Ophthalmol. 2008;146(4):496–500.
21. Nishida Y, Fujiwara T, Imamura Y, Lima LH, Kurosaka D, Spaide RF. Choroidal thickness and visual acuity in highly myopic eyes. Retina. 2012;32(7):1229–36.
22. Flores-Moreno I, Ruiz-Medrano J, Duker JS, Ruiz-Moreno JM. The relationship between retinal and choroidal thickness and visual acuity in highly myopic eyes. Br J Ophthalmol. 2013;97(8):1010–3.
23. Zaben A, Zapata MA, Garcia-Arumi J. Retinal sensitivity and choroidal thickness in high myopia. Retina. 2015;35(3):398–406.
24. Fujiwara T, Imamura Y, Margolis R, Slakter JS, Spaide RF. Enhanced depth imaging optical coherence tomography of the choroid in highly myopic eyes. Am J Ophthalmol. 2009;148(3):445–50.
25. El-Shazly AA, Farweez YA, ElSebaay ME, El-Zawahry WMA. Correlation between choroidal thickness and degree of myopia assessed with enhanced depth imaging optical coherence tomography. Eur J Ophthalmol. 2017;27(5):577–84.
26. Moussa M, Sabry D, Soliman W. Macular choroidal thickness in normal Egyptians measured by swept source optical coherence tomography. BMC Ophthalmol. 2016;5(16):138.
27. Ikuno Y, Kawaguchi K, Nouchi T, Yasuno Y. Choroidal thickness in healthy Japanese subjects. Invest Ophthalmol Vis Sci. 2010;51(4):2173–6.
28. Ding X, Li J, Zeng J, Ma W, Liu R, Li T, Yu S, Tang S. Choroidal thickness in healthy Chinese subjects. Invest Ophthalmol Vis Sci. 2011;52(13):9555–60.
29. Kim M, Kim SS, Koh HJ, Lee SC. Choroidal thickness, age, and refractive error in healthy Korean subjects. Optom Vis Sci. 2014;91(5):491–6.
30. Ruiz-Medrano J, Flores-Moreno I, Pena-Garcia P, Montero JA, Duker JS, Ruiz-Moreno JM. Macular choroidal thickness profile in a healthy population measured by swept-source optical coherence tomography. Invest Ophthalmol Vis Sci. 2014;55(6):3532–42.
31. Gupta P, Saw SM, Cheung CY, Girard MJ, Mari JM, Bhargava M, Tan C, Tan M, Yang A, Tey F, et al. Choroidal thickness and high myopia: a case-control study of young Chinese men in Singapore. Acta Ophthalmol. 2015;93(7):e585–92.
32. Wei WB, Xu L, Jonas JB, Shao L, Du KF, Wang S, Chen CX, Xu J, Wang YX, Zhou JQ, et al. Subfoveal choroidal thickness: the Beijing eye study. Ophthalmology. 2013;120(1):175–80.
33. Gupta P, Cheung CY, Saw SM, Koh V, Tan M, Yang A, Zhao P, Cheung CM, Wong TY, Cheng CY. Choroidal thickness does not predict visual acuity in young high myopes. Acta Ophthalmol. 2016;94(8):e709–15.
34. Gupta P, Thakku SG, Saw SM, Tan M, Lim E, Tan M, Cheung CMG, Wong TY, Cheng CY. Characterization of choroidal morphologic and vascular features in young men with high myopia using spectral-domain optical coherence tomography. Am J Ophthalmol. 2017;177:27–33.
35. Alzaben Z, Cardona G, Zapata MA, Zaben A. Interocular asymmetry in choroidal thickness and retinal sensitivity in high myopia. Retina; 2017. https://doi.org/10.1097/IAE.0000000000001756. [Epub ahead of print]

10

Short-term changes of choroidal vascular structures after phacoemulsification surgery

Haisong Chen[1], Zheming Wu[1], Yun Chen[1], Manshan He[1] and Jiawei Wang[2]*

Abstract

Background: To evaluate the changes of choroidal vascular structures in patients after phacoemulsification surgery.

Methods: A self-control study was conducted on 36 eyes of 36 patients who had uneventful phacoemulsification. Choroidal images were acquired preoperatively, 7 days (D7), 1 month (M1), and 3 months (M3) after surgery from enhanced depth imaging (EDI) optical coherence tomography (OCT) scans. Choroidal vascularity index (CVI) was used to assess vascular status of the choroid using image binarization by the Niblack method. The postoperative values of mean CVI were compared with baseline by paired t-test. Univariate and multiple linear regression analyses were performed to determine the associations between CVI and other factors.

Results: The mean age of the recruited patients was 63.1 ± 6.9 years. The mean CVI at baseline was $60.1 \pm 5.5\%$. After surgery, the CVI significantly increased to $61.7 \pm 5.3\%$ at D7, $63.6 \pm 4.4\%$ at M1 and $64.8 \pm 4.0\%$ at M3 ($p = 0.035$, 0.0006, < 0.0001, respectively). Univariate and multiple regression analysis revealed a positive association between CVI and subfoveal choroidal thickness (SFCT) at pre-operation and no significant association with age, axial length (AL), intraocular pressure (IOP) and gender at all timepoints.

Conclusions: Phacoemulsification induced increased CVI in patients diagnosed with cataract. Evaluation of the long-term change of CVI following surgery may provide valuable information for studying the relationship between phacoemulsification and disorders of the choroid.

Keywords: Choroid, Vascular structures, Phacoemulsification

Background

Cataract with phacoemulsification surgery is the most extensively performed eye surgery. There are more than 1300 cases per million people undergoing phacoemulsification surgery per year in China and greater than 5000 cases per million people per year in Europe, America and India [1]. Phacoemulsification surgery is safe and generally associated with successful visual outcomes.

Choroid, the highest blood circulation in the human body, is composed of blood vessels, connective tissues, nerves, melanocytes and extracellular fluid. A great deal of analysis and research indicates that even uncomplicated phacoemulsification induces disorders of the choroid, especially an increase in the choroid thickness [2–4]. However, only the choroidal thickness does not supply convincing evidence on what structures change, especially about the blood volume within the choroid in patients after Phacoemulsification surgery.

Further morphological and vascular analyses of the choroid may certify the change of choroidal blood volume in patients after Phacoemulsification surgery. With the advent of enhanced depth imaging (EDI) optical coherence tomography (OCT), it is possible to assess the choroidal stromal and vascular structures. Recently, application of image binarization of choroid structures has further provided a novel measure index for vascular status of the choroid [5]. To the best of our knowledge, there is no report about the change of choroidal vascular structures after Phacoemulsification surgery.

In the current study, we aimed to determine the influence of phacoemulsification on the proportion of choroidal vascular structures in patients after surgery. The choroidal vascularity index (CVI) from EDI-OCT scans will be used and we speculated that CVI may provide more additional information about the morphology and

* Correspondence: jiaweieye@yeah.net
[2]Eye Center of Shandong University, The Second Hospital of Shandong University, Shandong University, Jinan 250000, China
Full list of author information is available at the end of the article

physiology of the choroid and may be useful to interpret the disorders of the choroid after cataract surgery.

Methods

Thirty-six healthy patients undergoing uncomplicated Phacoemulsification surgery were recruited for this self-controlled case series study. All the patients were recruited consecutively (from October 2016 to December 2016) from the cataract department of Guangzhou Aier Eye Hospital and signed the consent form after a fullest explanation of the purpose and procedures of the study. The study was adhered to the provisions of the Declaration of Helsinki for research involving human subjects and was approved by the Ethical Review Committee of Guangzhou Aier Eye Hospital.

All the study participants were healthy individuals with no history of ocular disease or visual symptoms; aged at least 40 years; intraocular pressure (IOP) < 21 mmHg; normal appearance of optic nerve head; normal anterior chamber angles; Patients were excluded if they had glaucoma, high myopia or hyperopia (magnitude exceeding ±6 diopters (D) of spherical equivalent refraction), AMD, or other retinal diseases that could interfere the choroidal thickness. The diagnosis of glaucoma was based on the findings from gonioscopy, optic disc characteristics, and visual fields results. Patients with severe systemic diseases, such as diabetes mellitus, rheumatism, or malignant tumors, serious opacity of refractive media or unstable fixation that could prevent EDI-OCT measurement were also excluded.

All the patients underwent a comprehensive ophthalmologic examination, including IOP measurement using Goldmann applanation tonometry, autorefraction examination, measurement of visual acuity and a best-corrected visual acuity (BCVA), axial length using ocular biometry (IOL Master, Zeiss, Germany), fundus examination and EDI-OCT measurement (Spectralis, Heidelberg Engineering, Heidelberg, Germany) before surgery and postoperatively at 7 days (D7), month 1 (M1) and months 3 (M3).

All patients received standard phacoemulsification surgery through clear corneal incisions under superficial anesthesia (0.5% Proparacaine hydrochloride Eye Drops, Alcon, Fort Worth, TX). All phacoemulsification surgeries was performed by the same experienced surgeon (HSC) using the Infiniti system® (Alcon Labs Inc). In all cases, after removal of the lens cortex, a foldable intraocular lens was implanted uneventfully in the capsular bag. Within 1 month after surgery, Tobradex (0.3% tobramycin and 1% dexamethasone, Alcon, Fort Worth, TX) eye drops were applied four times a day, a non-steroidal anti-inflammatory eye drops (Pranoprofen Eye Drops, Senju Pharmaceutical Co.,Ltd. Osaka, Japan) were applied four times a day, and TobraDex eye ointment (Alcon, Fort Worth, TX) was applied once every evening before bed.

Image acquisition

EDI-OCT scans of the macular were performed for the operated eye using the EDI mode of SD-OCT (Spectralis, Heidelberg Engineering, Heidelberg, Germany). Horizontal 6-mm line scans centred on the fovea were acquired. Due to the diurnal variation of choroidal thickness, all the measurements were performed at the same time of the day (08:00 AM~ 12:00 AM) and accomplished in triplicate by two independent examiners. The sections going directly through the center of the fovea were selected for further analysis. The subfoveal choroidal thickness (SFCT) was measured using the in-built calipers tool. SFCT was defined as the vertical distance between the outer surface of the retinal pigment epithelium and the choroidal–sclera interface [6].

Procedures of image binarization

Image binarization of the subfoveal choroidal area was performed by one public domain software, Image J (version 1.47, provided in the public domain by the National Institutes of Health, Bethesda, MD, USA; http://imagej.nih.gov/ij/) [7, 8]. In brief, the images with one central scan passing through the fovea were chosen. The region of interest was manually selected using the polygon tool and added to ROI manager. After measuring the brightness of the selected luminal areas of the original OCT, the average brightness was set at the minimum value to minimize the noise in the OCT image. Then the original images were converted to 8 bits and adjusted by the Niblack Auto Local Threshold. The binarized image was converted to RGB (red, green, blue) image again, and the luminal area was determined using the Threshold Tool. After the image binarization, the total circumscribed area (TCA) and area of dark pixels were calculated. The dark pixels represent the luminal or vascular area (LA) and stromal or interstitial area (SA) was defined as the area of light pixels (Fig. 1). CVI was defined as the proportion of LA to TCA.

Inter-rater and intra-rater agreement

All the preoperative images were initially segmented by two graders to evaluate the inter-rater agreement (HSC and JWW). The same amount of images was segmented by one grader (JWW) after an interval of one week to determine intra-rater reliability. Absolute agreement model of the intra-class correlation coefficient (ICC) was used for the intra- and inter-rater reliability for the image binarization. ICC value of 0.81–1.00 indicates good agreement. The mean difference between the measurements was calculated by Bland-Altman plot analysis, which was constructed using MedCalc version 17.5.3 (Medcalc Statistical Software, Ostend, Belgium) software. After obtaining good inter-rater and intra-rater agreement,

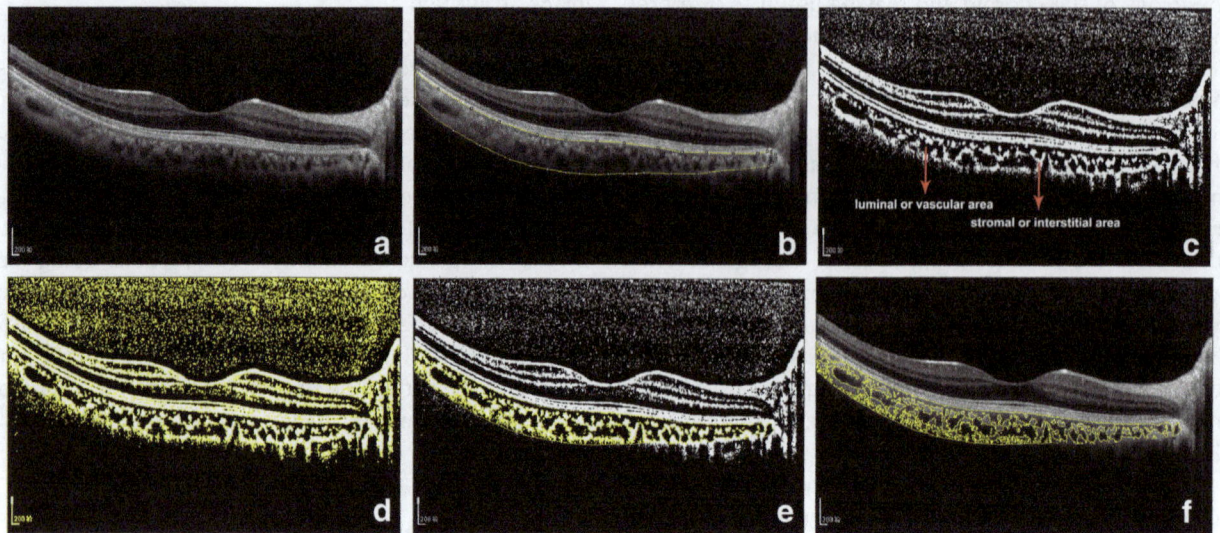

Fig. 1 Image binarization for choroid with Niblack auto local thresholding technique. **a** Original EDI-OCT scan image. **b** Manual segmentation of the choroidal area with one central scan passing through the fovea. **c** Conversion of the image with the Auto Local Threshold tool. **d** Clear segmentation of black and white areas on the choroid with Niblack autolocal threshold. **e** binarized image was reconverted back to RGB image. **f** binarized image over the original EDI-OCT scan

all the image binarization was performed by single author (JWW).

Statistical analysis

All statistical analyses were performed using SPSS software version 20.0 (IBM-SPSS, Chicago, Illinois, USA). Normally distributed data were expressed as mean ± standard deviation (SD). Each postoperative value was compared with baseline by paired t-test. Univariate and multiple linear regression analyses were performed to determine the associations between CVI and other factors. Values of $p < 0.05$ were considered to be statistically significant.

Results

A total of 36 patients (20 male and 16 female) were finally recruited for the current study and the demographic characteristics of the patients are shown in Table 1. Mean age of the volunteers was 63.1 ± 6.9 years (range, 49~ 78).

The inter-rater agreement for CVI was 0.932 (95% CI: 0.866–0.965) and the inter-rater reliability was 0.959 (95% CI: 0.920–0.979), which indicates excellentagreement for image binarization and CVI calculation. Bland Altman plot analysis was constructed to display the high agreement (Fig. 2).

The baseline CVI in patients was 60.1 ± 5.5%. After surgery, the CVI significantly increased to 61.7 ± 5.3% at D7, 63.6 ± 4.4% at M1 and 64.8 ± 4.0% at M3 ($p = 0.035$, 0. 0006, < 0.0001 for D7, M1 and M3 when compared with the preoperative values). The greatest progression of CVI was observed between D7 and M1 after surgery (Fig. 3).

Univariate linear regression analysis revealed a positive association between CVI and SFCT at baseline and M1 postoperative follow-up. Age was found to be related with CVI at W1 after surgery. However, in the multiple regression model, only SFCT was significantly associated with CVI. Univariate and multivariate linear regression analyses revealed no significant association of CVI with AL, IOP and gender (Table 2).

Table 1 Demographics characteristics of the recruited subjects

Characteristics	Mean ± SD			
	Baseline	D7	W1	W3
Axial length, mm	23.55 ± 1.58	23.37 ± 1.65	23.30 ± 1.58	23.11 ± 1.56
Intraocular pressure, mmHg	14.19 ± 2.13	13.18 ± 1.91	12.54 ± 1.62	11.93 ± 1.80
Subfoveal choroidal thickness (SFCT),um	234.8 ± 42.49	239.7 ± 40.61	266.6 ± 37.71	276.3 ± 36.20
Age, yrs	63.1 ± 6.9			
Gender, male (%)	20 (55.6%)			

Data were expressed as mean ± standard deviation (SD)

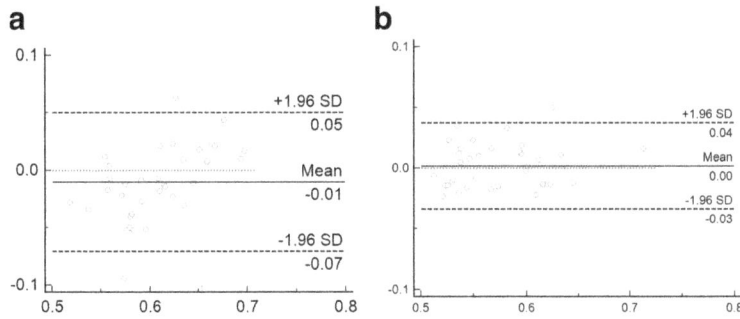

Fig. 2 Bland-Altman plot analysis of the intra- and inter-rater agreement. **a** and **b** shows the high reliability of the inter-rater and intra-rater agreement for the image binarization and CVI calculation

Discussion

A number of publications have reported the possible influence of cataract surgery on the choroid [2, 3, 9, 10]. Aslan BS et al. [9] have investigated the effects of uneventful phacoemulsification surgery on choroidal thickness using spectral domain optical coherence tomography (SD-OCT). They found that phacoemulsification may cause significant increase in choroid at all regions evaluated at 1 month postoperative follow-up. Yılmaz T et al. [10] have reported a long-term change in SFCT after cataract surgery. They have measured the SCT at baseline and postoperatively at week 1 and months 1, 3, 6 and 12 and the results indicated that uncomplicated phacoemulsification induced insignificant increases in SFCT and this did not return to baseline during follow-up. In our study, we found that the mean SFCT, as tested by EDI-OCT, significantly increased after surgery, which was consistent with the published literatures (Fig. 4). As well known, the choroid is predominantly composed of blood vessels surrounded by stromal tissue. Although many studies, including our study, have described the increased SCT after phacoemulsification, nobody really knows which

structures within the choroid increased. To answer this question, we used the binarization of EDI-OCT images and firstly attempted to assess the changes of choroidal vascular and stromal structures following cataract surgery.

With the advent of EDI-OCT, it is possible to analyze the structural changes allowing for quantitative measurements of choroidal vasculature in patients. Recently, an OCT based metric termed CVI has been used to assess the choroidal vascularity, using the image binarization technique for EDI-OCT scans [5]. CVI is more stable and less interferences from physiologic factors as opposed to the thickness of choroid [5, 7, 11]. In our previous study, we have found that SFCT is affected by many physiological factors, like AL and gender [12]. When comparing the factors influencing CVI, we found no significant association of CVI with AL, IOP and gender and there were positive associations between CVI and SFCT at pre-operation and 1 month postoperative follow-up. CVI was affected by few variables and demonstrated greater stability than SFCT. Measuring of the CVI would provide deeper understanding of the vascular structural changes in the process of choroid diseases, and therefore may be more informative compared to SFCT measurements alone.

By calculating the CVI, it is able to determine if there was an increase or decrease in vascularity and provide us more information on the proportion of vascularity in the choroid. Agrawal R and collaborators [13] found that eyes with acute central serous chorioretinopathy (CSC) had significantly higher CVI compared with their fellow eyes and age-matched healthy subjects. They demonstrated that CVI might be useful for the early diagnosis of CSC and to be a therapeutic index for the treatment response after laser photocoagulation or photodynamic therapy. In patients diagnosed with exudative age-related macular degeneration (AMD), there was a significantly lower CVI and CVI was probably a potential noninvasive tool for studying structural changes in choroid and exudative AMD development monitored [14]. Therefore, CVI is considered to be a relatively stable index to monitor the progression of choroidal diseases [15–17].

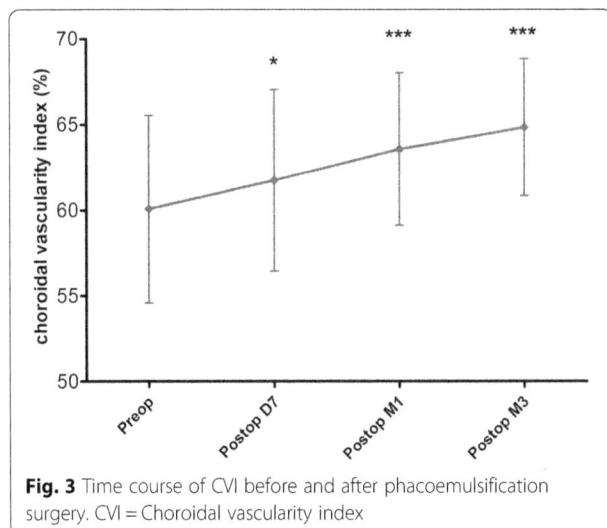

Fig. 3 Time course of CVI before and after phacoemulsification surgery. CVI = Choroidal vascularity index

Table 2 Univariate and multivariate linear regression analyses of age, gender and ocular factors associated with choroidal vascularity index

		Univariate			Multivariate		
		Unstandardized β	Standardized β	P-value	Unstandardized β	Standardized β	P-value
Age	Pre	0.053	0.067	0.698	0.092	0.115	0.462
	D7	0.032	0.041	0.810	0.048	0.062	0.721
	W1	0.225	0.346	0.039	0.163	0.251	0.119
	W3	0.015	0.026	0.880	0.024	0.041	0.818
Gender	Pre	3.520	0.324	0.054	3.307	0.305	0.057
	D7	3.056	0.291	0.085	2.246	0.214	0.234
	W1	0.349	0.040	0.819	−0.177	−0.020	0.898
	W3	0.237	0.030	0.862	0.487	0.062	0.725
Axial length, mm	Pre	−0.171	−0.288	0.775	−0.524	−0.204	0.202
	D7	0.550	0.171	0.317	0.660	0.206	0.271
	W1	0.424	0.151	0.380	0.579	0.206	0.231
	W3	−0.037	−0.014	0.933	−0.175	−0.069	0.706
IOP, mmHg	Pre	−0.575	−0.233	0.190	−0.524	−0.204	0.202
	D7	0.145	0.052	0.763	0.152	0.055	0.756
	W1	−0.731	−0.266	0.116	−0.518	−0.189	0.229
	W3	−0.702	−0.317	0.060	−0.743	−0.335	0.065
SFCT, μm	Pre	0.051	0.399	0.016	0.053	0.413	0.026*
	D7	0.029	0.223	0.190	0.033	0.253	0.168
	W1	0.044	0.372	0.025	0.048	0.406	0.02*
	W3	0.009	0.086	0.618	0.010	0.092	0.603

*Adjusted for variables with a p-value< 0.05 in the univariate analysis. β, regression coefcient

Phacoemulsification is the most frequently performed surgical intervention worldwide and considered to be safe and effective. However, in the past, concern has been raised about the association between cataract surgery with the incidence or progression of AMD. Disorders of the choroid after Phacoemulsification may cause

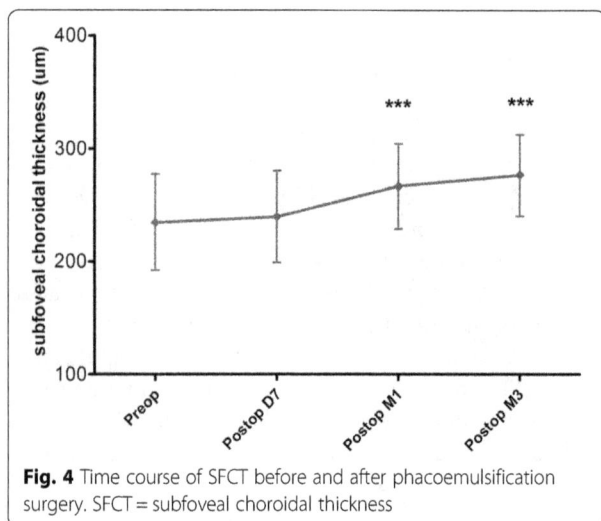

Fig. 4 Time course of SFCT before and after phacoemulsification surgery. SFCT = subfoveal choroidal thickness

the onset of many choroid diseases, including AMD. Some researchers have raised concerns that phacoemulsification may constitute a risk factor for the development of exudative AMD [18–20]. In contrast, recent evidence does not find the surgery to cause or worsen the progression of AMD [21–24]. In our study, the CVI was 60.1 ± 5.5% in the baseline and significantly increased D7, M1 and M3 after the surgery. The greatest progression of CVI was observed between D7 and M1 after surgery. Therefore, our data suggested that phacoemulsification seemed to be able to induce the expansion of choroidal vascular structures within 3 months after surgery. As a more stable parameter for disease monitoring, it will be very useful to evaluate CVI of patients after phacoemulsification at further follow-up over a longer period. Evaluation of CVI may provide further evidence about the relationship between phacoemulsification and AMD.

We found that phacoemulsification induced progressive increases in CVI. On the other hand, the surgery increased the proportion of vascular structures in the choroid. We suspect that the increased CVI may depend crucially on the choroidal inflammation induced by surgical trauma [25]. With the disruption to the blood-aqueous barrier, the inflammatory mediators in the aqueous humor pass through the vitreous to the retina and choroid, subsequently leading to the change of choroidal vascular structures. Another possibility is the IOP decrease after cataract surgery. The increased ocular perfusion pressure caused by reduced IOP may induce the increased CVI in the early period after phacoemulsification. However, the concrete mechanism has yet to be fully explained and further study is needed.

There are some limitations in the current study. Firstly, although this binarization technique is valid and widely used, there is no concrete evidence that the dark areas represented the vascular areas. Secondly, the postoperative anti-inflammatory eye drops may affect the CVI evaluation; Thirdly, the average ultrasonic emulsification time (UST) and the cumulative dissipated energy (CDE) were not recorded, which may also influence the CVI analysis. Lastly, the cohort of patients was not large enough and we only assessed the short-term changes of CVI after surgery. The future bigger sample research and longer follow-up periods are needed, especially to clarify the relationship between phacoemulsification and the frequency of disorders of the choroid such as AMD.

Conclusions

In the follow-up study, we firstly used CVI to assess the change of choroidal vascular structures in patients undergoing phacoemulsification surgery. Our results showed that the proportion of vascularity in the choroid, termed as CVI, significantly increased within 3 months following surgery. Evaluation of CVI may provide valuable information for studying the relationship between phacoemulsification and disorders of the choroid such as AMD.

Abbreviations
AL: Axial length; AMD: Age related macular degeneration; CSC: Central serous chorioretinopathy; CVI: Choroidal vascularity index; EDI: Enhanced depth imaging; IOP: Intraocular pressure; LA: Luminal or vascular area; OCT: Optical coherence tomography; SA: Stromal or interstitial area; SFCT: Subfoveal choroidal thickness; TCA: Total circumscribed area

Acknowledgements
Not applicable.

Funding
This study was supported by the National Natural Science Foundation of China (81700831), the Natural Science Foundation of Shandong province, China (ZR2017BH049) and the Medicine and Technology Program of Guangzhou, China (20161A011099).

Authors' contributions
All authors conceived of and designed the experimental protocol. HSC, YC, MSH and JWW collected the data and involved in the analysis and interpretation of the data. HSC wrote the first draft of the manuscript. JWW and ZMW reviewed and revised the manuscript and produced the final version. All authors read and approved the final manuscript.

Competing interests
The authors declare that they have no competing interests.

Author details
[1]Guangzhou Aier Eye Hospital, Guangzhou, China. [2]Eye Center of Shandong University, The Second Hospital of Shandong University, Shandong University, Jinan 250000, China.

References
1. Tan X, Lin H, Li Y, et al. Cataract screening in a rural area of southern China: a retrospective cohort study. Lancet. 2016;388(Suppl 1):S53.
2. Cheong KX, Tan CS. Long-term increase in subfoveal choroidal thickness after surgery for senile cataracts. Am J Ophthalmol. 2015;159(3):608–9.
3. Ohsugi H, Ikuno Y, Ohara Z, et al. Changes in choroidal thickness after cataract surgery. J Cataract Refract Surg. 2014;40(2):184–91.
4. Jiang H, Li Z, Sun R, Liu D, Liu N. Subfoveal choroidal and macular thickness changes after phacoemulsification using enhanced depth imaging optical coherence tomography. Ophthalmic Res. 2017; https://doi.org/10.1159/000480240.
5. Agrawal R, Salman M, Tan KA, et al. Choroidal vascularity index (CVI)–a novel optical coherence tomography parameter for monitoring patients with Panuveitis. PLoS One. 2016;11(1):e0146344.
6. Huang W, Wang W, Gao X, et al. Choroidal thickness in the subtypes of angle closure: an EDI-OCT study. Invest Ophthalmol Vis Sci. 2013;54(13):7849–53.
7. Agrawal R, Gupta P, Tan KA, Cheung CM, Wong TY, Cheng CY. Choroidal vascularity index as a measure of vascular status of the choroid: measurements in healthy eyes from a population-based study. Sci Rep. 2016;6:21090.
8. Agrawal R, Li LK, Nakhate V, Khandelwal N, Mahendradas P. Choroidal vascularity index in Vogt-Koyanagi-Harada disease: an EDI-OCT derived tool for monitoring disease progression. Transl Vis Sci Technol. 2016;5(4):7.
9. Aslan BS, Bayhan HA, Muhafiz E, Kırboğa K, Gürdal C. Evaluation of choroidal thickness changes after phacoemulsification surgery. Clin Ophthalmol. 2016; 10:961–7.
10. Yılmaz T, Karci AA, Yilmaz İ, Yılmaz A, Yıldırım Y, Sakalar YB. Long-term changes in subfoveal choroidal thickness after cataract surgery. Med Sci Monit. 2016;22:1566–70.
11. Agrawal R, Wei X, Goud A, Vupparaboina KK, Jana S, Chhablani J. Influence of scanning area on choroidal vascularity index measurement using optical coherence tomography. Acta Ophthalmol. 2017;95(8):e770–5.
12. Wang J, Gao X, Huang W, et al. Swept-source optical coherence tomography imaging of macular retinal and choroidal structures in healthy eyes. BMC Ophthalmol. 2015;15:122.
13. Agrawal R, Chhablani J, Tan KA, Shah S, Sarvaiya C, Banker A. Choroidal vascularity Index in central serous CHORIORETINOPATHY. Retina. 2016;36(9):1646–51.
14. Wei X, DSW T, Ng WY, Khandelwal N, Agrawal R, CMG C. CHOROIDAL VASCULARITY INDEX: A Novel Optical Coherence Tomography Based Parameter in Patients With Exudative Age-Related Macular Degeneration. Retina. 2017;37(6):1120–5.
15. LHL K, Agrawal R, Khandelwal N, Sai CL, Chhablani J. Choroidal vascular changes in age-related macular degeneration. Acta Ophthalmol. 2017;95(7):e597–601.
16. Tan KA, Laude A, Yip V, Loo E, Wong EP, Agrawal R. Choroidal vascularity index - a novel optical coherence tomography parameter for disease monitoring in diabetes mellitus. Acta Ophthalmol. 2016;94(7):e612–6.
17. Ng WY, Ting DS, Agrawal R, et al. Choroidal structural changes in myopic choroidal neovascularization after treatment with Antivascular endothelial growth factor over 1 year. Invest Ophthalmol Vis Sci. 2016;57(11):4933–9.
18. Freeman EE, Munoz B, West SK, Tielsch JM, Schein OD. Is there an association between cataract surgery and age-related macular degeneration? Data from three population-based studies. Am J Ophthalmol. 2003;135(6):849–56.
19. Cugati S, Mitchell P, Rochtchina E, Tan AG, Smith W, Wang JJ. Cataract surgery and the 10-year incidence of age-related maculopathy: the Blue Mountains eye study. Ophthalmology. 2006;113(11):2020–5.
20. Wang JJ, Klein R, Smith W, Klein BE, Tomany S, Mitchell P. Cataract surgery and the 5-year incidence of late-stage age-related maculopathy: pooled findings from the beaver dam and Blue Mountains eye studies. Ophthalmology. 2003;110(10):1960–7.

21. Chew EY, Sperduto RD, Milton RC, et al. Risk of advanced age-related macular degeneration after cataract surgery in the age-related eye disease study: AREDS report 25. Ophthalmology. 2009;116(2):297–303.

22. Ehmann DS, Ho AC. Cataract surgery and age-related macular degeneration. Curr Opin Ophthalmol. 2017;28(1):58–62.

23. Park SJ, Lee JH, Ahn S, Park KH. Cataract surgery and age-related macular degeneration in the 2008-2012 Korea National Health and nutrition examination survey. JAMA Ophthalmol. 2016;134(6):621–6.

24. Bockelbrink A, Rasch A, Roll S, Willich SN, Greiner W. What effects has the cataract surgery on the development and progression of Age-Related Macular Degeneration (AMD). GMS Health Technol Assess. 2006;2:Doc21.

25. Xu H, Chen M, Forrester JV, Lois N. Cataract surgery induces retinal pro-inflammatory gene expression and protein secretion. Invest Ophthalmol Vis Sci. 2011;52(1):249–55.

11

The fast exodrift after the first surgical treatment of exotropia and its correlation with surgical outcome of second surgery

Won Jae Kim and Myung Mi Kim[*]

Abstract

Background: To compare the rate of exodrift after a second surgery for recurrent exotropia, in patients grouped to fast versus slow exodrift after their first surgery. To determine whether there is a correlation with surgical outcome, and to evaluate the factors associated with fast exodrift.

Methods: Patients with recurrent intermittent exotropia, who underwent contralateral lateral rectus recession and medial rectus resection as the second surgery and were followed up for 24 months postoperatively between January 1991 and January 2013, were reviewed retrospectively. The patients were divided into two groups according to the rate of exodrift after the first surgery: Group F, patients exhibiting fast exodrift after the first surgery (> 10 prism diopters [PD] before postoperative month 6); and Group S, patients exhibiting slow exodrift after the first surgery ($\leq$10 PD before postoperative month 6). The difference in the clinical course over the 24 months after the second surgery between the two groups and factors associated with fast exodrift were analyzed.

Results: In total, 106 patients with recurrent exotropia were enrolled in this study. Of these, 68 (64.2%) and 38 (35.8%) patients were included in group F and S, respectively. Group F showed more exodrift compared with groups S over the 24-month postoperative period; however, there was no significant difference in the clinical course between the two groups during that time ($p = 0.54$, repeated-measure ANOVA). In logistic analysis, immediate postoperative deviation after the first surgery was associated with fast exodrift ($p <$ 0.001).

Conclusion: Although patients with recurrent exotropia had shown fast exodrift after the first surgery, no significant difference in the surgical outcome was observed after the second surgery according to the rate of exodrift after the first surgery.

Keywords: Recurrent exotropia, Exodrift, Surgical outcome

Background

Recurrent or persistent exodeviation may occur in patients with intermittent exotropia following surgical treatment [1–4]. Patients with intermittent exotropia who underwent surgical treatment generally experience postoperative exodrift over time [5]. When a patient who has undergone surgical treatment shows noticeable exodeviation in a short period of time, a second surgery would be considered to restore the ocular alignment. When planning the second surgery for patients with recurrent exotropia, one question frequently arises: do patients who experience a fast rate of exodrift after the first surgery also show fast exodrift after the second surgery? To the best of the authors' knowledge, there has been no study comparing the longitudinal clinical course of patients with recurrent exotropia after the second surgery according to the rate of exodrift after the first surgery. This study compared the surgical outcomes of patients with recurrent exotropia after the second surgery according to rate of exodrift after the first surgery to clarify whether patients with recurrent exotropia, who had experienced fast exodrift after the first surgery, will experience the same rate of exodrift after the second surgery. In addition, the factors associated with a fast rate of exodrift after the first surgery were also evaluated.

* Correspondence: mmk@med.yu.ac.kr
Department of Ophthalmology, Yeungnam University College of Medicine, 170, Hyeonchung-ro, Nam-gu, Daegu 42415, South Korea

Methods

This study was approved by the Institutional Review Board of Yeungnam University Hospital (IRB file number: 2015–11–044-007). Informed consent was waived by the board. A retrospective chart review was performed on patients with recurrent intermittent exotropia who had undergone contralateral lateral rectus recession and medial rectus resection (R&R) as a second surgery between January 1991 and January 2013. Patients who had undergone unilateral R&R as the first surgery were included in the study. Patients with at least a 24 months' follow-up after the second surgery were included. The basic type, which was defined when the difference between the distant and near angle was within 10 prism diopters (PD), was included in this study. Patients included in this study were divided into two subgroups according to the rate of exodrift after the first surgery: group F comprised patients with recurrent exotropia who exhibited fast exodrift after the first surgery (> 10 PD before postoperative month 6); and group S comprised patients with recurrent exotropia who exhibited slow exodrift after the first surgery (≤10 PD postoperative month 6).

The clinical characteristics and surgical outcomes after the second surgery were compared between group F and S. Patients with any other types of strabismus, such as oblique muscle dysfunction, dissociated vertical deviation, A-V pattern, and nystagmus, were excluded. Patients with previous intraocular surgery, any neurological impairments, such as cerebral palsy, or severe unilateral amblyopia were also excluded.

Patient evaluation and surgical plan

The patients underwent a complete ophthalmologic examination preoperatively and postoperatively, which included visual acuity testing, ocular alignment status, slit-lamp biomicroscopy, refraction, fundus examination, and stereoacuity test. The onset of exotropia was assessed using the parental or patients' report. The patients were asked to bring old photographs if they were unable to remember the onset of exotropia. The best-corrected visual acuity was measured where possible. Amblyopia was defined as an interocular difference in visual acuity of two or more lines. If amblyopia was detected, occlusion therapy was performed to treat the amblyopia as soon as possible before surgery. The angle of deviation was measured by alternate prism cover testing at 6 m (distance fixation) and 33 cm (near fixation) in cooperative children both pre- and postoperatively. An additional near measurement was made after 1 h of monocular occlusion of the non-dominant eye or by habitually deviating the eye to measure the largest angle of deviation. The post-occlusion near measurement was obtained with an additional + 3.00 diopters (D) sphere over each eye before allowing the patient to regain their binocular fusional ability. The stereoacuity was measured using the Lang I test (LANG-STEREOTEST AG, Küsnacht, Switzerland) and Stereo Fly Stereotest (Stereo Optical Co., Chicago, IL, USA) when the patient could cooperate and complete the test. All surgeries in this study were performed under general anesthesia. The R&R procedure was undertaken using the surgical dose at the authors' clinic (Table 1). The angle of deviation measured during the first follow-up visit within one week of surgery was defined as the immediate postoperative deviation. The patients were followed-up at postoperative month 1, 3, 6, and 12, and every 6 months thereafter. The postoperative angle of deviation was measured at each visit. To improve the statistical accuracy, patients who did not complete regular follow-ups during 24 postoperative months were excluded from study.

Statistical analysis

The continuous data are presented as the mean ± standard deviation, and the categorical data are presented as counts and percentages. Differences in the clinical course between the two groups over the 24-month postoperative period after the second surgery were analyzed using repeated measures ANOVA (rmANOVA). A univariate logistic regression test was conducted to examine the factors associated with fast exodrift after the first surgery. A p-value < 0.05 was considered as statistically significant.

Results

Demographic and clinical characteristics of the patients

A total of 231 patients with recurrent exotropia underwent contralateral R&R as the second surgery during the study period. Among these patients, 106 patients met the inclusion criteria. Of these, 68 patients (64.2%, 68/106) with recurrent exotropia exhibited fast exodrift after the first surgery and were included in group F. The remaining 38 patients (35.8%, 38/106) with recurrent exotropia exhibited slow exodrift after the first surgery and were included in group S. Therefore, approximately two-thirds of patients who underwent second surgery exhibited fast exodrift after the first surgery. The

Table 1 Surgical dose of LR recession and MR resection

Prism diopters	Recession amounts of LR	Resection amounts of MR
25	4	3
30	4	4
35	5	4
40	5	5
45	7	5
50	8	5

LR Lateral rectus muscle, MR medial rectus muscle

demographic and clinical characteristics of these patients are in Table 2. No significant differences in gender distribution, age at onset of exotropia, age at the first and second surgery, preoperative deviation at the first and second surgery, spherical equivalent refractive errors at the first and second surgery, and the result of the stereotest were observed between the two groups. The immediate postoperative deviation after the first surgery showed a significant difference between the two groups (Table 2, $p < 0.001$, unpaired t-test). The mean deviation at postoperative month 6 were 15.5 PD and 6.3 PD in group F and S, respectively. In group F, the mean deviation at postoperative month 6 was nearly one-half of mean preoperative deviation. The mean interval between the first and second surgery was 63.0 months in group F, which was shorter than that in group S (Table 2, $p = 0.009$). This may be because the fast rate of exodrift after the first surgery resulted in the earlier consideration of a second surgery.

Surgical outcome after second surgery according to the rate of exodrift after first surgery

The angle of deviation in the two groups over the 24 months after the second surgery are shown in Table 3. Group F showed more mean deviation compared with group S at all postoperative follows-ups over 24-month period. However, rmANOVA analysis revealed no significant difference in the group-by-time interaction in the postoperative angle of deviation between the two groups (Fig. 1, $p = 0.54$, rmANOVA). The clinical factors associated with fast exodrift after the first surgery were evaluated between two groups. The age at onset of exotropia, gender, age at the first surgery, preoperative deviation, spherical equivalent refractive errors, immediate postoperative deviation, and the results of the stereotest were analyzed by univariate logistic analysis. Immediate postoperative deviation was the only factor to show an association with the fast exodrift after the first surgery (odds ratio: 1.352, $p < 0.001$, logistic regression test).

Table 2 Demographic and clinical characteristics of the group F and S

	Group F (n = 68)	Group S (n = 38)	p-value
Gender (male: female)	30: 38	16: 22	0.503
Age at onset of exotropia, mo	21.3 ± 16.8 (65/68)	23.0 ± 13.5 (34/38)	0.617
Operated eye at first surgery (right: left)	32:36	18:20	0.568
First surgery			
Age at first surgery, yr	5.2 ± 1.6 (3–12)	5.3 ± 4.1 (3–29)	0.781
Preoperative distance deviation, PD	33.1 ± 5.1 (25–50)	32.7 ± 5.2 (25–50)	0.736
Preoperative near deviation, PD	33.4 ± 4.8 (25–50)	33.5 ± 5.6 (25–50)	0.926
SE refractive errors at first surgery, D			
Right eye	−0.13 ± 0.95	−0.32 ± 1.03	0.349
Left eye	−0.17 ± 1.04	−0.22 ± 1.05	0.807
Immediate postoperative deviation, PD	2.5 ± 3.3 (−4 to 10)	−0.4 ± 3.2 (−9 to 6)	< 0.001
6 months postoperatively deviation, PD	15.5 ± 3.9 (12–25)	6.3 ± 3.5 (0–10)	< 0.001
Interval from first to second surgery, mo	63.0 ± 19.0 (31–151)	80.0 ± 35.8 (33–202)	0.009
Second surgery			
Age at second surgery, yr	8.3 ± 2.1	10.2 ± 5.8	0.059
Preoperative distance deviation, PD	27.3 ± 3.2 (20–35)	27.9 ± 3.7 (23–35)	0.390
Preoperative near deviation, PD	28.0 ± 3.7 (20–35)	28.2 ± 3.7 (23–35)	0.815
SE refractive errors at second surgery, D			
Right eye	−0.97 ± 1.79	−1.53 ± 2.12	0.150
Left eye	−0.93 ± 1.57	−1.64 ± 2.31	0.094
Result of stereotest			
Lang I test, passed, (%)	56/66, (84.8)	32/36, (88.89)	0.256
Stereo Fly Stereotest ≤800 arcsec	20/25	11/14	0.611

Group F = patients with recurrent exotropia who exhibited fast exodrift (> 10 prism diopters [PD] before postoperative month 6) after the first surgery, Group S = patients with recurrent exotropia who exhibited slow exodrift (≤10 PD before postoperative month 6) after the first surgery, PD prism diopters, D dioptersm, SE spherical equivalent; arcsec; arcsecond

Table 3 The angle of deviation after the second surgery at each follow-up visits in group F and group S

	Group F (n = 68)	Group S (n = 38)
Immediate, PD	0.0 ± 3.7	−1.1 ± 4.1
1 mo	2.0 ± 4.3	1.1 ± 4.1
3 mo	3.5 ± 4.5	2.9 ± 4.7
6 mo	5.7 ± 5.8	3.5 ± 5.6
12 mo	7.5 ± 6.5	5.7 ± 6.8
18 mo	8.3 ± 7.1	6.0 ± 6.7
24 mo	9.4 ± 6.9	7.0 ± 6.9

Group F = patients with recurrent exotropia who exhibited fast exodrift (> 10 prism diopters [PD] before postoperative month 6) after the first surgery, Group S = patients with recurrent exotropia who exhibited slow exodrift (≤10 PD before postoperative month 6) after the first surgery, PD prism diopters

Discussion

The result of this study showed that patients exhibiting fast exodrift after the first surgery were not more likely to exhibit fast exodrift after the second surgery. Patients with exotropia usually experience postoperative exodrift over time. The rate of postoperative exodrift varies among patients, with some exhibiting faster exodrift than others [5–7]. Park and Kim [7] reported drift rates over 12 months of postoperative follow-up; they indicated that drift rate was fastest at postoperative weeks 1–3, and showed the strongest correlation with overall drift rate. Additionally, previous studies [8, 9] showed that more than one-half of the total amount of postoperative exodrift occurred during the first postoperative year. Therefore, fast postoperative exodrift would occur relatively early period after the surgical treatment of exotropia. Those results are consistent with the results of the present study, which showed that mean deviation observed at postoperative month 6 in group F was approximately one-half of the mean preoperative deviation.

If fast exodrift occurs after surgery, a second surgery to restore ocular alignment can be considered. Whether patients with recurrent exotropia who had experienced fast exodrift will exhibit fast exodrift after the second surgery is of concern; however, a search of the literature did not reveal any study that evaluated the surgical outcomes of recurrent exotropia after the second surgery according to the rate of exodrift after the first surgery. This study investigated the surgical outcome after the second surgery in patients with recurrent exotropia according to the rate of exodrift after the first surgery. The patients with recurrent exotropia were divided into two groups according to rate of exodrift after the first surgery. The fast exodrift after the first surgery was defined as more than 10 PD at 6 months after the first surgery. This value was selected because most studies evaluating surgical outcome of exotropia use 10 PD as the reference in their definition of successful alignment [2–4, 10]. Because patients with recurrent exotropia may exhibit exodrift over time after the second surgery [2, 3], this study included patients who were followed up for at least 24 months postoperatively to investigate long-term surgical outcomes after the second surgery and compare

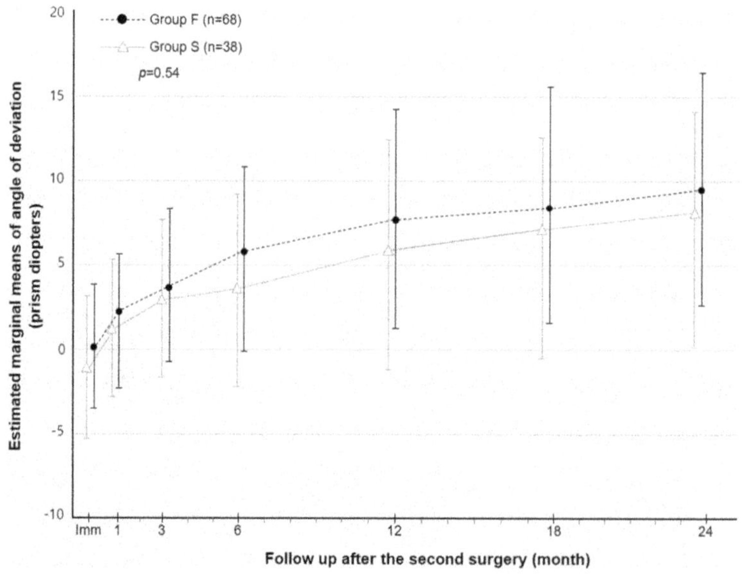

Fig. 1 Comparison of the angle of deviation after the second surgery between group F and group S over 24 months postoperatively. The repeated measures ANOVA analysis revealed no significant difference in the group-by-time interaction in the postoperative angle of deviation between the two groups ($p = 0.540$); Group F = patients with recurrent exotropia who exhibited fast exodrift (> 10 prism diopters [PD] before postoperative month 6) after the first surgery; Group S = patients with recurrent exotropia who exhibited slow exodrift (≤10 PD before postoperative month 6) after the first surgery; Imm, Immediate postoperative

these outcomes between patients with fast and slow exodrift after the first surgery.

In this study, there was no significant difference in the surgical outcome after the second surgery according to the rate of exodrift after the first surgery. Even when fast exodrift occurred after the first surgery, similar surgical outcomes were not necessarily seen after the second surgery. The results of the present study indicate that a second surgery may be considered for recurrent exotropia even though fast exodrift occurred after the first surgery. We suspect that both motor and sensory improvements after surgery were the reason that no significant differences in surgical outcomes were seen after the second surgery. From a motor perspective, the mechanical force from the resected medial rectus muscle in both eyes is considered one of the reasons for result of this study [11]. Kim and Kim [12] reported that the clinical course after a second surgery for recurrent exotropia was improved compared with the clinical course of both recurrent exotropia after the first of two surgeries and exotropia after a single surgery. From sensory perspective, even though fast exodrift occurred after the first surgery, it was assumed that there would be an improvement in the fusional ability compared with that before surgical treatment. Previous studies revealed an improvement in binocularity after surgical treatment in patients with exotropia, even constant exotropia [13–17]. These improvements in both motor and sensory aspects might lead to similar exodrift outcomes after the second surgery between the two groups.

Univariate analysis of the associated factors related to fast exodrift after the first surgery revealed its association with immediate postoperative deviation. This is consistent with a previous studies, which reported that the rate of exodrift correlated with the initial postoperative overcorrection [6, 7, 10]. However, the result of this study might be interpreted differently from previous studies, because previous studies evaluated exodrift in patients with exotropia who underwent a single surgery. This present study included only patients with recurrent exotropia who underwent a second surgery. The immediate deviation after the first surgery reached a statistical difference between the two groups, but these differences are very small from a clinical perspective. In group S, the mean deviation 6 months after first surgery progressed to 6.3 PD, only one-half of that in group F, but all included patients underwent a second surgery. Therefore, immediate postoperative deviation shows an association with fast exodrift after the first surgery, but it may not guarantee good surgical outcome over the long term.

The present retrospective study has some limitations. The mean interval between the first and second surgeries differed for each group, likely because fast exodrift after surgery can lead to earlier consideration of a second surgery. This study only included patients who underwent an R&R procedure as the first surgery. Another common surgery for the treatment of exotropia is the bilateral lateral rectus recession (BLR) procedure, and exodrift after the BLR procedure and its effect on surgical outcome after second surgery should also be determined. In addition, all surgeries were performed at the same institution and by the single surgeon. A future prospective study based on multiple institutions with a fixed interval between the first and second surgery and including both the R&R and the BLR procedure will provide more information on the clinical course of recurrent exotropia.

Conclusions

In conclusion, surgical outcomes in patients with recurrent exotropia who exhibited fast exodrift after the first surgery were not significantly different from the outcomes in those who exhibited slow exodrift after the first surgery. In addition, immediate postoperative deviation after the first surgery was associated with fast exodrift. These results will be helpful in explaining the expected prognosis after a second surgery to patients with recurrent exotropia who had previously experienced fast exodrift.

Abbreviations
BLR: Bilateral lateral rectus recession; R&R: Lateral rectus recession and medial rectus resection

Acknowledgements
Not applicable

Funding
Publication of this article was supported by a Yeungnam University research grant in 2015 (215A580081).

Authors' contributions
Involved in design of study (WJK, MMK); Conduct of study (WJK, MMK); Collection and management of data (WJK); Analysis and interpretation of data (WJK, MMK); Preparation of manuscript (WJK); and Review or approval of manuscript (MMK). Both authors read and approved the final manuscript.

Competing interests
All authors (WJK, MMK) declare no conflict of interests.

References

1. Joyce KE, Beyer F, Thomson RG, Clarke MP. A systematic review of the effectiveness of treatments in altering the natural history of intermittent exotropia. Br J Ophthalmol. 2015;99:440–50.

2. Lim SH, Hong JS, Kim MM. Prognostic factors for recurrence with unilateral recess-resect procedure in patients with intermittent exotropia. Eye (Lond). 2011;25:449–54.

3. Lim SH, Hwang BS, Kim MM. Prognostic factors for recurrence after bilateral rectus recession procedure in patients with intermittent exotropia. Eye (Lond). 2012;26:846–52.

4. Kim HJ, Choi DG. Clinical analysis of childhood intermittent exotropia with surgical success at postoperative 2 years. Acta Ophthalmol. 2016;94:e85–9.

5. Pukrushpan P, Isenberg SJ. Drift of ocular alignment following strabismus surgery. Part 1: using fixed scleral sutures. Br J Ophthalmol. 2009;93:439–42.

6. Choi J, Kim SJ, Yu YS. Initial postoperative deviation as a predictor of long-term outcome after surgery for intermittent exotropia. J AAPOS. 2011;15:224–9.

7. Park KH, Kim SY. Clinical characteristics of patients that experience different rates of exodrift after strabismus surgery for intermittent exotropia and the effect of the rate of exodrift on final ocular alignment. J AAPOS. 2013;17:54–8.

8. Kwon J, Kim SH, Cho YA. Postoperative stabilization of the strabismic angle in intermittent exotropia. Korean J Ophthalmol. 2012;26:446–50.

9. Park H, Kim WJ, Kim MM. The stabilization of postoperative Exo-drift in intermittent exotropia after surgical treatment. Korean J Ophthalmol. 2016;30:60–5.

10. Rajavi Z, Hafezian SF, Yaseri M, Sheibani K. Early postoperative alignment as a predictor of 6-month alignment after intermittent exotropia surgery. J Pediatr Ophthalmol Strabismus. 2014;51:274–82.

11. Rayner JW, Jampolsky A. Management of adult patients with large angle amblyopic exotropia. Ann Ophthalmol. 1973;5:95–9.

12. Kim WJ, Kim MM. The clinical course of recurrent intermittent exotropia following one or two surgeries over 24 months postoperatively. Eye (Lond). 2014;28:819–24.

13. Adams WE, Leske DA, Hatt SR, Mohney BG, Birch EE, Weakley DR Jr, et al. Improvement in distance stereoacuity following surgery for intermittent exotropia. J AAPOS. 2008;12:141–4.

14. Fatima T, Amitava AK, Siddiqui S, Ashraf M. Gains beyond cosmesis: recovery of fusion and stereopsis in adults with longstanding strabismus following successful surgical realignment. Indian J Ophthalmol. 2009;57:141–3.

15. Feng X, Zhang X, Jia Y. Improvement in fusion and stereopsis following surgery for intermittent exotropia. J Pediatr Ophthalmol Strabismus. 2015;52:52–7.

16. Gill LK, Arnoldi K. Binocular vision outcomes following surgery for long-standing large angle exodeviation. Strabismus. 2013;21:123–6.

17. Mets MB, Beauchamp C, Haldi BA. Binocularity following surgical correction of strabismus in adults. J AAPOS. 2004;8:435–8.

12

Decreased choroidal thickness in vitiligo patients

Serkan Demirkan[1]* iD, Zafer Onaran[2], Güzin Samav[1], Fatma Özkal[2], Erhan Yumuşak[2], Özgür Gündüz[1] and Ayşe Karabulut[1]

Abstract

Background: Vitiligo is a disease characterized by depigmented macules and patches that occur as a result of the loss of functional melanocytes from the affected skin through a mechanism which has not been elucidated yet. Destruction of pigment cells in vitiligo may not remain limited to the skin; the eyelashes, iris, ciliary body, choroid, retinal pigment epithelium and meninges may also be affected. This study aims to compare the choroidal thickness of patients with and without vitiligo using optical coherence tomography (OCT).

Methods: Spectral-domain optical coherence tomography (SD-OCT) (Retina Scan Advanced RS-3000 NIDEK, Japan) instrument (with $\lambda = 840$ nm, 27,000 A-scans/second and 5 μm axial resolution) was used for the imaging. Statistical analysis was performed using SPSS 21.0 software package.

Results: In all values except optic nevre area measurements, the choroidal thickness of all vitiligo patients was found out to be thinner compared to the control group.

Conclusions: In vitiligo, the choroidal thickness may be affected by the loss of melanocytes.

Keywords: Vitiligo, Choroidal thickness, OCT, VASI, Oculocutaneous disease

Background

Vitiligo is a disease characterized by depigmented macules and patches that occur as a result of the loss of functional melanocytes from the affected skin through a mechanism which has not been elucidated yet. The frequency of vitiligo throughout the world changes in the rate of 0.5–2% and does not vary depending on gender and race [1–3]. While vitiligo may occur at all ages soon after birth, the average age of onset is approximately 20 years [1–3].

The choroid is a vascularized and pigmented tissue which was first examined histologically in the 17th century and then tried to be visualized by various methods [4]. The choroid of the eye is a highly vascularized structure that supplies the outer retina and, histologically, consists of a thin choriocapillaris layer that is adjacent to the retinal pigment epithelium (RPE) and Bruch's membrane, medium- and large-caliber vessels (known as Sattler's and Haller's layers, respectively), and a suprachoroidal layer, all embedded within a collagenous and elastic stroma along with melanocytes [5]. The choroidal changes in many ocular pathological conditions such as polypoidal choroidal vasculopathy and age related macular degeneration were reported [6]. Choroidal thickness changes has also previously been observed in many systemic inflammatory disorders [6–9].

Melanocytes in the eyes consist of neural crest cells that have migrated ventrally. These melanocytes are located in the uveal tract (choroid, ciliary body, and the iris). Especially the stroma of the choroid layer consists of a high number of melanocytes [5]. The melanin, which is produced in melanocytes in the choroid layer, has an important function in an area starting from the retina and extending to the visual cortex of the brain. Melanin, which is produced in melanocytes in the eye and stored in melanosomes, has a very important role in the protection of the eye from the intraocular reflections of the light [5].

* Correspondence: serkan.demirkan@yahoo.com.tr
[1]Department of Dermatology and Venerology, Kirikkale University Faculty of Medicine, Yenisehir District, Tahsin Duru Avenue, No:14, Yahsihan, Kirikkale, Turkey
Full list of author information is available at the end of the article

Destruction of pigment cells in vitiligo may not remain limited to the skin; the eyelashes, iris, ciliary body, choroid, retinal pigment epithelium and meninges may also be affected [10]. Low choroidal thickness may be expected in vitiligo where melanocyte loss proceeds [10].

Although there have been many studies conducted to evaluate choroidal thickening in diseases that affected eye vasculature, limited research has been conducted on the diseases that affect melanocytes and another component of choroidal tissue, which remained under-researched. This study aims to compare the choroidal thickness of patients with and without vitiligo using optical coherence tomography (OCT).

Methods

This prospective clinical study addresses the examination of the bilateral eyes of (154 eyes). A total of 77 individuals, including 34 vitiligo and 43 non-vitiligo, were included in the study. This study was carried out between 2015 and 2016 in accordance with the tenets of the Declaration of Helsinki. The study protocol was approved by the Local Ethical Committee of the University of Kırıkkale. All patients and control subjects voluntarily participated in this study and signed an informed consent form.

Patients, who were diagnosed with vitiligo and were aged between 20 and 50 years, and non-vitiligo adults with similar characteristics participated in this study. VASI (vitiligo area severity index), which shows the depigmentation extent, was calculated in all vitiligo patients [11]. The percentage of the body area involved can be estimated by the so-called 1% rule or "palm method". In both children and adults, the palm of the hand, including the fingers, is approximately 1% of the total body surface area (TBSA), and it describes hand unit [11]. For each body region, the VASI was determined by the product of the area of vitiligo in hand units and the extent of depigmentation within each hand unit—measured patch (possible values of 0, 10, 25, 50, 75, 90% or 100%). The total body VASI was calculated using the following formula considering the contributions of all body regions (possible range, 0–100):

$$VASI = \sum \text{All Body Sites [Hand Units]} \times \text{[Residual Depigmentation]}$$

All participants had a thorough ophthalmologic examination, uncorrected visual acuity, best corrected visual acuity, manifest refraction, cycloplegic refraction and slit-lamp examination. Intraocular pressures were measured with an air-puff tonometer. Dilated fundus examinations were performed using a 78 D lens.

Individuals with poor OCT quality having a history that may have affected the choroidal thickness, such as diabetes, cigarette use, hypertension, antihypertensive drug use, known atherosclerotic disease, pregnancy, macular degenerations, previous ocular surgery, choroidal pathology, glaucoma, high refractive error (patients with more than +6 and −6 diopters as cycloplegic spherical equivalent), best corrected visual acuity below 20/25, and patients with a systemic other disease were not included in this study. Spectral-domain optical coherence tomography (SD-OCT) (Retina Scan Advanced RS-3000 NIDEK, Japan) instrument (with λ = 840 nm, 27,000 A-scans/second and 5 μm axial resolution) was used for the imaging.

Before evaluation, using EDI-OCT scanning, the central macular thickness was measured in the right eye of each patient. Choroidal and scleral boundaries were drawn with the assistance of software programs. Choroidal thickness was measured at the center of the fovea (SubF), and 500 μm nasally, temporally, superiorly and inferiorly (N1, T1, S1, I1), and 1500 μm (N2, T2, S2, I2) from the center of the fovea. The peripapillary region was measured 500 μm (N, T, S, I) from the center of the optic nerve. The averages of upper hemifield, lower hemifield, and whole hemifield of the peripapillary region were also measured (Fig. 1a, b). The foveal and parafoveal choroidal thickness was determined by measuring the region between the outer border of the retinal pigment epithelium layer and the sclero-choroidal interface manually. Measurements in the peripapillary area were carried out automatically with the instrument. The values of the right and left eyes of the patient and control group were separately specified and compared. All measurements are presented with median, minimum and maximum values.

Statistical analysis was performed using SPSS 21.0 software package. Descriptive statistics were presented as a mean ± standard deviation. In comparisons between patient and control groups, the student's t-test was applied to numerical data that followed a normal distribution, while the Mann-Whitney U test was applied to data that did not follow a normal distribution. The Pearson correlation test was applied to normally distributed measurements, and the Spearman correlation test was applied to data that did not follow a normal distribution. The statistical significance value was accepted as $p < 0.05$.

Results

Thirty four vitiligo patients and 43 individuals without vitiligo diagnosis were included in the study. The mean age of the vitiligo patients was 39.2 years, and the average age of the individuals in the control group was 39.3 years. Table 1 shows the age and sex distrubation, intraocular pressure, axial length, visual acuity, and refraction defect values of the patients and control group.

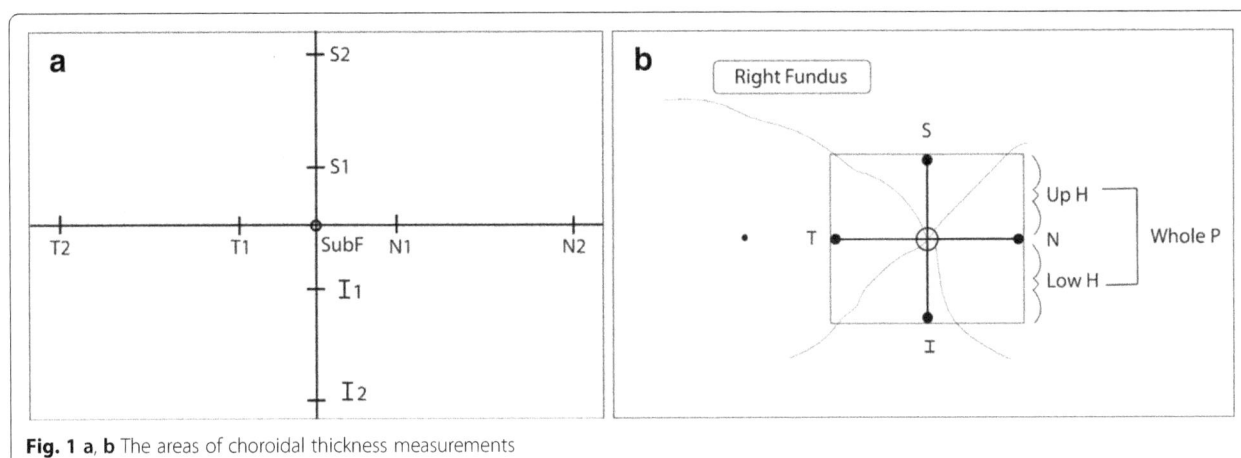

Fig. 1 a, b The areas of choroidal thickness measurements

In all values except optic nerve area measurements, the choroidal thickness of all vitiligo patients was found out to be thinner compared to the control group (Table 2). Correlation between VASI values of vitiligo patients and age, duration of disease, and choroidal thickness were signed in Table 3.

There was a negative correlation between age and choroidal thickness in some areas in patients. In patients and control groups, gender had an effect on the choroidal difference in none of the measured regions ($p > 0.05$). There was no correlation between duration of disease and choroidal thickness in all areas.

In those with higher VASI value, periorbital involvement was significantly more frequent. ($p = 0.029$). The frequency of periorbital involvement increased with the duration of the disease ($p < 0.001$). The periorbital involvement did not have an effect on choroidal thickness in patients with vitiligo. There was no statistically significant difference between those with and without periorbital involvement concerning age ($p = 0.300$).

Discussion

The stroma of the choroid layer consists of a high number of melanocytes [5]. Destruction of pigment cells in vitiligo may not remain limited to the skin; the eyelashes, iris, ciliary body, choroid, retinal pigment epithelium and meninges may also be affected [10]. A low choroidal thickness may be expected in vitiligo where melanocyte loss proceeds [10]. To our knowledge, this is the first study that examined the relation between choroidal changes and vitiligo in adulthood.

The choroid covers the outer retina and is among the most vascularized tissues in the body. This tissue supplies oxygen and nutrition to and provides temperature regulation for the retina. Also, choroid-containing melanocytes prevent intraocular reflections. In the eye, choroidal thickness may be affected by several factors, such as age, axial length, and refractive errors [12, 13]. A number of studies have found that choroidal thickness plays a prognostic or predictive role in various local (e.g., diabetic retinopathy), and systemic diseases (e.g., hypertension, anemia, rheumatoid arthritis and obesity) [14–20].

Table 1 Age and sex distrubation, intraocular pressure, axial length, visual acuity, refraction defect values of the patients and control group

	Patients (n:34) (mean±)	Control group (n:43) (mean±)	P value
Age	39.2 ± 16.14	39.3 ± 12.51	0.101*
Sex(F/M)	15:19 (44%:56%)	20:23 (46%:54%)	
Right intraocular pressures	14.20 ± 3.31	15.00 ± 2.23	0.105*
Left intraocular pressures	14.55 ± 2.83	14.76 ± 2.09	0.347*
Axial length	23.57 ± 1.04	23.58 ± 1.22	0.960*
Right eyes visual acuity	0.07 ± 0.21	−0.01 ± 0.26	0.330*
Left eyes visual acuity	0.08 ± 0.22	0.06 ± 0.40	0.845*
Right eye refraction defect	− 0.37 ± 1.00	0.00 ± 0.92	0.184*
Left eyes refraction defect	−0.21 ± 0.97	− 0.01 ± 0.98	0.702*

*…Student's t test

Table 2 Mean choroidal thickness in vitiligo patients and control group individuals

	Patient (n:34)				Control (n:43)				P value
	Mean ± SD	Minimum	Median	Maximum	Mean ± SD	Minimum	Median	Maximum	
Right, SubF	220.2 ± 39.8	170	224	290	261.4 ± 31.1	168	256	305	< 0.001**
Right, N1	223.6 ± 42.1	163	220	276	258.4 ± 32.5	190	248	302	< 0.001**
Right, N2	226.0 ± 39.2	130	220	340	261.5 ± 37.4	200	265	361	< 0.001*
Right, T1	220.5 ± 39.9	143	224	303	257.9 ± 34.2	139	257.5	311	< 0.001**
Right, T2	225.2 ± 41.1	109	220	280	253.4 ± 32.3	200	250	327	0.001*
Right, S1	222.9 ± 44.6	142	219	296	268.7 ± 38.1	198	271	289	< 0.001**
Right, S2	217.8 ± 40.8	151	219	301	259.1 ± 33.4	201	261	306	< 0.001**
Right, I1	223.4 ± 45.2	119	221	289	266.3 ± 37.0	136	264	321	< 0.001**
Right, I2	224.5 ± 45.2	117	226	340	265.9 ± 34.9	200	260	360	< 0.001*
Right optic nerve, LowH	95.0 ± 15.4	34	96	138	97.5 ± 7.9	80	97	118	0.429*
Right optic nerve, UpH	80.2 ± 16.8	43	81	128	77.1 ± 16.8	41	79	135	0.418**
Right optic nerve, WholP	98.9 ± 15.2	47	97	134	100.5 ± 8.1	54	101	126	0.805*
Right optic nerve, N	80.2 ± 16.8	54	77.5	126	77.1 ± 16.8	33	75	117	0.418**
Right optic nerve, T	68.9 ± 14.1	45	68	104	68.4 ± 15.5	29	69	99	0.689*
Right optic nerve, S	128.9 ± 25.3	59	132	168	129.4 ± 16.5	95	129	175	0.712*
Right optic nerve, I	118.9 ± 23.6	21	125.5	175	125.6 ± 17.0	79	125	165	0.230*
Left, SubF	222.7 ± 37.3	118	223	296	269.1 ± 31.0	129	267	305	< 0.001**
Left, N1	223.7 ± 38.5	105	224	301	271.7 ± 36.1	119	269	301	< 0.001**
Left, N2	228.2 ± 39.6	106	227	298	265.4 ± 35.8	129	267	311	< 0.001**
Left, T1	227.2 ± 42.2	164	226.5	380	308.2 ± 30.8	210	265	291	< 0.001*
Left, T2	235.4 ± 38.3	131	234	324	272.7 ± 35.7	176	275	329	< 0.001**
Left, S1	215.3 ± 40.2	126	216	305	257.2 ± 35.2	161	254	298	< 0.001**
Left, S2	220.0 ± 37.6	137	219	299	249.5 ± 48.2	148	251	324	0.005**
Left, I1	216.5 ± 38.0	139	218	301	262.3 ± 31.7	167	264	341	< 0.001**
Left, I2	222.2 ± 37.1	170	220	344	262.8 ± 31.9	210	260	350	< 0.001*
Left optic nerve, LowH	94.8 ± 12.2	59	95	141	95.5 ± 11.0	48	97	173	0.955*
Left optic nerve, UpH	122.6 ± 19.5	75	96	124	127.3 ± 16.3	77	93	125	0.255**
Left optic nerve, WholP	98.1 ± 12.0	70	99	125	100.2 ± 11.7	79	101	133	0.655*
Left optic nerve, N	75.6 ± 21.6	30	78	126	82.1 ± 23.7	27	78	174	0.432*
Left optic nerve, T	66.0 ± 18.1	35	61.5	106	65.0 ± 14.3	38	66	95	0.782*
Left optic nerve, S	128.4 ± 19.9	81	131.5	162	128.6 ± 20.5	76	131	178	0.951*
Left optic nerve, I	122.6 ± 19.5	89	122	169	127.3 ± 16.3	97	127	174	0.310*

*…Mann Whitney U test
**…Student's t test

In oculocutaneous albinism patients with melanocyte absence, the choroidal thickness in the subfoveal area was found to be significantly lower compared to the control group. However, no difference was found in the peripapillary region compared to the control group [21]. Choroidal thickness measurement was compared in a much higher number of regions in our study compared to the aforementioned study in which the lower choroidal thickness is also expected in vitiligo, which is another disease that proceeds with melanocyte loss [21].

Vogt-Koyanagi-Harada Diseaseis a bilateral granulomatous panuveitis associated with autoimmunity developed against melanocytes [22]. Patients with VKH increased choroidal thickness, which is probably due to exudation with inflammatory processes [23]. Invitiligo patients, the inflammatory process is chronic and exudative is not observed. Therefore, despite the presence of melanocyte destruction as it is in VKH, the increase in choroidal thickness of vitiligo patients is not expected.

The study conducted by Bulbul-Baskan et al. showed that eye pathology was observed in 10 of the 45 vitiligo

Table 3 Correlation between VASI values of vitiligo patients and age, duration of disease, and choroidal thickness

	VASI	r	p
Age	Weak correlation	0.349[a]	0.043
Duration of disease	Moderate correlation	0.555[a]	< 0.001
Right fovea, horizontal	Negative correlation	−0.417[a]	0.014
Right nasal 500	Negative correlation	− 0561[a]	0.001
Right nasal 1500	Negative correlation	−0.381[b]	0.026
Left fovea, vertical	Negative correlation	−0.437[a]	0.010
Left superior 500	Negative correlation	−0.481[a]	0.004
Left inferior 500	Negative correlation	−0.484[a]	0.004
Left superior 1500	Negative correlation	−0.356[a]	0.039
Left inferior 1500	Negative correlation	−0.380[a]	0.027

[a]…Pearson correlation test
[b]Spearman correlation test

patients. Their findings revealed that iris involvement in one patient, ring-like peripapillary atrophy around the optic nerve in seven patients, hyperpigmented rim in the left top segment of the retinal pigment epithelium in addition to peripapillary atrophy in one patient, focal hypopigmented dots in the temporal retinal area in one patient, and diffuse hypopigmentation in onepatient were observed [24]. Another study carried out with black patients with vitiligo, thin and dot-like pigmentary disturbances were identified in four of the 17 patients [25].

In the current study, we observed a significant reduction in OCT in all areas except optic nerve regions in the vitiligo patients. When we reviewed the relevant literature on this subject, we have not seen any published studies that would allow us to make a direct comparison regarding our findings. The lack of differences between the vitiligo patients and the control group in optic nerve regions may be because melanocytes occupy less space in the histological structure in the optic nerve regions.

Some studies maintained that gender and hormonal status may influence choroidal blood flow and lead to change in the choroidal thickness [26, 27]. However, in our study, it was observed that gender resulted the difference in choroidal thickness neither in the vitiligo patients group nor the control group.

Many authors have reported that the reasons for the differences in the choroidal thickness results between studies are different software programs for measurement, differences in the light source of the OCT, ethnic differences, differences in the age, refraction defects and axial length in the patient profile [14–20]. However, since a comparison was made with the control group, and the characteristics of the patient and control group were similar, the findings suggest that comparison of the measurements resulted in useful data.

Conclusion

Melanin, which is produced in melanocytes in the eye and stored in melanosomes, has a very important role in the protection of the eye from the intraocular reflections of light. In this study, in all values except optic nerve area measurements, the choroidal thickness of all vitiligo patients was found out to be thinner compared to the control group.

The melanocyte amount in the choroidal layer in vitiligo should be studied in the future postmortem and in vivo studies.

Abbreviations
CT: Choroidal thickness; EDI-OCT: Enhanced-depth imaging optical coherence tomography; I: Choroidal thickness at 500 μm inferior to the fovea; I1: Choroidal thickness at 500 μm inferior to the fovea; I2: Choroidal thickness at 1500 μm inferior to the fovea; LowH: LowerHemifield; N: Choroidal thickness at 500 μm nasal to the fovea; N1: Choroidal thickness at 500 μm nasal to the fovea; N2: Choroidal thickness at 1500 μm nasal to the fovea; OCT: Optical coherence tomography; RPE: Retinal pigment epithelium; S: Choroidal thickness at 500 μm superior to the fovea; S1: Choroidal thickness at 500 μm superior to the fovea; S2: Choroidal thickness at 1500 μm superior to the fovea; SD-OCT: Spectral-domain optical coherence tomography; SubF: Choroidal thickness at fovea; T: Choroidal thickness at 500 μm temporal to the fovea; T1: Choroidal thickness at 500 μm temporal to the fovea; T2: Choroidal thickness at 1500 μm temporal to the fovea; UpH: Upper Hemifield; VASI: Vitiligo area severity index; VKH: Vogt-Koyanagi-Harada; WholP: Whole peripapillary

Authors' contributions
SD, GS, ÖGand AAK collected patients and control group for the study.ZO, FÖ, and EY made eye measurements.SD wrote and edited the manuscript. All authors read and approved the final manuscript.

Competing interests
The authors declare that they have no competing interests.

Author details
[1]Department of Dermatology and Venerology, Kirikkale University Faculty of Medicine, Yenisehir District, Tahsin Duru Avenue, No:14, Yahsihan, Kirikkale, Turkey. [2]Department of Ophtalmology, Kirikkale University Faculty of Medicine, Yenisehir District, Tahsin Duru Avenue, No:14, Yahsihan, Kirikkale, Turkey.

References
1. Alikhan A, Felsten LM, Daly M, Petronic-Rosic V. Vitiligo: a comprehensive overview part I. Introduction, epidemiology, quality of life, diagnosis, diferantial diagnosis, associations, histopathology, etiology, andwork-up. J Am Acad Dermatol. 2011;65(3):473–91.
2. Ortonne JP, Passeron T. Vitiligo and other disorders of hypopigmentation. In: Bolognia JL, Jorizzo JL, Schaeffer JV, editors. Dermatology. 3rd ed. Philedelphia: Elsevier Saunders; 2012. p. 1023–30.
3. Taieb A, Alomar A, Böhm M, Dell'anna ML, De Pase A, Eleftheriadou V, et al. Guidelines for the management of vitiligo: the European dermatology forum consensus. Br J Dermatol. 2013;168(1):5–19.
4. Ryan SJ. Retina, vol. 1. 4th ed. Philadelphia: Elsevier Mosby; 2006.
5. Nickla DL, Wallman J. The multifunctional choroid. Prog Retin Eye Res. 2010; 29:144–68.
6. Chung SE, Kang SW, Lee JH, et al. Choroidal thickness in polypoidal choroidal vasculopathy and exudative age-related macular degeneration. Ophthalmology. 2011;118:840–5.

7. Kurt A, Kurt EE, Kılıç R, Öktem C, Tuncay F, Erdem HR. Is choroidal thickness related with disease activity and joint damage in patient with rheumatoid arthritis. Bratisl Lek Listy. 2017;118(1):23–7.

8. Kılıç R, Kurt A, Acer E, Öktem Ç, Kocamış Ö. Choroidal thickness in psoriasis. Int Ophthalmol. 2017;37(1):173–7.

9. Kola M, Kalkisim A, Karkucak M, et al. Evaluation of choroidal thickness in ankylosing spondylitis using optical coherence tomography. Ocul Immunol Inflamm. 2014;22:434–8.

10. Örnek N, Onaran Z, Koçak M, Örnek K. Retinal nerve fiber layer thickness in vitiligo patients. J Res Med Sci. 2013;18(5):405–7.

11. Hamzavi I, Jain H, McLean D, Shapiro J, Zeng H, Lui H. Parametric modeling of narrowband UV-B phototherapy for vitiligo using a novel quantitative tool: the vitiligo area scoring index. Arch Dermatol. 2004;140(6):677–83.

12. Ikuno Y, Kawaguchi K, Nouchi T, Yasuno Y. Choroidal thickness in healthy Japanese subjects. Invest Ophthalmol Vis Sci. 2010;51:2173–6.

13. Agawa T, Miura M, Ikuno Y, Makita S, Fabritius T, Iwasaki T, et al. Choroidal thickness measurement in healthy Japanese subjects by three-dimensional high-penetration optical coherence tomography. Graefes Arch Clin Exp Ophthalmol. 2011;249(10):1485–92.

14. Yiu G, Chiu SJ, Petrou PA, Stinnett S, Sarin N, Farsiu S, et al. Relationship of central choroidal thickness with age-related macular degeneration status. Am J Ophthalmol. 2015;159(4):617–26.

15. Sanchez-Cano A, Orduna E, Segura F, Lopez C, Cuenca N, Abecia E, Pinilla I. Choroidal thickness and volume in healthy young white adults and the relationships between them and axial length, ammetropy and sex. Am J Ophthalmol. 2014;158(3):574–83.

16. Akay F, Gundogan FC, Yolcu U, Toyran S, Uzun S. Choroidal thickness in systemic arterial hypertension. Eur J Ophthalmol. 2016;26(2):152–7.

17. Sizmaz S, Küçüker Dönmez C, Pinarci EY, Karalezli A, Canan H, Yilmaz G. The effect of smoking on choroidal thickness measured by optical coherence tomography. Br J Ophthalmol. 2013;97:601–4.

18. Duru N, Altinkaynak H, Erten Ş, Can ME, Duru Z, Uğurlu FG, Çağıl N. Thinning of choroidal thickness in patients with rheumatoid arthritis unrelated to disease activity. Ocul Immunol Inflamm. 2015;31:1–8.

19. Ingegnoli F, Gualtierotti R, Pierro L, Del Turco C, Miserocchi E, Schioppo T, ACUTE study group, et al. Choroidal impairment and macular thinning in patients with systemic sclerosis: the acute study. Microvasc Res. 2015;97:31–6.

20. Pekel G, Alur I, Alihanoglu YI, Yagci R, Emrecan B. Choroidal changes after cardiopulmonary bypass. Perfusion. 2014;29:560–6.

21. Karabas L, Esen F, Celiker H, Elcioglu N, Cerman E, Eraslan M, Kazokoglu H, Sahin O. Decreased subfoveal choroidal thickness and failure of emmetropisation in patients with oculocutaneous albinism. Br J Ophthalmol. 2014;98:1087–90.

22. Bordaberry MF. Vogt-Koyanagi-Harada disease: diagnosis and treatments update. Curr Opin Ophthalmol. 2010;21:430–5.

23. Nakayama M, Keino H, Okada AA, Watanabe T, Taki W, Inoue M, Hirakata A. Enhanced depth imaging optical coherence tomography of the choroid in Vogt-Koyanagi-Harada disease. Retina. 2012;32:2061–9.

24. Bulbul-Baskan E, Baykara M, Ercan İ, Tunali S, Yucel A. Vitiligo and ocular findings: a study on possible associations. J Eur Acad Dermatol Venereol. 2006;20:829–33.

25. Ayotunde A, Olakunle G. Ophthalmic assessment in black patients with vitiligo. J Natl Med Assoc. 2005;97(2):286–7.

26. Kavroulaki D, Gugleta K, Kochkorov A, et al. Influence of gender and menopausal status on peripheral and choroidal circulation. Acta Ophthalmol. 2010;88:850–3.

27. Centofanti M, Bonini S, Manni G. Do sex and hormonal status influence choroidal circulation? Br J Ophthalmol. 2000;84:786–7.

13

Trachoma in Yunnan province of southwestern China: findings from trachoma rapid assessment

Min Wu[1,2*†], Zhu Lin Hu[1,2*†], Dan He[1,2], Wen Rong Xu[1,2] and Yan Li[1,2]

Abstract

Background: To understand the situation of active trachoma among children aged 6 to 8 years old and scarring trachoma among those aged 15 and over in Yunnan Province, South-western China.

Methods: A rapid assessment of trachoma was conducted to determine the presence or absence of trachoma in Yunnan. Through risk assessment, 9 sites in 8 suspected trachoma epidemic counties were selected. Trachoma Rapid Assessment was conducted in these areas afterwards. Within each sites, 50 students from grade one in local primary school and adults aged 15 and above with suspected scarring trachoma were examined by survey teams.

Results: A total of 450 children aged 6–8 years and 160 adults aged 15 and above were screened in 9 sites of 8 counties. Only 1 case of active trachoma was found. Detection rate of active trachoma in children was 0.2%(1/450) in all sites and 2% (1/50)in Pingbian County. Out of 150 adults only 1 case of TT and 1 case of CO were found in all the highest at risk communities. People with scarring trachoma were aged over 60 years.

Conclusions: The active trachoma was rarely seen and trachoma is unlikely to be a significant public health problem in Yunnan Province, South-western China.

Keywords: Trachoma, Rate, Trachomatous folliculs, Trachomatous trichiasis, Corneal opacity

Background

It is well known that trachoma is an infectious chronic infectious ocular surface disorder caused by the bacterium Chlamydia trachomatis, and one of the main blinding diseases, especially in Africa. An estimated 2.2 million persons are visually impaired due to trachoma, among which 1.2 million are blind [1, 2]. Conjuctival inflammation is the main characteristic in primary infection of trachoma. As a result of repeated infection, trichiasis and corneal scar may present at late stage which can cause irreversible visual loss [3]. Trachoma is more common in communities with underdeveloped economy, drought and poor sanitation [4, 5]. Data from the Ministry of Health in China showed that the prevalence of trachoma ranged from 63.0%~ 98.0% in 1958 [6]. In the first national survey of blindness and low vision in China, trachoma was the second cause of visual impairment [7, 8]. Trachoma interventions were implemented in China for decades. Following the WHO recommendations to reach the target of WHA51.11 Global elimination of blinding trachoma [9], a trachoma rapid assessment (TRA) was carried out in 14 provinces in P. R.China as a key activity to determine the current situation of trachoma and provide information for future planning. Yunnan province locates in the southwest border of China and is at the far eastern edge of the Himalayan uplift. Yunnan has an area of 394,100 km^2, 4.1% of the nation's total, and shares a border of 4060 km with Myanmar, Laos and Vietnam. Mountain land accounts for almost 94% of its total area. The elevation ranges from 76.4 to 6740 m and the average annual rainfall ranges from 584 to 2300 mm. Because of diverse climate and poor traffic conditions, economic development level in Yunnan is relatively backward with more poverty-stricken

* Correspondence: ynwumin@126.com; hzl77@263.net
†Equal contributors
[1]Department of Ophthalmology, Yunnan Key Laboratory for prevention and treatment of eye diseases, Yunnan Innovation Team for Cataract and Ocular fundus Disease (2017HC010), Yunnan Eye Institute, Yunnan Eye Hospital, The 2nd People's Hospital of Yunnan Province, Kunming, China
Full list of author information is available at the end of the article

counties. The prevalence of trachoma was as high as 63.1% in Yunnan Province in 1963 [10]. In 1987, trachoma was reported as one of the three leading causes of blindness in the National survey of blindness in Yunnan. Among 109,181 participants, 107 people were blind caused by trachoma (0.098%) [8]. In 1999, the government of China included Yunnan as one of 12 provinces in which trachoma was still believed to be present [11]. In recent years, trachoma continued to be reported in school health reports [12–14]. Severe drought in recent years led to a shortage of drinking water in 7.42 million people. In the majority of mountainous and the mid-altitude level districts across the province, it is common practice for the whole family to use the same basin of water for face washing. Yunnan Province has been assumed by the government as a region in which trachoma was a public health problem. However, a large scale prevalence survey has so far not been carried out in Yunnan Province and assumptions are commonly based on clinical reports only. As part of a number of TRAs conducted across the country, a TRA was also conducted in Yunnan Province. Purpose of the survey was to assess the presence of active disease, defined as trachomatous inflammation, follicular (TF) and/or trachomatous inflammation, intense (TI) among children aged from 6 to 8 and trachomatous trichiasis (TT) and/or trachoma-related corneal opacity (CO) among those aged 15 and over.

Methods
Ethical considerations
The protocol for this trachoma survey was approved by the Ethical Committee of The 2nd People's Hospital of Yunnan Province, China. During the survey, informed consent was given by every adult and the parents of all enrolled children. The study procedure was explained to the parents, teachers and students by survey staff. The guidelines of the Declaration of Helsinki were strictly followed during the survey.

Study sites
The WHO recommended standard methodology for TRA [15, 16] was followed in this survey, including purposive sampling of choosing villages/communities where trachoma is likely to exist. A first phase of investigation was carried out to gather evidence of trachoma, its complications and socioeconomic information in Yunnan. According to the national population census in 2010, the total population in Yunnan Province was 45.9 million. Yunnan Province was divided into 230 districts consisting of populations between 150,000 to 200,000 people. The suspected trachoma epidemic areas were determined within all districts based on the following factors: 1) geographically remote; 2) poor economic development; 3) poor access to water; 4) known high-epidemic and endemic trachoma areas; 5) poor access to

health care; and 6) low socio-economic status. Evidence of known endemic trachoma areas, e.g. The number of trichiasis surgical cases performed annually and number of corneal opacity cases seen in recent 5 years, was collected from two sources: literature review and key informants, such as eye doctors, ophthalmic nurses and public health workers. Based on this information, eight counties were identified as suspected trachoma epidemic areas: Daguan, Binchuan, Fuyuan, Mojiang, Shuangjiang, Pingbian, Xichou, and Yuanmou county (See Fig. 1). Nine towns with poor socio-economic status (environmental, sanitation and water supply were also considered) in eight counties were defined as survey clusters.

Participants
Target population of the survey included the children aged 6 to 8 years for active trachoma and adults aged 15 years and over for blinding trachoma (TT and CO). The gross enrollment rates of primary education in China was estimated as 99.8% in 2014 [17]. Thus for children, a school-based survey was applied. With the help of the local Education Bureau, a list of primary schools in the selected towns was generated and one primary school per town was randomly selected for screening of active trachoma. One class of grade one students in the defined primary school was selected randomly. If the number of students in the class was more than 50, the first 50 students were documented as participants in the survey. When the number of students in the class was less than 50, more students would be recruited from the neighboring class until 50 students were examined. Adult participants were recruited via pre-screening by key informants. One week before the survey team arrived, local village leaders, teachers and village/township doctors etc., were requested to identify adults aged ≥15 years old with trichiasis and corneal opacity door to door. People identified were invited to the township hospital and confirmed by survey team.

Trachoma grading
Two survey teams were organized and each team included 1 ophthalmologist, 1 field assistant (local ophthalmologist) and 1 driver. One ophthalmologists in each survey team was trained by World Health Organization (WHO) experts during a workshop held by the China Ministry of Health in Beijing. The WHO simplified grading system was taught and applied to identify trachoma. The two trained ophthalmologists led the survey teams. Trachoma was categorized into five grades according to the WHO trachoma grading system [18]: trachomatous inflammation, follicular (TF), trachomatous inflammation, intense (TI), trachomatous trichiasis (TT), trachomatous scarring (TS) and corneal opacity(CO). TF is defined as five or more off-white follicles

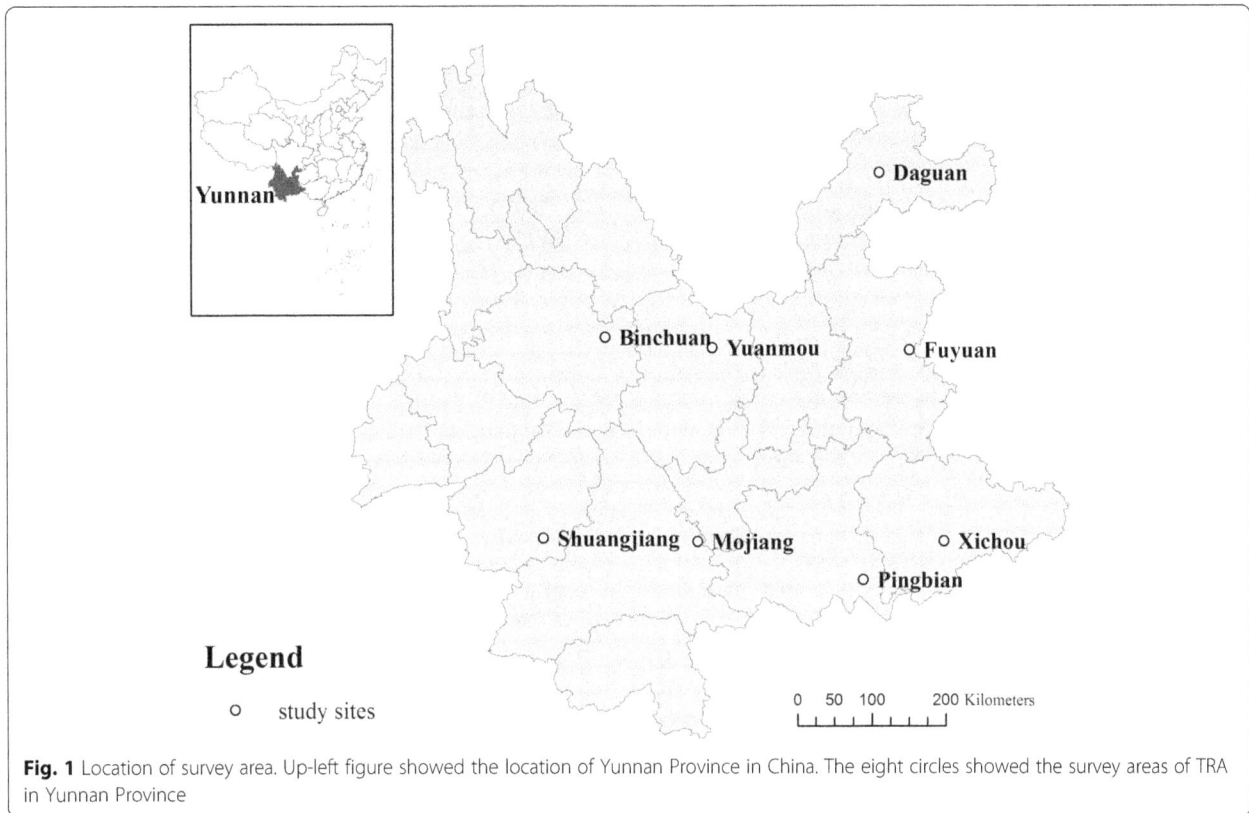

Fig. 1 Location of survey area. Up-left figure showed the location of Yunnan Province in China. The eight circles showed the survey areas of TRA in Yunnan Province

of 0.5–2.0 mm on the upper tarsal conjunctiva; TI is defined as inflammatory thickening of the upper tarsal conjunctival tissues obscuring more than half the deep tarsal vessels; TS is defined as small scarring in tarsal conjunctiva forming dense fibrotic tissue and distortion of normal lid architecture; TT is defined as at least one eyelash ingrown and touching the globe; CO is defined as corneal opacity which covers part of pupil margin as a result of ingrown eyelashes or secondary bacterial infections. "Active trachoma" was defined as TF and/or TI in either eye. "Scarring trachoma" was defined as TS, TT and/or CO in either eye. A WHO trachoma grading card and slides were carried by survey team.

Examination of trachoma
After written informed consent was obtained from parents, all the students were examined by trained ophthalmologists using a torch and a 2.5× magnifying binocular loupe. The examiner sat opposite to the student, examining for signs of inflammation (TF and TI) on the upper conjunctiva after turning of upper lid. Between examinations, hand disinfectant was applied to clean the examiners' hands. Once TF or TI was detected in any student, single dose of Azithromycin was prescribed. Health education information including face washing and strategies against infection was given to students, teachers and parents.

If active trachoma case was detected in non-boarding schools of any survey site, at least 50 children including the siblings of detected case would be examined in the community. If the case was detected in a boarding school, at least 50 students in the same school would be examined for trachoma.

All the adults aged 15 and above screened with suspected TT and/or CO were informed and gathered in the township hospital on the survey day. The survey team examined everyone following the same procedure used in children screening. People with TS, TT and/or CO were documented and people with TT and/or CO were referred to the county hospital for further treatment. Other people with treatable diseases were also referred to the county hospital.

Data analysis
Double entry of data were performed by two survey staff at the end of each survey day using Microsoft Office Excel 2010(Microsoft Corporation, USA). Integrity of data and consistency check were conducted. Statistical analysis was conducted using SPSS 16.0 software (SPSS Corporation, USA). The percentage of active and scarring trachoma was calculated. The association between risk factors and rate of trachoma was analyzed using Univariate analysis method.

Results

Detection rate of trachoma

In total, 450 eligible children and 165 people aged 15 and above were examined in this survey. The response rate in students was 100.0%(450/450) and 96.97% in people aged 15 and above (160/165). The female to male ratio in children and adults examined was 0.95:1 and 1.96:1, respectively. All the children screened were aged from 6 to 8 years old. In adults aged ≥15 years old, the age ranged 15 to 88 years, with a median age of 59 years. In children, 1 case of TF was detected in Pingbian County and oral azithromycin tablets was prescribed. No case of TI was detected. The percentage of TF was 0.2% (95%CI: 0.04–1.2%)(1/450) in total and 2% (95%CI:0.4–10.5%)(1/50) in Pingbian County. In people aged 15 and above, the percentage of TS, TT and CO in "trachoma suspects" was 3.1% (95% CI: 1.3–7.1%)(5/160), 0.6% (95%CI: 0.1–3.5%)(1/160) and 0.6% (95%CI: 0.1–3.5%)(1/160), respectively. The overall detection rate of active trachoma and scarring trachoma was 0.2% and 4.4%, respectively. The detection rate of active and scarring trachoma by survey sites is shown in Table 1. No trachoma was detected in all the remaining survey sites. People detected with TS, TT or CO were aged from 63 to 80 years with median age of 70 years. Within scarring trachoma cases, the CO case was male (14.3%) and other cases of TT or TS were female (85.7%). Although the detection rate of scarring trachoma in females was higher than that in males, there was no statistically significant association between sex and scarring trachoma ($p = 0.85$).

Further investigation of school where TF case was detected

Since one student with TF was found in Pingbian county, the details of the student were investigated. This student was a 7 year old boy and studied in grade one of a boarding school. The dormitory, water supply and environment were inspected in the school. The school had sufficient clean water supply and children could wash face using clean water every day and take shower once a week. The dormitory accommodated 15 students from different classes of grade one or two. 76 students in grade one and in the same or neighboring dormitory were examined by the

survey team. One student with TF was detected in this group and oral azithromycin tablets was prescribed. This student was the first detected TF child's roommate and shared the same towel. Health education on "F" strategy was given to the children, teachers and parents.

Discussion

The WHO led Global Alliance for the Elimination of Trachoma (GET2020) aims to elimination the disease as a public health problem in the world by 2020. The key trachoma control strategy is SAFE strategy endorsed by WHO: "surgery" for patients with advanced disease, "antibiotics" azithromycin or tetracycline eye ointment for active trachoma, "facial" cleanliness and "environmental" improvement on water supply and sanitation [4, 5]. In spite of implementation of SAFE strategy, data from Ethiopia [19], Sudan [20], India [21, 22] and countries in Pacific island [23] indicated trachoma is epidemic. The rate of active trachoma ranged from 25.2%–71.0% [19–23]. Trachoma was endemic and the second cause of blindness in China, also in Yunnan Province [6–8, 10]. School health reports showed that the detection rate of active trachoma in primary and middle school students was 29.56% and 18.24% in Fuyuan County in year 2000 [10], and 5.21% in BinChuan County in 2004 [12]. To reduce the trachoma, Ministry of Health in China had launched trachoma intervention programs nationwide since 1960s'. With the intervention of SAFE strategy, findings from several population-based epidemiological studies revealed that trachoma was no longer main cause of blindness in China, including Yunnan Province [24–29]. In our TRA in Yunnan Province, only one case of TF was detected out of 450 6–8 years children and the detection rate of active trachoma was only 0.2% in all the nine survey sites. Hence we conclude that active trachoma is sporadic in Yunnan Province nowadays. The finding is comparable with the findings of very low detection rate of active trachoma from TRA studies in the neighboring Sichuan province, Hainan province and Shandong province [30–32]. The improvement of school environment and general hygiene in community likely contributed to a decrease of trachoma. In the past, almost every village had one primary school. However, most of the schools had very poor infrastructure and

Table 1 Detection rate of trachoma in all the survey sites

County	Survey site	No. of children examined	No. of adults ≥15 years old examined	Active trachoma(%)		Scarring trachoma(%)		
				TI(%)	TF(%)	TS(%)	TT(%)	CO(%)
Fuyuan	Dahe	50	29	0(0.0%)	0(0.0%)	3(10.3%)	0(0.0%)	0(0.0%)
Pingbian	Baihe	50	21	0(0.0%)	1(2.0%)	0(0.0%)	0(0.0%)	0(0.0%)
Shuangjiang	Bangbing	50	23	0(0.0%)	0(0.0%)	2(8.7%)	1(4.3%)	1(4.3%)
Other 4 counties	4 sites	300	87	0(0.0%)	0(0.0%)	0(0.0%)	0(0.0%)	0(0.0%)
Total		450	160	0(0.0%)	1(0.2%)	5(3.1%)	1(0.6%)	1(0.6%)

insufficient water supply. During the past 10 years, merging of primary schooling had been completed. Small schools in villages were merged into one central school in town. As a result of increased governmental input to the central schools, the school environment, including water supply, was improved.

Out of 450 children and 150 adults only 1 case of TF, 1 case of TT and 1 case of CO were found in the highest at risk communities. Our study proposes that trachoma is unlikely to be a significant public health problem in Yunnan Province. The presence of blinding trachoma in elderly people aged over 60 years could be a sequelae of high epidemic active trachoma in several decades ago. Screening of scarring trachoma suspect people recommended by key informants would be a realistic solution to find people with TT and/or CO who need surgical services. People aged ≥60 years should be the target population for finding scarring trachoma suspect.

TRA is a cost-effective fast survey method recommended by WHO and validated in many countries worldwide. The applications of TRA comprised determining the presence or absence of endemic trachoma, whether or not trachoma is a blinding disease, or prioritizing communities with trachoma for treatment [33]. The TRA was completed in the mountainous region within one month by six survey staffs. It covered 9 sites in 8 counties, which spread in the different directions of Yunnan Province. The longest travel distance was 800 km from the capital city to the survey site. It shows that TRA is an useful tool which can provide an overview of presence or absence of trachoma, even in a mountainous region.

There are some limitations in this study: (1) During screening of scarring trachoma, survey teams did not look for cases using door to door method, but only examined suspected people in township hospitals. There might be selection bias in this process. Some adults with scarring trachoma could be missed when key informants screened in community. For the children, we did school-based survey only. Considering the enrollment rate of primary school in Yunnan Province was 99.5% in 2013, the school children are likely to be good representatives. (2) Microbiological investigation was not conducted in the detected TF case. However the clinical signs in the only TF case fulfilled WHO grading system.

Conclusion

Active trachoma is a rare condition and scarring trachoma is mainly found in people aged over 60 years old. Trachoma is unlikely to be a significant public health problem in Yunnan Province. Large scale of population-based survey and trachoma prevention program are not necessary. Efforts should be input to find possible blinding trachoma (TT and/or CO) in limited regions and surgical services for trichiasis should be provided when necessary.

Abbreviations
ASTRA: Acceptance sampling trachoma rapid assessment; CO: Trachoma-related corneal opacity; CRS: cluster random sampling; ENT: Ear, nose & throat; SAFE: Surgery for people at immediate risk of blindness; Antibiotic therapy to treat individual active cases and reduce the community reservoir of infection; Facial cleanliness and improved hygiene to reduce transmission; Environmental improvements to make living conditions better so that the environment no longer facilitates the maintenance and transmission of trachoma; TF: Trachomatous follicular; TI: Trachomatous inflammation intense; TRA: Trachoma rapid assessment; TT: Trachomatous trichiasis; WHO: World Health Organization

Acknowledgments
Sincerely acknowledgments should be given to the Health & Family Planning Committee of Yunnan Province, health workers and school staff in all the eight survey sites for the strong support in this survey. We also would like to thank Hai Liu, Jia Gao,Yuan Fang, Chun Li Li and all the investigators in this survey for their devotion. Deeply acknowledgement should be given to Professor Andreas Mueller for revising the paper.

Funding
This study is supported by Sight First China Action Project(SFCA-26-2013-01).

Authors' contributions
WM carried out the study design, acquisition of data, analysis and interpretation of data and drafted the manuscript. HZL contributed to the study design, revising and give the final approval of the version. HD participated in the design of the study. XWR and LY participated in the data acquisition. All authors read and approved the final manuscript.

Competing interests
The authors declare that they have no competing interests.

Author details
[1]Department of Ophthalmology, Yunnan Key Laboratory for prevention and treatment of eye diseases, Yunnan Innovation Team for Cataract and Ocular fundus Disease (2017HC010), Yunnan Eye Institute, Yunnan Eye Hospital, The 2nd People's Hospital of Yunnan Province, Kunming, China. [2]Department of Ophthalmology, The 4th Affiliated Hospital of Kunming Medical University, Kunming, Yunnan, China.

References
1. World Health Organization. Global data on visual impairment 2010. http://www.who.int/blindness/GLOBALDATAFINALforweb.pdf?ua=1) Accessed 24 June 2015.
2. World Health Organization. Global alliance for the elimination of blindng trachoma by 2020. Wkly Epidemiol Rec. 2013;88(24):241–56.
3. Hu VH, Harding-Esch EM, Burton MJ, Bailey RL, Kadimpeul J, et al. Epidemiology and control of trachoma: systematic review. Tropical Med Int Health. 2010;15:673–91.
4. Stocks ME, Ogden S, Haddad D, Addiss DG, McGuire C, Freeman MC. Effect of water, sanitation, and hygiene on the prevention of trachoma: a systematic review and meta-analysis. PLoS Med. 2014;11(2):e1001605.

5. Dye C, Mertens T, Hirnschall G, Mpanju-Shumbusho W, Newman RD, Raviglione MC, Savioli L, Nakatani H. WHO and the future of disease control programmes. Lancet. 2013;381:413–8.

6. Medical Prevention Buearu, Ministry of Health of China. Data compilation of National Trachoma prevention on-site meeting. Beijing: People's Health Publisher; 1959. p. 40–59.

7. Zhang SY, Zou LH, Gao YQ, Di Y, Wang XD. National epidemiological survey of blindness and low vision in China. Chin Med J(Engl)[JJ]. 1992;105(7):603–8.

8. Shang CX, Zhang XM, Pan X. The epidemiological study of blindness and low vision in Yunnan Province. Chin J. Ophthalmology. 1988;24:331–3.

9. WHA 51.11 Global elimination of blinding trachoma, 16 May 1998. (http://www/who.int/blindness/causes/WHA 51.11/en/index.html, Accessed Sept 2015.).

10. Sanitation and antiepidemic station of Wenshan Region in Yunnan Province. The survey of trachoma in rural area of Wenshan Zhuang and Miao autonomous region in Yunnan Province. Chin J Ophthalmology. 1965;12(4):303–4.

11. WHO Programme for the Prevention of Blindness and Deafness. First national workshop on the assessment and management of trachoma in the People's Republic of China: Kunming, Yunnan Province, People's Republic of China, 1-4 November 1999 : conclusions and recommendations. Geneva; World Health Organization; 2000. p. 28.

12. Gao GS. The survey of common diseases in students in Fuyuan County. Chin J School Health. 2000;21(6):472.

13. Zhang JJ, Pu GM, Fu X. The epidemiological survey of blindness and low vision in Pingbian Miao minority Autonomous County, Yunnan Province. Med J Chin People's Armed Police Forces. 2002;13(10):598–601.

14. He X, Yang RT, Wu HF, Yang JX. Status of common diseases in primary and middle school students in Binchuan County. Chin J School Health. 2005; 26(9):763–4.

15. Negrel AD, Mariotti SP. Trachoma rapid assessment: rationale and basic principles. Community Eye Health. 1999;12(32):51–3.

16. World Health Organization. London School of Hygiene of tropical medicine, International Trachoma Initiative. Trachoma control-a guide for programme managers. Geneva: World Health Organization, London School of Hygiene of tropical medicine, International Trachoma Initiative; 2006.

17. Yuan LS, He TT, Li ZY. Estimating the 2000–2014 gross enrollment rates of primary and secondary education in China. China Econ Educ Rev. 2017;3:3–19.

18. Baneke A. Review: targeting trachoma: strategies to reduce the leading infectious cause of blindness. Travel Med Infect Dis. 2012;10(2):92–6. Br J Ophthalmol, 2012, 10(2):92–96

19. Ejigu M, Kariuki MK, Ilako DR, Gelaw Y. Rapid trachoma assessment in Kersa District, Southwest Ethiopia. Ethiop J Health Sci. 2013;23(1):1–9.

20. Edwards T, Smith J, Sturrock HJW, Kur LW, Sabasio A, Finn TP, Lado M, Haddad D, Kolaczinshi JH. Results from a large-scale population-based survey and potential implications for further surveys. PLoS Negl Trop Dis. 2012;6(4):e1585.

21. Khanduja S, Jhanji V, Sharma N, Vshist P, Murthy GVS, Gupta SK, et al. Trachoma prevalence in women living in rural northern India: rapid assessment findings. Ophthalmic Epidemiol. 2012;19(4):216–20.

22. Vashist P, Gupta N, Rathore AS, Shah A, Singh S. Rapid assessment of trachoma in underserved population of car-nicobar island, India. PLoS One. 2013;8(6):e65918.

23. Mathew AA, Keeffe JE, Mesurier RTL, Taylor HR. Trachoma in the Pacific Islands: envidence from trachoma rapid assessment. Br J Ophthalmo. 2009; 93:866–70.

24. Tang Y, Wang Y, Wang J, Huang W, Gao Y, Luo Y, Lu Y. Prevalence and causes of visual impairment in a Chinese adult population: the Taizhou eye study. Ophthalmogy. 2015;122(7):1480–8.

25. Yao Y, Shao J, Sun W, Zhu J, Hong FD, Guan H, Liu Q. Prevalence of blindness and causes of visual impairment among adults aged 50 years or above in southern. Jiangsu Province of China. Pak J Med Sci. 2013;29(5):1203–7.

26. Wu M, Yip J, Kuper H. Rapid assessment of avoidable blindness in Kunming. China Opthalmol. 2008;115(6):965–74.

27. Cai N, Yuan YS, Zhao JL, Zhong H, Ellwein LB, Chen MM, et al. Prevalence and causes of blindness and moderate and severe visual impairment among adults aged 50 years or above in Luxi County of Yunnan Province: the China Nine-Province survey. Zhonghua Yan Ke Za Zhi. 2013;49(8):901–6.

28. Cheng JW, Cheng SW, Cai JP, Li Y, Wei RL. The prevalence of visual impairment in older adults in mainland China: a systematic review and meta-analysis. Ophthalmic Res. 2013;49(1):1–10.

29. Li X, Zhou Q, Sun L, Wang Z, Han S, Wu S, Wang N. Prevalence of blindness and low vision in a rural population in northern China: preliminary results from a population-based survey. Ophthalmic Epidemiol. 2012;19(5):272–7.

30. Chen H, Wu X, Wei M, Eichner JE, Fan Y, Zhang Z, Lei C, Stone DU, Yang J. Changes in the prevalence of visual impairment due to blinding trachoma in Sichuan Province, China: a comparative study between 1987 and 2006. Ophthalmic Epidemiol. 2012;19(1):29–37.

31. Liu H, Ou B, Paxton A, et al. Rapid assessment of trachoma in Hainan Province, China: validation of the new World Health Organization methodology. Ophthalmic Epidemiol. 2002;9:97–104.

32. Qu Y, Bi H, Wen Y, Li C, Wu H. Trachoma rapid assessment in Shandong province of China. Chin Med J(Engl). 2014;127(14):2668–71.

33. Ngondi J, Reacher M, Matthews F, Brayne C, Emerson P. Trachoma survey methods: a literature review. Bull World Health Organ. 2009;87(2):143–51.

14

Development of macular retinoschisis long after the onset of retinal arterial occlusion (RAO): a retrospective study

Norihiko Ishizaki[1,2], Teruyo Kida[2*], Masanori Fukumoto[2], Takaki Sato[2], Hidehiro Oku[2] and Tsunehiko Ikeda[2]

Abstract

Background: To describe a retrospective study of macular retinoschisis that developed long after the onset of retinal artery occlusion (RAO) using optical coherence tomography (OCT).

Methods: We describe changes in macular findings and visual acuity (VA) of 29 patients (21 males and 8 females, mean age: 66.1 ± 16.9 years) with RAO (18 branch RAOs [BRAOs] and 11 central RAOs [CRAOs] who visited Osaka Medical College Hospital over an 8-year period based on a medical chart review.

Results: The mean VA (logMAR) increased from 1.06 ± 1.08 (CRAO: 2.04 ± 0.99; BRAO: 0.37 ± 0.40) at the first visit to 0.71 ± 0.87 (CRAO: 1.46 ± 0.86; BRAO: 0.18 ± 0.30) at the final visit. Macular OCT revealed swelling or hyper-reflectivity of the inner retina in the early phase of RAO and retinal thinning in the late phase. Among the 29 patients, two patients (a patient with BRAO and a patient with CRAO) developed macular retinoschisis about 1 year after RAO onset. The VA of the patient with BRAO was 20/300 at the first visit, and it improved to 20/25 two days after onset following eye massage and anterior chamber paracentesis. However, his VA worsened, declining from 20/25 to 20/50, and retinoschisis occurred 13 months after RAO onset. The patient with CRAO showed macular changes including small cystoids at the first follow-up visit more than 3 weeks after onset and developed retinoschisis 11 months after the first visit. In addition, two patients with BRAO and one patient with CRAO developed macular changes including small cystoids 3 weeks after onset, with the BRAO complicated by retinal vein occlusion. In the CRAO patient, the cystoid macular edema was resolved 1 month after the first visit.

Conclusions: Macular retinoschisis is unusual, but a possible complication of RAO that can develop long after the onset of the occlusion, potentially resulting in renewed VA deterioration.

Keywords: Retinal artery occlusion (RAO), Optical coherence tomography (OCT), Macula, Retinoschisis

Background

Retinal artery occlusion (RAO) is induced by emboli and usually occurs suddenly. Systemic diseases, such as systemic hypertension, myocardial infarction, carotid artery stenosis, and diabetes mellitus, can be risk factors for RAO [1–4]. The diagnosis of RAO is based on sudden visual loss and characteristic fundus findings [5]. The ophthalmoscopic findings of acute-phase and late-phase RAO have been described in detail elsewhere [6].

Optical coherence tomography (OCT), which is a non-invasive technology, can be used to produce in vivo cross-sectional images of the retinal microstructure [7]. Macular OCT findings are helpful for determining the degree of retinal damage and predicting the prognosis of visual acuity (VA) in early- and late-stage RAO. A previous study reported that macular OCT showed swelling or hyper-reflectivity of the inner retina in the early phase of RAO, followed by retinal thinning in the late stage [8]. Such macular OCT findings are seen in most RAO cases.

In this retrospective study, we describe macular retinoschisis and macular changes including small cystoids detected by OCT long after the onset of RAO.

* Correspondence: opt038@osaka-med.ac.jp
[2]Department of Ophthalmology, Osaka Medical College, 2-7 Daigaku-machi, Takatsuki, Osaka 569-8686, Japan
Full list of author information is available at the end of the article

Methods

This retrospective study was approved by the Institutional Review Board (IRB) (the Ethics Committee of the Osaka Medical College (No. 2034)), and the tenets of the Declaration of Helsinki were followed.

For this retrospective study, we reviewed our medical charts of RAO patients who visited Osaka Medical College hospital from April 2008 to May 2016. In the initial examination, each patient underwent a comprehensive ophthalmic examination that included the measurement of their best-corrected visual acuity (VA) using a Landolt chart and retinal findings using fundus biomicroscopy with a non-contact lens. In each follow-up visit, patients underwent a comprehensive ophthalmologic examination that included the measurement of their best-corrected VA, color fundus photography, and macular OCT examination; an additional fluorescein angiography (FA) was performed if deemed necessary.

Results

Changes in macular findings and visual acuity (VA) of 29 patients (21 males and 8 females; mean age: 66.1 ± 16.9 years) with RAO (18 branch RAOs [BRAOs] and 11 central RAOs [CRAOs]) were investigated in this study. Systemic complications were as follows: systemic hypertension ($n = 17$, 54.8%), myocardial infarction ($n = 7$, 22.6%), diabetes mellitus ($n = 5$, 16.1%), stenosis of the carotid artery ($n = 5$, 16.1%), cerebral infarction ($n = 4$, 12.9%), postsurgery heart valve replacement ($n = 4$, 12.9%), atrial fibrillation ($n = 2$, 6.5%), atherosclerotic obstruction ($n = 2$, 6.5%),

postsurgery synthetic blood vessel graft in the aorta ($n = 1$, 3.3%), and anemia ($n = 1$, 3.3%). Macular findings were assessed by optical coherence tomography (OCT) (Spectralis, Heidelberg, Germany). The mean VA (logMAR) improved from 1.06 ± 1.08 (2.04 ± 0.99 for CRAO and 0.37 ± 0.40 for BRAO) at the first visit to 0.71 ± 0.87 (1.46 ± 0.86 for CRAO and 0.18 ± 0.30 for BRAO) at the final visit. The macular OCT findings showed swelling or hyper-reflectivity of the inner retina in the early phase of RAO, followed by thinning of retina in the late phase.

Of the 29 patients, two patients (a patient with BRAO and a patient with CRAO) developed macular retinoschisis about 1 year after RAO onset. In the patient with BRAO, his VA was 20/300 at the first visit, and it improved to 20/25 two days after the onset, following eye massage and anterior chamber paracentesis performed at the first visit. Figure 1 shows the macular changes revealed by fundus photography and macular OCT at the first visit. However, the patient's VA worsened, declining from 20/25 to 20/50, and retinoschisis recurred 13 months after onset. The retinoschisis remained 16 months after the first visit.

In the patient with CRAO (Fig. 2), macular change including a small cyst was observed at the first follow-up visit 3 weeks after onset, and his VA was remained 30 cm according to the finger counting test. Eleven months after the first visit, the patient developed retinoschisis, and his VA was 20/1000. The retinoschisis disappeared 22 months after the first visit, but the patient's VA did not improve.

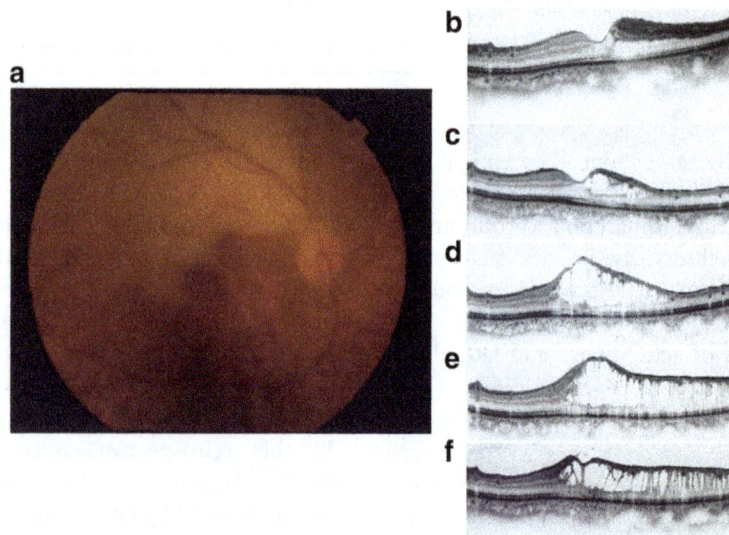

Fig. 1 A case of BRAO with retinoschisis. a Fundus photograph at the first visit. b Macular OCT image 1 month after the patient's first visit. The patient's VA was 20/25, and hyper-reflectivity of the inner retina was observed. The outer nuclear layer and Henle's layer were detached. c 9 months: Retinoschisis and thinning of the inner retina were observed. The VA was 20/25. d 13 months: Retinoschisis had spread and involved the fovea. The VA had dropped to 20/40. e 15 months: Retinoschisis was widespread. The VA was 20/40. f 16 months: The VA was unchanged

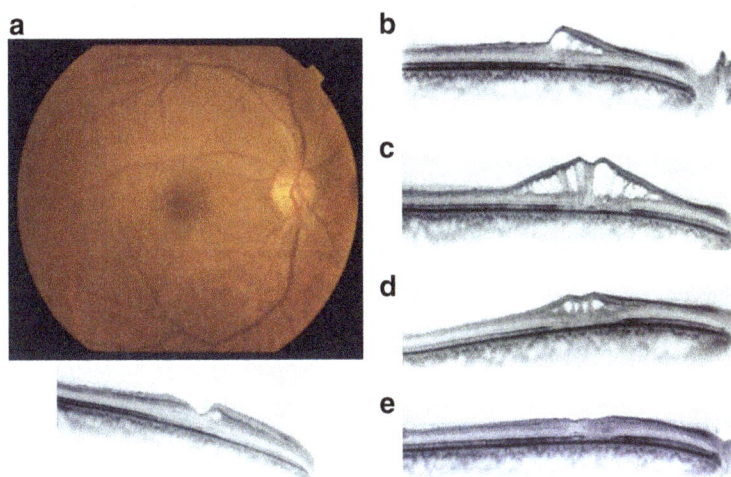

Fig. 2 A case of CRAO, with macular change including a small cystoid. **a** Fundus photograph and macular OCT image at the first visit. The VA was 30 cm according to the finger-counting method. A small cystoid was observed in macular OCT 3 weeks after onset. **b** 11 months: Retinoschisis developed following the macular change including a small cystoid. The VA was 20/1000. **c** 18 months: Retinoschisis had spread. The VA was unchanged. **d** 19 months: Retinoschisis had decreased. The VA was unchanged (20/1000). **e** 22 months: Retinoschisis was resolved, but the VA was not improved. This figure was previously published in *Ganka Rinsho Kiyo* [18]. Ganka Rinsho Kiyo-kai granted permission

In addition, two patients with BRAO and one patient with CRAO showed cystoid macular changes 3 weeks after onset. Two of these BRAOs were complicated by retinal vein occlusion. In the CRAO patient, cystoid macular edema was observed at the first visit (Fig. 3). The patient visited our outpatient clinic for a second opinion. His VA was 20/300. The cystoid macular edema resolved 1 month after the first visit. However, his VA had deteriorated (20/300 at the first visit and 20/600 at the final visit). We have obtained consent to publish from the three patients described above.

Discussion
Herein, we described the development of macular retinoschisis in patients long after the onset of RAO. The findings in this retrospective study indicate that

some kind of macular changes may occur in some patients with RAO, even after retinal thinning has occurred in late-stage RAO. They also indicate that VA may deteriorate in BRAO patients, despite an initial improvement, due to the occurrence of macular retinoschisis. Clinicians should be aware of the various presentations of macular changes on OCT findings during the acute and late stages of RAO.

There are rare, but a few case reports of paracentral acute middle maculopathy (PAMM) due to CRAO [9]. PAMM is the term recently used to describe the spectral-domain OCT finding of band-like hyper-reflectivity at the level of the inner nuclear layer associated with retinal vascular diseases. In this retrospective study, we had no case of only PAMM, and macular OCT findings in all of our cases showed hyper-reflectivity and/or swelling of

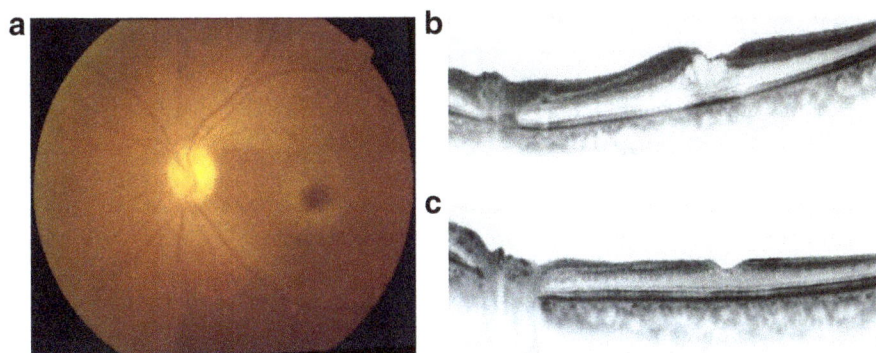

Fig. 3 A case of CRAO with cystoid macular edema. **a** Fundus photograph at the first visit. **b** Macular OCT image at the first visit. At least more than 3 weeks had passed from the onset. Cystoid macular edema was observed, and the VA was 20/300. **c** 1 month: The cystoid macular edema had disappeared, but the VA had dropped to 20/600

the inner retina in the early phase of RAO, followed by thinning of retina in the late phase. Some cases of PAMM might be included; however, the details are unknown because we could not analyze layer-by-layer findings of macular OCT from our every case from 2008 to 2016. This is a limitation of this retrospective study.

There have been a few reports of macular findings of retinoschisis in the late phase of RAO. Pathologically, retinal changes were observed soon after occlusion of the central retinal artery, in addition to necrosis of the nerve fibers, ganglion cells, inner nuclear layer, and inner plexiform layer after a short period of anoxia [10]. In experimental occlusion of the central retinal artery using rhesus monkeys, occlusion for up to 90 min did not result in significant permanent neural damage [11]. However, occlusion of the central retinal artery for 105 min or longer produced irreversible permanent neural damage. Research also showed that neuroglia can be damaged after RAO and that necrotic tissue may be ingested by macrophages and moved through the outer retina, choroid, or recanalized retinal vessels [12]. Müller cells are the primary glial cells of the retina. They extend longitudinally through the retina from the outer nuclear layer to the border of the retina and vitreous [13]. Experimental embolization of the central retinal artery in the owl monkey led to various types of intraretinal schisis [14, 15]. These findings suggest that the formation of retinoschisis in patients with late-stage RAO may be the result of damage to Müller cells and nerve fibers.

In the present study, macular changes including small cystoids were detected in subacute-stage RAO. Such macular findings are uncommon but have been described in earlier case reports [16, 17]. Cystoid macular edema, which is extracellular arising between the inner nuclear and outer plexiform layer, resulting in a "flower petal" appearance, can be seen in acute phase of RAO. Ng WY et al. described that the outer retinal layer is involved as well in CRAO [16]. The pathomechanism is unclear; however, the occurrence of cystoid macular edema means that CRAO does not only affect the inner retina but the outer retinal layer and outer blood-retinal barrier. In the present study, two patients with late-stage RAOs developed retinoschisis following macular changes including small cystoids. In both patients, these changes occurred within 1 month after onset. These changes may be the result of necrosis in the inner retina. All the patients in this retrospective study showed thinning of the retina in late-stage RAO. OCT findings of retinoschisis after RAO are relatively rare. Clinicians should be aware of retinoschisis in cases of late-stage RAO, as it may result in deterioration of VA.

Conclusion

We described a retrospective study of macular retinoschisis that developed long after the onset of retinal artery occlusion (RAO). Macular retinoschisis is unusual, but a possible complication of RAO that can develop long after the onset of the occlusion, potentially resulting in renewed VA deterioration.

Abbreviations
BRAO: Branch retinal artery occlusion; CRAO: Central retinal artery occlusion; FA: Fluorescein angiography; OCT: Optical coherence tomography; PAMM: Paracentral acute middle maculopathy; RAO: Retinal artery occlusion; VA: Visual acuity

Acknowledgments
None.

Funding
Not applicable.

Authors' contributions
TK contributed the conception and design of this study. NI, TK drafted the manuscript, NI, TK, TS collected the data, and MF, TS, HO, TI reviewed the literature. NI, MF analyzed and interpreted the data, and NI, HO, TI critically reviewed the manuscript. TK, HO, TI reviewed the final manuscript. All authors read and approved the final manuscript.

Competing interests
All the authors declare that they have no competing interests.

Author details
[1]Department of Ophthalmology, Yao Tokushukai General Hospital, 1-17 Wakakusa-cho, Yao, Japan. [2]Department of Ophthalmology, Osaka Medical College, 2-7 Daigaku-machi, Takatsuki, Osaka 569-8686, Japan.

References
1. Bhargava M, Ikram MK, Wong TY. How does hypertension affect your eyes? J Hum Hypertens. 2012;26:71–83. https://doi.org/10.1038/jhh.2011.37.
2. Wong T, Mitchell P. The eye in hypertension. Lancet. 2007;369:425–35. https://doi.org/10.1016/s0140-6736(07)60198-6.
3. Appen RE, Wray SH, Cogan DG. Central retinal artery occlusion. Am J Ophthalmol. 1975;79:374–81.
4. Gass JD. A fluorescein angiographic study of macular dysfunction secondary to retinal vascular disease. VI. X-ray irradiation, carotid artery occlusion, collagen vascular disease, and vitritis. Arch Ophthalmol. 1968;80:606–17.
5. Ikeda Y, Sano I, Fujihara E, Tanito M. Periarteriolar-sparing retinal edema in acute central retinal artery occlusion. Case Rep Ophthalmol. 2015;6:390–3. https://doi.org/10.1159/000442175.
6. Hayreh SS, Zimmerman MB. Fundus changes in central retinal artery occlusion. Retina. 2007;27:276–89. https://doi.org/10.1097/01.iae.0000238095.97104.9b.
7. Ahn SJ, Woo SJ, Park KH, Jung C, Hong JH, Han MK. Retinal and choroidal changes and visual outcome in central retinal artery occlusion: an optical coherence tomography study. Am J Ophthalmol. 2015;159:667–76. https://doi.org/10.1016/j.ajo.2015.01.001.
8. Chen H, Xia H, Qiu Z, Chen W, Chen X. Correlation of optical intensity on optical coherence tomography and visual outcome in central retinal artery occlusion. Retina DOI. 2016; https://doi.org/10.1097/iae.0000000000001017.
9. Christenbury JG, Klufas MA, Sauer TC, Sarraf D. OCT angiography of paracentral acute middle maculopathy associated with central retinal artery occlusion and deep capillary ischemia. Ophthalmic Surg Lasers Imaging Retina. 2015;46:579–81. https://doi.org/10.3928/23258160-20150521-11.
10. Dahrling BE 2nd. The histopathology of early central retinal artery occlusion. Arch Ophthalmol. 1965;73:506 10.

11. Hayreh SS, Weingeist TA. Experimental occlusion of the central artery of the retina. I. Ophthalmoscopic and fluorescein fundus angiographic studies. Br J Ophthalmol. 1980;64:896–912.
12. Wolter JR. Pathology of Henle's fibre layer after occlusion of the central retinal artery. Br J Ophthalmol. 1967;51:169–72.
13. Bringmann A, Pannicke T, Grosche J, Francke M, Wiedemann P, Skatchkov SN, Osborne NN, Reichenbach A. Muller cells in the healthy and diseased retina. Prog Retin Eye Res. 2006;25:397–424. https://doi.org/10.1016/j.preteyeres.2006.05.003.
14. Algvere P. Dissociation of the vitreo-retinal junction following experimental embolization of retinal circulation. Albrecht Von Graefes Arch Klin Exp Ophthalmol. 1977;201:229–35.
15. Algvere P. Retinal detachment and pathology following experimental embolization of choroidal and retinal circulation. Albrecht Von Graefes Arch Klin Exp Ophthalmol. 1976;201:123–34.
16. Ng WY, Wong DW, Yeo IY, Han DC. Cystoid macular edema in acute presentation of central retinal artery occlusion. Case Rep Ophthalmol Med. 2012;2012:530128. https://doi.org/10.1155/2012/530128.
17. Friberg TR, Landers MB 3rd. Aphakic cystoid macular edema after branch artery occlusion. Ophthalmic Surg. 1980;11:192–3.
18. Kawano K, Tanaka K, Murakami F, Ohba N. Congenital hereditary retinoschisis: evolution at the initial stage. Albrecht Von Graefes Arch Klin Exp Ophthalmol. 1981;217:315–23.

15

Prevalence of refractive errors in Tibetan adolescents

Xuehan Qian[1], Beihong Liu[2], Jing Wang[3], Nan Wei[1], Xiaoli Qi[1], Xue Li[1], Jing Li[1], Ying Zhang[1], Ning Hua[1], Yuxian Ning[1], Gang Ding[1], Xu Ma[2*] and Binbin Wang[2*]

Abstract

Background: The prevalence of adolescent eye disease in remote areas of the Qinghai-Tibet Plateau has rarely been reported. To understand the prevalence of common eye diseases in Tibet, we performed ocular-disease screening on students from primary and secondary schools in Tibet, and compared the prevalence to that in the Central China Plain (referred to here as the "plains area").

Methods: The refractive status of students was evaluated with a Spot™ vision screener. The test was conducted three or fewer times for both eyes of each student and results with best correction were recorded.

Results: A total of 3246 students from primary and secondary schools in the Tibet Naidong district were screened, yielding a refractive error rate of 28.51%, which was significantly lower than that of the plains group (28.51% vs. 56.92%, $p < 0.001$). In both groups, the prevalence of refractive errors among females was higher than that among males.

Conclusions: We found that Tibetan adolescents had a lower prevalence of refractive errors than did adolescents in the plains area, which may be related to less intensive schooling and greater exposure to sunlight.

Keywords: Refractive errors, Tibet, Abnormal rate, Myopia

Background

In recent years, with the increasing educational pressure on adolescents, the incidence of eye disorders such as myopia, hyperopia and astigmatism is increasing. These common conditions can cause many inconveniences for people. Visual impairment at birth or during childhood can affect learning, communication, employment, health and quality of life, and the effects are often life-long [1]. According to a survey by Pi et al. [2], 20% of individuals with visual impairment, worldwide, are children. With the increasing prevalence of visual impairment among young people, more attention is being paid to it. In fact, it is a priority of the World Health Organization's VISION 2020 program to control visual impairment and blindness in children [3].

Tibet is located in the southwest of China's Qinghai-Tibet plateau. It is characterized by its high elevation (an average

of > 3500 m), low air pressure and large climatic differences. There are great differences between Tibet and China's inland cities in regional environment and eating habits. It is known that living at altitudes above 3000 m has effects on the human body [4, 5]. Accordingly, congenital heart disease, high blood pressure and other diseases in Tibet have high incidence and regional characteristics.

In the Tibetan plateau region, the incidence of eye diseases in adolescents also showed certain geographical characteristics. We found that in China, people in the plains pay more attention to the development of visual impairment than do people in Tibet and other plateau areas. Therefore, we conducted a screening study to understand the ocular health status of school-age children living on the Tibetan plateau.

Methods
Participants
A total of 3248 students in Tibet were enrolled in the screening. The students were from 7 primary schools and 1 secondary school in Naidong district, which

* Correspondence: Nicgr@263.net; wbbahu@163.com
2Department of Genetics, Center for Genetics, National Research Institute for Family Planning, 12 Dahuisi Road, Haidian, Beijing 100081, China
Full list of author information is available at the end of the article

averages about 3500 m above sea level. The participants in the Tibetan region are referred to as the "plateau group".

We have included ocular screening data from 11,102 students from Tianjin Dagang as a control ("plains") group. The average elevation of the Tianjin Dagang area is 6 m.

Detection of ocular abnormalities

The refractive status of all students was evaluated with the Spot™ vision screener(Welch Allyn, Skaneateles Falls, NY). The screener is held approximately 1 m from the subject while they observe the display of twinkling lights and sounds. The screen reports when the subject is too far away, or too close, and shows a spinning circle and the child's face when data acquisition is occurring. Data acquisition is usually complete within approximately 2 s. On each test, the screener measures the student's pupil diameter, ocular alignment, binocular refraction and astigmatism axis, and stores the data. The test was conducted less than 3 times for both eyes of each student and results with best correction were recorded. The final result was determined by the instrument. The vision screener can accurately detect myopia without mydriation, so the children were not cyclopleged. Our diagnostic criteria for various eye disorders are listed in Table 1.

Statistical analysis

The crude rates of myopia, hypermetropia and anisometropia were determined using direct standardization (both age and sex). Means ± standard deviation (SD), frequencies, and percentages were used to summarize the characteristics of the research subjects. The rate of each type of abnormality was compared between the two groups, using chi-square tests. The Cochran–Armitage test for trend was used to determine whether there was an association between participant age and the prevalence of disorders. All statistical analyses were performed using IBM SPSS Statistics software (version 22.0). P-values less than 0.05 were considered statistically significant.

Results

We conducted eye examinations on 3248 students from primary and secondary schools in Tibet (the "plateau group"). Excluding the 19 students for whom data were missing, the plateau group had 2129 males and 1982 females. There was no significant difference in the distribution of sexes between the plateau and plains group. The mean age (± SD) in the plateau group was 12.69 (±2.88) years, which is higher than that of the plains group (see Table 2).

The screening results were abnormal for 926 students in the plateau group (28.51% of the total). Compared with the anomaly rate of 56.93% in the plains group, the anomaly rate of the plateau group was significantly lower. Analysis of the two groups by sex showed that the anomaly rate for males in the plateau group was significantly lower than that in the plains group; the same was true for females. Finally, both groups had higher rates of anomalies among females than males.

Due to the limitations of environment and equipment, our investigation mainly focused on 6 common ophthalmic disorders: anisocoria, anisometropia, astigmatism, gaze, hyperopia and myopia. In the plateau group, there were 26 students with anisocoria (0.80%), 127 with anisometropia (3.91%), 138 with astigmatism (4.25%), 62 with gaze (1.91%), 23 with hyperopia (0.71%) and 774 with myopia (23.83%). The prevalences of anisometropia, astigmatism, gaze and myopia were significantly lower in the plateau group than in the plains group, whereas the prevalence of anisocoria in the plateau group was higher than that in the plains group. However, there was no significant difference between the two groups in the prevalence of hyperopia (Table 3).

Discussion

It is known that living at altitudes above 3000 m has biological effects on humans [4, 5]. The unique plateau environment comprises low air pressure, reduced oxygen, dryness, cold weather, sunshine and exposure time, intense solar infrared light, intense ultra-violet radiation, and long winters, which all have effects on the human

Table 1 Diagnostic criteria for various eye disorders

Age (months)	6–12	12–36	36–72	72–240	240–1200
Anisocoria	1	1	1	1	1
Anisometropia	1.5	1	1	1	1
Astigmatism	2.25	2	1.75	1.5	1.5
Hyperopia	3.5	3	2.5	2.5	1.5
Myopia	2	2	1.25	1	0.75
Vertical gaze	8	8	8	8	8
Nasal gaze	5	5	5	5	5
Radiant gaze	8	8	8	8	8
Gaze asymmetry	8	8	8	8	8

Table 2 Participant demographics

	Plateau group	Plains group
Total	3248	11,102
Gender		
Female	1558	5274
Male	1671	5740
Age (average ± SD, year)	12.69 (±2.88)	11.94 (±3.13)
Eye examination		
Normal	2322	4782
Abnormal	926	6320

Table 3 Ocular abnormalities in the two groups

Type of disorder	Plateau group (n,%)	Plains group (n,%)	X^2	p value
Anisocoria	26(0.80)	25(0.23)	23.485	$p < 0.001$
Anisometropia	127(3.91)	1652(14.88)	278.448	$p < 0.001$
Astigmatism	138(4.25)	1290(11.62)	152.348	$p < 0.001$
Gaze	62(1.91)	791(7.12)	122.280	$p < 0.001$
Hyperopia	23(0.71)	104(0.94)	1.498	$P = 0.221$
Myopia	774(23.83)	5487(49.42)	669.251	$p < 0.001$

body, in general, and on the eyes in particular [6, 7]. Because Tibet is located on the high-altitude Qinghai-Tibet plateau, the environment could be expected to affect the ocular health of people living there, but not much is known about the rates of eye diseases in the plateau region. We therefore conducted this study and used the data from the plains group to study the characteristics of common refractive errors in Tibet by comparing results between the two groups.

We found that myopia was the most prevalent abnormality in the plateau group, as well as in the plains group. In recent years, the incidence of myopia has gradually increased, attracting more attention from researchers and the public. Myopia has a serious impact on society, including on education and the economy, and it also can cause great inconvenience for patients [8]. Previous studies have shown that the prevalence of myopia in various regions of the world varies widely. In Western populations, myopia (nearsightedness) is found in one out of every three individuals [9–11]; in contrast, in selected regions of Asia, its prevalence is as high as 80% [12, 13]. High school is the high time of myopia. During this period, students can have a great deal of schoolwork to do, and previous researchers have shown that the intensity of studying closely relates to the incidence of myopia, so that could account for the high incidence of myopia in adolescents. Studies have also shown that, within a certain range, the longer the exposure to outdoor sunlight, the lower the incidence of myopia [14]. In the plateau region,, there are more hours of sunlight, and, because of the lower pressure on students, time for outdoor activities can be greater. Therefore, the students in the plateau group may be exposed to longer periods of sunshine, which could explain their lower prevalence of myopia.

Despite the high altitude of the plateau region, in the present study, the prevalence of eye disorders in Tibet was significantly lower than that in Tianjin Dagang. We hypothesize that this may be because the Tibetan children have less homework and lower scholastic pressure. The level of education in Tibet is lagging behind that in Tianjin, and students would have fewer hours in school and more time outdoors. Previous studies have shown

that advising children to go outdoors at rest (for about 80 min a day) can decrease their myopia by half in 1 year [15]. Although there is no proven connection between refractive errors and educational methods or the environment, a relaxed lifestyle is likely beneficial to ocular health. In both the plateau and plains groups, the prevalence of refractive errors was higher for females than males, which may be due to girls performing fewer outdoor activities than boys do.

There are some limitations to our study. Due to logistical constraints, we could only test for common refractive errors and did not obtain information on other eye disorders or diseases. In additional, when screening for myopia, we did not have specialized inspection shadow diopter examination or clinical diagnoses. Thus we may be overestimating the prevalence of myopia, so that the rate reported here should be referred to as a "suspected myopia" rate. Finally, we did not record the children's family relationships, so we do not know if there were cases of multiple children from the same family. Children in the same family share many lifestyle factors, which could have biased the results of the present study [2].

Conclusion

In this high-altitude region in Tibet, the prevalence of refractive errors in adolescents was significantly lower than that in adolescents living in the plains region, which may be related to easier schooling and more exposure to sunlight.

Acknowledgements
We thank all of the students for participating in the study.

Funding
This project was supported by the National Key Research and Development Program of China (No. 2016YFC1000307-6), the Natural Science Foundation of Tibet Autonomous Region (Medical support), National Science and Technology Basic Work(2014FY130100) and the National Infrastructure of Chinese Genetic Resources (YCZYPT[2017]01).

Authors' contributions
XHQ performed the data analysis and participated in article writing. BL was responsible for the data collection and drafting the manuscript. JW, NW

and XLQ revised the manuscript and gave final approval. XL, JL and YZ also collected data. NH, YN and GD processed the data. XM participated in both designing the experiment and analyzing the data. BW guided the experimental design and conducted the study. All authors have read and approved the manuscript.

Competing interests
The authors declare that they have no competing interests.

Author details
[1]Department of Strabismus and Pediatric Ophthalmology, Tianjin Medical University Eye Hospital, Tianjin, China. [2]Department of Genetics, Center for Genetics, National Research Institute for Family Planning, 12 Dahuisi Road, Haidian, Beijing 100081, China. [3]Department of Medical Genetics and Developmental Biology, School of Basic Medical Sciences, Capital Medical University, Beijing, China.

References
1. Brown MM, Brown GC, Sharma S, Busbee B. Quality of life associated with visual loss: a time tradeoff utility analysis comparison with medical health states. Ophthalmology. 2003;110(6):1076–81.
2. Pi LH, Chen L, Liu Q, Ke N, Fang J, Zhang S, Xiao J, Ye WJ, Xiong Y, Shi H, et al. Prevalence of eye diseases and causes of visual impairment in school-aged children in western China. Journal of epidemiology. 2012;22(1):37–44.
3. Gilbert C, Foster A. Childhood blindness in the context of VISION 2020–the right to sight. Bull World Health Organ. 2001;79(3):227–32.
4. Wang GQ, Bai ZX, Shi J, Luo S, Chang HF, Sai XY. Prevalence and risk factors for eye diseases, blindness, and low vision in Lhasa, Tibet. International journal of ophthalmology. 2013;6(2):237–41.
5. Gallagher RP, Lee TK. Adverse effects of ultraviolet radiation: a brief review. Prog Biophys Mol Biol. 2006;92(1):119–31.
6. Guo B, Lu P, Chen X, Zhang W, Chen R. Prevalence of dry eye disease in Mongolians at high altitude in China: the Henan eye study. Ophthalmic Epidemiol. 2010;17(4):234–41.
7. Bali J, Chaudhary KP, Thakur R. High altitude and the eye: a case controlled study in clinical ocular anthropometry of changes in the eye. High altitude medicine & biology. 2005;6(4):327–38.
8. Saw SM, Katz J, Schein OD, Chew SJ, Chan TK. Epidemiology of myopia. Epidemiol Rev. 1996;18(2):175–87.
9. Kempen JH, Mitchell P, Lee KE, Tielsch JM, Broman AT, Taylor HR, Ikram MK, Congdon NG, O'Colmain BJ. Eye diseases prevalence research G: the prevalence of refractive errors among adults in the United States, Western Europe, and Australia. Arch Ophthalmol. 2004;122(4):495–505.
10. Lee KE, Klein BE, Klein R, Wong TY. Changes in refraction over 10 years in an adult population: the beaver dam eye study. Invest Ophthalmol Vis Sci. 2002;43(8):2566–71.
11. Chang PY, Yang CM, Yang CH, Huang JS, Ho TC, Lin CP, Chen MS, Chen LJ, Wang JY. Clinical characteristics and surgical outcomes of pediatric rhegmatogenous retinal detachment in Taiwan. Am J Ophthalmol. 2005;139(6):1067–72.
12. Shimizu N, Nomura H, Ando F, Niino N, Miyake Y, Shimokata H. Refractive errors and factors associated with myopia in an adult Japanese population. Jpn J Ophthalmol. 2003;47(1):6–12.
13. Wong TY, Foster PJ, Hee J, Ng TP, Tielsch JM, Chew SJ, Johnson GJ, Seah SK. Prevalence and risk factors for refractive errors in adult Chinese in Singapore. Invest Ophthalmol Vis Sci. 2000;41(9):2486–94.
14. Wang Y, Ding H, Stell WK, Liu L, Li S, Liu H, Zhong X. Exposure to sunlight reduces the risk of myopia in rhesus monkeys. PLoS One. 2015;10(6):e0127863.
15. Wu PC, Tsai CL, Wu HL, Yang YH, Kuo HK. Outdoor activity during class recess reduces myopia onset and progression in school children. Ophthalmology. 2013;120(5):1080–5.

16

High incidence of rainbow glare after femtosecond laser assisted-LASIK using the upgraded FS200 femtosecond laser

Yu Zhang and Yue-guo Chen*

Abstract

Background: To compare the incidence of rainbow glare (RG) after femtosecond laser assisted-LASIK (FS-LASIK) using the upgraded FS200 femtosecond laser with different flap cut parameter settings.

Methods: A consecutive series of 129 patients (255 eyes) who underwent FS-LASIK for correcting myopia and/or astigmatism using upgraded WaveLight FS200 femtosecond laser with the original settings was included in group A. Another consecutive series of 129 patients (255 eyes) who underwent FS-LASIK using upgraded WaveLight FS200 femtosecond laser with flap cut parameter settings changed (decreased pulse energy, spot and line separation) was included in group B. The incidence and fading time of RG, confocal microscopic image and postoperative clinical results were compared between the two groups.

Results: There were no differences between the two groups in age, baseline refraction, excimer laser ablation depth, postoperative uncorrected visual acuity and refraction. The incidence rate of RG in group A (35/255, 13.73%) was significantly higher than that in group B (4/255, 1.57%) ($P < 0.05$). The median fading time was 3 months in group A and 1 month in group B ($P > 0.05$).The confocal microscopic images showed wider laser spot spacing in group A than group B. The incidence of RG was significantly correlated with age and grouping ($P < 0.05$).

Conclusions: The upgraded FS200 femtosecond laser with original flap cut parameter settings could increase the incidence of RG. The narrower grating size and lower pulse energy could ameliorate this side effect.

Keywords: Rainbow glare, Incidence, Fs-LASIK, FS200 femtosecond laser

Background

Femtosecond laser-assisted flap creation in LASIK surgery has rapidly become popular with increasing safety and efficacy over time [1–4]. When using femtosecond laser for flap creation, each pulse of the laser causes the generation of a small amount of microplasma at its focal point in the corneal tissue leading to formation of microscopic gas bubbles and cavitations, which then dissipate into surrounding tissue [5, 6]. Compared with mechanical microkeratome for making flaps, a key benefit of femtosecond laser technology is to provide a more precision, predictable flap and less vision threatening flap complications [7, 8]. However, the femtosecond laser technique, as the resulting laser pattern may act as

an optical grating, could be a major drawback. Previous studies indeed reported on perceptions of rainbow glare (RG) as a mild side effect of FS-LASIK and was verified on a model eye [9–11].

WaveLight FS200 femtosecond laser system (Alcon Laboratories Inc., Fort Worth, TX) is a high pulse frequency (repetition rate of 200 kHz) and comparatively lower pulse energy system that can produce flaps in a shorter period of time, around 6 s. Flaps created using FS200 demonstrated both precision and reproducibility with minimal side effects [12–14]. Only two previous studies reported two cases of unilateral RG following FS-LASIK with the WaveLight FS-200 femtosecond laser [15, 16]. To our knowledge, there is no published study on incidence rate and alleviating management of RG when using FS200 femtosecond laser. In this retrospective study, we reported a high incidence of RG after FS-

* Correspondence: chenyueguo@263.net; 1494867399@qq.com
Department of Ophthalmology, Peking University Third Hospital, 49 North Huayuan Road, Haidian District, Beijing 100191, China

LASIK using the upgraded FS200 and evaluated the alleviative effect of adjustment of flap cut parameter settings.

Methods

Subjects

This was a retrospective cohort study conducted at Peking University Third Hospital from December 2015 to May 2017. It was carried out in accordance with the tenets of the Declaration of Helsinki and approved by the Ethics Committee of Peking University Third Hospital. An informed consent was obtained from each subject.

A consecutive series of 129 patients (255 eyes) who underwent FS-LASIK for correcting myopia and/or myopic astigmatism using upgraded WaveLight FS200 femtosecond laser with original flap cut parameter settings was included in group A. Another consecutive series of 129 patients (255 eyes) who in the period immediately following group A underwent FS-LASIK using same laser platform with flap cut parameter setting changed was included in group B.

Surgical procedures

All surgical procedures were performed by the same surgeon (Yue-guo Chen). All flaps were created by the WaveLight FS200 laser. The flap/canal/hinge parameters were as followed: flap thickness, 110 μm; flap diameter, 8.5 mm to 9.0 mm; side-cut angle, 90°; hinge angle, 50°; canal width, 1.5 mm. For group A, after FS200 laser was upgraded, the energy and laser separations settings were the same to the original one: side-cut pulse energy, 0.8 μJ; bed cut pulse energy, 0.8 μJ; stromal bed cut spot separation, 8 μm; line separation, 8 μm; side cut bed separation, 5 μm; and line separation, 3 μm (Fig. 1). For group B, all settings was the same to group A except for

side-cut and bed cut pulse energy, 0.6 μJ; stromal bed cut spot separation and line separation, 6 μm (Fig. 2). Every flap was superiorly hinged, with a superior gas canal. Flaps were lifted immediately after flap creation to perform ablation using the Allegretto EX500 excimer laser (Alcon Laboratories Inc., Fort Worth, TX).

Postoperative care and follow-up

The standard postoperative regimen included one drop each of 0.5% levofloxacin (Cravit, Santen, Inc.) and 0.1% fluorometholone (FML, Allergan, Inc.) QID for 2 weeks. Each patient was followed up at days 1 and 7, and months 1, 3, 6 and 12 after surgery. The follow-up examinations involved measurements of uncorrected visual acuity (UCVA), slit-lamp examination, subjective refraction, best corrected visual acuity, corneal topography (Sirius, CSO, Italy), and HRT II confocal microscope (Heidelberg Engineering, GmbH, Dossenheim, Germany). The acquired two- dimensional image by HRT II is defined by 384 × 384 pixels covering an area of 400 × 400 μm with lateral digital resolution of 1 μm/pixel and digital depth resolution of 2 μm/pixel.

Determination of rainbow glare symptom

During follow-up, the patients complained seeing a spectrum of colored bands radiating from a white-light source when viewed in a dark environment and could match the sample pictures of rainbow glare described by Krueger RR et al [9]. Then determination of the presence of RG was made.

Statistical analysis

Data were analyzed using SPSS 21.0 (SPSS Inc., Chicago, Illinois). Independent-samples t test (normal distribution), independent-samples Mann-Whitney U test (non-normal distribution), Pearson Chi-Square test and Kaplan-Meier

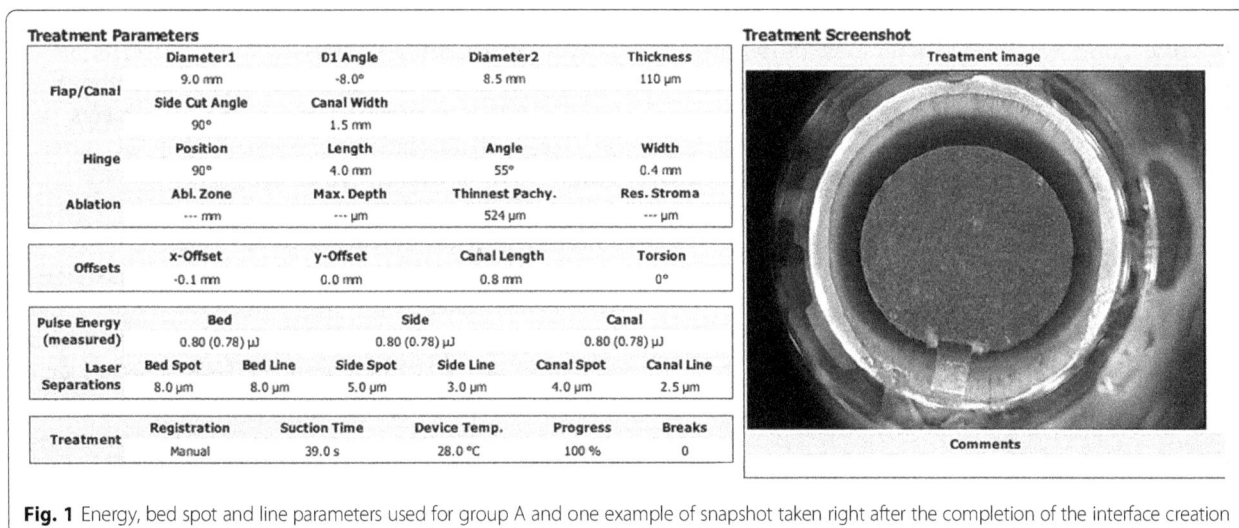

Fig. 1 Energy, bed spot and line parameters used for group A and one example of snapshot taken right after the completion of the interface creation

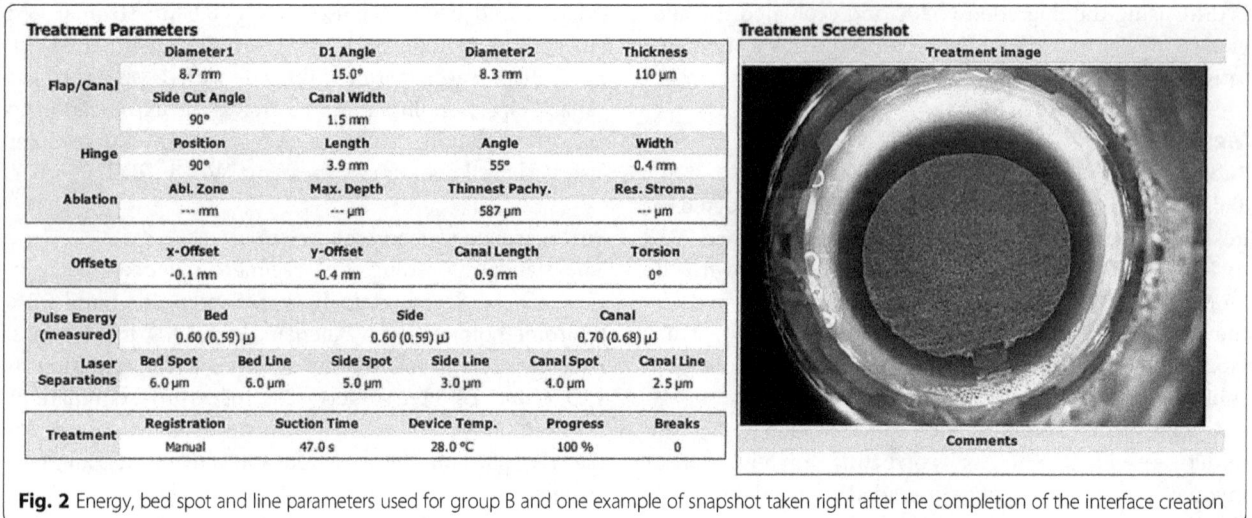

Treatment Parameters				
Flap/Canal	Diameter1	D1 Angle	Diameter2	Thickness
	8.7 mm	15.0°	8.3 mm	110 µm
	Side Cut Angle	Canal Width		
	90°	1.5 mm		
Hinge	Position	Length	Angle	Width
	90°	3.9 mm	55°	0.4 mm
Ablation	Abl. Zone	Max. Depth	Thinnest Pachy.	Res. Stroma
	--- mm	--- µm	587 µm	--- µm

Offsets	x-Offset	y-Offset	Canal Length	Torsion
	-0.1 mm	-0.4 mm	0.9 mm	0°

Pulse Energy (measured)	Bed		Side		Canal	
	0.60 (0.59) µJ		0.60 (0.59) µJ		0.70 (0.68) µJ	
Laser Separations	Bed Spot	Bed Line	Side Spot	Side Line	Canal Spot	Canal Line
	6.0 µm	6.0 µm	5.0 µm	3.0 µm	4.0 µm	2.5 µm

Treatment	Registration	Suction Time	Device Temp.	Progress	Breaks
	Manual	47.0 s	28.0 °C	100 %	0

Treatment Screenshot

Fig. 2 Energy, bed spot and line parameters used for group B and one example of snapshot taken right after the completion of the interface creation

analysis were used to compare data between the two groups. Spearman bivariate correlation was used to analyze the correlative factors of rainbow glare. A P value < 0.05 was considered statistically significant.

Results

Visual acuity and refractive results

There were no significant differences between the two groups in age, preoperative refraction, and excimer laser ablation depth (Table 1). At postoperative 1, 3, 12-month, there were no significant differences in UCVA and spherical equivalence (SE) between the two groups ($P > 0.05$).

Incidence of rainbow glare

Eighteen patients (35 eyes: 17 bilateral; 1 unilateral) complained RG in group A. However, only two patients (4 eyes) reported RG in group B. The difference in the incidence rate of rainbow glare between the two groups was statistically significant ($P < 0.05$) (Fig. 3). The symptom arose within one week among most of the patients (18/20, 90%).

Fading time of rainbow glare

Rainbow glare faded away as time went by. In group A, all the patients experienced complete resolution of

symptom by the 16th postoperative month. In group B, rainbow glare faded away by the 6th postoperative month (Fig. 4). The median fading time was 3 months in group A and 1 month in group B. However, there was no significant difference in fading time between the two groups (Log Rank, $\chi^2 = 0.044$, $P = 0.834$).

Confocal microscopic results

HRT II confocal microscope equipped with the Rostock corneal module showed the femtosecond laser spots, spot spacing and grating pattern clearly at approximately 100~110 µm level below the anterior corneal surface. The images showed comparatively wider laser spot spacing in a patient of group A (Fig. 5a) and narrower spot spacing in a patient of group B (Fig. 5b). Although much more undistinguishable with time, this phenomenon could be found even at 12 months after surgery.

Comparison between eyes with RG and eyes without RG

Among all the 510 eyes, no significant differences in refraction, UCVA and ablation depth were found between eyes with RG (39 eyes) and eyes without RG (471 eyes). However, the mean age of subjects with RG was significantly older than that of subjects without RG ($P < 0.05$). (Table 2).

Correlative factors of rainbow glare

In all the 510 eyes, the occurrence of RG was significantly correlated with age ($r = 0.115$, $P < 0.05$) and grouping ($r = 0.229$, $P < 0.001$), but not with baseline SE, baseline cylinder or excimer laser ablation depth ($P > 0.05$).

Discussion

LASIK is the main stream refractive surgery procedure for correction of myopia and myopic astigmatism

Table 1 Refraction and demographic data of the two groups ($\bar{x} \pm s$/ M)

	Group A	Group B	t / Z	P
Age (years)	27.62±6.25	26.24±7.02	1.597	0.111
SE(D)	−6.36±2.04	−6.47±2.26	0.617	0.535
Cyl(D)	−0.75 (0~ − 3.25)	−0.75 (0~ − 4.25)	2.143	0.062
AD (µm)	92.06±21.02	94.71±22.20	−1.43	0.153

SE spherical equivalent, *Cyl* cylinder, *AD* excimer laser ablation depth

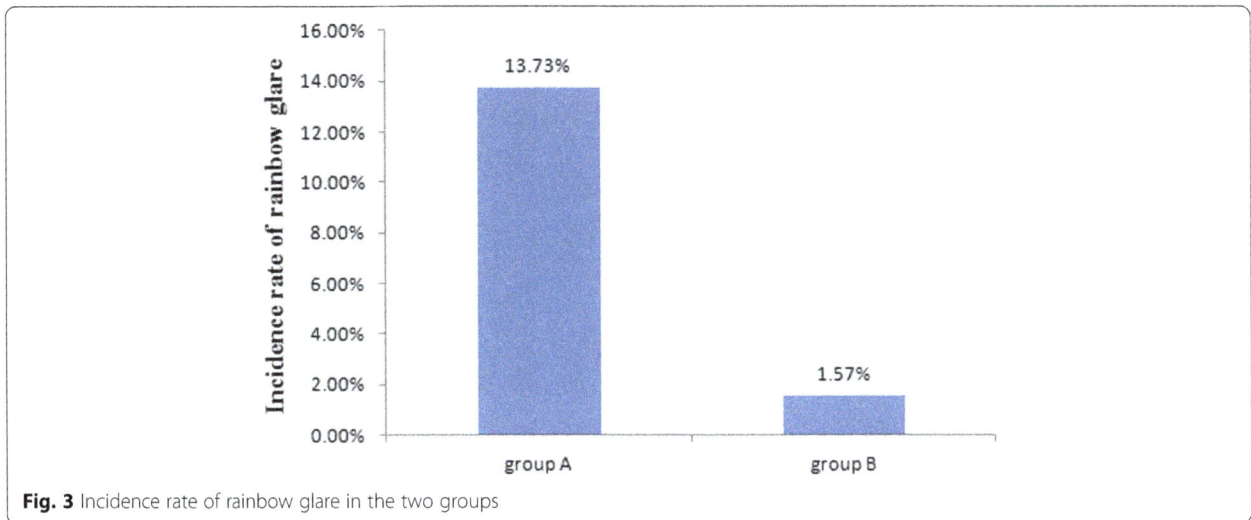

Fig. 3 Incidence rate of rainbow glare in the two groups

worldwide. The introduction of the femtosecond laser in LASIK enabled the creation of lamellar corneal flaps in a more accurate, more stable, evener and safer manner. Even though RG which was first reported in 2008 by Krueger et al. is a mild and temporary optical side effect of FS-LASIK [9], it may disturb patients' night driving and decrease their satisfaction [9, 10]. The cause of RG was defined as the diffraction of light from the grating pattern created on the back surface of the LASIK flap

after femtosecond laser exposure [17]. The first clinical study describing RG found an incidence rate of 19.07% with an older high pulse energy, low frequency (15 kHz) IntraLase femtosecond laser model [9]. A subsequent study reported an incidence of rainbow glare of 5.8% with a newer generation of lower pulse energy, higher frequency (60 kHz) IntraLase model [10].

Since low pulse energy and high frequency femtosecond laser system was applied, less incidence of RG has

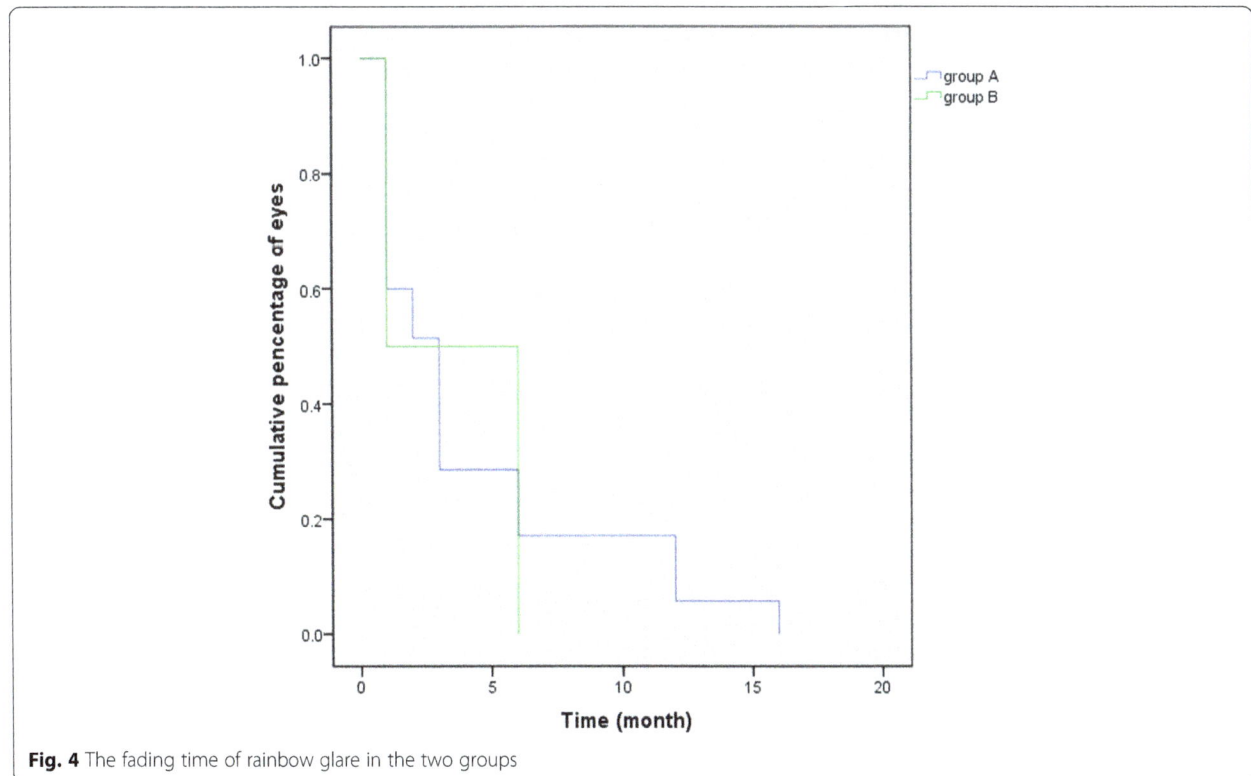

Fig. 4 The fading time of rainbow glare in the two groups

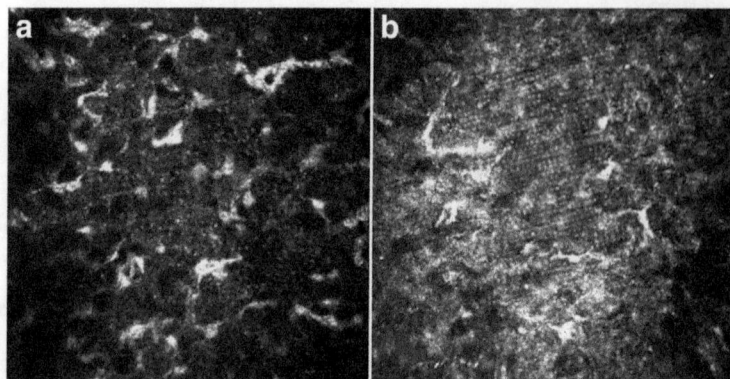

Fig. 5 Three months post-operation, HRT II corneal confocal microscopy showed comparatively wider laser spot spacing in a group A patient (**a**) and narrower spot spacing in a group B patient (**b**) (original magnification 400 × 400 μm)

been reported. The first case of RG with WaveLight FS200 femtosecond laser platform, the lower pulse energy and higher frequency system, was reported by Gatinel D, et al. in 2013 [15]. We have used the Wave-Light FS200 femtosecond laser platform (≤0.8 μJ pulse energy for flap, 200 kHz frequency) for performing FS-LASIK since 2011 with the recommended optimized cut settings of 0.80 μJ pulse energy, 8.00 μm spot and line separations for stromal bed cut and barely heard complaining of the RG symptom until the laser platform was upgraded to "Green" version in December, 2015. As we understood, "Green" brought only new features of software, such as patient data management, docking guidance system and flap position registration on the basis of pupil center for more convenient without changing any laser parameter settings. After the high incidence of RG was noted, we got a new recommendation of optimized cut settings of 0.60 μJ pulse energy, 6.00 μm spot and line separations, the tolerable arrangement of former version, for stromal bed cut. Since then, the incidence rate of RG had decreased to 1.57% among the following consecutive series cases.

Up to date, the reason why the incidence of RG significantly increased after machine being upgraded has still been unclear. The quality of the focused laser beam and numerical aperture of the focusing optics appears to be

the most significant factor in minimizing the diffractive dispersion of light that leads to RG [9, 10]. Otherwise, the relationship between length of time between service calls and the incidence of RG emphasized the importance of a proper maintenance and alignment of the optical components used to focus the beam [10].

Gatinel D, et al. calculated a grating pattern spacing of 7.90μm was the cause of rainbow glare [15]. This value was very close to 8.0μm in group A of the present study. It might seem that reducing the spot/line separation could increase the angle of the spectral pattern sufficient enough to avoid photodetection by the retina altogether [17]. Correlative results in the present study showed that less laser pulse energy and narrower spot/line separations might play an important role in decreasing the incidence of RG. With the settings changed, the energy intensity and the flap cutting time (from 6 to 7 s to 12–13 s) increased, which may induce more corneal lamellar tissue reaction and should be observed for longer time.

With intensively in vivo confocal microscope scan, at around the 110 μm depth level from the anterior corneal surface of almost all the cases after FS-LASIK in this study, no matter whether RG existed or not, the hyper-reflective spots could be found in an equidistant grid-like pattern with HRT II confocal microscope. The spot pattern matched the laser spots/lines separation of

Table 2 Comparison between eyes with rainbow glare and eyes without rainbow glare ($\bar{x}\pm s$ / M)

	With RG (39 eyes)	Without RG (471 eyes)	t / Z	P
Age (years)	29.97±5.01	26.75±6.76	2.584	0.013
Baseline SE (D)	−6.34±2.13	− 6.42±2.16	0.232	0.816
Baseline Cyl (D)	−0.75 (0~ − 3.50)	−0.75 (0~ − 4.25)	0.113	0.984
AD (μm)	90.59±22.96	93.57±21.53	−0.827	0.409
1 M UCVA(LogMAR)	−0.04(− 0.15~ 0.15)	−0.04(− 0.18~ 0.22)	0.206	0.955
1 M SE (D)	0.00 (0.00~ 1.00)	0.13 (− 1.00~ 1.00)	0.198	0.961

SE spherical equivalent, *Cyl* cylinder, *AD* excimer laser ablation depth, *RG* rainbow glare, *1 M UCVA* uncorrected visual acuity at postoperative 1 month

8.0μm or 6.0μm programmed in the FS200 femtosecond laser. There was a report of successful RG correction using undersurface ablation of the LASIK flap [16]. We considered that it was not necessary to do so if merely the symptom of RG existed, because the symptom of RG disappeared with time in all the subjects of the present study, even when the hyper-reflective spots were still visible under confocal microscopy. In this aspect, the patients' individual variation of sensitivity and self-adaption might play a pivotal role.

Krueger et al. found an increased degree of myopic correction was associated with an increased incidence of RG [9]. However, the present study did not found correlation between initial SE or ablation depth and the incidence of RG, which was consistent with the study of Bamba et al [10]. The present study first found that older age was a correlative factor of RG. Only one previous report studied the relationship between age and the incidence of RG and found negative result [10]. Different race of subjects and femtosecond laser machine might lead to the reverse results. RG was subjective feeling, and older subjects might have more need in night vision, such as driving in the night, which might cause more older subjects felt and reported RG to the doctor. More prospective large-sample studies are needed in future to explore the risk or correlative factors of RG.

Conclusions

In conclusion, the upgrade of WaveLight FS200 femtosecond laser with original flap cut parameter settings could increase the incidence of RG. After the pulse energy, spot/line separations for stromal bed cut was adjusted, the incidence of RG decreased significantly. RG did not influence postoperative visual acuity or refractive results. It faded away as time went by. Narrower grating size and lower pulse energy could significantly ameliorate this side effect after FS-LASIK when using WaveLight FS200 femtosecond laser.

Abbreviations
FS-LASIK: femtosecond laser assisted-laser in situ keratomileusis; RG: rainbow glare; SE: spherical equivalence; UCVA: uncorrected visual acuity

Acknowledgements
Not applicable.

Funding
The authors declare that they have no funding.

Authors' contributions
YZ analyzed and interpreted the patient data, and wrote the manuscript. YC designed the study, collected data and revised the manuscript. All authors read and approved the final manuscript.

Competing interests
The authors declare that they have no competing interests.

References
1. Salomao MQ, Wilson SE. Femtosecond laser in laser in situ keratomileusis. J Cataract Refract Surg. 2010;36:1024–32.
2. Farjo AA, Sugar A, Schallorn SC, Majmudar PA, Tanzer DJ, Trattler WB, et al. Femtosecond lasers for LASIK flap creation: a report by the American Academy of ophthalmology. Ophthalmology. 2013;120:e5-e20.
3. Lubatschowski H. Overview of commercially available femtosecond lasers in refractive surgery. J Refract Surg. 2008;24:S102–7.
4. Kymionis GD, Kontadakis GA, Naoumidi I, Kankariya VP, Panagopoulou S, Manousaki A, et al. Comparative study of stromal bed of LASIK flaps created with femtosecond lasers (IntraLase FS150, WaveLight FS200) and mechanical microkeratome. Br J Ophthalmol. 2014;98:133–7.
5. Chung SH, Mazur E. Surgical applications of femtosecond laser. J Biophotonics. 2009;210:557–72.
6. Kurtz RM, Liu X, Elner VM, Squier JA. Du D, Mourou GA. Photodisruption in the human cornea as a function of laser pulse width. J Refract Surg. 1997; 13:653–8.
7. Reinstein DZ, Archer TJ, Gobbe M, Johnson N. Accuracy and reproducibility of Artemis central flap thickness and visual outcomes of LASIK with the Carl Zeiss Meditec VisuMax femtosecond laser and MEL80 excimer laser platforms. J Refract Surg. 2010;26:107–19.
8. Zhang Y, Chen YG, Xia YJ. Comparison of corneal flap morphology using AS-OCT in LASIK with the WaveLight FS200 femtosecond laser versus a mechanical microkeratome. J Refract Surg. 2013;29:320–4.
9. Krueger RR, Thornton IL, Xu M, Bor Z, van den Berg TJ. Rainbow glare as an optical side effect of IntraLASIK. Ophthalmology. 2008;115:1187–95.
10. Bamba S, Rocha KM, Ramos-Esteban JC, Krueger RR. Incidence of rainbow glare after laser in situ keratomileusis flap creation with a 60 kHz femtosecond laser. J Cataract Refract Surg. 2009;35(6):1082.
11. Kamm A, Tünnermann A, Merker M, Kamm A, Tünnermann A, Nolte S. Optical side-effects of fs-laser treatment in refractive surgery investigated by means of a model eye. Biomedical Optics Express. 2013;4:220–9.
12. Mochen M, Wüllner C, Krause J, Klafke M, Donitzky C, Seiler T. Technical aspects of the WaveLight FS200 femtosecond laser. J Refract Surg. 2010;26: 833–40.
13. Kanellopoulos AJ, Asimellis G. Refractive and keratometric stability in high myopic LASIK with high-frequency femtosecond and excimer lasers. J Refract Surg. 2013;29:832–7.
14. Kanellopoulos AJ, Asimellis G. Digital analysis of flap parameter accuracy and objective assessment of opaque bubble layer in femtosecond laser-assisted LASIK: a novel technique. Clin Ophthalmol. 2013;7:343–51.
15. Gatinel D, Saad A, Guilbert E, Rouger H. Unilateral rainbow glare after uncomplicated Femto-LASIK using the FS-200 femtosecond laser. J Refract Surg. 2013;29:498–501.
16. Gatinel D, Saad A, Guilbert E, Rouger H. Simultaneous correction of unilateral rainbow glare and residual astigmatism by undersurface flap photoablation after femtosecond laser-assisted LASIK. J Refract Surg. 2015; 31:406–10.
17. Moshirfar M, Desautels JD, Quist TS, Skanchy DF, Williams MT, Wallace RT. Rainbow glare after laser-assisted in situ keratomileusis: a review of literature. Clin Ophthalmol. 2016;10:2245–9.

17

Visual outcomes and prognostic factors in open-globe injuries

Azusa Fujikawa[1], Yasser Helmy Mohamed[1,2]* , Hirofumi Kinoshita[1], Makiko Matsumoto[1], Masafumi Uematsu[1], Eiko Tsuiki[1], Kiyoshi Suzuma[3] and Takashi Kitaoka[1]

Abstract

Background: Ocular trauma is an important cause of visual loss worldwide. Improvements in our knowledge of the pathophysiology and management of ocular trauma during the past 30 years, in conjunction with advances in the instrumentation and techniques of ocular surgery, have improved the efficacy of vitreoretinal surgery in injured eyes. The aim of the current study was to determine the visual outcomes and prognostic factors of open-globe injuries in the Japanese population.

Methods: Retrospective study of 59 eyes of 59 patients presented with open globe injuries between September 2008 and March 2014 at Nagasaki University Hospital was conducted.

Demographic factors including age, gender, and clinical data such as cause of injury, presenting visual acuity (VA), location of injury, type of injury, lens status, presence of intraocular foreign body, types of required surgeries, and final VA were recorded. According to the classification of Ocular Trauma Classification Group, wound location was classified into three zones. Chi-square test was used to compare presented data.

Results: Out of the 59 patients, 46 were placed in the Light Perception (LP) group, and 13 were placed in the No Light Perception (NLP) group. Work-related trauma was the most common cause (27 eyes) followed by falls (19eyes). Work-related trauma was common in males ($P = 0.004$), while falls was significantly common in females ($P = 0.00001$). Zone III injuries had statistically significantly poor prognostic factor compared to other zones ($P = 0.04$). All cases of NLP group (100%) presented with rupture globe. Poor VA at first visit ($P = 0.00001$), rupture globe ($P = 0.026$), history of penetrating keratoplasty (PK) ($P = 0.017$), retinal detachment (RD) ($P = 0.0001$), vitreous hemorrhage (VH) ($P = 0.044$), and dislocation of crystalline lens ($P = 0.0003$) were considered as poor prognostic factors.

Conclusion: Poor VA at first visit, rupture globe, zone III injuries, history of penetrating keratoplasty, RD, VH, and dislocation of crystalline lens were found to be poor prognostic factors. PPV had a good prognostic value in open globe injuries associated with posterior segment involvement.

Keywords: Open-globe injury, Vitrectomy, Retinal detachment, Penetrating keratoplasty

Background

Ocular trauma is a prominent cause of visual disability and, depending on the sample population, can contribute up to 65% of the cases of unilateral blindness worldwide. The burden of blindness is related to both its inevitable effect on the quality of life and the loss of productivity that subsequently occurs in these subjects [1, 2]. Mechanical trauma to the eye has been classified by the Birmingham Eye Trauma Terminology (BETT) and Ocular Trauma Classification Group and subdivided it into open and closed globe injuries [3].

An open-globe injury is defined as a full thickness wound of the eye wall (full injury of the sclera, cornea, or both) with this vision-threatening condition often leading to blindness. Although there has been considerable effort to prevent this type of blindness, it remains common around the world, with an annual global

* Correspondence: yasserhelmy@nagasaki-u.ac.jp
[1]Department of Ophthalmology and Visual Sciences, Graduate School of Biomedical Sciences, Nagasaki University, 1-7-1 Sakamoto, Nagasaki, Nagasaki 852-8501, Japan
[2]Department of Ophthalmology, EL-Minia University Hospital, EL-Minia, Egypt
Full list of author information is available at the end of the article

incidence rate of 3.5/100,000 persons [4]. There is worldwide interest in the epidemiology of ocular trauma [2]. Different studies have reported varying proportions of open versus closed globe injury [5–7]. Although public health campaigns have been organized to prevent eye injuries, unfortunately, open-globe injuries are still too frequent. Moreover, it has been shown that open-globe injuries result in more hospitalization and a poorer visual outcome compared to closed globe injuries [8, 9].

Improvements in our knowledge of the pathophysiology and management of ocular trauma during the past 30 years, in conjunction with advances in the instrumentation and ocular surgery techniques, have improved the efficacy of vitreoretinal surgery in injured eyes [10].

Achieving or maintaining useful vision is dependent upon several prognostic factors, such as the severity of the initial trauma, involvement of ocular structures, preoperative visual acuity, and both a timely diagnosis and treatment [10, 11].

The aim of the current study was to determine the visual outcomes and prognostic factors of open-globe injuries in the Japanese population.

Methods

This retrospective study reviewed the records of all subjects who sustained an open-globe injury and were examined at Nagasaki University Hospital between September 2008 and March 2014.

Reviews of the patients' medical charts included the initial ophthalmology consultation notes, hospital records, details of the primary and subsequent surgical interventions, and outpatient follow-up records. During the review of the records, demographics, including age and gender, wound characteristics (i.e., mechanism, causes, sizes, and locations), and visual acuity (VA) (presenting and final VA), were collected. The final VA was defined as the VA at the end of the follow-up. Associated ocular damage (i.e., vitreous hemorrhage (VH), retinal detachment (RD), intraocular foreign body (IOFB), lens status, and endophthalmitis) was also evaluated.

Based on the Birmingham Eye Trauma Terminology, the mechanisms of injury were classified as rupture, penetration, IOFB, perforation, and mixed injury [3]. In cases in which there was a high clinical suspicion of an IOFB that could not be confirmed by clinical examination or in which the media opacity prohibited any examination of intraocular structures, ancillary testing with X-rays, computed tomography, or echography were used to classify the injuries.

Patients were divided into groups according to the real size of the wound (in mm). The 4 classifications used included wounds that were smaller than 5 mm, 5–10 mm, 10–15 mm, and larger than 15 mm.

Distance VA was tested using a Landolt C acuity chart. If the VA improved when using a pinhole, this was recorded as the VA at the initial examination. Details of the

primary and subsequent treatments and final VAs were also collected. The initial VA was divided into the following 6 categories: acuity 20/40 or better, between 20/40 to 20/400, between 20/400 to counting fingers (CF), hand movement (HM), light perception (LP), and no light perception (NLP). The outcome, which was defined as the VA measured at the last visit, was divided into 2 categories: ocular survival (with VA ranging between 20/20 and LP) (LP group) and NLP (NLP group). The visual acuity of NLP was confirmed using a bright light source, such as an indirect ophthalmoscope. This light source was set at the highest intensity during which time the fellow eye was completely occluded. A cross-sectional analysis was performed on all patient data in order to investigate the correlation between the initial and final VA. As part of this investigation, we used a value of 1/400 VA (logMAR = 2.6) to represent the vision of the CF patients, with the extrapolated values of 2.7, 2.8, and 2.9 logMAR used to represent HM, LP, and NLP, respectively.

Wound locations were classified according to the Ocular Trauma Classification Group [3]. Zone I injuries were confined to the cornea and limbus, zone II injuries involved the anterior 5 mm from the limbus (not extending into the retina), and zone III injuries extended to the posterior by more than 5 mm from the limbus. In cases of multiple corneoscleral openings, the zone was defined according to the most posterior opening. In cases of IOFBs, the zone was defined at the specific entry site. For perforating injuries, however, the zone was defined by the most posterior defect, which was generally the exit site. While all of the zones of the injury were determined at the time of the initial examination, in some cases, the exact extent of the injury was more accurately determined during the surgical intervention, which led to further identification and revision of the zone of injury.

After collecting all of the records, the data were evaluated for the influences of the initial VA, wound location and size, mechanism of injury, and associated ocular tissue damage on the visual survival rates. This study was approved by the Institutional Review Board (IRB) of the Nagasaki University Hospital and adhered to the tenets of the Declaration of Helsinki.

Statistical Methods:

A Student's two-tailed t-test was used to compare the quantitative variables, while the chi-square test was used to compare the categorical data. Values of $p < 0.05$ were considered statistically significant.

Results

Patient demographics

This study evaluated 59 patients (46 in the LP group and 13 in the NLP group). The mean age was 56.7 ± 21.8 years in the LP group and 62.3 ± 21.7 years in the NLP group, with no significant difference found between the two groups ($p = 0.21$). Figure 1 presents the details for the age

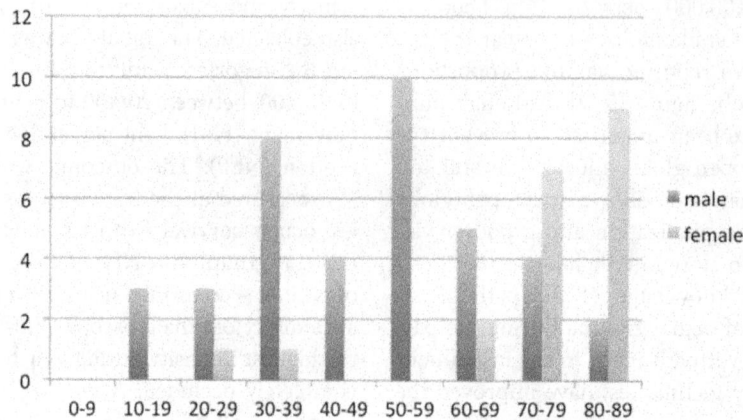

Fig. 1 Sex and age distribution of the patients with open-globe injury. The patient group consisted of 39 (66.1%) males and 20 (33.9%) females, with a male:female ratio of nearly 2:1

and gender distribution. Only 1 case was younger than the age of 16 years. The patient group included 39 (66.1%) males and 20 (33.9%) females, resulting in a ratio of nearly 2:1.

None of the patients presented with a bilateral open-globe injury. The injuries occurred in 27 right eyes and in 32 left eyes, with no significant difference with regard to the side.

Cause of injury
Work-related trauma (27 [45.8%] eyes) was the most common cause of the injury, which was followed by falls (19 [32.2%] eyes). Work-related trauma was common in males ($p = 0.004$), while falls were common in females ($p = 0.00001$) (Fig. 2). The mean ages were 51.3 ± 18.1 years for the work-related trauma and 61.1 ± 8.8 years for the falls. There were 6 (10.2%) eye injuries related to sports injuries, and 2 (3.4%) eye injuries caused by car accidents.

Mechanism of injury
All 13 (100%) eyes in the NLP group and 28 (60.8%) eyes in the LP group presented with a ruptured globe.

Ruptured globe was a statistically significant poor prognostic factor ($p = 0.026$) (Table 1).

Posterior segment IOFBs were observed in 12 (20.3%) eyes, with all of these patients belonging to the LP group (26.1%). A metallic IOFB was found in 11 cases, while 1 case had a concrete IOFB. In these patients, IOFB removal was the primary procedure performed, with 3 IOFBs located in the anterior chamber, 2 in the vitreous cavity, 6 in the peripheral retina, and 1 nasal relative to the optic disc in the posterior pole of the eye. IOFB removal was successful in all cases.

Penetrating trauma occurred in the remaining 6 eyes of the LP group (13.1%). However, neither penetrating trauma nor IOFB exhibited any significant predictive factors.

Location of injury
Zone III injuries were more common in the eyes with a final VA of NLP (4 [30.8%] of 13 eyes) as compared to eyes with a final VA of LP or better (4 [8.7%] of 46 eyes). Zone III injuries were found to be a statistically significant poor prognostic factor for visual outcome

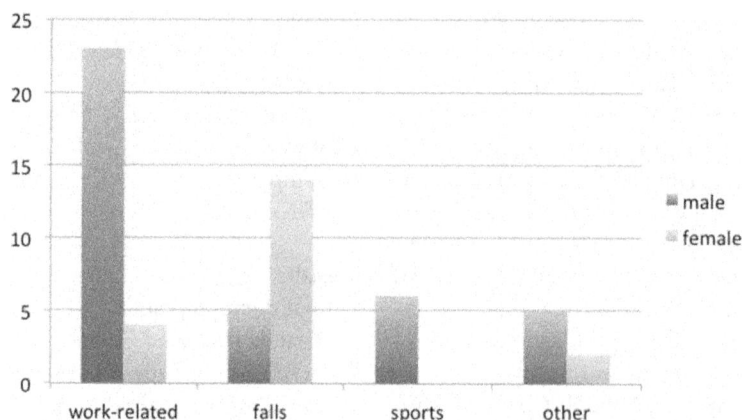

Fig. 2 Cause of injury: Work-related trauma was more common in males ($p = 0.004$), while falls were more common in females ($p = 0.00001$)

Table 1 Final visual outcomes and prognostic factors

Final VA	LP	NLP	Total	P value
n	46	13	59	
Age	56.7	62.3		0.21
Sex				
Male	30	9	39	0.67
Female	16	4	20	
Trauma eye				
Right	23	4	27	0.22
Left	23	9	32	
Type of injury				
Penetrating	6	0	6	0.026
Rupture	28	13	41	
Foreign body	12	0	12	
Location				
Zone I	21	4	25	0.34
Zone II	21	5	26	0.64
Zone III	4	4	8	0.04
Initial Visual Acuity				
20/40 ≤	5	0	5	0.0001
20/400 < 20/40	3	0	3	
CF < 20/400	5	0	5	
HM	12	0	12	
LP	20	5	25	
NLP	1	8	9	
Size of injury				
≤ 5 mm	17	0	17	0.0078
5–10 mm	21	6	27	
10–15 mm	8	6	14	
15 < mm	0	1	1	
Status of the lens				
Aphakia	2	2	4	0.34
Phakia	31	7	38	
Pseudophakia	13	4	17	
Dislocation of the lens				
Yes	5	6	11	0.00025
No	26	1	27	
History of PKP				
Yes	3	4	7	0.017
No	43	9	52	
Retinal detachment				
Yes	10	10	20	0.0001
No	36	1	37	
Unknown	0	2	2	

Table 1 Final visual outcomes and prognostic factors *(Continued)*

Final VA	LP	NLP	Total	P value
Vitreous Hemorrhage				
Yes	27	10	37	0.0443
No	19	1	20	
Unknown	0	2	2	
Primary operation with PPV				
Yes	26	3	29	0.033
No	20	10	30	

All 13 (100%) eyes in the NLP group and 28 (60.8%) eyes in the LP group presented with a ruptured globe. Ruptured globe was a statistically significant poor prognostic factor (p = 0.026)
VA Visual acuity, *LP* Light perception, *NLP* No light perception, *CF* counting fingers, *HM* hand movement, *PK* Penetrating Keratoplasty, *RD* Retinal detachment, *VH* Vitreous hemorrhage, *PPV* Pars plana vitrectomy

($p = 0.04$). Zone I injuries were found in 25 (42.4%) eyes (21 in the LP group and 4 in the NPL group), while zone II injuries occurred in 26 (44.1%) eyes (21 in the LP group and 5 in the NPL group). There were no statistically significant predictive factors for visual outcomes found for zones I and II.

Size of the injury
Patients with a wound that was smaller than 5 mm had a statistically significant better prognosis than patients with wounds that were larger than 5 mm ($p = 0.0078$).

Associated ocular damage
Crystalline lens expulsion, which occurred in 11 eyes (5 in the LP group and 6 in the NLP group), was a poor prognostic factor for visual outcome ($p = 0.0003$). However, results showed that phakia, aphakia, and pseudophakia were not significant predictive factors for visual outcome.

A history of penetrating keratoplasty (PK) was found in 4 (30.8%) of 13 eyes in the NLP group (30.8%) and in 3 (6.5%) eyes in the LP group. A past history of PK was a statistically significant poor prognostic factor for visual outcome ($p = 0.017$).

Both RD and VH were statistically significant poor prognostic factors for visual outcome ($p = 0.0001$ and $p = 0.044$, respectively). Pars plana vitrectomy (PPV) was performed in 11 RD cases. Retinal re-attachment with a good visual outcome was found in 8 cases (LP group), while 3 cases (NLP group) failed to obtain a good visual outcome primarily due to a severely torn retina. PPV was additionally performed as the primary procedure in 22 cases that presented with VH. Of these, 3 cases (NLP group) failed to gain a good visual outcome, while 19 cases (LP group) did achieve a good visual outcome after the procedure.

Our results also showed that there were no significant predictive factors or any statistically significant differences between the two groups in this study for other associated ocular damage, such as choroidal hemorrhage and hyphema. In addition, we did not find a single case of traumatic or postoperative endophthalmitis in this study.

PPV

PPV was performed as the primary operation in 29 (49.2%) cases. The most common indications were VH (22 [75.9%] of 29 eyes) and RD (11 [37.9%] of 29 eyes), with 26 (56.5%) patients undergoing the procedure in the LP group and 3 (23.0%) patients in the NLP group. Eyes that underwent PPV were significantly more likely to achieve a final vision of LP or better as compared to those that did not ($p = 0.033$). Furthermore, in the eyes that achieved a final VA of LP or better, those that underwent PPV were found to have slightly better visual outcomes (0.81 logMAR) versus those that did not undergo the procedure (1.1 logMAR). In 2 cases where the globes were severely disorganized in addition to a fear of the subsequent occurrence of sympathetic ophthalmia, enucleation was performed as the primary procedure.

Visual acuity

Poor VA at the first visit ($p = 0.00001$), a ruptured globe ($p = 0.026$), history of PK ($p = 0.017$), zone III injuries ($p = 0.04$), RD ($p = 0.0001$), VH ($p = 0.044$), and expulsion of the crystalline lens ($p = 0.0003$) were all determined to be poor prognostic factors. Patients with a wound that was smaller than 5 mm had a significantly better VA than those groups that had wounds that were larger than 5 mm ($p = 0.0078$). Eyes that were first treated with PPV were significantly more likely to achieve a final vision of LP or better ($p = 0.033$). Figure 3 shows the correlation between

the initial and final VA. As seen in this figure, even if the initial VA was poor, there was variation in the final VA.

Discussion and conclusion

This study evaluated the visual outcomes after open-globe injuries in Japanese patients and tried to identify the possible risk factors and the prognostic factors responsible for the final visual outcomes. To the best of our knowledge, this is the first study that has examined the prognostic factors of open-globe injuries in the Japanese population.

The mean age of our study populations was 56.7 ± 21.8 years in the LP group and 62.3 ± 21.7 years in the NLP group. These values are higher than those that have been reported in other studies [11–14]. Additionally, the mean age of the work-related trauma group was 51.3 ± 18.1 years while that for the falls group was 61.1 ± 8.8 years. This variability may be due to inter-population differences in the culture, lifestyle, mean lifespan, occupation, and socioeconomic status. Unlike other studies that have reported finding a prevalence of children with eye traumas [11–14], we only encountered 1 case of a patient who was younger than 16 years of age.

The male predominance (male:female = 2:1) observed in our current study is in agreement with the results of several previous studies [12, 14–17]. As previously speculated, this most likely indicates that males probably have a higher risk of being exposed to dangerous situations in the workplace or during outdoor activities, as well during gender-based behavior [16].

Occupational injuries predominate in older age groups, with work-related trauma (27 [45.76%] eyes) followed by falls at home (19 [32.2%] eyes) the most common causes of trauma that result in open-globe injuries. In the relatively younger age groups, the trauma was related to sports injuries (6 [10.2%] eyes).

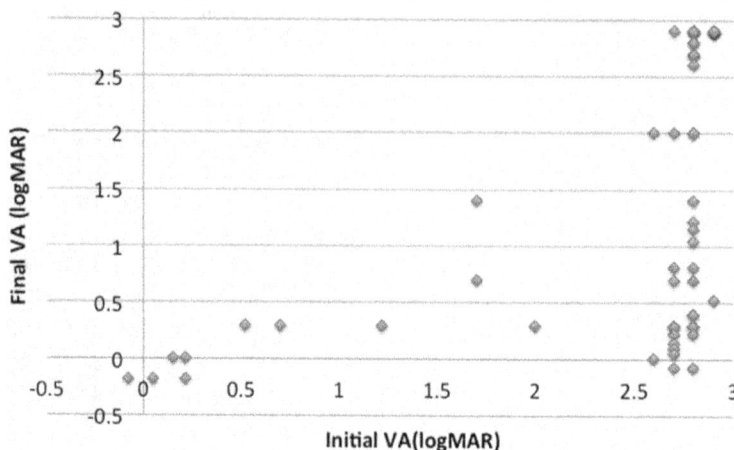

Fig. 3 Correlation between the initial and final VA. Even when the initial VA was poor, there was variation in the final VA

In line with our results, the previous literature has also reported that the most frequently associated cause of trauma was occupational injury [11, 13, 18, 19]. Other studies have confirmed that the majority of open-globe injuries occur in the home, ranging from 38 to 71% of the cases [20, 21]. However, Tok et al. [22] and El-Sebaity et al. [5] reported that injuries at home were less prevalent than those outside the home in pediatric cases. However, work-related trauma remains an important cause of avoidable and predominantly monocular visual morbidity, due to the fact that the majority of injuries are the result of not following proper safety precautions. Although the use of safety precautions had no effect on the final visual acuity, safety precautions are advised for all practical purposes as a means of preventing injuries, ocular or otherwise [18].

Although one of the important causes of open-globe is related to car accidents, our current study found that only 2 (3.4%) cases were due to an automobile accident. Thevi et al. confirmed that road accidents are the second cause of open-globe injuries ($n = 17$, 32.7%) [18].

The most frequent mechanism of injury was rupture injury (69.5%), which was followed by IOFBs (20.3%) and penetrating injury (10.2%). All 13 (100%) eyes in the NLP group presented with a ruptured globe, which was a poor prognostic factor ($p = 0.026$). All cases of IOFB and penetrating injuries were related to the LP group and had a better prognosis than rupture injury.

All 12 of the IOFB cases occurred in the workplace, with 11 cases due to metal origin and 1 case due to concrete. IOFB removal was successful in all cases. A study by Madhusdhan et al. reported that the cases were predominantly penetrating injuries and that the mechanism of injury was not significantly associated with the final visual acuity [11]. Our study confirmed that rupture was a mechanism of injury with a poor prognosis for the visual outcome ($p = 0.026$), which is in agreement with other studies that showed rupture was associated with a lower rate of both visual function and functional success rates than laceration [12, 23]. Additionally, these studies confirmed that both IOFB (other than metal pellets fired from a BB gun) and penetrating injuries resulted in better visual results and prognoses [12, 23]. Perforating injuries from explosions and gunshots were not observed in our current cases, as these are rare in the Japanese community.

In our study, patients with wounds that were smaller than 5 mm had a good prognosis for the visual outcome compared to patients with wounds that were larger than 5 mm ($p = 0.0078$), which is in accordance with several previous reports [14, 17, 18, 24, 25]. A larger wound reflects more extensive ocular tissue damage and a higher likelihood of posterior involvement. Additionally, Rofail et al. demonstrated that a laceration larger than 10 mm had a 14.49-fold risk of attaining a final VA of CF or worse compared with lacerations that were 1 to 5 mm [14].

Han and Yu established that a larger wound (> 10 mm) was related to a poorer final visual acuity [12]. These findings suggested that the size of the laceration had both therapeutic and prognostic implications, with an increase in the laceration length significantly correlated to a worse visual outcome ($p < 0.001$).

Our results also demonstrated that the zone of the injury was associated with the visual outcome. Wounds involving zone III had significantly poorer visual outcomes versus those involving zones I or II. This result is supported by previous studies, which reported a significant association between the posterior extension of the wound and a worse final VA [3, 11, 12, 18, 26–28]. Madhusudhan et al. reported that subjects with a wound extending posterior to the equator had 20 times the risk of having a final visual acuity less than 3/60 as compared to patients whose wounds were anterior to the recti insertions or restricted to the cornea [11].

Our study showed that a poor VA at the first visit was an important prognostic factor ($p = 0.00001$). A good initial VA was the strongest prognostic factor of a favorable final VA in both the univariate and multivariate analyses, similar to that reported by other numerous studies [4, 11–18, 23–25].

Han and Yu performed a multivariate analysis and demonstrated that an initial VA of LP or better resulted in an 18.2-fold chance of attaining visual survival, while CF or better resulted in a 2.81-fold chance of achieving functional success. This result suggests that a better initial VA reflects milder ocular tissue damage, which ensures a better visual outcome. In contrast, an initial VA of NLP suggests serious ocular tissue destruction, particularly of the retina and optic nerve [12].

Many previous studies have reported finding a significant correlation between the lenticular involvement and the visual outcome [12, 15, 23, 24, 29]. In our study, crystalline lens expulsion was observed in 11 eyes (5 in the LP group and 6 in the NLP group) and this group had a significantly poor prognosis for the visual outcome ($p = 0.0003$). In contrast, phakia, aphakia, and pseudophakia were not significant predictive factors for the visual outcome. Thus, expulsion of the crystalline lens can be used to document the degree or extensiveness of the injury and determine if it will affect other important structures in the eye, thereby leading to a worse visual outcome.

Our study found a history of PK in 4 (30.8%) of the 13 eyes in the NLP group and in 3 (6.5%) of the cases in the LP group. To the best of our knowledge, this is the first study to clarify that PK is a poor prognostic factor for open-globe injuries, and that there is a statistically significant association with the visual outcome ($p = 0.017$).

As previously discussed, we evaluated 12 IOFB cases that all occurred in the workplace. In all cases, the IOFB removal was successful, with 11 cases due to a metal origin and 1 cased due to concrete. All of these IOFB cases belonged to the LP group, and they did not show that the group had a poor predictive effect on the visual outcome. This may be due to the location of the IOFB, as only 1 case was present at the posterior pole nasal to the optic disc, while all of the others were distributed in the anterior chamber (3 cases), vitreous (2 cases), and peripheral retina (6 cases). Although we did not find the IOFB to be a significant predictive factor, its prevalence as the second major mechanism of injury suggest that it should carefully evaluated, especially if it is a preventable cause. Though there are mandatory regulations that have been designed to reduce the incidence of eye trauma, such as the use of protective glasses in the workplace, many people simply ignore these precautions. Thus, there needs to be a widespread increased public awareness about eye injuries, IOFB complications, and measures that can be taken in order to prevent eye trauma, especially among those workers who are exposed to such dangers during their normal workdays.

Our current study showed that both RD and VH were significantly poor prognostic factors for visual outcomes. These findings are in agreement with previous studies that also reported RD to be a poor prognostic factor for visual outcome [3, 12, 15, 30, 31]. Additionally, other previous studies have found VH to be a poor predictive factor for visual outcome [15, 23, 24, 29–31]. However, there were no cases of endophthalmitis in our current study, which may be due to the early closure of the wound and prompt initiation of antibiotics that was performed in all of our cases.

One of the challenges in the treatment of open-globe injuries is identifying the optimal timing for the ultimate reconstruction, namely vitrectomy. While it is clear that suture-closure of the wound for open-globe injuries should be performed as soon as possible, it is less clear whether vitrectomy should be performed during the same surgical session (primary comprehensive reconstruction) or deferred until a later time (staged approach) [32].

In this study, we concluded that eyes that underwent PPV as the primary procedure were significantly more likely to achieve a final vision of LP or better versus those that did not undergo the procedure ($p = 0.033$). PPV was the primary operation used in 29 (49.2%) of the cases, with 26 (89.7%) exhibiting a good visual outcome (LP group) and 3 (10.4%) failing to achieve a gain in their vision (NLP group). This is in agreement with previous studies that have demonstrated the efficacy of vitreoretinal surgery for treating open-globe injuries [12, 33–35]. In a retrospective, matched cohort study,

De Juan et al. found no benefit of vitrectomy in the management of penetrating ocular injury [29]. It should be noted, however, that this is a relatively old study that was performed in 1983, which was well before the marked improvement of the PPV techniques and instrumentation that are currently available.

Another important feature in our current versus the previous studies is that we evaluated the number of open-globe injuries over a period of more than 5 years. The number of these injuries was less than one patient per month (59 cases/66 months), which indicates an awareness by the Japanese population with regard to the use of protective measures for preventing open-globe injuries.

The limitation of our study is related to insufficient documentation, especially with regard to the presence or absence of a relative afferent papillary defect (RAPD).

In conclusion, improvements in our knowledge of the pathophysiology of eye trauma and its prognostic factors, as well as advances in diagnostic and therapeutic techniques, have greatly improved the success rates for managing open-globe injuries. A better understanding of these prognostic factors may help provide our patients with better and more realistic expectations of their final VA. This study demonstrated that a poor VA at the first visit, a ruptured globe, zone III injuries, PK, RD, VH, and expulsion of the crystalline lens are considered to be poor prognostic factors for open-globe injuries. Patients with a wound smaller than 5 mm had a significantly better VA than the other groups with wounds larger than 5 mm. When patients with open-globe injuries had posterior segment involvement, PPV proved to be a good prognostic factor.

Acknowledgements
Not applicable.
We confirm that we have given due consideration to the protection of intellectual property associated with this work and that there are no impediments to publication, including the timing of publication, with respect to intellectual property. In so doing we confirm that we have followed the regulations of our institutions concerning intellectual property. We understand that the Corresponding Author is the sole contact for the Editorial process (including Editorial Manager and direct communications with the office). He is responsible for communicating with the other authors about progress, submissions of revisions and final approval of proofs. We confirm that we have provided a current, correct email address which is accessible by the Corresponding Author and which has been configured to accept email from (yasserhelmy@nagasaki-u.ac.jp) Corresponding Author signature on behave of all Authors: Yasser Helmy Mohamed.

Funding
We wish to confirm that we have no funding support to report. We wish also to confirm that all authors have no financial disclosures in medicine to report ("No financial disclosures") associated with this publication and there has been no significant financial support for this work that could have influenced its outcome.

Authors' contributions

All authors except YM carried out the surgical operations to reconstruct globes after trauma. YM and AF participated in the sequence alignment and drafted the manuscript. AF and TK participated in the design of the study and performed the statistical analysis. All authors conceived of the study, and participated in its design and coordination and helped to draft the manuscript. All authors read and approved the final manuscript.

Competing interests

The authors declare that they have no competing interests.

Author details

[1]Department of Ophthalmology and Visual Sciences, Graduate School of Biomedical Sciences, Nagasaki University, 1-7-1 Sakamoto, Nagasaki, Nagasaki 852-8501, Japan. [2]Department of Ophthalmology, EL-Minia University Hospital, EL-Minia, Egypt. [3]Department of Ophthalmology and Visual Sciences, Graduate School of Medicine Kyoto University, Kyoto, Japan.

References

1. Eballe AO, Epee E, Koki G, Bella L, Mvogo CE. Unilateral childhood blindness: a hospital based study in Yaounde, Cameroon. Clin Ophthalmol. 2009;3:461–4.
2. May DR, Kuhn FP, Morris RE, Witherspoon CD, Danis RP, Matthews GP, Mann L. The epidemiology of serious eye injuries from the United States eye injury registry. Graefes Arch Clin Exp Ophthalmol. 2000;238(2):153–7.
3. Pieramici DJ, Sternberg P, Jr., Aaberg TM, Sr., Bridges WZ, Jr., Capone A, Jr., Cardillo JA, de Juan E, Jr., Kuhn F, Meredith TA, Mieler WF, Olsen TW, Rubsamen P, Stout T. A system for classifying mechanical injuries of the eye (globe). The Ocular Trauma Classification Group Am J Ophthalmol 1997;123(6):820–831.
4. Negrel AD, Thylefors B. The global impact of eye injuries. Ophthalmic Epidemiol. 1998;5(3):143–69.
5. El-Sebaity DM, Soliman W, Soliman AM, Fathalla AM. Pediatric eye injuries in upper Egypt. Clin Ophthalmol. 2011;5:1417–23.
6. Khatry SK, Lewis AE, Schein OD, Thapa MD, Pradhan EK, Katz J. The epidemiology of ocular trauma in rural Nepal. Br J Ophthalmol. 2004;88(4):456–60.
7. Soylu M, Sizmaz S, Cayli S. Eye injury (ocular trauma) in southern Turkey: epidemiology, ocular survival, and visual outcome. Int Ophthalmol. 2010;30(2):143–8.
8. Onakpoya OH, Adeoye A, Adeoti CO, Ajite K. Epidemiology of ocular trauma among the elderly in a developing country. Ophthalmic Epidemiol. 2010;17(5):315–20.
9. Kadappu S, Silveira S, Martin F. Aetiology and outcome of open and closed globe eye injuries in children. Clin Exp Ophthalmol. 2013;41(5):427–34.
10. Heidari E, Taheri N. Surgical treatment of severely traumatized eyes with no light perception. Retina. 2010;30(2):294–9.
11. Madhusudhan AL, Evelyn-Tai LM, Zamri N, Adil H, Wan-Hazabbah WH. Open globe injury in Hospital Universiti Sains Malaysia - A 10-year review. Int J Ophthalmol. 2014;7(3):486–90.
12. Han SB, Yu HG. Visual outcome after open globe injury and its predictive factors in Korea. J Trauma. 2010;69(5):E66–72.
13. Yalcin Tok O, Tok L, Eraslan E, Ozkaya D, Ornek F, Bardak Y. Prognostic factors influencing final visual acuity in open globe injuries. J Trauma. 2011;71(6):1794–800.
14. Rofail M, Lee GA, O'Rourke P. Prognostic indicators for open globe injury. Clin Exp Ophthalmol. 2006;34(8):783–6.
15. Schmidt GW, Broman AT, Hindman HB, Grant MP. Vision survival after open globe injury predicted by classification and regression tree analysis. Ophthalmology. 2008;115(1):202–9.
16. Rahman I, Maino A, Devadason D, Leatherbarrow B. Open globe injuries: factors predictive of poor outcome. Eye (Lond). 2006;20(12):1336–41.
17. Entezari M, Rabei HM, Badalabadi MM, Mohebbi M. Visual outcome and ocular survival in open-globe injuries. Injury. 2006;37(7):633–7.
18. Thevi T, Mimiwati Z, Reddy SC. Visual outcome in open globe injuries. Nepal J Ophthalmol. 2012;4(2):263–70.
19. Altintas L, Altintas O, Yuksel N, Pirhan D, Ozkan B, Caglar Y. Pattern of open eye injuries in Northwest Turkey: a retrospective study. Ulus Travma Acil Cerrahi Derg. 2011;17(4):334–9.
20. Framme C, Roider J. Epidemiology of open globe injuries. Klin Monatsbl Augenheilkd. 1999;215(5):287–93.
21. Falcao M, Camisa E, Falcao-Reis F. Characteristics of open-globe injuries in northwestern Portugal. Ophthalmologica. 2010;224(6):389–94.
22. Tok O, Tok L, Ozkaya D, Eraslan E, Ornek F, Bardak Y. Epidemiological characteristics and visual outcome after open globe injuries in children. J AAPOS. 2011;15(6):556–61.
23. Pieramici DJ, MacCumber MW, Humayun MU, Marsh MJ, de Juan E. Open-globe injury. Update on types of injuries and visual results. Ophthalmology. 1996;103(11):1798–803.
24. Sternberg P Jr, de Juan E Jr, Michels RG, Auer C. Multivariate analysis of prognostic factors in penetrating ocular injuries. Am J Ophthalmol. 1984;98(4):467–72.
25. Gilbert CM, Soong HK, Hirst LW. A two-year prospective study of penetrating ocular trauma at the Wilmer Ophthalmological institute. Ann Ophthalmol. 1987;19(3):104–6.
26. Soni NG, Bauza AM, Son JH, Langer PD, Zarbin MA, Bhagat N. Open globe ocular trauma: functional outcome of eyes with no light perception at initial presentation. Retina. 2013;33(2):380–6.
27. Knyazer B, Levy J, Rosen S, Belfair N, Klemperer I, Lifshitz T. Prognostic factors in posterior open globe injuries (zone-III injuries). Clin Exp Ophthalmol. 2008;36(9):836–41.
28. Al-Mezaine HS, Osman EA, Kangave D, Abu El-Asrar AM. Prognostic factors after repair of open globe injuries. J Trauma. 2010;69(4):943–7.
29. De Juan E Jr, Sternberg P Jr, Michels RG. Penetrating ocular injuries. Types of injuries and visual results. Ophthalmology. 1983;90(11):1318–22.
30. Brinton GS, Aaberg TM, Reeser FH, Topping TM, Abrams GW. Surgical results in ocular trauma involving the posterior segment. Am J Ophthalmol. 1982;93(3):271–8.
31. Groessl S, Nanda SK, Mieler WF. Assault-related penetrating ocular injury. Am J Ophthalmol. 1993;116(1):26–33.
32. Kuhn F. The timing of reconstruction in severe mechanical trauma. Ophthalmic Res. 2014;51(2):67–72.
33. Sheard RM, Mireskandari K, Ezra E, Sullivan PM. Vitreoretinal surgery after childhood ocular trauma. Eye (Lond). 2007;21(6):793–8.
34. Erakgun T, Egrilmez S. Prognostic factors in vitrectomy for posterior segment intraocular foreign bodies. J Trauma. 2008;64(4):1034–7.
35. Szijarto Z, Gaal V, Kovacs B, Kuhn F. Prognosis of penetrating eye injuries with posterior segment intraocular foreign body. Graefes Arch Clin Exp Ophthalmol. 2008;246(1):161–5.

18

Schnyder corneal dystrophy and associated phenotypes caused by novel and recurrent mutations in the *UBIAD1* gene

Cerys J. Evans[1†], Lubica Dudakova[2†], Pavlina Skalicka[2,3], Gabriela Mahelkova[4], Ales Horinek[5,6], Alison J. Hardcastle[1], Stephen J. Tuft[7] and Petra Liskova[2,3*]

Abstract

Background: The purpose of this study was to identify the genetic cause and describe the clinical phenotype of Schnyder corneal dystrophy (SCD) in six unrelated probands.

Methods: We identified two white Czech, two white British and two South Asian families with a clinical diagnosis of SCD. Ophthalmic assessment included spectral domain optical coherence tomography (SD-OCT) of one individual with advanced disease, and SD-OCT and confocal microscopy of a child with early stages of disease. *UBIAD1* coding exons were amplified and Sanger sequenced in each proband. A fasting serum lipid profile was measured in three probands. Paternity testing was performed in one family.

Results: A novel heterozygous c.527G>A; p.(Gly176Glu) mutation in *UBIAD1* was identified in one Czech proband. In the second Czech proband, aged 6 years when first examined, a previously described de novo heterozygous c.289G>A; p.(Ala97Thr) mutation was found. Two probands of South Asian descent carried a known c.305G>A; p.(Asn102Ser) mutation in the heterozygous state. Previously reported heterozygous c.361C>T; p.(Leu121Phe) and c.308C>T; p.(Thr103Ile) mutations were found in two white British families. Although crystalline deposits were present in all probands the affected area was small in some individuals. Corneal arcus and stromal haze were the most prominent phenotypical feature in two probands. In the Czech probands, SD-OCT confirmed accumulation of reflective material in the anterior stroma. Crystalline deposits were visualized by confocal microscopy. Mild dyslipidemia was found in all three individuals tested.

Conclusion: Although de novo occurrence of mutations in *UBIAD1* is extremely rare, SCD should be considered in the differential diagnosis of bilateral corneal haze and/or crystal deposition, especially in children.

Keywords: Schnyder corneal dystrophy, *UBIAD1*, Novel mutation, De novo, Crystalline deposits, Confocal microscopy, Spectral domain optical coherence tomography

Background

Schnyder corneal dystrophy (SCD; MIM #121800) is a rare autosomal dominant disorder characterized by bilateral corneal opacification due to an accumulation of unesterified cholesterol and phospholipids in the corneal stroma [1].

* Correspondence: petra.liskova@lf1.cuni.cz
†Cerys J. Evans and Lubica Dudakova contributed equally to this work.
²Research Unit for Rare Diseases, Department of Paediatrics and Adolescent Medicine, First Faculty of Medicine, Charles University and General University Hospital in Prague, Ke Karlovu 2, 128 08 Prague 2, Czech Republic
³Department of Ophthalmology, First Faculty of Medicine, Charles University and General University Hospital in Prague, Prague, Czech Republic
Full list of author information is available at the end of the article

Approximately 50% of individuals have crystalline deposits [2]. An association with genu valgum and systemic hyperlipidemia has also been reported [3].

SCD is caused by mutations in the *UBIAD1* gene (MIM *611632), encoding a membrane-embedded UbiA prenyltransferase domain-containing protein which catalyses the Mg^{2+}-dependent transfer of a hydrophobic polyprenyl chain onto a variety of acceptor molecules, including vitamin K and coenzyme Q [1, 4, 5]. At least 26 mutations that cause SCD have been identified to date [6].

In this study we report the clinical and genetic investigation of six probands of white and South Asian origin.

Methods

Clinical examination

The study was approved by the relevant research ethics committees and adhered to the tenets of the Helsinki Declaration. Previously unreported probands from six families with a clinical diagnosis of SCD were investigated; two were recruited in the Czech Republic and four in the UK (Table 1). Family history of SCD was documented and available family members were invited to participate.

Ophthalmic examination included best corrected Snellen visual acuity (BCVA) converted to decimal values, intraocular pressure, and fundal examination after pupil dilation. We performed corneal imaging of probands 1 and 2 using spectral domain optical coherence tomography (SD-OCT) (Spectralis; Heidelberg Engineering GmbH). Proband 2 also underwent scanning slit confocal microscopy equipped with a non-applanating 40× immersion objective lens (Confoscan 3.0; Nidek Technologies, Viconza, Italy) [7].

We measured the fasting serum lipid profile of three probands and recorded the levels of total cholesterol, high and low-density lipoproteins, and triglycerides. The presence of joint deformity, scoliosis or learning difficulty was based on self-reported symptoms.

Molecular genetic analysis

Genomic DNA from probands and any additional available family members was extracted from venous blood samples using a Gentra Puregene blood kit (Qiagen, Hilden, Germany) or from saliva using an Oragene kit (Oragene OG-300, DNA Genotek, Canada). We then performed PCR amplification and Sanger sequencing of the two UBIAD1 coding exons and exon/intron boundaries (primer sequences and conditions are listed in Table 2). Variants were annotated against the reference sequence for transcript NM_013319.2. Mutation description followed standard nomenclature guidelines (http://varnomen.hgvs.org/) starting with nucleotide numbering c.1 at the A of the ATG translation initiation codon. Pathogenicity was evaluated in silico by six different algorithms (PROVEAN [8], SNPs&GO [9], MutPred [10], SIFT [11], PolyPhen-2 [12] and MutationTaster [13]). We also performed paternity testing in family 2, using a previously published set of markers [14]. The population frequency of variants was determined by the Genome Aggregation Database (gnomAD), which provides sequencing data from more than 123,136 exomes and 15,496 genomes from unrelated individuals of various ethnic backgrounds [15], and 2500 Czech control chromosomes available through the next generation sequencing projects of the Czech National Center for Medical Genomics (https://ncmg.cz/en).

Table 1 Demographic and clinical data of six probands with Schnyder corneal dystrophy

No	Ethnicity	Family history	UBIAD1 mutation	Age (when recruited)/gender	BCVA LE	BCVA RE	Corneal phenotype	Chol (mmol/l)	HDL (mmol/l)	LDL (mmol/l)	TG (mmol/l)	Other relevant clinical data
1	White Czech	Y	c.527G>A p.(Gly176Glu)	36/M	0.6	0.7	Subepithelial central and mid-peripheral crystals in a ring pattern, minimal corneal arcus	**5.72**	1.58	**3.21**	1.51	
2	White Czech	N	c.289G>A p.(Ala97Thr)	6/F	0.6	0.5	Subepithelial mid-peripheral and mid-stromal crystals in a ring pattern	**4.89**	1.31	2.66	**2.05**	
3	White British	Not known	c.361C>T p.(Leu121Phe)	10/M	0.3	0.3	Mid-stromal central crystals	**5.00**	1.90	UA	1.80	Amblyopia in BE Lamellar keratoplasty in RE and LE at the age of 10 and 12 years
4	White British	Y	c.308C>T p.(Thr103Ile)	54/F	0.5	0.66	Central stromal haze, arcus, few mid-peripheral subepithelial crystals	**UA***	UA	UA	UA	
5	South Asian	Y	c.305G>A p.(Asn102Ser)	37/F	0.66	0.66	Diffuse stromal haze, few subepithelial mid-peripheral crystals	UA	UA	UA	UA	Knee deformities, scoliosis, learning difficulties
6	South Asian	Y	c.305G>A p.(Asn102Ser)	40/F	0.5	0.66	Central stromal haze, arcus, few subepithelial mid-peripheral crystals	UA	UA	UA	UA	

BCVA best corrected visual acuity, LE left eye, RE right eye, BE both eyes, M male, F female, Chol total cholesterol, HDL high density lipoprotein, LDL low density lipoprotein, TG triglycerides, *- elevated but value not known, UA unavailable data
Elevated values are shown in bold

Table 2 Primer sequences and condition used for PCR and Sanger sequencing of *UBIAD1* gene

Target	Forward primer	Reverse Primer	Size (bp)	Enzyme	Annealing Temp
exon 1	CCGTCCTTCCTCCTTCCC	AAGCCACCTTTGACATCCCT	700	GoTaqGreen	65 ℃
exon 2	CCACCTGCACAGTCTAAGGA	CTGCCAAATCACATTCCTTCCT	689	GoTaqGreen	60 ℃

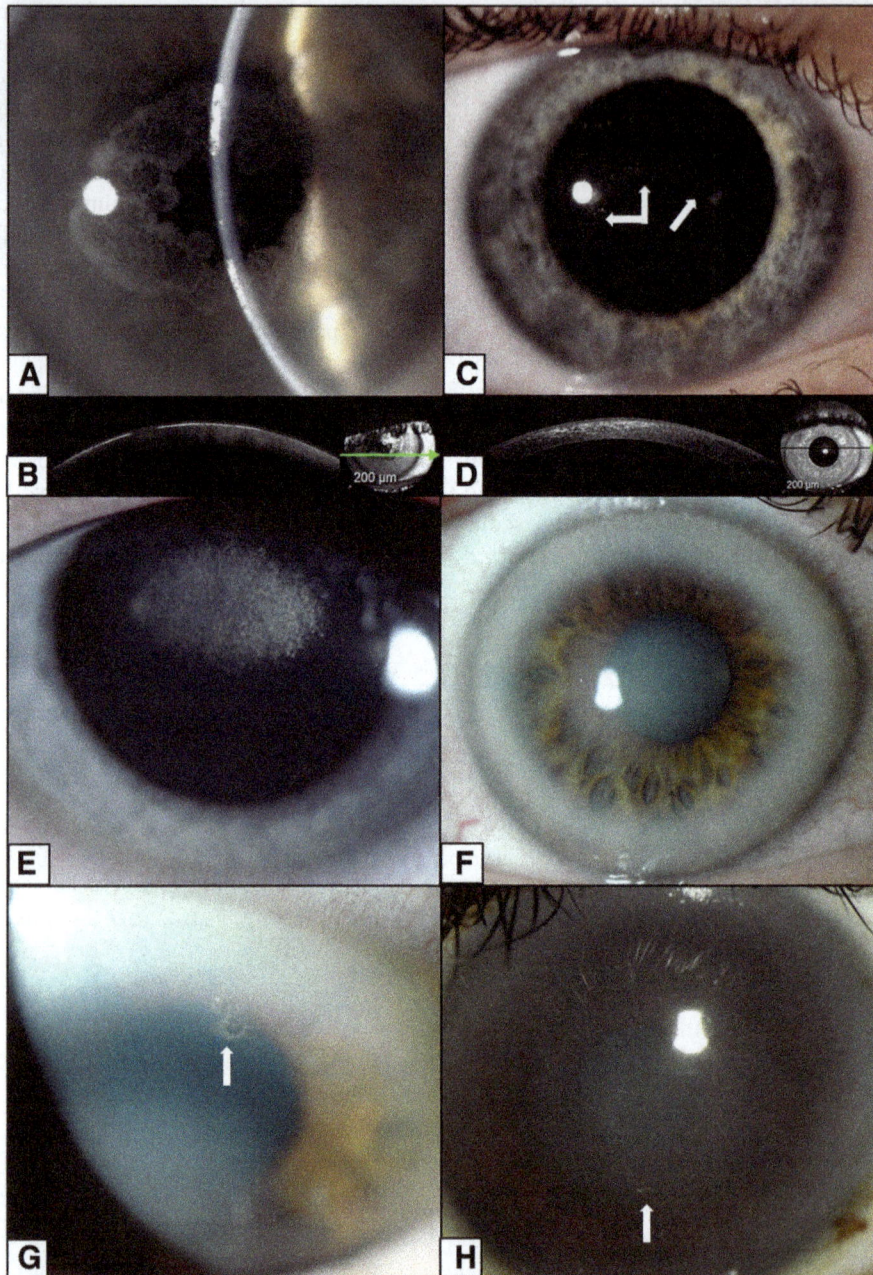

Fig. 1 Corneal phenotype observed in five probands with Schnyder corneal dystrophy. Ring of prominent superficial crystalline deposits in proband 1 aged 36 years (**a**), also documented by SD-OCT as a discontinuous hyper-reflective line beneath the epithelium and within the anterior corneal stroma (**b**). Discrete crystalline deposits in proband 2 aged 8 years (**c**) and more scattered opacities on SD-OCT (**d**). Central mid-stromal crystalline deposits in proband 3 aged 10 years (**e**). Diffuse stromal haze with prominent arcus in proband 4 aged 54 years (**f**, **g**) and proband 5 aged 37 years (**h**). Corneal crystals (arrows) were present in all probands, although in proband 2 they were a minor feature (**b**), corresponding to an early stage of the disease, and in probands 4 and 5 (**g**, **h**) they were present in only a very small area (arrows). All images show findings in the right eye

Results

Clinical, demographic and genotype data for all six probands are summarized in Table 1. There was no family history of SCD in two pedigrees; however, in family 3 the disease status of the proband's mother was unavailable. The corneal phenotypes were diverse and included anterior and mid-stromal crystalline deposits, diffuse stromal haze and arcus lipoides (Fig. 1). There was an incremental accumulation of corneal deposits with age, and the corneal changes were symmetric in all individuals. There were corneal crystals in all probands, although these deposits were minimal in some individuals (Fig. 1 g, h). Corneal crystals were present at slit lamp examination of proband 2 at age 6 years, but neither parent had signs of corneal disease. The patient was re-examined at the age 8 years, when an increase in the corneal crystals was noted (Fig. 1b), but the visual acuity had remained unchanged (Table 1).

Corneal imaging highlighted the presence of crystals. With SD-OCT there were highly reflective deposits in the anterior stroma of probands 1 and 2 (Fig. 1c, d), with confocal microscopy there were bright reflective crystalline deposits identified in the anterior stroma of proband 2 (Fig. 2e). On confocal microscopy small round deposits were also identified in the superficial epithelial cells (Fig. 2a), in and around anterior stromal keratocytes (Fig. 2d) and in mid-stroma (Fig. 2f). The basal epithelial cells, sub-epithelial nerves, posterior stroma and corneal endothelium all appeared normal (Fig. 2b, c, g, h).

Coexisting systemic disease was present in some probands. Proband 5 and her affected sister both had bilateral knee deformities, although their affected mother was normal (Fig. 3). In proband 1 a fasting lipid profile showed high levels of total cholesterol (5.72 mmol/l; normal values in adults < 5.17 mmol/l) [16] and in probands 2 and 3 there was a borderline elevation of total cholesterol to 4.89 mmol/l and 5.00 mmol/l, respectively (normal values in children < 4.40 mmol/l) [17].

A novel c.527G>A; p.(Gly176Glu) variant, predicted to be pathogenic or probably pathogenic by all six bioinformatic tools (Table 3), was identified in proband 1 of Czech origin. The amino acid residue Gly-176 is highly conserved and located in the transmembrane domain of *UBIAD1*, therefore a mutation is likely to disrupt the transmembrane helices and active site [18]. Czech proband 2 harboured a known *UBIAD1* c.289G>A; p.(Ala97Thr) mutation. This variant was absent in both parents, suggesting a de novo origin that was confirmed by paternity testing. The white British probands had previously reported mutations c.361C>T; p.(Leu121Phe) [19] and c.308C>T; p.(Thr103Ile) [6]. Two reportedly unrelated British families of South Asian origin, both harboured a known c.305G>A; p.(Asn102Ser) mutation [19–21]. Pedigrees and segregation of the respective

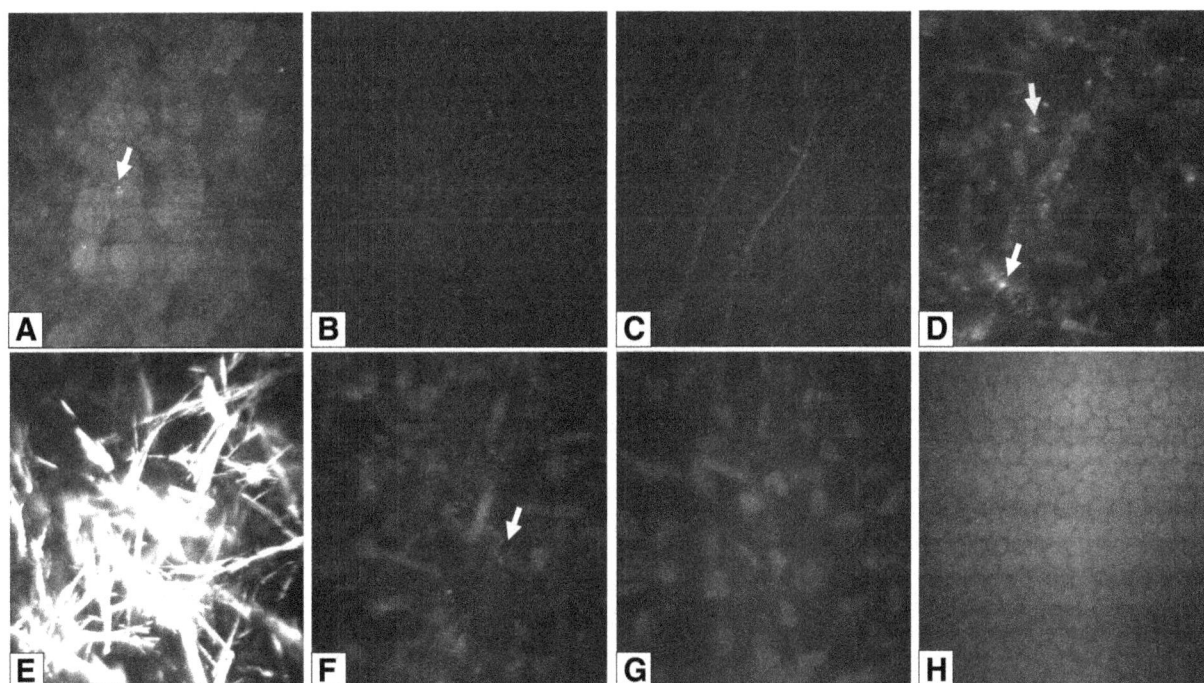

Fig. 2 Corneal confocal microscopy imaging in an 8-year old child with Schnyder corneal dystrophy. Superficial epithelial cells with small round hyperreflective deposits (arrows) in the left eye (**a**). Normal appearance of the basal epithelial cell layer (**b**), and subepithelial nerve plexus in the right eye (**c**). Hyper-reflective deposits within and around keratocytes (arrows) (**d**) and needle-shaped crystals in anterior stroma of the left eye (**e**). Hyper-reflective deposits in mid-stroma in the left eye (**f**), but with unaffected posterior stroma (**g**) and endothelium in the left eye (**h**)

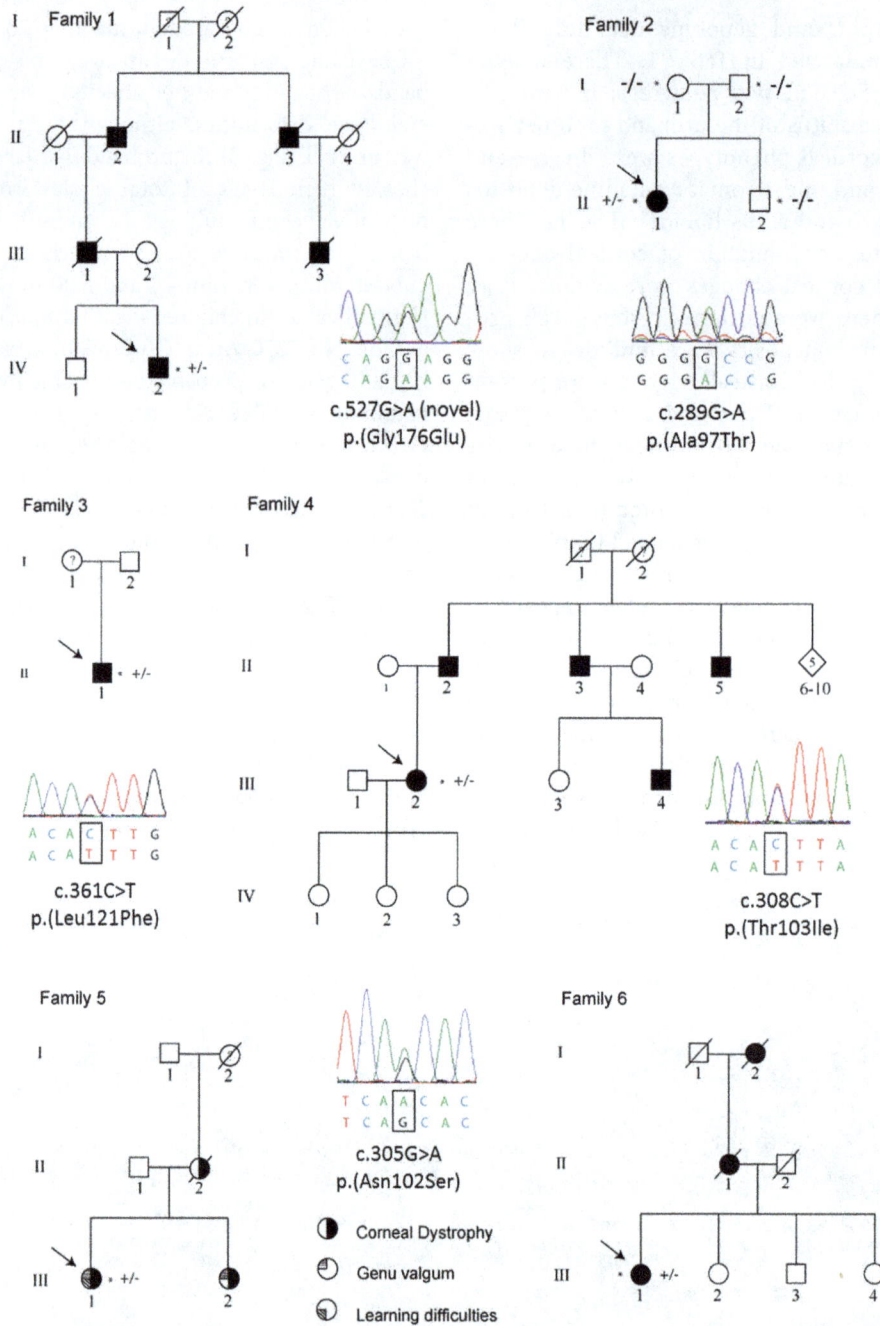

Fig. 3 Pedigrees of the six families with Schnyder corneal dystrophy. Sequence electropherograms of the identified heterozygous mutations in *UBIAD1* are also shown. The mutation arose de novo in family 2. Probands are indicated by an arrow and examined individuals by an asterisk. Mutation status in tested subjects is shown +/− for those who are heterozygous for a mutation in *UBIAD1* and −/− for those who do not carry the pathogenic variant. Individuals known to be affected by Schnyder corneal dystrophy are shown in black, whereas a question mark indicates that the disease status of the individual was unknown

heterozygous *UBIAD1* mutations are shown in Fig. 3. None of the *UBIAD1* pathogenic changes found in the current study were observed in the gnomAD dataset or in the Czech control population. All of the in silico algorithms predicted that the detected mutations were pathogenic or likely pathogenic, except for SNP&GO

prediction for previously reported variant c.361C>T; p.(Leu121Phe) [19] (Table 3).

Discussion

In this study we report the phenotype and genotype of six families with SCD. Five different *UBIAD1* mutations were

Table 3 In silico analysis of *UBIAD1* missense variants identified in patients with Schnyder corneal dystrophy in the current study

	MutPred	Polyphen2	PROVEAN	SNP&GO	SIFT	MutationTaster
p.(Ala97Thr)	Disease	Probably damaging	Disease	Disease	Disease	Disease
p.(Leu121Phe)	Disease	Probably damaging	Disease	Benign	Disease	Disease
p.(Thr103Ile)	Possibly damaging	Probably damaging	Disease	Disease	Disease	Disease
p.(Asn102Ser)	Disease	Probably damaging	Disease	Disease	Disease	Disease
p.(Gly176Glu)	Possibly damaging	Probably damaging	Disease	Disease	Disease	Disease

Six different algorithms were used; tolerated and neutral scores are indicated in green as benign; yellow indicates a possibly damaging variant, and red was used for a probably damaging and disease-causing mutation

As for MutPred an overall probability score > 0.5 was considered possibly damaging and a score > 0.75 was considered as disease-causing. NM_013319.2, NP_037451.1 and ENST00000376810.5 were used as reference sequences

identified in a heterozygous state, of which one, c.527G>A; p.(Gly176Glu), was novel. The youngest proband was found to harbour a de novo c.289G>A; p.(Ala97Thr) mutation, previously identified in an Irish-French family [18]. To the best of our knowledge, this is only the second observation of a spontaneously occurring mutation in an SCD patient [6]. The family history provided by proband 3 also indicated possible de novo occurrence of the identified mutation, but unfortunately this could not be confirmed as parental DNA samples were unavailable.

The c.305G>A; p.(Asn102Ser) mutation, identified in two South Asian probands, is the most frequently occurring *UBIAD1* mutation. It has been reported in several populations including the Czech Republic, Poland, Taiwan and China, supporting the hypothesis that it is a mutation hotspot [19–22]. One white British proband had a c.361C>T; p.(Leu121Phe) mutation, previously observed in three SCD families from the UK, America and Saudi Arabia [19, 23]. The c.308C>T; p.(Thr103Ile) mutation, detected in one white British individual, has previously been described in a proband of Japanese-European descent [6].

The clinical course of SCD is associated with characteristic corneal opacities that increase with age. Initially, central corneal haze and/or crystals are present; this was observed in our youngest proband, who was 6 years old when first examined. Arcus lipoides typically develops in the third decade, followed by mid-peripheral corneal haze in the late fourth decade [24], as documented in the current case series (probands 1, 4–5). Corneal crystals are present in approximately 50% of patients with SCD [2]. Interestingly, crystals were found in all six of our probands, although in two probands the area of crystal deposit was very small. However, the number of individuals we examined is relatively low compared with prior studies [2].

Confocal microscopy has previously been performed in two children with SCD, both at a similar age as our proband 2 [25]. Our findings corroborate observations of accumulation of crystal/reflective material in anterior stroma, both intra- and extracellularly. Interestingly, unlike the previous study, subepithelial nerves appeared normal and we were able to detect tiny reflective deposits in the corneal epithelium. Electron microscopy of corneas with SCD has also documented lipid accumulation inside epithelial cells [26, 27].

The differential diagnosis of crystalline corneal deposition includes monoclonal gammopathy and cystinosis. These conditions should be considered in any individual with corneal crystals who does not have a family history of SCD. Laboratory investigation should be guided by the presence of associated symptoms and patient age.

Dyslipidemia and genu valgum have been reported to be associated with SCD [3, 28]. Three of the six probands in this study had fasting serum lipid testing. Total cholesterol was elevated in one proband and borderline levels were found in the other two probands. Self-reported knee deformities were only present in proband 5 and her sister, although their mother was not affected, which may indicate that other genetic or environmental factors influence the expression of this trait.

Conclusions

SCD should be considered in the differential diagnosis of any unexplained corneal haze and/or crystal deposition, even in the absence of a family history of corneal disease.

Abbreviations

BCVA: Best corrected visual acuity; gnomAD: Genome Aggregation Database; MIM: Mendelian Inheritance in Man; SCD: Schnyder corneal dystrophy; *UBIAD1*: UbiA prenyltransferase domain-containing protein

Acknowledgements

We thank The Czech National Center for Medical Genomics (https://ncmg.cz/en) (LM2015091) for providing ethnically matched population frequency data (project CZ.02.1.01/0.0/0.0/16_013/0001634).

Funding

This work was supported by UNCE 204064 and PROGRES-Q26/LF1 programs of the Charles University, Fight for Sight, Moorfields Eye Charity, Rosetrees Trust, and the National Institute for Health Research Biomedical Research Centre based at Moorfields Eye Hospital NHS Foundation Trust and UCL Institute of Ophthalmology. PS was supported by GAUK 250361/2017, SVV 260367/2017 and PROGRES Q25/LF1/2. GM was supported by MH CZ – DRO, Motol University Hospital, Prague, Czech Republic 00064203. The views expressed are those of the authors and not necessarily those of the NHS, the NIHR or the Department of Health. This work was performed within the framework of ERN-EYE.

Authors' contributions

CJE and LD provided molecular genetic analysis, paternity testing was done by AH. PS, GM, SJT and PL contributed in clinical data collection and analysis AJH, SJT and PL contributed to study design and writing. All authors read and approved the final manuscript.

Competing interests

The authors declare that they have no competing interests.

Author details

[1]UCL Institute of Ophthalmology, London, UK. [2]Research Unit for Rare Diseases, Department of Paediatrics and Adolescent Medicine, First Faculty of Medicine, Charles University and General University Hospital in Prague, Ke Karlovu 2, 128 08 Prague 2, Czech Republic. [3]Department of Ophthalmology, First Faculty of Medicine, Charles University and General University Hospital in Prague, Prague, Czech Republic. [4]Department of Ophthalmology, Second Faculty of Medicine, Charles University and Motol University Hospital, Prague, Czech Republic. [5]3rd Department of Medicine, Department of Endocrinology and Metabolism, First Faculty of Medicine, Charles University and General University Hospital in Prague, Prague, Czech Republic. [6]Institute of Biology and Human Genetics, First Faculty of Medicine, Charles University and General University Hospital in Prague, Prague, Czech Republic. [7]Moorfields Eye Hospital, London, UK.

References

1. Weiss JS, Kruth HS, Kuivaniemi H, Tromp G, White PS, Winters RS, et al. Mutations in the UBIAD1 gene on chromosome short arm 1, region 36, cause Schnyder crystalline corneal dystrophy. Invest Ophthalmol Vis Sci. 2007;48:5007–12.
2. Weiss JS, Moller HU, Aldave AJ, Seitz B, Bredrup C, Kivelä T, et al. IC3D classification of corneal dystrophies--edition 2. Cornea. 2015;34:117–59.
3. Hoang-Xuan T, Pouliquen Y, Gasteau J. Schnyder's crystalline dystrophy. II. Association with genu valgum. J Fr Ophtalmol. 1985;8:743–7.
4. Orr A, Dube MP, Marcadier J, Jiang H, Federico A, George S, et al. Mutations in the UBIAD1 gene, encoding a potential prenyltransferase, are causal for Schnyder crystalline corneal dystrophy. PLoS One. 2007;2:e685.
5. Li W. Bringing bioactive compounds into membranes: the UbiA superfamily of intramembrane aromatic prenyltransferases. Trends Biochem Sci. 2016;41: 356–70.
6. Lin BR, Frausto RF, Vo RC, Chiu SY, Chen JL, Aldave AJ. Identification of the first de novo UBIAD1 gene mutation associated with Schnyder corneal dystrophy. J Ophthalmol. 2016;2016:1968493.
7. Mahelkova G, Filous A, Odehnal M, Cendelin J. Corneal changes assessed using confocal microscopy in patient with unilateral buphthalmos. Invest Ophthalmol Vis Sci. 2013;54:4048–53.
8. Choi Y, Sims GE, Murphy S, Miller JR, Chan AP. Predicting the functional effect of amino acid substitutions and indels. PLoS One. 2012;7:e46688.
9. Calabrese R, Capriotti E, Fariselli P, Martelli PL, Casadio R. Functional annotations improve the predictive score of human disease-related mutations in proteins. Hum Mutat. 2009;30:1237–44.
10. Li B, Krishnan VG, Mort ME, Xin F, Kamati KK, Cooper DN, et al. Automated inference of molecular mechanisms of disease from amino acid substitutions. Bioinformatics. 2009;25:2744–50.
11. Kumar P, Henikoff S, Ng PC. Predicting the effects of coding non-synonymous variants on protein function using the SIFT algorithm. Nat Protoc. 2009;4:1073–81.
12. Adzhubei IA, Schmidt S, Peshkin L, Ramensky VE, Gerasimova A, Bork P, et al. A method and server for predicting damaging missense mutations. Nat Methods. 2010;7:248–9.
13. Schwarz JM, Rodelsperger C, Schuelke M, Seelow D. MutationTaster evaluates disease-causing potential of sequence alterations. Nat Methods. 2010;7:575–6.
14. Evans CJ, Liskova P, Dudakova L, Hrabcikova P, Horinek A, Jirsova K, et al. Identification of six novel mutation in ZEB1 and description of the associated phenotypes in patients with posterior polymorphous corneal dystrophy 3. Ann Hum Genet. 2015;79:1–9.
15. Lek M, Karczewski KJ, Minikel EV, Samocha KE, Banks E, Fennell T, et al. Analysis of protein-coding genetic variation in 60,706 humans. Nature. 2016; 536:285–91.
16. Expert panel on detection, evaluation, and treatment of high blood cholesterol in adults. Executive summary of the third report of the National Cholesterol Education Program (NCEP) expert panel on detection, evaluation, and treatment of high blood cholesterol in adults (adult treatment panel III). JAMA. 2001;285:2486–97.
17. American Academy of Pediatrics. Committee on nutrition. Cholesterol in childhood. Pediatrics. 1998;101:141–7.
18. Nickerson ML, Bosley AD, Weiss JS, Kostiha BN, Hirota Y, Brandt W, et al. The UBIAD1 prenyltransferase links menaquinone-4 [corrected] synthesis to cholesterol metabolic enzymes. Hum Mutat. 2013;34:317–29.
19. Weiss JS, Kruth HS, Kuivaniemi H, Tromp G, Karkera J, Mahurkar S, et al. Genetic analysis of 14 families with Schnyder crystalline corneal dystrophy reveals clues to UBIAD1 protein function. Am J Med Genet A. 2008;146A:271–83.
20. Du C, Li Y, Dai L, Gong L, Han C. A mutation in the UBIAD1 gene in a Han Chinese family with Schnyder corneal dystrophy. Mol Vis. 2011;17:2685–92.
21. Nickerson ML, Kostiha BN, Brandt W, Fredericks W, Xu KP, Yu FS, et al. UBIAD1 mutation alters a mitochondrial prenyltransferase to cause Schnyder corneal dystrophy. PLoS One. 2010;5:e10760.
22. Nowinska AK, Wylegala E, Teper S, Lyssek-Boron A, Aragona P, Roszkowska AM, et al. Phenotype-genotype correlation in patients with Schnyder corneal dystrophy. Cornea. 2014;33:497–503.
23. Al-Ghadeer H, Mohamed JY, Khan AO. Schnyder corneal dystrophy in a Saudi Arabian family with heterozygous UBIAD1 mutation (p.L121F). Middle East Afr J Ophthalmol. 2011;18:61–4.
24. Weiss JS, Khemichian AJ. Differential diagnosis of Schnyder corneal dystrophy. Dev Ophthalmol. 2011;48:67–96.
25. Vesaluoma MH, Linna TU, Sankila EM, Weiss JS, Tervo TM. In vivo confocal microscopy of a family with Schnyder crystalline corneal dystrophy. Ophthalmology. 1999;106:944–51.
26. Rodrigues MM, Kruth HS, Krachmer JH, Willis R. Unesterified cholesterol in Schnyder's corneal crystalline dystrophy. Am J Ophthalmol. 1987;104:157–63.
27. Rodrigues MM, Kruth HS, Krachmer JH, et al. Cholesterol localization in ultrathin frozen sections in Schnyder's corneal crystalline dystrophy. Am J Ophthalmol. 1990;110:513–7.
28. Kohnen T, Pelton RW, Jones DB. Schnyder corneal dystrophy and juvenile, systemic hypercholesteremia. Klin Monatsbl Augenheilkd. 1997;211:135–7.

19

Intermittent high glucose-induced oxidative stress modulates retinal pigmented epithelial cell autophagy and promotes cell survival via increased HMGB1

Wei Zhang[†], Jian Song[†], Yue Zhang[†], Yingxue Ma, Jing Yang, Guanghui He and Song Chen[*]

Abstract

Background: In this study, we evaluated the effects of intermittent high glucose on oxidative stress production in retinal pigmented epithelial (RPE) cells and explored whether the mechanisms of autophagy and apoptosis in oxidative stress are associated with high-mobility group box 1 (HMGB1) protein.

Methods: Cultured human RPE cell line ARPE-19 cells were exposed to intermittent high glucose-induced oxidative stress. Reactive oxygen species (ROS) was determined by 2′, 7′-dichlorofluorescin diacetate (DCFH-DA); and malonyldialdehyde (MDA), superoxide dismutase (SOD) by commercial kits. Transmission electron microscopy was used to observe the generation of autophagosome. And MTT assay was used to examine the effect of autophagy on cell viability. For the inhibition experiments, cells were pre-incubated with lysosomal inhibitors NH4Cl or N-acetyl cysteine (NAC).Western blot was used to measure the expression patterns of autophagic markers, including LC3 and p62. The expression of HMGB1 was detected by immunohistochemistry.Cells were pre-incubated with HMGB1 inhibitor ethyl pyruvate (EP) ,then detected the expression pattern of autophagic markers and level of cellular ROS.

Results: We found that intermittent high glucose significantly increased oxidative stress levels (as indicated by ROS, MDA, SOD), increased in the generation of autophagosome, decreased the level of p62, induced conversion of LC3 I to LC3 II. We further demonstrated that the NH4Cl/NAC inhibited intermittent high glucose-induced autophage by altered level of LC3 and p62. Intermittent high glucose-induced autophagy is independent of HMGB1 signaling, inhibition of HMGB1 release by EP decreased expression pattern of autophagic markers and level of cellular viability.

Conclusions: Under intermittent high glucose condition, autophagy may be required for preventing oxidative stress-induced injury in RPE. HMGB1 plays important roles in signaling for both autophagy and oxidative stress.

Keywords: Intermittent high glucose, HMGB1, Oxidative stress, Autophagy, Retinal pigment epithelium cell

Background

Diabetic retinopathy (DR) is the main cause of visual loss in the adults. Increased retinal inflammatory cytokines are closely related to retinal pathologies in DR. The injury and cell apoptosis of retinal pigment epithelial (RPE) cells are considered to be happened in DR. RPE is a monolayer of pigmented cells that separates the neural retina from a network of fenestrated vessels called the choriocapillaris, which serves as the major blood supply for the photoreceptors, and therefore the RPE constitutes the outer blood-retinal barrier (BRB). Impairment of the outer BRB is increasingly recognized to play an important role in the initiation and progression of early DR. [1, 2] Oxidative stress and impaired protein degradation in RPE cells may result in RPE damage and dysfunction [3]. Although the mechanism of RPE cells injury induced by diabetes is not yet clear, studies show that fluctuating glucose is more harmful to RPE cells than constantly high glucose concentration [4, 5].

* Correspondence: chensong20@hotmail.com
[†]Wei Zhang, Jian Song and Yue Zhang contributed equally to this work.
Tianjin Eye Hospital, Tianjin Key Lab of Ophthalmology and Visual Science, Tianjin Eye Institute, Clinical College of Ophthalmology Tianjin Medical University, No. 4, Gansu Road, Tianjin 300020, China

Furthermore, fluctuating glucose promotes a greater increase in inflammatory cytokine production from retinal endothelial cells than constantly high glucose through release of reactive oxygen species (ROS) which is another important trigger for DR pathogenesis [6]. In addition, ROS can further exaggerate inflammation in the pathogenesis of DR.

Autophagy is a process of catabolic reaction that involves the mechanical degradation of cellular components through lysosomes [7]. Autophagy plays a key role in the growth, development, and homeostasis of cells by maintaining the balance between the synthesis, degradation, and recirculation of cellular components [8]. Autophagy is also the key to RPE homeostasis because the RPE has high metabolic activity under a highly oxidative environment. ROS can induce autophagy through several different mechanisms including catalase, autophagy related gene 4 (ATG4) [9]. Therefore, the damaged autophagy or lysosome activity may lead to insufficiently remove the intracellular organelles or protein aggregates of oxidative damage, which leads to the accumulation of toxic substances within and outside the cells and damages the RPE function during DR.

Thus, autophagy could be regulated and executed, which is crucial for maintaining cellular homeostasis, as a key adaptive mechanism against multiple cellular stress situation. However, the function of autophagy in RPE is remain unclear on glucose fluctuation stress. Moreover, we recently demonstrated that oxidative stress is implicated in retinal inflammation during DR. [10] In this study, we evaluated the effects of intermittent high glucose on oxidative stress production in RPE cells and explored whether the mechanisms of autophagy and apoptosis in oxidative stress are associated with high-mobility group box 1 (HMGB1) protein.

Methods
Cell culture
Human cell line, ARPE-19 cells was obtained from the American Type Culture Collection. The cells were cultured in DMEM medium containing 10% Foetal bovine serum (FBS) and 1% penicillin/streptomycin. ARPE-19 cells were chosen as monolayers, they express all the signature genes of human RPE cells. Cells were exposed to the following experimental conditions for 48hs: 1) normal glucose (5 mM, Control); 2) constant high glucose (25 mM, HG); 3) normal and high glucose alternating every 3 h (HG-Int). Medium were collected and cells harvested for analysis.

Proliferation assay
Proliferation was analysed by MTT (Becton Dickinson, Bedford, MA, USA) as previously described [11]. In short, we seeded ARPE-19 cells in 96-well plates with 6×10 [3] cells/well and cultured them at 37 °C with 5% CO_2 for 24 h. Second, added 10 μl of MTT solution (5 mg/ml) to each well, incubating ARPE-19 cells for 4 h at 37 °C. After the formation of a crystal, discarded MTT medium and replaced with 150 μl of dimethyl sulfoxide (DMSO) (Sigma Chemical Co., USA) to dissolve crystal. Then, the plates were shaken for 5 min. The absorbance of each well was recorded by a microplate spectrophotometer at 570 nm.

Detection of reactive oxygen species (ROS)
The concentration of ROS in ARPE-19 cells was detected by measuring the fluorescent signal from the DCFDA (redox-sensitive-fluoroprobe- 2′, 7′-dichlorofluorescein--diacetate). In short, ARPE-19 cells were cultured in phenol red-free DMEM in 12-well plates, and then incubated with the following experimental conditions: 1) normal glucose (5 mM, Control); 2) constant high glucose (25 mM, HG); 3) normal and high glucose alternating every 3 h (HG-Int). Washed the cells in PBS buffer, and then added DCFDA (10 mM) in serum-free medium at 37 °C for 30 min. The fluorescence of DCF in the ARPE-19 cells was detected with 525 nm as an emission wavelength and 485 nm as an excitation wavelength.

Malondialdehyde (MDA) was an end product of lipid peroxidation, which was detected to detect the levels of lipid peroxidation by a MDA assay kit (Sigma Chemical Co., USA). The results were shown to be nM/mg protein. WST-1 was used to detect the content of superoxide dismutase (SOD) in the lysis solution. The SOD WST-1 kit was purchased (Coherent, Santa Clara, CA, USA) and used based on the manufacturer's instructions.

Electron microscopy
Autophagosome in RPE, was characterized by transmission electron microscope FEI Tecnai G2 Spirit by a digital camera Morada. The cell was washed again and stained for 5 min in 2.5% aqueous uranyl acetate. The sample was dehydrated with graded alcohol and embedded in Epon resin. Images were acquired in the AC mode using a silicon tip with a typical resonance frequency of 300 kHz and a radius smaller than 10 nm. Autophagosome was identified under the microscope solely based on size and morphology.

Treatment with inhibitors and western blot analysis
For the inhibition experiments, ARPE-19 cells were pre-incubated for 1 h with each inhibitor, such as lysosomal inhibitors NH4Cl, antioxidant N-acetyl cysteine (NAC) or HMGB1 inhibitor ethyl pyruvate (EP). Cells were washed in PBS and immediately lysed in RIPA buffer (Thermo, Carlsbad, CA, USA) supplemented with phosphatase/protease inhibitor cocktail (Thermo). The lysate was centrifuged at 15000 g for 20 min, and the

supernatant was further used for analysis. Using bovine serum albumin as the standard to detect the protein concentration. The protein (40 μ g/well) was loaded and separated by SDS-PAGE and transferred to the nitrocellulose membrane. The membrane was coated with 5% non-fat skim milk in TBST (150 mM NaCl, 10 mM Tris-HCl [pH 8.0], 0.02% Tween20) for 1 h at 15 °C, and then probed overnight at 4 °C with primary antibodies. Primary antibodies used were LC3 (DAB; Sigma Chemical Co., USA), p62 (DAB; Sigma Chemical Co., USA) and β-actin (C DAB; Sigma Chemical Co., USA).

Immunocytochemistry

Immunocytochemistry was also performed on ARPE-19 cells grown as monolayers on transwell plates, fixed in 4% paraformaldehyde. After extensive washing, cells were incubated either in rabbit polyclonal antibodies recognizing anti-HMGB1 (1:200; Invitrogen, Carlsbad, CA, USA) in blocking solution (0.5% Triton-X in tris buffered saline with 10% goat serum), and followed by Alexa Fluor 488 (1:500; Sigma Chemical Co., USA) as the secondary antibody. Staining was examined via fluorescence microscopy (Zeiss, USA) equipped with a digital camera.

Statistical analysis

The data were presented as the mean ± SEM, and the data were compared using one-way analysis of variance (ANOVA). A p-value < 0.05 was considered statistically significant. All analyses were performed using a statistical software package (SPSS 15.0, Chicago, IL, USA).

Results

Intermittent high glucose induces significant oxidative stress and inhibits proliferative activity in ARPE-19 cells

In this study, we exposed ARPE-19 cells to intermittent and constant high glucose to make an oxidative stress injury model. To prove that intermittent and constant high glucose could affect cell oxidative stress and survival, we first treated ARPE-19 cells with high glucose for 48 h and then detected cell proliferation by MTT assay. We found that proliferative activity was decreased in both constant high glucose-treated cells (0.613 ± 0.077 OD) and intermittent high glucose-treated cells (0.527 ± 0.045 OD) compared with cells exposed to normal glucose (0.714 ± 0.089 OD) ($p < 0.05$) (Fig. 1a). Intermittent glucose could greatly decrease the proliferative activity compared with constant high glucose ($p < 0.05$) (Fig. 1a), indicative of an inhibitory effect of proliferative activity on ARPE-19 cells. In following experiments using DCFDA,

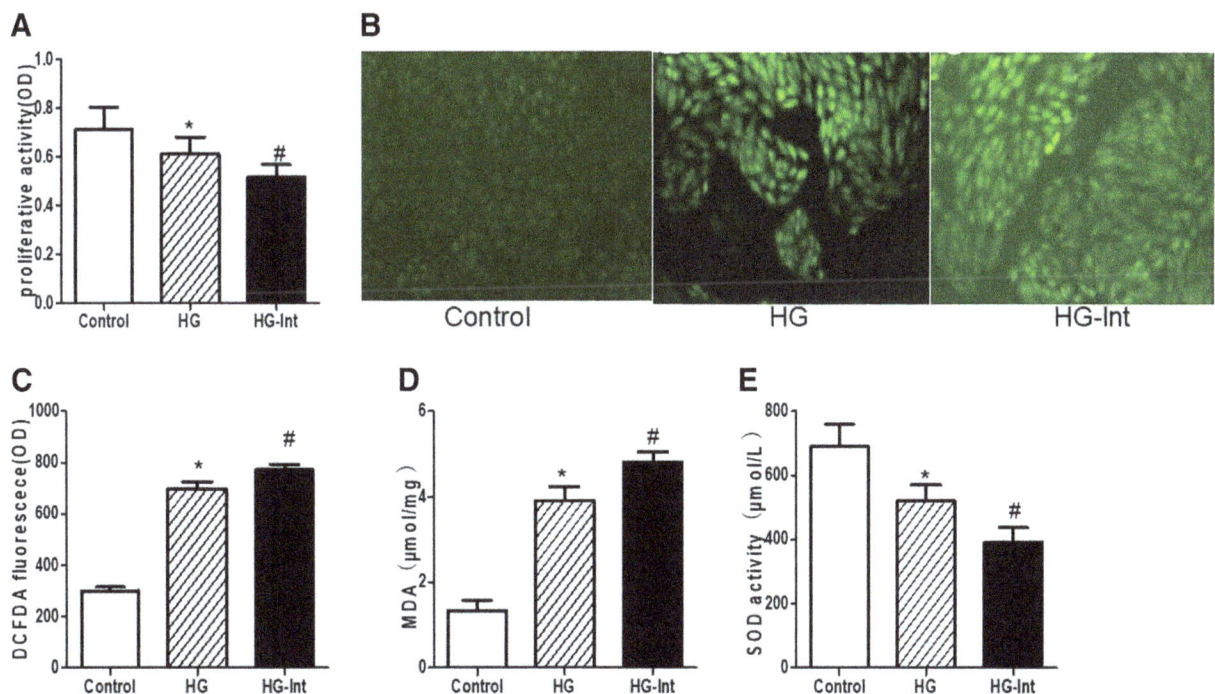

Fig. 1 Intermittent high glucose induces significant oxidative stress and inhibits proliferative activity in ARPE-19 cells. **a**: Proliferative activity was decreased in both constant high glucose-treated cells and Intermittent glucose induced a more remarkable decrease in proliferative activity when compared to constant high glucose. **b-c**: Intermittent high glucose resulted in dramatic significantly higher fluorescence of cellular ROS marker DCFDA than constant high glucose and normal glucose. **d**: MDA concentrations of intermittent high glucose-treated cells was higher than that of constant high glucose and normal glucose. **e**: SOD concentrations in intermittent high glucose-treated cells was lower than that in constant high glucose and normal glucose. (*$p < 0.05$ vs. control, #$p < 0.05$ vs. HG)

MDA and SOD assays, we found that intermittent high glucose resulted in dramatic significantly higher fluorescence of cellular ROS marker DCFDA (772.41 ± 20.352 OD) than constant high glucose (697.98 ± 27.798 OD) and normal glucose(300.04 ± 14.503 OD) (Fig. 1b, c). Similarly, MDA concentrations of intermittent high glucose-treated cells (4.818 ± 0.236 μmol/mg) was higher than that of constant high glucose (3.913 ± 0.317 μmol/mg) and normal glucose (1.338 ± 0.228 μmol/mg) ($p < 0.05$) (Fig. 1d). However, SOD concentrations in intermittent high glucose-treated cells (392.7 ± 47.5 μmol/L) was lower than that in constant high glucose (525.1 ± 51.2 μmol/L) and normal glucose (695.3 ± 73.4 μmol/L) ($p < 0.05$) (Fig. 1e), suggested that the oxidative stress increased in intermittent high glucose-treated cells. Taken together, these data suggested that intermittent high glucose could induce significant oxidative damage and inhibit proliferative activity than constant high glucose in ARPE-19 cells.

Intermittent high glucose induces RPE autophagy and alters the expression pattern of autophagic markers

In order to determine the effect of intermittent high glucose on autophagy, ARPE-19 cells were seeded in the medium containing normal glucose (5 mM) or high glucose (25 mM) alternating every 3 h. Transmission electron microscopy examination revealed that intermittent high glucose lead to increasing of double-membrane vacuoles, which was a typical of autophagosomes (Fig. 2a). LC3 was processed from LC3-I to LC3-II, which could incorporate into vacuoles. In Fig. 2b, western blot results showed that intermittent high glucose lead to a significant increase in conservation of LC3-II (Fig. 2c), indicating that intermittent high glucose could induce RPE autophagy. P62 selectively incorporates into autophagosomes with the direct binding to LC3, which is ultimately degraded by autophagy [12]. Therefore, the amount of p62 was negatively correlated with autophagic activity. Our results showed that compared with LC3-II level, intermittent high glucose resulted in a marked decrease in p62 protein level (Fig. 2d). Collectively, the level of LC3-II/LC3-I and p62 suggests that intermittent high glucose induced autophagy in ARPE-19 cells.

Effect of lysosomal inhibitors and antioxidant on intermittent high glucose-induced RPE autophagy and proliferative activity

NH4Cl as a lysosomal inhibitor can interrupt the lysosome-autophagosome fusion. N-acetylcysteine (NAC) was a molecule with antioxidant properties, which possessed a sulfhydryl group and acted as the source of

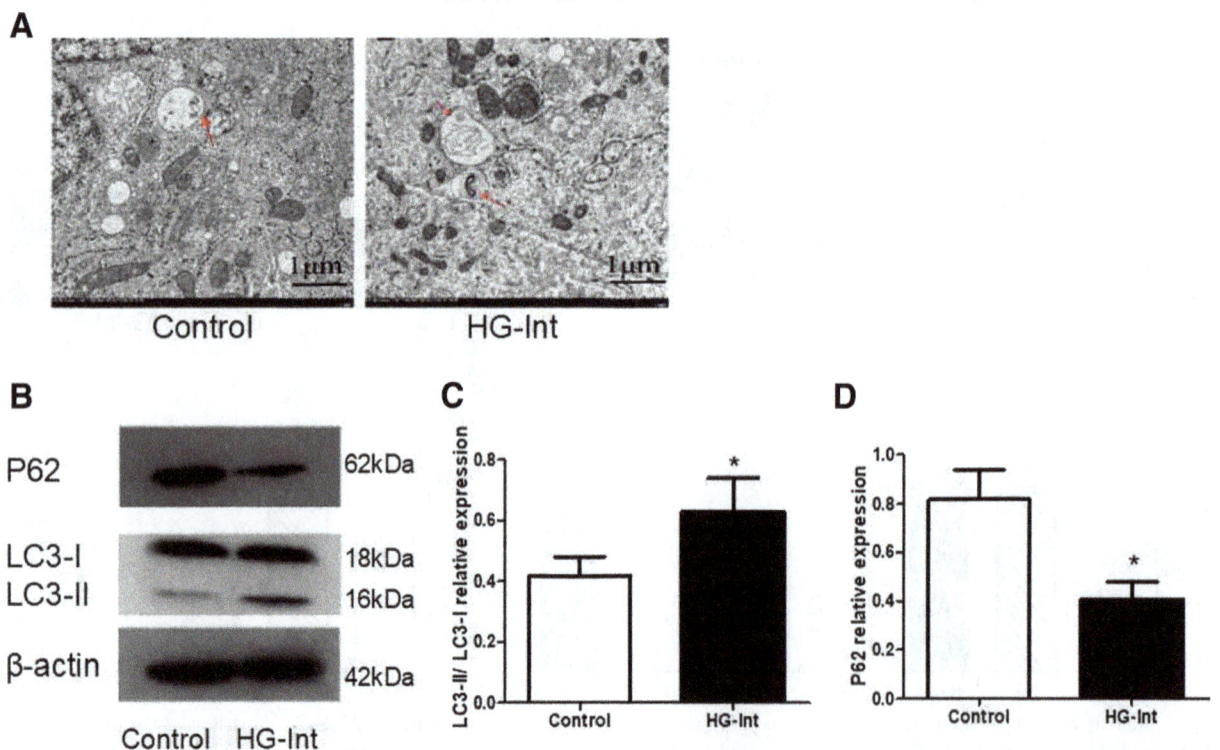

Fig. 2 Intermittent high glucose induces RPE autophagy and alters the expression pattern of autophagic markers. **a**: Transmission electron microscopy examination revealed that intermittent high glucose lead to an increase in the number of double-membrane vacuoles, which was a typical of autophagosomes. **b-d**: Western blot results showed that intermittent high glucose lead to a significant increase in conservation of LC3-II. Intermittent high glucose resulted in a marked decrease in p62 protein expression. (*$p < 0.05$ vs. control, #$p < 0.05$ vs. HG)

cysteine to glutathione synthesis. To determine the effect of NH4Cl and NAC on intermittent high glucose-induced RPE autophagy, we measured the level of LC3-II/LC3-I in the presence of either NH4Cl or NAC. Intermittent high glucose treatment in the presence of either NH4Cl or NAC decreased the level of LC3-II/LC3-I in ARPE-19 cells (Fig. 3a, b, d, e), indicating that intermittent high glucose-induced increasing of LC3-II was blocked in the presence of either NH4Cl or NAC. Similaly, we found that compared with LC3-II/LC3-I level, p62 protein has an opposite expression trend. Intermittent high glucose treatment in the presence of either NH4Cl or NAC resulted in a marked increase in p62 protein level (Fig. 3c, f). Collectively, the level of LC3-II and p62 indicates that NH4Cl and NAC could inhibit intermittent high glucose induce autophagy in RPE.

We used MTT method to measure the RPE viability under intermittent high glucose stress. We showed that compared with the HG-Int group (0.498 ± 0.038 OD), intermittent high glucose treatment in the presence of either NH4Cl (0.365 ± 0.051 OD) or NAC (0.417 ± 0.053 OD) resulted in an obvious reduction in proliferative activity ($p < 0.05$) (Fig. 3g, h), suggesting that autophagy has a protective effect on RPE under intermittent high glucose stress.

HMGB1 mediates intermittent high glucose-induced autophagy

HMGB1 is a rich nuclear protein with pro-inflammatory activity dependent on its extra-nuclear function [13]. The distribution of HMGB1 was detected under intermittent high glucose condition, and ARPE-19 cells were stained with specific anti-HMGB1 antibody. ARPE-19 cells were mainly expressed as nuclear localization of HMGB1in the normal glucose condition. However, in ARPE-19 cells treated with intermittent high glucose, the proportion of HMGB1 in the cytoplasm was increased (Fig. 4a, b).

To detect if HMGB1 affects the expression of autophagy in response to intermittent high glucose condition, we examined the autophagic flux in the presence of HMGB1 inhibitor ethyl pyruvate (EP). Our results showed that EP could inhibite intermittent high

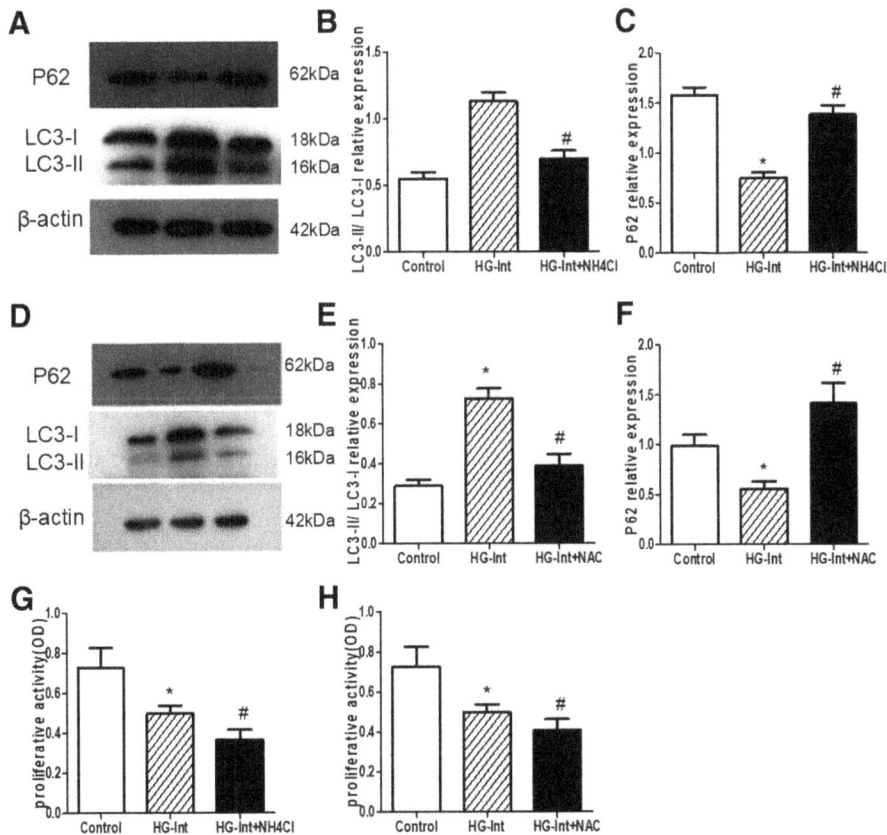

Fig. 3 Effect of lysosomal inhibitors and antioxidant on intermittent high glucose-induced RPE autophagy and proliferative activity. **a, b, d, e**: Intermittent high glucose treatment in the presence of either NH4Cl or NAC decreased the level of LC3-II/LC3-I in ARPE-19 cells. **c, f**: Intermittent high glucose treatment in the presence of either NH4Cl or NAC resulted in a marked increase in p62 protein expression. **g-h**: Compared with the HG-Int group, intermittent high glucose treatment in the presence of either NH4Cl or NAC resulted in an obvious reduction in proliferative activity. (*$p < 0.05$ vs. control, #$p < 0.05$ vs. HG)

glucose-induced LC3-II level (Fig. 4c, d), indicating an important role of HMGB1 in the regulation of intermittent high glucose-induced autophagy. In addition, EP could increase the level of p62 protein under conditions of intermittent high glucose (Fig. 4e), suggesting that the degradation is dependent upon HMGB1 mediated autophagy. Overall, our results suggest that HMGB1 is essential for autophagy induced by intermittent high glucose.

In following experiments using MTT assays, we found that loss of HMGB1 under intermittent high glucose condition resulted in dramatic significantly reduction in proliferative activity (0.277 ± 0.044 OD) than intermittent high glucose (0.492 ± 0.048 OD) and normal glucose (0.719 ± 0.078 OD) ($p < 0.05$) (Fig. 4f), suggesting that HMGB1 mediated autophagy has a protective effect on RPE under intermittent high glucose stress.

Discussion

More evidences from cell culture and animal models show that oxidative stress is an important cause of RPE damage diabetic macular edema [14]. We found that intermittent high glucose induced autophagic flux in RPEs, which seems to have a protective effect on intermittent high glucose-induced RPE damage. It is possible that the repeated shift from normal glucose to high

glucose during glucose fluctuation may lead to oxidative stress. Recent studies showed that autophagy plays a key regulator in the RPE and is a crucial role in protection against oxidative stress [15, 16]. In our study, we show that p62 is dramatically down-regulated under intermittent high glucose condition, which is related to enhanced autophagic flux in ARPE-19 cells and that lysosomal inhibitors NH4Cl or antioxidant NAC make ARPE-19 cells more susceptible to oxidative stress. Consistently, we demonstrated that NH4Cl or NAC decreases both p62 and autophagic flux. We also showed that autophagy may be required for preventing oxidative stress-induced injury in RPE under intermittent high glucose condition, while HMGB1 plays important roles in signaling for both autophagy and oxidative stress in ARPE-19 cells.

Autophagy is the conservative mechanism for the degeneration of cellular components in the cytoplasm [17]. It is shown that autophagy is a double-edged sword for cell physiology [18]. Autophagy acts as a cell survival mechanism under oxidative stress condition, and plays a key role in cell apoptosis [19]. p62/ Sequestosome1 (SQSTM1) is a multifunctional scaffold protein, which acts a key role in different cellular signaling pathways and plays an adaptive role in various cellular processes [20, 21]. It is shown that the inhibition of proteasoome

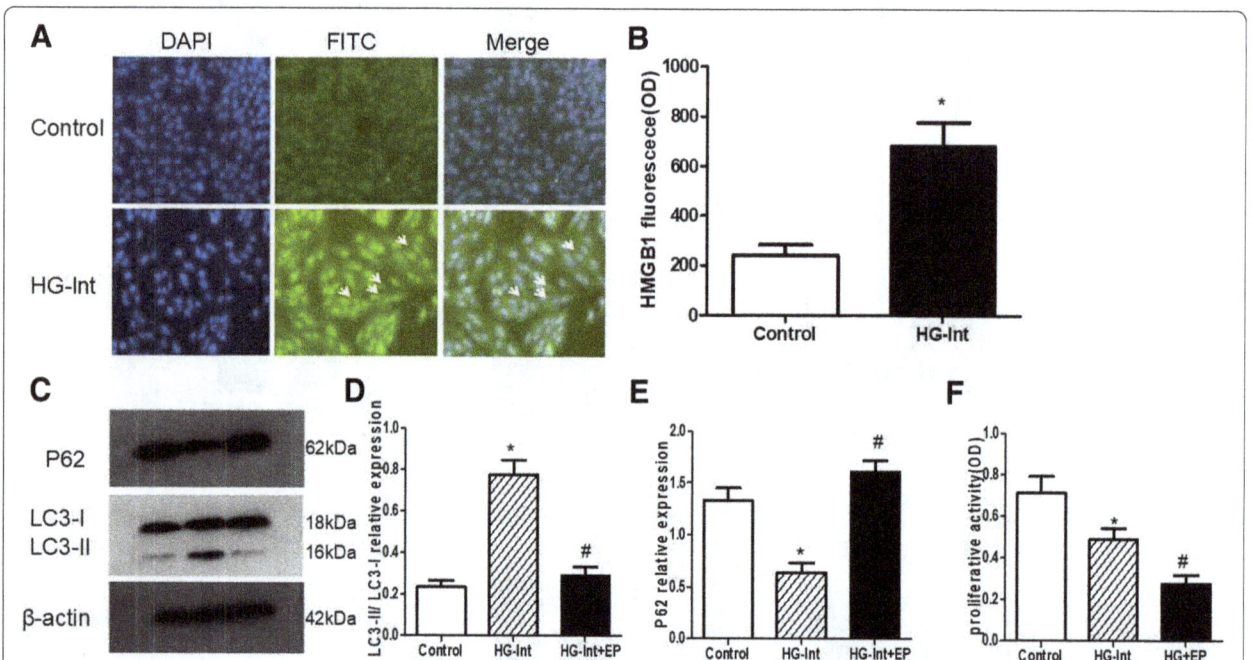

Fig. 4 HMGB1 mediates intermittent high glucose-induced autophagy. DAPI was used to stain the nuclei. **a-b**: Immunohistochemistry showed that the normal glucose ARPE-19 cells were mainly expressed as nuclear localization of HMGB1. However, in ARPE-19 cells treated with intermittent high glucose, the proportion of HMGB1 in the cytoplasm was increased. **c-d**: EP could inhibit intermittent high glucose-induced LC3-II expression. **e**: EP could increase the expression of p62 protein under conditions of intermittent high glucose. **f**: Loss of HMGB1 under intermittent high glucose condition resulted in dramatic significantly reduction in proliferative activity than intermittent high glucose and normal glucose(*$p < 0.05$ vs. control, #$p < 0.05$ vs. HG)

caused elevated p62 level in RPE cells [16]. Our data indicates that intermittent high glucose induces expression of p62 in the ARPE-19 cells, which starts the autophagic pathway and considers as a protective response against high glucose induced oxidative stress. Previous researches have shown that high glucose promoted autophagy in endothelial cells by inhibiting PI3K/AKT signaling [7]. While in RPE cells, autophagy can prevent the oxidative damage caused by diabetes [22]. We have revealed that autophagy has a positive effect on RPEs under intermittent high glucose condition. In contrast, Yang F et al. showed an opposite phenomenon that inhibition of autophagy has a protective effect on high glucose-induced cardiac vascular endothelial cells injury [23]. These results emphasize the fact that autophagy may be either protective or harmful, which depends on cell types and cell environments. Therefore, the function of autophagy should be discussed separately under different pathological conditions [24].

HMGB1 protein is a chromatin-binding nuclear protein. It is a part of damage-related molecular patterns and has an important effect on oxidative stress response and cell death signals, involving autophagy and apoptosis [25]. Recent researches have showed that autophagy regulates the release of selective HMGB1 in endothelial cells that are destined to death [26, 27]. On the contrary, autophagy induced by exogenous HMGB1 could promote chemotherapeutic resistance in leukemia cells [28]. It is noteworthy that our experimental data show HMGB1 could be a regulator of high glucose-induced autophagy, the reasons as follow: 1) HMGB1 could regulate the turnover of LC3-II/ LC3-I. Under in which autophagy is increased, such as exposure to intermittent high glucose condition, HMGB1 regulated LC3-positive punctae is apparent. Correspondingly, without HMGB1 inhibited intermittent high glucose condition-induced LC3-positive punctae, suggesting HMGB1 regulated the LC3 reaction [29]. 2) HMGB1 can regulate the p62 autophagic degradation. The accumulation of p62 was found in the cells withoutHMGB1 deficient after oxidative stress, suggesting that the autophagic degradation or defects in autophagic degradation of p62 in the present of EP. It is important that continuous expression of p62 induced by autophagy defects is sufficient to alter NF-kB regulation, and then reduce the proliferation activity of ARPE-19 cells [30]. 3) Loss of HMGB1 in RPE cells promotes the production of ROS. The targeted inhibition of HMGB1 increased the production of ROS and reduced autophagy with oxidative stress, which indicates that the role of HMGB1 is the upstream of oxidative stress [31]. These results show a key signaling pathway that relates intermittent high glucose-induced RPE autophagy to dysregulation of HMGB1.

Conclusions
Our data clearly indicate that activation of autophagy may be required for preventing oxidative stress-induced injury in RPE under intermittent high glucose condition by activation of HMGB1. Autophagy participates in oxidative stress induced by mitochondrial dysfunction. Foresti R et al. [32] found that RPEs in HG did not affect the activation of the Nrf2/heme axis but affected the oxidative and mitochondrial-dependent cellular functions. The inhibition of autophagy by blockage of HMGB1 suggests that HMGB1 may be suitable target for a protective therapy for DR. Understanding the role of intermittent high glucose condition-induced stimulation of autophagy in the RPE cells will provide new sight for the pathogenesis of DR.

Abbreviations
DR: Diabetic retinopathy; HMGB1: High-mobility group box 1; MDA: Malonyldialdehyde; NAC: N-acetyl cysteine; ROS: Reactive oxygen species; RPE: Retinal pigmented epithelial; SOD: Superoxide dismutase

Funding
This work was supported by Tianjin Science and Technology Project of China (No. 14JCYBJC27400) and the National Natural Science Foundation of China (No. 81700846) and the China Scholarship Council (CSC).

Authors' contributions
SC and WZ conceived and designed the experiments; WZ, JS, and YZ performed the experiments and prepared tables and figures; YM, JY and GH collected the sample data; WZ contributed to the writing of the manuscript; SC reviewed the manuscript; all authors contributed to the writing of the manuscript and discussed the manuscript at various stages. All authors read and approved the final manuscript.

References
1. Xu HZ, Le YZ. Significance of outer blood-retina barrier breakdown in diabetes and ischemia. Invest Ophthalmol Vis Sci. 2011;52(5):2160–4.
2. Pittalà V, Fidilio A, Lazzara F, et al. Effects of novel nitric oxide-releasing molecules against oxidative stress on retinal pigmented epithelial cells. Oxidative Med Cell Longev. 2017;2017:1420892.
3. Hu W, Wang R, Li J, Zhang J, Wang W. Association of irisin concentrations with the presence of diabetic nephropathy and retinopathy. Ann Clin Biochem. 2016;53:67–74.
4. de Carlo TE, Bonini Filho MA, Baumal CR, et al. Evaluation of Preretinal neovascularization in proliferative diabetic retinopathy using optical coherence tomography angiography. Ophthalmic surgery, lasers & imaging retina. 2016;47:115–9.
5. Shin JH, Bae DJ, Kim ES, et al. Autophagy regulates formation of primary cilia in Mefloquine-treated cells. Biomol Ther. 2015;23:327–32.
6. Shtir C, Aldahmesh MA, Al-Dahmash S, et al. Exome-based case-control association study using extreme phenotype design reveals novel candidates with protective effect in diabetic retinopathy. Human genetics. 2016;135: 193–200.
7. Mitter SK, Song C, Qi X, et al. Dysregulated autophagy in the RPE is associated with increased susceptibility to oxidative stress and AMD. Autophagy. 2014;10:1989–2005.
8. Abebe T, Mahadevan J, Bogachus L, et al. Nrf2/antioxidant pathway mediates beta cell self-repair after damage by high-fat diet-induced oxidative stress. JCI insight. 2017;2(24).

9. Diaz-Morales N, Iannantuoni F, Escribano-Lopez I, et al. Does Metformin Modulate Endoplasmic Reticulum Stress and Autophagy in Type 2 Diabetic Peripheral Blood Mononuclear Cells? Antioxid Redox Signal. 2018;28(17):1562–69.

10. Zhang W, Wang Y, Kong J, Dong M, Duan H, Chen S. Therapeutic efficacy of neural stem cells originating from umbilical cord-derived mesenchymal stem cells in diabetic retinopathy. Sci Rep. 2017;7:408.

11. Zhang W, Yan H. Dysfunction of circulating endothelial progenitor cells in type 1 diabetic rats with diabetic retinopathy. Graefes Arch Clin Exp Ophthalmol = Albrecht Von. 2013;251:1123–31.

12. Hou B, Qiang G, Zhao Y, et al. Salvianolic acid a protects against diabetic nephropathy through ameliorating glomerular endothelial dysfunction via inhibiting AGE-RAGE signaling. Cell Physiol Biochem. 2017;44:2378–94.

13. Chen Y, Zhou X, Qiao J, Bao A. MiR-142-3p overexpression increases chemo-sensitivity of NSCLC by inhibiting HMGB1-mediated autophagy. Cell Physiol Biochem. 2017;41:1370–82.

14. Shi H, Zhang Z, Wang X, et al. Inhibition of autophagy induces IL-1beta release from ARPE-19 cells via ROS mediated NLRP3 inflammasome activation under high glucose stress. Biochem Biophys Res Commun. 2015; 463:1071–6.

15. Chai P, Ni H, Zhang H, Fan X. The evolving functions of autophagy in ocular health: a double-edged sword. Int J Biol Sci. 2016;12:1332–40.

16. Guha S, Liu J, Baltazar G, Laties AM, Mitchell CH. Rescue of compromised lysosomes enhances degradation of photoreceptor outer segments and reduces lipofuscin-like autofluorescence in retinal pigmented epithelial cells. Adv Exp Med Biol. 2014;801:105–11.

17. Song C, Mitter SK, Qi X, et al. Oxidative stress-mediated NFkappaB phosphorylation upregulates p62/SQSTM1 and promotes retinal pigmented epithelial cell survival through increased autophagy. PLoS One. 2017;12: e0171940.

18. Fu D, Yu JY, Connell AR, et al. Beneficial effects of Berberine on oxidized LDL-induced cytotoxicity to human retinal Muller cells. Invest Ophthalmol Vis Sci. 2016;57:3369–79.

19. Fu D, Yu JY, Yang S, et al. Survival or death: a dual role for autophagy in stress-induced pericyte loss in diabetic retinopathy. Diabetologia. 2016;59: 2251–61.

20. Fung FK, Law BY, Lo AC. Lutein attenuates both apoptosis and autophagy upon cobalt (II) chloride-induced hypoxia in rat Muller cells. PLoS One. 2016; 11:e0167828.

21. Lopes de Faria JM, Duarte DA, Montemurro C, Papadimitriou A, Consonni SR, Lopes de Faria JB. Defective autophagy in diabetic retinopathy. Invest Ophthalmol Vis Sci. 2016;57:4356–66.

22. Wei Y, Gao J, Qin L, et al. Curcumin suppresses AGEs induced apoptosis in tubular epithelial cells via protective autophagy. Exp Ther Med. 2017;14:6052–8.

23. Yang F, Zhang L, Gao Z, et al. Exogenous H2S protects against diabetic cardiomyopathy by activating autophagy via the AMPK/mTOR pathway. Cell Physiol Biochem. 2017;43:1168–87.

24. Zhang M, Wang S, Cheng Z, et al. Polydatin ameliorates diabetic cardiomyopathy via Sirt3 activation. Biochem Biophys Res Commun. 2017; 493:1280–7.

25. Yin H, Yang X, Gu W, et al. HMGB1-mediated autophagy attenuates gemcitabine-induced apoptosis in bladder cancer cells involving JNK and ERK activation. Oncotarget. 2017;8:71642–56.

26. Huang J, Yang J, Shen Y, et al. HMGB1 mediates autophagy dysfunction via perturbing Beclin1-Vps34 complex in dopaminergic cell model. Front Mol Neurosci. 2017;10:13.

27. Gao D, Lv AE, Li HP, Han DH, Zhang YP. LncRNA MALAT-1 elevates HMGB1 to promote autophagy resulting in inhibition of tumor cell apoptosis in multiple myeloma. J Cell Biochem. 2017;118:3341–8.

28. Liu L, Ren W, Chen K. MiR-34a promotes apoptosis and inhibits autophagy by targeting HMGB1 in acute myeloid leukemia cells. Cell Physiol Biochem. 2017;41:1981–92.

29. Ou Z, Chen Y, Niu X, et al. High-mobility group box 1 regulates cytoprotective autophagy in a mouse spermatocyte cell line (GC-2spd) exposed to cadmium. Ir J Med Sci. 2017;186:1041–50.

30. Petrovic A, Bogojevic D, Korac A, et al. Oxidative stress-dependent contribution of HMGB1 to the interplay between apoptosis and autophagy in diabetic rat liver. J Physiol Biochem. 2017;73:511–21.

31. Song E, Jahng JW, Chong LP, et al. Lipocalin-2 induces NLRP3 inflammasome activation via HMGB1 induced TLR4 signaling in heart tissue of mice under pressure overload challenge. Am J Transl Res. 2017;9:2723–35.

32. Foresti R, Bucolo C, Platania CM, et al. Nrf2 activators modulate oxidative stress responses and bioenergetic profiles of human retinal epithelial cells cultured in normal or high glucose conditions. Pharmacol Res. 2015;99:296–307.

20

Ocular changes during hemodialysis in patients with end-stage renal disease

Hejun Chen[1], Xi Zhang[2] and Xi Shen[1*] (iD)

Abstract

Background: To explore ocular changes during hemodialysis (HD) in chronic renal failure patients and to determine the effects of different causes of renal failure during HD.

Methods: A total of 90 eyes from 45 end-stage renal disease (ESRD) patients undergoing HD were evaluated in this study. All ophthalmological examinations were conducted within 1 h before and after a single HD session. The HD patients were divided into primary kidney disease (KD), hypertensive KD, diabetic KD (DM-KD) and unknown etiology subgroups according to the primary etiology of renal failure. The statistics of 38 eyes from 19 healthy people were set as normal control.

Results: Tear break-up time (TBUT) ($P = 0.020$), Schirmer's I test results ($P = 0.030$), anterior chamber depth (ACD) ($P = 0.006$), lens thickness (LT) ($P < 0.001$) and choroidal thickness (CHT) ($P < 0.001$)decreased significantly after a single HD. The retinal nerve fiber layer (RNFL) thickness and average retinal thickness (RT) increased after HD, especially in the nasal inner macula (NIM) subfield ($P < 0.001$), the inferior inner macula (IIM) subfield ($P = 0.004$) and the superior outer macula (SOM) subfield ($P = 0.012$). TBUT, Schirmer's I test, IOP, RT, and CHT were correlated with one or more parameters. All ESRD patients regardless of etiology had the same trend for most parameters during HD, with the exception of the logMAR of BCVA, central corneal thickness, RNFL thickness and CHT.

Conclusions: HD may affect a range of ocular parameters in ESRD patients. Dry eye parameters, RT and CHT exhibited the most obvious changes. Different etiologies tended to have similar trends in ocular parameter changes during HD.

Keywords: End-stage renal disease, Hemodialysis, Ocular changes

Background

End-stage renal disease (ESRD), with a glomerular filtration rate lower than 15 ml/ (min*1.73 m^2), is the 5th stage of disease and the final outcome of disease progression in chronic kidney disease (CKD) patients. At this stage, a variety of clinical manifestations, such as hypertension, anemia, and edema, and metabolic and endocrine disorders can occur; thus, renal replacement therapy, such as hemodialysis (HD), is needed to remove excess water and metabolic wastes from the extracorporeal blood and to maintain the electrolyte and acid-base balance [1].

The negative impact of CKD on the patient's eye is complex and diverse. Studies have shown that HD, as a relief and treatment of CKD, can improve certain ocular symptoms in ESRD patients. It has been reported that best corrected visual acuity (BCVA) improves after a single HD session, and patients with diabetes tend to have more obvious improvements [2, 3]. Other researchers have reported that HD can relieve macular edema in patients with kidney failure caused by diabetes [4]. However, in most cases, the negative impact of hemodialysis on the eye in CKD patients seems to be far beyond its positive impact. Aktas et al. [5] found aggravation of dry eye syndrome after a single session of HD. Moreover, it has been observed since the early sixties that HD can change the level of intraocular pressure (IOP). Different studies have shown IOP to increase [6–8], decrease [9] or remain unchanged [10]. The effects of HD on the posterior pole include changes in

* Correspondence: carl_shen2005@126.com

Hejun Chen and Xi Zhang are first authors.

Hejun Chen and Xi Zhang contributed equally to this work.

[1]Ruijin Hospital Affiliated to Shanghai Jiao Tong University School of Medicine, No. 197 Rui Jin Er Road, Shanghai 200025, China

Full list of author information is available at the end of the article

retinal thickness, retinal nerve fiber layer (RNFL) thickness, and choroidal thickness. Significant differences in these parameters have been reported in some studies, although others hold different views [11–13].

Since most of the effects of HD on ophthalmological parameters remain unclear and because no studies have reported the effects of HD on different etiologies, we conducted this study including a total of 45 patients with ESRD who underwent HD and analyzed the changes of both laboratory test and ocular parameters after HD to investigate the effects of the hemodialysis on the eye.

Methods
Subjects
CKD stage 5 patients undergoing hemodialysis treatment for at least 3 months at the Blood Purification Center of Ruijin Hospital affiliated with Shanghai Jiao Tong University from February 2014 to October 2014 were enrolled in this study. Hemodialysis was performed 3 times a week, each lasting 3–5 h.

The inclusion criteria were visual acuity over 20/200 as well as Oculus Pentacam® anterior segment analyzer (Oculus Inc., Wetzlar, Germany) results and OCT reports of acceptable quality. The exclusion criteria were a history of surgical or laser-based operations to the eye, other ocular diseases such as corneal scarring, uveitis, macular holes, and other conditions, or a history of renal replacement therapy, including peritoneal dialysis and kidney transplantation.

The hemodialysis group was divided into primary kidney disease (KD), hypertensive KD and diabetic KD (DM-KD) subgroups strictly according to the initial etiology of renal insufficiency. When patients failed to provide reliable supporting materials or when two or more etiologies were suspected, the patients were included in the etiology unknown subgroup. Nineteen healthy people without HD history were set as normal control.

This study adhered to the Declaration of Helsinki and was approved by the institutional review board of Shanghai Ruijin Hospital. Informed consent was obtained from the subjects after verbal and written explanations of the nature and possible consequences of the study were provided.

Protocol
Blood reports, including urea, creatinine, uric acid, serum electrolytes (Na, K, Ca, P, Mg), parathyroid hormone (PTH), and fasting blood glucose levels, were collected before hemodialysis.

Blood pressure and detailed ophthalmological examinations, including spherical and cylinder powers, BCVA, IOP, dry eye analysis, corneal endothelial measurements, central corneal thickness (CT), anterior chamber depth (ACD), lens measurements, retinal thickness (RT) around the fovea, RNFL thickness, and choroidal thickness (CHT), were performed. BCVA was examined using a standard vision chart, and the logarithmic minimum angle of resolution (logMAR) was recorded. Refractive parameters were measured by a full auto ref-keratometer (Canon, Japan). IOP was measured by non-contact tonometer (NCT) (Canon, Japan). Dry eye syndrome was estimated by the tear break-up time (TBUT) and Schirmer's I test. Endothelial cell density (ECD), the average endothelial cell size (ECS), and the endothelial cell size variation coefficient (ECSCV) were obtained using a Tomey EM-3000 non-contact specular microscope corneal endothelial cell counter. The CT, ACD and lens thickness (LT) were automatically calculated using a Pentacam® anterior segment analyzer (Oculus Inc., Wetzlar, Germany). The RT and RNFL thickness was measured using Cirrus HD-OCT (Carl Zeiss Meditec, Inc., Dublin CA, United States) under the Macular Cube 512×128 mode. The RT was defined as the average thickness of the 6 mm × 6 mm scan. The nine subfields of the RT map were measured separately. The inner, intermediate, and outer rings had radii of 1 mm, 3 mm, and 6 mm, respectively. The average thickness within the inner ring was defined as the central foveal subfield (CSF) thickness [14]. The average CHT was measured in the EDI mode of OCT. The subfoveal, nasal and temporal choroidal thicknesses were each measured 1 mm and 2 mm away from the center of the macula, averaged, and recorded as the average thickness of the choroid.

All examinations were measured within an hour before and after a single session of hemodialysis.

Statistical analysis
Paired t-tests were used for indexes measured before and after HD if homogeneity of variance was verified. If homogeneity of variance was not verified, then a non-parametric test was used. Multiple linear regression analyses were conducted to identify correlations between parameters. Then, single factor analysis of variance (one-way ANOVA) and least-significant difference (LSD) tests were performed to determine parameters with significant changes during HD among subgroups according to their etiological classification. Lastly, one-way ANOVA was used to compare parameters with significant changes. A box plot was drawn, and Tukey's test was used to isolate data with large deviations. The P-values, Estimated Marginal Means and their standard errors (SEs) were calculated by General Estimating Equations (which automatically take into account paired eye data from the same subject) after adjusting for age, sex, eyes, measurement times, HD duration, and primary diseases.

SPSS22.0 software was used to analyze the data. Statistical significance was considered when $P < 0.05$. All data are presented as the means ± standard deviation (means ± SD). All values are expressed as the means ± SD.

Table 1 Demographic characteristics of the hemodialysis group (pre HD) and the control group: comparison of basic situation and baseline data (Mean ± SD)

Pre HD	HD Group	Control Group	P value
Male [eyes (percentage)]	54 (60.00%)	60 (63.83%)	0.593
Female [eyes (percentage)]	36 (40.00%)	34 (36.17%)	
Age (year)	57.78 ± 13.57	54.90 ± 17.60	0.239
Systolic pressure (mmHg)	147.14 ± 22.43	133.65 ± 18.64	0.016*
Diastolic pressure (mmHg)	83.75 ± 16.03	75.28 ± 11.79	0.022*
Urea (mmol/L)	24.330 ± 7.853	5.275 ± 0.936	< 0.001**
Creatinine (umol/L)	891.10 ± 70.78	77.00 ± 20.38	< 0.001**
Uric acid (umol/L)	427.50 ± 79.78	367.88 ± 85.441	0.012*
Na (mmol/L)	138.20 ± 2.64	142.00 ± 2.45	< 0.001**
K (mmol/L)	4.860 ± 0.920	4.191 ± 0.217	< 0.001**
Ca (mmol/L)	2.279 ± 0.206	2.283 ± 0.070	0.908
P (mmol/L)	1.849 ± 0.542	1.160 ± 0.180	< 0.001**
Mg (mmol/L)	1.050 ± 0.129	0.873 ± 0.035	< 0.001**
PTH (ng/L)	479.70 ± 419.20	40.30 ± 12.45	< 0.001**
Fasting plasma glucose (mmol/L)	7.725 ± 3.356	5.433 ± 0.695	< 0.001**
Spherical power (D)	0.088 ± 0.508	−2.4011 ± 3.7786	0.012*
Cylinder power (D)	−0.857 ± 0.138	−0.6711 ± 0.6071	0.070
logMAR of BCVA	0.100 ± 0.0282	− 0.0205 ± 0.2344	0.345
TBUT(s)	6.957 ± 0.861	9.171 ± 5.801	0.949
Schirmer's I test (mm)	12.014 ± 2.020	16.934 ± 9.617	0.309
IOP (mmHg)	12.855 ± 0.420	15.01 ± 3.69	0.073
ACD (mm)	2.642 ± 0.073	2.783 ± 0.481	0.082
CT (μm)	575.18 ± 5.859	549.11 ± 38.67	0.650
ECD (cell/mm²)	2758.47 ± 35.494	2707.46 ± 194.91	0.055
ECS (μm²)	363.16 ± 6.577	371.34 ± 29.27	0.132
ECSCV	40.717 ± 1.573	40.88 ± 7.35	0.381
LT (mm)	4.146 ± 0.064	3.979 ± 0.460	0.120
CSF (μm)	244.36 + 4.464	249.68 ⊥ 32.75	0.080
SIM (μm)	312.22 ± 2.912	323.45 ± 22.49	0.350
NIM (μm)	310.28 ± 2.904	322.13 ± 21.33	0.220
IIM (μm)	311.14 ± 3.990	316.29 ± 17.85	0.022*
TIM (μm)	302.88 ± 4.233	310.79 ± 19.39	0.030*
SOM (μm)	276.82 ± 3.915	280.42 ± 16.98	0.475
NOM (μm)	289.25 ± 2.368	294.61 ± 19.35	0.428
IOM (μm)	267.27 ± 5.037	266.45 ± 19.31	0.204
TOM (μm)	259.62 ± 5.432	262.37 ± 20.73	0.290
Average RT (μm)	273.40 ± 3.302	276.39 ± 17.37	0.164
RNFL thickness (μm)	90.65 ± 1.829	96.24 ± 23.06	0.669
CHT (μm)	289.55 ± 11.385	232.87 ± 65.23	0.302

PTH Parathyroid hormone, *TBUT* Tear break-up time, *logMAR* Logarithmic minimum angle of resolution, *BCVA* Best corrected visual acuity, *IOP* Intraocular pressure, *ACD* Anterior chamber depth, *LT* Lens thickness, *CT* Corneal thickness, *ECD* Endothelial cell density, *ECS* Endothelial cell size, *ECSCV* Endothelial cell size variation coefficient, *CSF* Central subfield, *SIM* Superior inner macula, *NIM* Nasal inner macula, *IIM* Inferior inner macula, *TIM* Temporal inner macula, *SOM* Superior outer macula, *NOM* Nasal outer macula, *IOM* Inferior outer macula, *TOM* Temporal outer macula, *MV* Macular volume, *RNFL* Retinal nerve fiber layer, *CHT* Choroidal thickness, *: $P < 0.05$; **: $P<0.01$

Results

Demographic characteristics of the HD patients and healthy controls

A total of 90 eyes from both sides of 45 HD patients were included in the study, including 27 pairs of male eyes (60.00%) and 18 pairs of female eyes (40.00%). The average age was 57.48 ± 13.57 years. The mean dialysis time was 70.09 ± 58.03 months. The patients were divided into 3 subgroups: the primary KD subgroup, the hypertensive KD subgroup and the DM-KD subgroup. No differences were found in age ($P = 0.639$) or dialysis time ($P = 0.270$) among the 3 subgroups.

Thirty-eight eyes from 19 healthy people were set as normal control. The blood pressure (both systolic and diastolic), urea, creatinine, uric acid, Na, K, P, Mg, PTH, fasting plasma glucose were found statistically different from the pre-HD ESRD patients. However, most of the ocular parameters, except for Spherical power and a few part of the retinal thickness showed no statistical difference (Table 1).

A comparison of blood pressure during HD

The average systolic pressure (SP) before HD was 147.14 ± 22.43 mmHg, which increased to 136.09 ± 24.37 mmHg after HD ($P = 0.001$). The mean diastolic blood pressure (DP) decreased from 83.75 ± 16.03 mmHg to 76.48 ± 13.47 mmHg ($P = 0.006$).

Conjunctival and corneal calcification

Visible calcium deposits were spotted on the cornea or conjunctiva in 22 (48.89%) of the 45 hemodialysis patients. These deposits were located in the nasal and/or temporal side of the cornea, conjunctiva and limbus. They were either white or gray and were point-, line- or block-shaped (Fig. 1).

A comparison of the ocular surface, BCVA, and refractive parameters during HD

After HD, the TBUT decreased from 6.957 ± 0.861 s to 5.205 ± 0.670 s ($P = 0.020$), and the Schirmer's I test results decreased from 12.014 ± 2.020 mm to 9.964 ± 1.912 mm ($P = 0.030$). However, no significant change was observed in the BCVA ($P = 0.880$), spherical power ($P = 0.442$) or cylinder power ($P = 0.937$) measurements during HD (Table 2).

A significant positive correlation was found between the TBUT change within each HD session and the duration of all HD treatments ($B = 0.040$, $T = 3.670$, $P = 0.001$). Meanwhile, the change in the Schirmer's I test results ($B = -0.566$, $T = -5.121$, $P < 0.001$) and blood urea levels ($B = -0.271$, $T = -2.179$, $P = 0.036$) were negatively correlated.

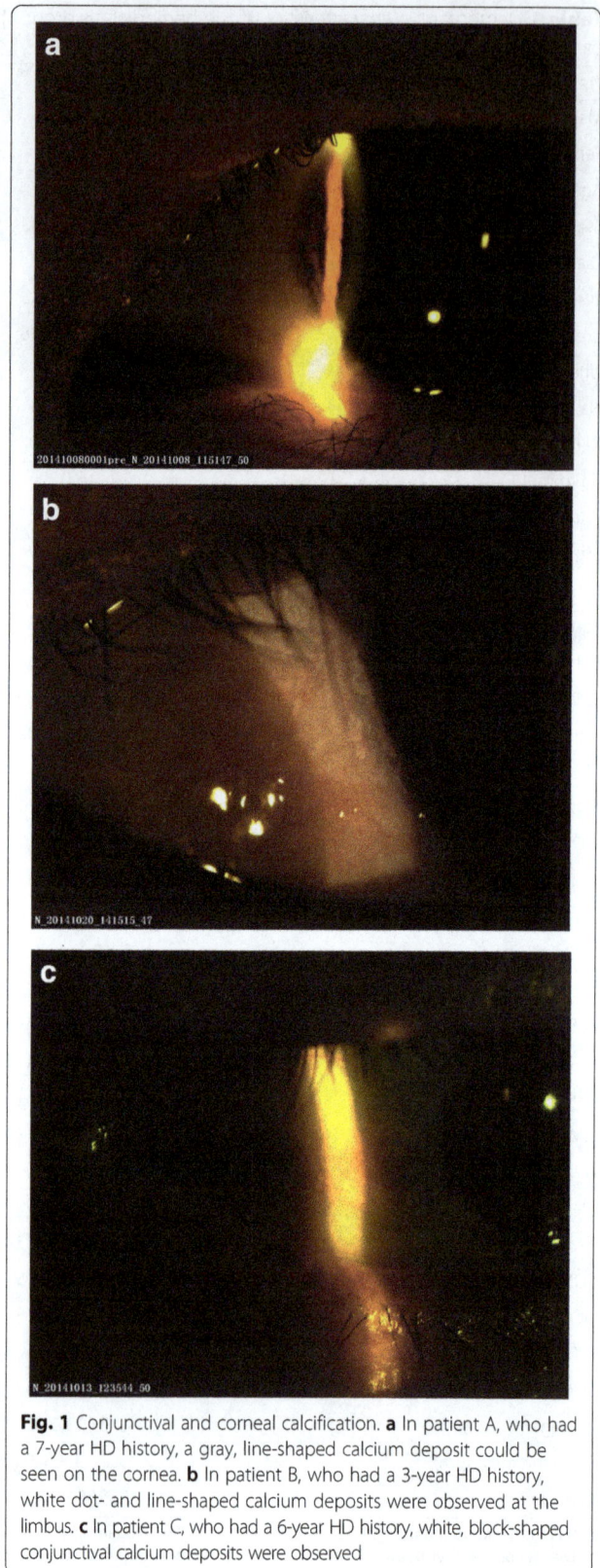

Fig. 1 Conjunctival and corneal calcification. **a** In patient A, who had a 7-year HD history, a gray, line-shaped calcium deposit could be seen on the cornea. **b** In patient B, who had a 3-year HD history, white dot- and line-shaped calcium deposits were observed at the limbus. **c** In patient C, who had a 6-year HD history, white, block-shaped conjunctival calcium deposits were observed

Table 2 Comparison of the ocular surface, BCVA, and refractive parameters during HD

HD group parameters	Pre (Estimated Marginal Mean ± SE)	Post (Estimated Marginal Mean ± SE)	P value
TBUT (s)	6.957 ± 0.861	5.205 ± 0.670	0.020*
Schirmer's I test (mm)	12.014 ± 2.020	9.964 ± 1.912	0.030*
logMAR of BCVA	0.100 ± 0.0282	0.099 ± 0.027	0.880
Spherical power (D)	0.088 ± 0.508	0.032 ± 0.498	0.442
Cylinder power (D)	−0.857 ± 0.138	− 0.863 ± 0.148	0.937

TBUT Tear break-up time, *logMAR* Logarithmic minimum angle of resolution, *BCVA* Best corrected visual acuity, *: P < 0.05
The P-values, Estimated Marginal Means and their standard errors (SEs) were calculated by General Estimating Equations after adjusting for age, sex, eyes, measurement times, HD duration, and primary diseases

Comparison of the IOP and anterior segment parameters during HD

The ACD decreased from 2.642 ± 0.073 mm to 2.613 ± 0.077 mm after HD ($P = 0.006$). The mean LT dropped from 4.153 ± 0.413 mm to 4.056 ± 0.389 mm ($P < 0.001$). No significant differences were observed in IOP ($P = 0.113$), CT ($P = 0.643$), ECD ($P = 0.807$), ECS ($P = 0.164$), or ECSCV ($P = 0.348$) during HD (Table 3).

We found a negative correlation between changes in IOP during HD and diastolic pressure ($B = -0.068$, $T = -3.606$, $P = 0.001$).

A comparison of the posterior segment parameters during HD

The average retinal thickness increased from 273.40 ± 3.302 μm to 275.60 ± 3.180 μm ($P = 0.071$), especially in the nasal inner macula (NIM) subfield ($P < 0.001$), the inferior inner macula (IIM) subfield ($P = 0.004$) and the superior outer macula (SOM) subfield ($P = 0.012$). The remaining subfields had no significant differences. The RNFL thickness increased from 90.65 ± 1.829 μm to 93.18 ± 1.974 μm ($P = 0.001$). The CHT decreased from 289.55 ± 11.385 μm to 254.134 ± 11.46 μm ($P < 0.001$) (Table 4).

A positive correlation was found between the average RT change and the central corneal thickness ($B = 0.130$, $T = 5.127$, $P < 0.001$) and the potassium level ($B = 3.950$, $T = 2.650$, $P = 0.012$) before HD. The choroidal thickness change was positively related to TBUT ($B = 3.120$, $T = 3.637$, P = 0.001) and was negatively correlated with sodium level (B = − 4.163, $T = -2.241$, $P = 0.031$) and ACD (B = − 30.190, $T = -2.356$, $P = 0.024$) before HD.

Comparison of parameters between subgroups according to the original cause of HD

Both eyes of all HD patients were divided into 4 subgroups according to the etiology of ESRD: the primary kidney disease (KD) subgroup ($n = 27$), the hypertensive KD subgroup ($n = 9$), the diabetic mellitus KD (DM-KD) subgroup ($n = 6$) and the etiology unknown subgroup ($n = 3$). The 3 etiology unknown patients were not included in the following analysis (Table 5).

There were no differences in the sex, age and HD duration among the 3 subgroups. However, four parameters, logMAR of BCVA, CT, RNFL thickness and CHT, were significantly different among subgroups (Fig. 2).

In summary, primary KD, hypertension and diabetes mellitus are three conditions that affect eye examination results during HD to a certain degree. However, the different causes of CRF requiring hemodialysis tend to have the same overall trend in most parameter changes except the logMAR of the BCVA, CT, RNFL thickness and CHT. Lower BCVA, increased central corneal thickness, and decreased RNFL thickness and CHT were observed in the DM-KD patients.

Table 3 Comparison of the IOP and anterior segment parameters during HD

HD group parameters	Pre (Estimated Marginal Mean ± SE)	Post (Estimated Marginal Mean ± SE)	P value
IOP (mmHg)	12.855 ± 0.420	12.292 ± 0.476	0.113
ACD (mm)	2.642 ± 0.073	2.613 ± 0.077	0.006*
LT (mm)	4.146 ± 0.064	4.049 ± 0.063	< 0.0001*
CT (μm)	575.18 ± 5.859	579.62 ± 5.427	0.643
ECD (cells/mm²)	2758.47 ± 35.494	2766.55 ± 41.074	0.807
ECS (μm²)	363.16 ± 6.577	359.36 ± 5.120	0.164
ECSCV	40.717 ± 1.573	40.073 ± 1.306	0.348

IOP Intraocular pressure, *ACD* Anterior chamber depth, *LT* Lens thickness, *CT* Corneal thickness, *ECD* Endothelial cell density, *ECS* Endothelial cell size, *ECSCV* Endothelial cell size variation coefficient, *: P < 0.05
The P-values, Estimated Marginal Means and their SEs were calculated by General Estimating Equations after adjusting for age, sex, eyes, measurement times, HD duration, and primary diseases

Table 4 Comparison of the posterior segment parameters during HD

HD group parameters	Pre (Estimated Marginal Mean ± SE)	Post (Estimated Marginal Mean ± SE)	P value
Average RT (μm)	273.40 ± 3.302	275.60 ± 3.180	0.071
CSF (μm)	244.36 ± 4.464	246.56 ± 4.575	0.308
SIM (μm)	312.22 ± 2.912	312.43 ± 2.717	0.895
NIM (μm)	310.28 ± 2.904	313.21 ± 3.037	< 0.001*
IIM (μm)	311.14 ± 3.990	313.53 ± 4.090	0.004*
TIM (μm)	302.88 ± 4.233	304.58 ± 3.889	0.150
SOM (μm)	276.82 ± 3.915	282.49 ± 4.127	0.012*
NOM (μm)	289.25 ± 2.368	291.42 ± 2.636	0.064
IOM (μm)	267.27 ± 5.037	266.69 ± 4.816	0.570
TOM (μm)	259.62 ± 5.432	261.21 ± 4.707	0.409
RNFL thickness (μm)	90.65 ± 1.829	93.18 ± 1.974	0.001*
CHT (μm)	289.55 ± 11.385	254.134 ± 11.46	< 0.001*

CSF Central subfield, SIM Superior inner macula, NIM Nasal inner macula, IIM Inferior inner macula, TIM Temporal inner macula, SOM Superior outer macula, NOM Nasal outer macula, IOM Inferior outer macula, TOM Temporal outer macula, MV Macular volume, RNFL Retinal nerve fiber layer, CHT Choroidal thickness, *: $P < 0.05$
The P-values, Estimated Marginal Means and their SEs were calculated by General Estimating Equations after adjusting for age, sex, eyes, measurement times, HD duration, and primary diseases

Discussion

All patients showed significant changes in dry eye parameters, RT and CHT. Different etiologies tended to exhibit similar trends in ocular parameter changes during HD.

HD is the process of clearing excess body water and metabolic waste. Therefore, body fluid volume, solute concentration, and crystal osmotic pressure decrease after HD. Our study shows that, consistent with most studies [2, 15], the TBUT and Schirmer's test results significantly decrease during HD. Aggravation of dry eye syndromes may be the result of less body fluid and tear secretion. Although toxins are removed from patients during HD, these patients still resemble secretion-deficient dry eye patients after treatment and are in need of ophthalmic artificial tear replacement. Moreover, a positive correlation was found between the TBUT reduction and HD duration, indicating the cumulative effect of HD on the patients' dry eye conditions. Dry eye symptoms

Table 5 Demographic characteristics of the 3 etiological ESRD subgroups

Characteristics	Primary KD n = 45
Number of eyes (eyes)	90
Men, n (%)	27 (60.0%)
Age (years)	57.78 ± 13.57
HD duration (months)	70.09 ± 58.03
Primary Diseases, n (%)	27 (60.0)
Hypertensive KD, n (%)	9 (20.0)
DM-KD, n (%)	6 (13.3)

KD Kidney disease, DM Diabetes mellitus

can be observed immediately (within an hour) after a single HD session. Both the long-term and short-term effects of HD should be fully considered to relieve symptoms of dry eye.

Over the years, there have been a number of studies on HD, leading to changes in IOP. However, the conclusions of different scholars vary. Overall, the factors associated with post-HD IOP change are mainly measurement techniques and the anterior chamber angle. Findings obtained using the Goldmann tonometer tended to find reductions; the use of NCT resulted in opposite findings in that increased IOP is more likely to take place in a narrow and obstructive anterior chamber angle and tends to decline at an opposite angle [2, 9–11, 16, 17]. Our study suggested that the IOP has no significant change after HD regardless of the etiology of the ESRD. A negative correlation was observed between the changes in the IOP and diastolic pressure. IOP might be related not only to measurement method and anterior chamber angle, but also to blood pressure.

Early researchers believed that after HD, the ACD would either decline [2] or would not change [16]. In our study, the ACD significantly declined after HD. With the reductions in body fluid volume and osmotic pressure caused by HD, the amount of aqueous humor declined. Moreover, because this decrease is mainly due to changes in the crystal osmotic pressure rather than the colloid osmotic pressure, the latter increases after HD, and it can result in the aqueous humor flowing into the blood via the anterior chamber angle trabecular meshwork. This mechanism also contributes to reduced intraocular pressure. However, in patients with narrow or obstructive angles, this process is hampered, and due

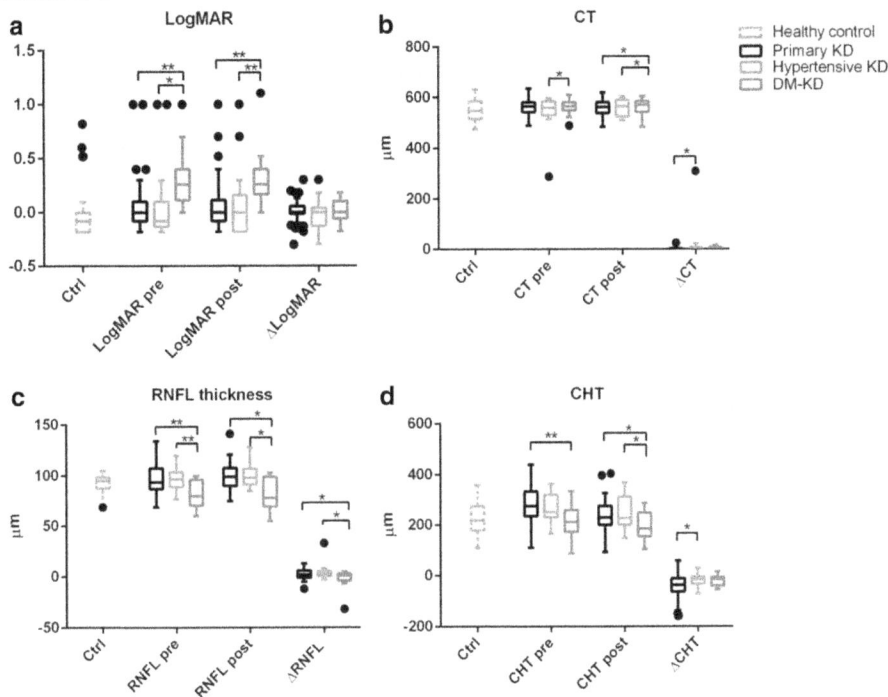

Fig. 2 Comparison of the logMAR of the BCVA, central corneal thickness (CT), RNFL thickness and choroid thickness (CHT) among the primary KD, hypertensive KD, and DM-KD subgroups. **a** The logMAR of the BCVA of the DM-KD subgroup was significantly higher than that of the primary KD subgroup and the hypertensive KD subgroup before and after HD. **b** The CT of the DM-KD subgroup was significantly higher before and after HD. **c** The average RNFL thickness of the DM-KD subgroup was significantly lower than that of the other 2 subgroups both before and after HD, and a lower change of RNFL thickness of the DM-KD was found compared to the other 2 subgroups. The 3 bars are from left to right: the primary kidney disease (KD) subgroup ($n = 27$), the hypertensive KD subgroup ($n = 9$), the diabetic mellitus KD (DM-KD) subgroup ($n = 6$). **d** The CHT in the DM-KD subgroup was lower than that of the other 2 subgroups before and after HD. Δ value (change of value) was defined as the value after HD minus the value before HD. *: $P < 0.05$; **: $P < 0.01$

to the decline in the plasma crystal osmotic pressure, body fluid moves along the concentration gradient into the anterior chamber; this process may lead to increased IOP and even acute angle-closure glaucoma [17]. Based on this conclusion, we should consider IOP, gonioscopy, and visual field tests for HD patients. For those with a high risk of anterior chamber obstruction, more detailed follow-ups should be conducted to determine any possible existence of glaucoma. These patients are classified as high risk patients, and preventative measures should be taken in the hemodialysis unit.

During HD, retinal thickness tended to increase in different locations and different layers of the retina, including the RNFL. Different etiologies did not affect the degree of change in these parameters. However, previous research found no statistically significant differences before and after HD in terms of the macular thickness [13, 18], the thickness of the surrounding macular areas [13], the macular volume [12] or the layer of retinal ganglion cells [11, 12]. Our conclusion is not yet supported by other studies, so we propose the following hypothesis: HD reduces the plasma crystal osmotic pressure such that the

liquid goes into the layers of the retina along the concentration gradient, thickening the retina and leading to edema. The specific mechanisms of our hypothesis await verification from follow-up studies.

Many studies have shown that the subfoveal, nasal, temporal and average choroidal thicknesses can be significantly reduced by HD [13, 19]. Our conclusion is the same as those of previous studies in that the average CHT significantly decreased after HD; this was especially the case in patients with DM, in whom the CHT was significantly smaller both before and after HD. The CHT change was positively related to the TBUT before HD because HD removes excess body liquid and reduces the blood volume. Thus, the choroidal vascular layer significantly "shrinks," and the choroidal thickness is reduced. These changes are associated with certain indicators that reflect the body fluid volume. Earlier research found that the peak systolic flow velocity (PSV) and end diastolic flow velocity (EDV) both significantly decline in the temporal posterior ciliary artery (TPCA) and the central retinal artery (CRA) [20] after HD. Combined with the findings of our study, we suggest that optic blood vessels can be considered to provide relatively insufficient blood supply after hemodialysis. Therefore, in this phase, clinical physicians should pay special attention to the prevention and treatment of ocular ischemic diseases.

No obvious change in BCVA occurred after HD. Moreover, no change in vision was related to the etiology of ESRD, leading to the conclusion that HD cannot directly affect vision. A previous study suggested that HD can improve BCVA [21], although some scholars hold the opposite view, particuarly for patients with DM-KD [10]. Similarly, we found that visual acuity before and after HD in patients with DM was significantly worse than in patients with other etiologies. Diabetes may be an important factor leading to reduced visual acuity because diabetes can cause and aggravate lens turbidity.

The central CT and endothelial number and form remained unchanged after HD, and the subgroup analysis showed that CT during HD in the DM-KD subgroup was significantly greater than that in the other two subgroups. However, previous studies have found that the CT was significantly reduced [2, 5, 11, 13] or remained unchanged [12, 22] after HD; this phenomenon is related to dehydration but is not correlated with DM. Our study differed in that we first used the Oculus Pentacam Anterior Segment Analyzer to measure the CT, and we recorded the corneal vertex thickness (Pachy apex) as the central CT. We used this approach because the Pentacam measurement principle is based on using the point at the Pachy apex as a benchmark, and the remaining points are obtained relative to this point. The different conclusions between previous studies and our present study require further research.

HD failed to change the spherical and cylinder power in our study, as Çaliṣkan et al. [16] concluded. However, the HD procedure significantly changed the average lens thickness and density. We believe that the process of HD partially dehydrated lens so that after HD, the average thickness of the lens decreased, and the relative density increased. Although the lens thickness change was highly significant, but the change was small, just about 2% in lens thickness. As mentioned above, the BCVA of the DM-KD subgroup was significantly worse than that of the other two subgroups. Therefore, in patients with CRF, particularly those with diabetic nephropathy, early screening and treatment for vision loss should be conducted.

Conclusions

In conclusion, renal failure patients undergoing HD may be at increased risk of developing vision-threatening complications, and both physicians of the hemodialysis unit and ophthalmologists should be made aware of this risk.

Abbreviations

ACD: Anterior chamber depth; AVG: Average cell size; BCVA: Best corrected visual acuity; CD: Endothelial cell density; CHT: Choroidal thickness; CSF: Central subfield; CT: Corneal thickness; CV: Cell size variation coefficient; DM: Diabetes mellitus; ESRD: End-stage renal disease; HD: Hemodialysis; IIM: Inferior inner macula; IOM: Inferior outer macula; IOP: Intraocular pressure; KD: Kidney disease; logMAR: Logarithmic minimum angle of resolution; LT: Lens thickness; NIM: Nasal inner macula; NOM: Nasal outer macula; RNFL: Retinal nerve fiber layer; SIM: Superior inner macula; SOM: Superior outer macula; TBUT: Tear break-up time; TIM: Temporal inner macula; TOM: Temporal outer macula

Acknowledgments
We would like to thank all the patients and personnel of the HD unit of Ruijin hospital affiliated with the Shanghai Jiao Tong University School of Medicine for their kind cooperation.

Funding
This work was supported by grant from Shanghai Hospital Development Center (SHDC12016116) Shanghai Key Laboratory of Visual Impairment and Restoration.

Authors' contributions
XS and HJC conceived and designed the study. HJC performed the experiments and wrote the paper. XS reviewed and edited the manuscript. XZ redid all the statistical calculations according to the reviewers' suggestions. All authors read and approved the manuscript.

Competing interests
The authors declare that they have no competing interests.

Author details
[1]Ruijin Hospital Affiliated to Shanghai Jiao Tong University School of Medicine, No. 197 Rui Jin Er Road, Shanghai 200025, China. [2]Xinhua Hospital Affiliated to Shanghai Jiao Tong University School of Medicine, No.1665 Kongjiang Road, Shanghai 200092, China.

References
1. National Kidney Foundation. K/DOQI clinical practice guidelines for chronic kidney disease: evaluation, classification, and stratification. Am J Kidney Dis. 2002;39:S1–266.
2. Jung JW, Yoon MH, Lee SW, Chin HS. Effect of hemodialysis (HD) on intraocular pressure, ocular surface, and macular change in patients with chronic renal failure. Effect of hemodialysis on the ophthalmologic findings. Graefes Arch Clin Exp Ophthalmol. 2013;251:153–62.
3. Ghasemi H, Afshar R, Zerafatjou N, Abdi S, Davati A, Askari MK, et al. Impact of hemodialysis on visual parameters in patients with end-stage renal disease. Iran J Kidney Dis. 2012;6:457–63.
4. Evans RD, Rosner M. Ocular abnormalities associated with advanced kidney disease and hemodialysis. Semin Dial. 2005;18:252–7.
5. Aktas Z, Ozdek S, Dinc UA, Akyurek N, Atalay V, Guz G, et al. Alterations in ocular surface and corneal thickness in relation to metabolic control in patients with chronic renal failure. Nephrology. 2007;12:380–5.
6. Mullaem G, Rosner MH. Ocular problems in the patient with end-stage renal disease. Semin Dial. 2012;25:403–7.
7. Tovbin D, Belfair N, Shapira S, Rosenthal G, Friger M, Feldman L, et al. High postdialysis urea rebound can predict intradialytic increase in intraocular pressure in dialysis patients with lowered intradialytic hemoconcentration. Nephron. 2002;90:181–7.
8. Nongpiur ME, Wong TY, Sabanayagam C, Lim SC, Tai ES, Aung T. Chronic kidney disease and intraocular pressure: the Singapore malay eye study. Ophthalmology. 2010;117:477–83.
9. Tokuyama T, Ikeda T, Sato K. Effect of plasma colloid osmotic pressure on intraocular pressure during haemodialysis. Br J Ophthalmol. 1998;82:751–3.
10. Pelit A, Zumrutdal A, Akova Y. The effect of hemodialysis on visual field test in patients with chronic renal failure. Curr Eye Res. 2003;26:303–6.

11. Dinc UA, Ozdek S, Aktas Z, Guz G, Onol M. Changes in intraocular pressure, and corneal and retinal nerve fiber layer thickness during hemodialysis. Int Ophthalmol. 2010;30:337–40.
12. Yang SJ, Han YH, Song GI, Lee CH, Sohn SW. Changes of choroidal thickness, intraocular pressure and other optical coherence tomographic parameters after haemodialysis. Clin Exp Optom. 2013;96:494–9.
13. Ulas F, Dogan U, Keles A, Ertilav M, Tekce H, Celebi S. Evaluation of choroidal and retinal thickness measurements using optical coherence tomography in non-diabetic haemodialysis patients. Int Ophthalmol. 2013;33:533–9.
14. Meshi A, Goldenberg D, Armarnik S, Segal O, Geffen N. Systematic review of macular ganglion cell complex analysis using spectral domain optical coherence tomography for glaucoma assessment. World J Ophthalmol. 2015;5:86–98.
15. Aktas S, Sagdik HM, Aktas H, Gulcan E, Tetikoglu M, Cosgun S, et al. Tear function in patients with chronic renal failure undergoing hemodialysis. Ren Fail. 2015;37:245–8.
16. Caliskan S, Celikay O, Bicer T, Ayli MD, Gurdal C. Effect of hemodialysis on intraocular lens power calculation. Ren Fail. 2016;38:209–13.
17. Hu J, Bui KM, Patel KH, Kim H, Arruda JA, Wilensky JT, et al. Effect of hemodialysis on intraocular pressure and ocular perfusion pressure. JAMA Ophthalmol. 2013;131:1525–31.
18. Ishibazawa A, Nagaoka T, Minami Y, Kitahara M, Yamashita T, Yoshida A. Choroidal thickness evaluation before and after hemodialysis in patients with and without diabetes. Invest Ophthalmol Vis Sci. 2015;56:6534–41.
19. Jung JW, Chin HS, Lee DH, Yoon MH, Kim NR. Changes in subfoveal choroidal thickness and choroidal extravascular density by spectral domain optical coherence tomography after haemodialysis: a pilot study. Br J Ophthalmol. 2014;98:207–12.
20. Yakut ZI, Karadag R, Akcay A, Bavbek N, Akay H, Koktener A. Effect of dialysis type on orbital vascular flow in patients with end-stage renal disease. Ren Fail. 2012;34:691–6.
21. Zhao HL, Qi XH, Shen W, Ye MX, Wu MQ. Investigation of changes in the biometric structure of the anterior chamber and intraocular pressure in patients with chronic renal failure after hemodialysis. Chin J Optom Ophthalmol Vis Sci. 2011;13:140–3.
22. Ohguro N, Matsuda M, Fukuda M. Corneal endothelial changes in patients with chronic renal failure. Am J Ophthalmol. 1999;128:234–6.

21

Utility of the optical quality analysis system for decision-making in cataract surgery

Jin Sun Hwang, Yoon Pyo Lee, Seok Hyun Bae, Ha Kyoung Kim, Kayoung Yi and Young Joo Shin[*]

Abstract

Background: A cataract is a common cause of vision impairment that requires surgery in older subjects. The Optical Quality Analysis System (OQAS, Visiometrics SL, Terrassa, Spain) assesses the optical quality of the eye in cataract patients. This study shows the role of the optical quality evaluation system for decision-making in cataract surgery. We investigated the clinical utility of the OQAS for decision-making in cataract surgery.

Methods: Sixty-seven eyes from 67 patients undergoing cataract surgery and 109 eyes from 109 control subjects were compared. The best corrected visual acuity (BCVA) was measured. The objective scatter index (OSI), modulation transfer function (MTF), Strehl ratio, predicted visual acuity (PVA) 100%, PVA 20%, and PVA 10% were measured using the OQAS. The sensitivity and specificity of the different parameters were analyzed using the receiver operating characteristic (ROC) curve. The main parameters measured were sensitivity and specificity.

Results: The BCVA, OSI, PVA 100%, PVA 20%, and PVA 10% were higher in the cataract group compared to those in the control group, while the MTF and Strehl ratios were lower ($p < 0.001$ for all). ROC analysis showed that the OSI had the largest area under the curve and that the sensitivity and specificity of the OSI were 83.9 and 84.6%, respectively, at the optimal cut-off point of 2.35.

Conclusion: The MTF, OSI, Strehl ratio, PVA 100%, PVA 20% and PVA 10% may be useful parameters for preoperative decision-making in cataract surgery. The OSI appears to be the most effective parameter for this purpose.

Keywords: Optical quality analysis system, Cataract, Objective scatter index, Modulation transfer function, Strehl ratio, Predicted visual acuity

Background

Cataracts are a common cause of vision impairment in the older population, affecting the quality of vision and visual acuity and negatively impacting daily activities [1–3]. Although age-related cataracts progress slowly, cataract surgery is ultimately required [4]. The timing of surgery depends on weighing the benefits of surgery against the risks [5]. Advances in cataract surgery and intraocular lenses have improved surgical outcomes, promoted early visual rehabilitation, and reduced complications [4, 5]. These advances have led healthcare professionals to recommend cataract surgery to patients in early stages of the disease [4–6]. However, cataract surgery performed on eyes with good preoperative visual acuity has been linked to adverse visual results [5].

Visual functions, including visual acuity, glare and visual difficulties with daily activity, should be considered in the preoperative decision-making process for cataract surgery [7]. An accurate assessment of visual function facilitates the preoperative decision-making process for cataract surgery, resulting in a minimization of visual discomfort for patients. Indeed, the optical quality impairment caused by cataracts has become one of the major indications for cataract surgery [5].

The Lens Opacities Classification System III (LOCS III) is a nuclear opalescence grading system that is used to assess nuclear cataracts and has been shown to be a convenient and effective method in several studies [8–10]. However, this method is not able to provide information regarding optical quality or assess the visual quality impairment caused by cataracts [11]. The Optical Quality Analysis System (OQAS, Visiometrics, Terrassa, Spain) is based on the double-pass (DP) technique and

* Correspondence: schinn@hanmail.net
Department of Ophthalmology, Hallym University Medical Center, Hallym University College of Medicine, 948-1 Daerim1-dong, Youngdeungpo-gu, Seoul 150-950, Korea

was developed to evaluate vision quality objectively [12, 13]. The OQAS allows an objective assessment of intraocular scattering [14] and objectively measures the effect of optical aberrations and the loss of ocular transparency on the optical quality of the eye [15]. It provides optical quality parameters, such as the objective scatter index (OSI), modulation transfer function (MTF), Strehl ratio, and predicted visual acuity (PVA). However, a study of the utility of the OQAS for decision-making in cataract surgery has not been reported, and the most appropriate parameter for facilitating the decision-making process for cataract surgery has not been determined. Thus, in the present study, we investigated the usefulness of the OQAS for decision-making in cataract surgery.

Methods

This study was a retrospective cross-sectional observational series. This study was approved by the Institutional Review Board (IRB) of Hallym University Kangnam Sacred Heart Hospital and adhered to the tenets of the Declaration of Helsinki for research involving human subjects. This study received a waiver of informed consent from the IRB of Hallym University Kangnam Sacred Heart Hospital because this study was a retrospective chart review study. The medical charts of patients who planned to undergo cataract surgery at Hallym University's Kangnam Sacred Heart Hospital between October 1, 2014 and August 31, 2015 and those of the control subjects were retrospectively reviewed. Data from all patients were collected and analyzed. The cataract group included the patients who needed cataract surgery and planned to undergo the procedure because they had a decrease in vision due to the cataracts. They wished to undergo the cataract surgery, had a visual acuity less than 20/30, had any type of cataract greater than grade 2, or had a cataract that affected the patient's lifestyle. They had normal retinal and corneal findings. The patients in the cataract group discussed the risks and benefits of cataract surgery with the surgeon, and then they decided to undergo the cataract surgery. During the same period, a gender-matched control group was included. The control group consisted of patients who visited the clinic for routine eye examinations, had minimal opacities in the lens, and normal retinal and corneal findings. Patients who had undergone additional intraocular procedures and patients with corneal abnormalities were excluded.

The best corrected visual acuity (BCVA) was assessed using the Hans visual acuity chart and refractive error with an auto kerato-refractometer (KR-8100, Topcon, Tokyo). Cataracts were classified using the LOCS III [8]. For this analysis, each subject was allocated an LOCS III grade based on the single highest score reported in each of the following categories: nuclear cataract (NC; on a scale from I to VI), cortical cataract (CC; on a scale from I to V), and posterior subcapsular cataract (PSC; on a scale from I to V) [8–10]. Mixed cataract was defined as a combination of any two types of opacity [9, 10].

Using an artificial pupil of 4.0 mm in diameter under mesopic conditions, the optical quality of the eyes was measured using the OQAS, which is an instrument based on the DP technique. The subject was asked to put his or her chin on the chinrest and fix the center of a figure. The examiner aligned the optical axis of the instrument with the subject's pupil center. During the measurements, spherical errors were corrected by an incorporated optometer in the DP system, while external lenses were used to correct cylindrical errors $\geq -0.50D$ [12]. The MTF, OSI, Strehl ratio, PVA 100%, PVA 20%, and PVA 10% were all measured using the OQAS. The MTF curve displays the percentage reduction of retinal image contrast at a variety of resolutions. The OSI quantifies the degree of ocular scattering caused by the loss of transparency in ocular structures, such as corneal haze, cataract, and vitreous opacities [16]. The acuity calculated using the OQAS represented optical characteristics of the eye, including aberrations and ocular scatter [16]. The maximum visual acuity was predicted for objects with 100, 20, and 10% contrast [16].

Statistics

A two-sample t-test was used to compare the patients undergoing cataract surgery to the control subjects. The similarities and differences between cataract classification groups were determined using the Kruskal-Wallis test following the Mann-Whitney U test. Statistical significance was based on two-tailed statistical analyses, and probability values < 0.05 were considered statistically significant. Visual acuity was measured in terms of the logarithm of the minimum angle of resolution (log-MAR). Receiver operating characteristic (ROC) analysis was used to calculate test sensitivity and specificity using SPSS 23.0 for Windows (IBM Corp., Chicago, IL). Comparison of the ROC curves was performed using the DeLong method from MedCalc version 11.4.4 statistical software (MedCalc Software, Mariakerke, Belgium).

Results

Data were analyzed from 29 men and 38 women in the cataract group and 33 men and 76 women in the control group ($p = 0.079$, chi-square test). The mean age was 67.34 ± 8.18 years in the cataract group and 59.45 ± 10.53 years in the control group ($p < 0.001$, t-test). The mean logMAR visual acuity was 0.48 ± 0.41 in the cataract group and 0.08 ± 0.23 in the control group ($p < 0.001$, t-test). The lens opacity grade using the LOCS III was 0.31 ± 0.47 for NC, 0.19 ± 0.44 for CC, and 0.00 ± 0.00 for PSC in the control group and 1.75 ± 1.03 for NC, 1.79 ± 1.30 for CC and 0.68 ± 1.17 for PSC in the cataract group ($p < 0.001$ between cataract group and control group for all, t-test).

Table 1 shows clinical findings for the subjects, including age, gender, and symptoms. There was no difference in gender between the control and cataract groups ($p = 0.104$, chi-square test). The control group was comprised of 109 eyes, while the cataract group was comprised of 67 eyes (from 67 patients). The BCVA (logMAR) was worse in the cataract group (0.48 ± 0.41) compared to that in the control group (0.08 ± 0.23; $p < 0.001$). Measurements obtained from the OQAS were compared between the cataract group and the control group (Fig. 1). The MTF was lower in the cataract group (11.38 ± 8.13) compared to that in the control group (22.14 ± 11.17; $p < 0.001$). The OSI was higher in the cataract group (6.23 ± 3.75) compared to that in the control group (1.75 ± 1.51; $p < 0.001$). The Strehl ratio was lower in the cataract group (0.08 ± 0.04) compared to that in the control group (0.13 ± 0.07; $p < 0.001$). The PVA 100% (logMAR) was higher in the cataract group (0.55 ± 0.32) compared to that in the control group (0.19 ± 0.26; $p < 0.001$). The PVA 20% (logMAR) was also higher in the cataract group (0.62 ± 0.34) compared to that the control group (0.31 ± 0.28; $p < 0.001$). Finally, the PVA 10% (logMAR) was higher in the cataract group (0.83 ± 0.21) compared to that in the control group (0.53 ± 0.29; $p < 0.001$).

Cataracts were classified into 4 types (Table 1). As a percentage of total cataracts studied, 29.9% were NC, 26.9% were CC, 13.4% were PSC, and 29.9% were mixed cataracts. There was no difference in gender between subgroups ($p = 0.394$, chi-square test). The Kruskal-Wallis analysis of the data grouped according to the cataract type revealed no significant differences in the BCVA, MTF, Strehl ratio, PVA 100%, PVA 20%, and PVA 10% between cataract types, whereas there was a significant difference in the OSI according to cataract type ($p < 0.001$; Fig. 2). The MTF was lower in the NC, PSC and Mixed groups compared to that in the CC group ($p = 0.041, 0.035$ and 0.048, respectively, Mann-Whitney U test). The OSI was higher in the NC, PSC and Mixed groups, compared to that in the CC group ($p < 0.001, 0.001$, and 0.001, respectively). The Strehl ratio was lower in the PSC group compared to that in the CC group ($p = 0.046$). The PVA 100% was higher in the NC and PSC groups compared to that in the CC group ($p = 0.048$ and 0.035, respectively). The PVA 20% was higher in the NC group compared to that in the CC group ($p = 0.022$). No difference in the BCVA and PVA 10% was observed between cataract types.

According to the ROC curve analysis (Fig. 3), the area under the curve (AUC) was 0.900 (0.847–0.953) for the BCVA, 0.805 (0.733–0.876) for the MTF, 0.902 (0.853–0.951) for the OSI, 0.800 (0.727–0.873) for the Strehl ratio, 0.828 (0.761–0.896) for the PVA 100%, 0.749 (0.6669–0.833) for the PVA 20%, and 0.791 (0.720–0.862) for the PVA 10%. Overall, the OSI had the largest AUC. The AUC for the OSI was larger compared to that for the MTF, Strehl ratio, PVA 20% and PVA 10% ($p < 0.001$ for all, DeLong's method). The sensitivity and specificity of the OQAS parameters for facilitating preoperative decision-making in cataract surgery are shown in Table 2. The sensitivity and specificity of the OSI at the optimal cut-off point of 2.35 were 83.9 and 84.61%, respectively.

Table 1 Comparison between control and cataract groups

| | Control group | Cataract group | | | | | | |
		Total	p-value	CC	NC	PSC	Mixed	p-value
N (eyes)	109	67		18	20	9	20	
Age (year)	59.45 ± 10.53	67.34 ± 8.18	< 0.001*	63.39 ± 6.75	66.35 ± 11.34	69.67 ± 8.53	68.15 ± 5.23	< 0.001*
Male: female	33:76	29:38	†0.079	8:10	7:13	4:5	10:10	†0.408
Eye laterality								
Right: left	54:55	34:33	0.877	10:8	12:8	1:8	11:9	0.185
SE (D)	−0.01 ± 1.71	− 0.25 ± 3.28	0.522	0.87 ± 1.52	−1.00 ± 3.00	− 1.514 ± 7.36	0.05 ± 0.92	0.062
BCVA (logMAR)	0.08 ± 0.23	0.48 ± 0.41	< 0.001*	0.43 ± 0.46	0.54 ± 0.43	0.68 ± 0.61	0.44 ± 0.47	< 0.001*
MTF	22.14 ± 11.17	11.38 ± 8.13	< 0.001*	15.17 ± 8.94	9.68 ± 5.39	8.48 ± 6.03	10.98 ± 9.65	< 0.001*
OSI	1.75 ± 1.51	6.23 ± 3.75	< 0.001*	2.99 ± 1.35	7.58 ± 3.38	8.82 ± 4.10	6.61 ± 3.70	< 0.001*
Strehl ratio	0.13 ± 0.07	0.08 ± 0.04	< 0.001*	0.09 ± 0.03	0.08 ± 0.03	0.07 ± 0.027	0.08 ± 0.05	< 0.001*
PVA 100% (logMAR)	0.19 ± 0.26	0.55 ± 0.323	< 0.001*	0.36 ± 0.24	0.61 ± 0.30	0.67 ± 0.31	0.59 ± 0.35	< 0.001*
PVA 20% (logMAR)	0.31 ± 0.28	0.62 ± 0.34	< 0.001*	0.48 ± 0.29	0.72 ± 0.26	0.64 ± 0.42	0.62 ± 0.40	< 0.001*
PVA 10% (logMAR)	0.53 ± 0.29	0.83 ± 0.21	< 0.001*	0.78 ± 0.20	0.86 ± 0.18	0.90 ± 0.17	0.85 ± 0.24	< 0.001*

NC nuclear cataract, CC cortical cataract, PSC posterior subcapsular cataract, SE spherical equivalent, BCVA best corrected visual acuity, MTF modulation transfer function, OSI objective scatter index, PVA predicted visual acuity
*statistically significant using Student's t-test, † the Pearson chi-square test

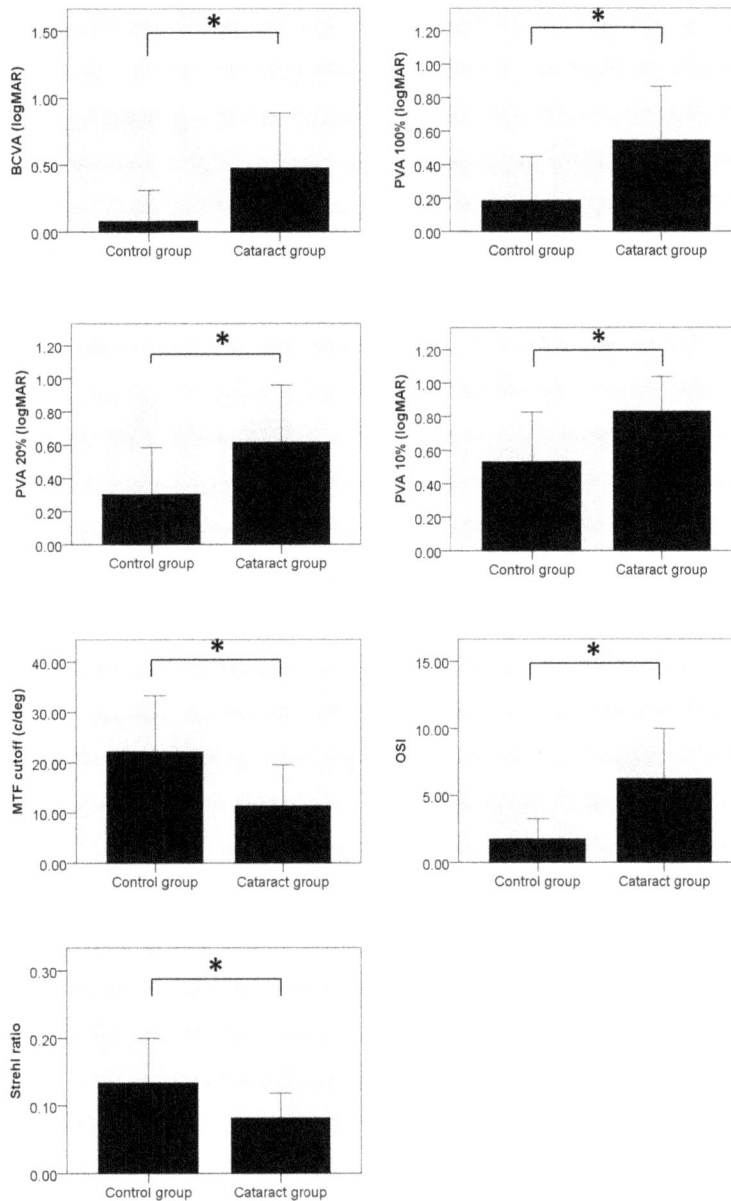

Fig. 1 The Optical Quality Analysis System (OQAS) parameters in cataract and control groups are shown. Best corrected visual acuity (BCVA), predicted visual acuity (PVA) 100%, PVA 20%, PVA 10%, and objective scatter index (OSI) were higher in the cataract group than in the control group ($p < 0.001$ for all, t-test). The modulation transfer function (MTF) and Strehl ratio were lower in the cataract group compared to that in the control group ($p < 0.001$ for all, Student's t-test). * statistically significant using Student's t-test

Discussion

Prior to cataract surgery, an assessment of the patient's discomfort resulting from the cataract and an objective evaluation of the consequent visual impairment are essential [5]. Optical quality has become an important factor for consideration during decision-making in cataract surgery because it has an effect on the quality of life [4]. The OQAS has been shown to provide robust and fully objective measurements of optical quality; i.e., not depending on subjective decisions [11]. Furthermore, the

OQAS has previously been suggested to be helpful when used in combination with standard methods to improve cataract surgery scheduling [11]. This study investigated the usefulness of different optical quality measurements obtained using the OQAS in the preoperative decision-making process for cataract surgery.

In this study, measurements obtained from the OQAS were compared between the cataract group and a control group. The BCVA, PVA 100%, PVA 20%, PVA 10%, and OSI were higher in the cataract group than in the

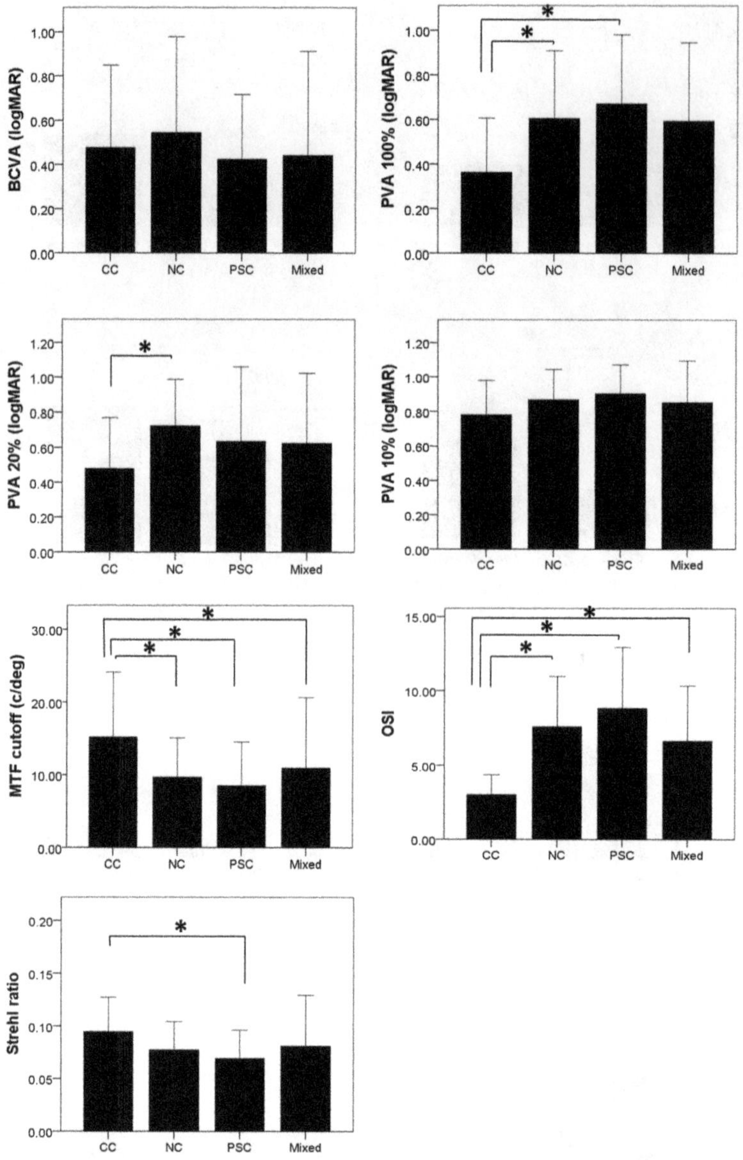

Fig. 2 The Optical Quality Analysis System (OQAS) parameters grouped according to cataract classification are shown. The Kruskal-Wallis analysis of the data grouped according to cataract type revealed significant differences in best corrected visual acuity (BCVA), modulation transfer function (MTF), objective scatter index (OSI), Strehl ratio, predicted visual acuity (PVA) 100%, PVA 20%, and PVA 10% among the cataract types ($p < 0.001$ for all). The MTF was lower in the NC, PSC and Mixed groups compared to that in the CC group ($p = 0.041$, 0.035 and 0.048, respectively, Mann-Whitney U test). The OSI was higher in the NC, PSC and Mixed groups compared to that in the CC group ($p < 0.001$, 0.001, and 0.001, respectively). The Strehl ratio was lower in the PSC group compared to that in the CC group ($p = 0.046$). The PVA 100% was higher in the NC and PSC groups compared to that in the CC group ($p = 0.048$ and 0.035, respectively). The PVA 20% was higher in the NC group compared to that in the CC group ($p = 0.022$). No difference in the BCVA and PVA 10% was observed between cataract types. * statistically significant using the Mann-Whitney U test

control group ($p < 0.001$ for all, t-test). In contrast, the MTF and Strehl ratio were lower in the cataract group compared to that in the control group ($p < 0.001$ for all, Student's t-test). It is important to note that these parameters were also different among cataract types. According to previous reports, the MTF cut-off frequency and the Strehl ratio decreased, while the OSI increased with aging [17]. The optical quality of a patient's eyes has been shown to degrade with cataract grade [18]. The

MTF was determined from an iTrace and a DP system from the OQAS and differed significantly in a comparison between subjects with early cataract development and normal controls [19]. However, the correlations of the MTF with visual performance were higher for the OQAS system. Thus, the MTF derived from the OQAS has been suggested to be useful as an indicator of visual performance in eyes with cataracts [19]. The OSI, another parameter obtained using the DP system, has been

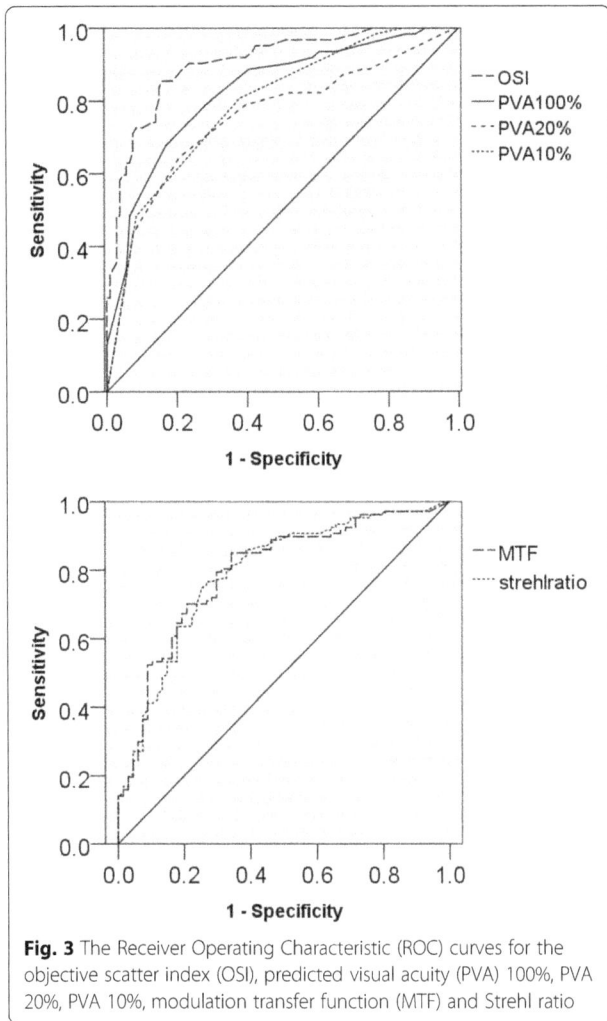

Fig. 3 The Receiver Operating Characteristic (ROC) curves for the objective scatter index (OSI), predicted visual acuity (PVA) 100%, PVA 20%, PVA 10%, modulation transfer function (MTF) and Strehl ratio

reported that several objective measurements obtained using the OQAS, including the MTF cut-off, OSI and Strehl ratio, differ between eyes with cataracts and control eyes [11, 16, 20, 21]. The MTF curve, computed from the point spread function (PSF), displays the percentage reduction of the contrast of the retinal image at various spatial resolutions and represents the combined effects of high-degree optical aberrations and scatter [16]. It is the ability of a lens or ocular structure to transfer the object contrast to the image. It has been suggested that the MTF plots are associated with the subsystems that make up a complete electro-optical or photographic system [22]. The MTF is associated with tear film stability [23] or the type of intraocular lens [24]. The OSI is defined as the ratio between the integrated light intensity in the periphery and that around the central peak of the double-pass image [11]. The OSI reflects the degree of scattering caused by the loss of transparency in the cornea or lens [16]. The OSI gradation relates directly to the extent of visual degradation (forward scatter) [11]. The higher OSI value represents a higher level of intraocular scattering [16]. The OSI has been found to correlate with NC and PSC severity [16, 25]. The Strehl ratio is defined as the ratio of the peak intensity of a measured PSF to that of a perfect optical system [26, 27]. The Strehl ratio expresses the ability of the eye to form a point image on the retina when a point object is seen [28]. It is related to wavefront errors [29], aging [17] and characteristics of the intraocular lens [24].

In this study, the MTF was lower in the NC, PSC and Mixed groups compared to that in the control, and the OSI was higher in the NC, PSC and Mixed groups compared to that in the control and CC groups. Optical quality by OQAS was measured in a pupil diameter of 4 mm [30]. The NC and PSC are located at the center of the lens and disturb visual quality [31]. Thus, central opacity of the lens may have a greater effect on optical quality [30]. A CC may have less effect on optical quality of the lens because a CC affects the periphery of the lens [8, 32]. The PVA 100% and PVA 20% were higher in the

shown to be correlated with the Scheimpflug-measured lens density, subjective lens grading, and cumulative dissipated energy. The measurement of the OSI may improve the preoperative evaluation of nuclear cataracts and help predict phacodynamics in cataract surgery [20].

Using ROC curve analysis, this study found that the AUC was the largest for the OSI. It has previously been

Table 2 Receiver operating characteristic curves for the OSI, PVA100%, PVA20%, PVA10%, MTF and Strehl ratio

	Cut-off point	Sensitivity	Specificity	J-index	AUC (95% CI)	p-value
BCVA (logMAR)	0.2600	70.6%	95.2%	0.650	0.900 (0.847–0.953)	< 0.001*
MTF	16.15	79.3%	72.1%	0.514	0.805 (0.733–0.876)	< 0.001*
OSI value	2.35	83.9%	84.6%	0.685	0.902 (0.853–0.951)	< 0.001*
Strehl ratio	0.0955	71.0%	78.8%	0.498	0.800 (0.727–0.873)	< 0.001*
PVA100% (logMAR)	0.2600	79.0%	71.7%	0.507	0.828 (0.761–0.896)	< 0.001*
PVA20% (logMAR)	0.4600	64.5%	79.2%	0.437	0.749 (0.666–0.833)	< 0.001*
PVA10% (logMAR)	0.6600	80.6%	62.3%	0.429	0.791 (0.720–0.862)	< 0.001*

AUC area under the curve, *95% CI* 95% confidence interval, *BCVA* best corrected visual acuity, *MTF* modulation transfer function, *OSI* objective scatter index, *PVA* predicted visual acuity
*statistically significant

NC, PSC and Mixed groups compared to that in the control group. An NC has opacities in the center, which may have an impact on the PVA 100% and PVA 20%.

Although the LOCS III grading system is still an economical and effective way to evaluate the severity of lens opacities, the OSI can be useful to assess the impact of cataracts on a patient's vision objectively when there is a difference between patient symptoms and ocular examination findings [21]. It is suggested that OSI scores ≥3.0 can be helpful as a possible cut-off for preoperative decision making [21]. In contrast to this previous study, we employed an ROC analysis to determine the cut-off value for the decision-making process in cataract surgery. The use of ROC analysis to evaluate diagnostic tests is widespread [33].

According to the ROC curve analysis, the OSI had the largest AUC. The AUC for the OSI was larger compared to that of the MTF, Strehl ratio, PVA 20%, and PVA 10% ($p < 0.001$ for all, DeLong's method). The AUC is an effective tool to assess sensitivity and specificity of diagnostic tests. The AUC summarizes the entire location of the ROC curve rather than depending on a specific operating point [34]. Thus, the OSI is the most accurate test for decision-making in cataract surgery. The Youden index (J-index) is used to determine the optimal cut-off point [35]. In our study, the sensitivity and specificity of the OSI were 83.9 and 84.6%, respectively, at the optimal cut-off point of 2.35. These results provided the rationale that cataract surgery may be postponed in eyes with low OSI scores, whereas cataract surgery is necessary in the eyes with high OSI scores. Visual functions should be considered in the preoperative decision-making process for cataract surgery [7]. The OQAS parameters directly relate with the visual degradation in any type of cataract [11, 13]. Because the cataract observed in a slit lamp examination is not always predictive of the actual visual impact, the OQAS parameters have the advantage of being able to predict the quality of the patient's vision and provide it to the operator.

One limitation of this study is that the quality of life was not measured even though a discussion occurred between the patients and the doctor in determining the cataract surgery. Further study is necessary to evaluate the quality of life in the decision-making process for cataract surgery. Another limitation was that the control group was younger compared to the age of the cataract group. The change in the OQAS due to aging is mainly associated with a decrease in optical quality secondary to cataract formation or lens changes [36]; cataracts increase with aging [37]. Therefore, the age of the cataract group was higher in the normal group. Another source of optical quality changes due to aging is corneal changes. The high order aberration of the cornea due to aging is increased [38], which can be reflected in the change in optical quality [39]; however, it does not have much effect. In this study, the cornea could not have affected the optical quality because all subjects had normal corneal findings.

In this study, the cataract group consisted of the patients with cataracts requiring cataract surgery. Although the difference in the OQAS between nonsurgical cataracts and cataracts were previously evaluated [40], further study including the patients with early cataract development is needed to increase the clinical significance of the decision-making process.

Conclusion
The MTF, OSI, Strehl ratio, PVA 100%, PVA 20% and PVA 10%, measured by the OQAS may be useful for preoperative decision-making in cataract surgery. Among these, the OSI is the most effective parameter for use in the decision-making process for the determination of the suitability of cataract surgery.

Abbreviations
BCVA: best corrected visual acuity; CC: cortical cataract; DP: double-pass; LOCS III: Lens Opacities Classification System III; logMAR: logarithm of the minimum angle of resolution; MTF: modulation transfer function; NC: nuclear cataract; OQAS: Optical Quality Analysis System; OSI: objective scatter index; PSC: posterior subcapsular cataract; PVA: predicted visual acuity; ROC: receiver operating characteristic

Funding
This study was supported by the National Research Foundation (NRF) grant (NRF-2015R1D1A1A09058505) funded by the Korea government and Hallym University Research Fund.

Authors' contributions
HKK, KY and YJS were responsible for the conception and design of this study. JSH, YPL and SHB acquired, analyzed and interpreted the data. JSH and YJS drafted the manuscript. All authors have read and approved the final manuscript and agree to be accountable for all aspects of the work in ensuring that questions related to the accuracy or integrity of any part of the work are appropriately investigated and resolved. All of the authors read and approved the final manuscript.

Competing interests
The authors declare that they have no competing interests.

References
1. Owsley C, McGwin G Jr, Sloane ME, Stalvey BT, Wells J. Timed instrumental activities of daily living tasks: relationship to visual function in older adults. Optom Vis Sci. 2001;78:350–9.
2. Klaver CC, Wolfs RC, Vingerling JR, Hofman A, de Jong PT. Age-specific prevalence and causes of blindness and visual impairment in an older population: the Rotterdam study. Arch Ophthalmol. 1998;116:653–8.
3. Morris D, Fraser SG, Gray C. Cataract surgery and quality of life implications. Clin Interv Aging. 2007;2:105–8.
4. Asbell PA, Dualan I, Mindel J, Brocks D, Ahmad M, Epstein S. Age-related cataract. Lancet. 2005;365:599–609.
5. Lundstrom M, Goh PP, Henry Y, et al. The changing pattern of cataract surgery indications: a 5-year study of 2 cataract surgery databases. Ophthalmology. 2015;122:31–8.

6. Javadi MA, Zarei-Ghanavati S. Cataracts in diabetic patients: a review article. J Ophthalmic Vis Res. 2008;3:52–65.

7. Schein OD, Katz J, Bass EB, et al. The value of routine preoperative medical testing before cataract surgery. Study of medical testing for cataract surgery. N Engl J Med. 2000;342:168–75.

8. Chylack LT Jr, Wolfe JK, Singer DM, et al. The Lens opacities classification system III. The longitudinal study of cataract study group. Arch Ophthalmol. 1993;111:831–6.

9. Pei X, Bao Y, Chen Y, Li X. Correlation of lens density measured using the Pentacam Scheimpflug system with the Lens opacities classification system III grading score and visual acuity in age-related nuclear cataract. Br J Ophthalmol. 2008;92:1471–5.

10. Grewal DS, Brar GS, Grewal SP. Correlation of nuclear cataract lens density using Scheimpflug images with Lens opacities classification system III and visual function. Ophthalmology. 2009;116:1436–43.

11. Artal P, Benito A, Perez GM, et al. An objective scatter index based on double-pass retinal images of a point source to classify cataracts. PLoS One. 2011;6:e16823.

12. Tian M, Miao H, Shen Y, Gao J, Mo X, Zhou X. Intra- and intersession repeatability of an optical quality and intraocular scattering measurement system in children. PLoS One. 2015;10:e0142189.

13. Guell JL, Pujol J, Arjona M, Diaz-Douton F, Artal P. Optical quality analysis system; Instrument for objective clinical evaluation of ocular optical quality. J Cataract Refract Surg. 2004;30:1598–9.

14. Diaz-Douton F, Benito A, Pujol J, Arjona M, Guell JL, Artal P. Comparison of the retinal image quality with a Hartmann-shack wavefront sensor and a double-pass instrument. Invest Ophthalmol Vis Sci. 2006;47:1710–6.

15. Kamiya K, Shimizu K, Igarashi A, Kobashi H, Ishii R, Sato N. Clinical evaluation of optical quality and intraocular scattering after posterior chamber phakic intraocular lens implantation. Invest Ophthalmol Vis Sci. 2012;53:3161–6.

16. Cabot F, Saad A, McAlinden C, Haddad NM, Grise-Dulac A, Gatinel D. Objective assessment of crystalline lens opacity level by measuring ocular light scattering with a double-pass system. Am J Ophthalmol. 2013;155:629–35. 35 e1–2

17. Kamiya K, Umeda K, Kobashi H, Shimizu K, Kawamorita T, Uozato H. Effect of aging on optical quality and intraocular scattering using the double-pass instrument. Curr Eye Res. 2012;37:884–8.

18. Ortiz D, Alio JL, Ruiz-Colecha J, Oser U. Grading nuclear cataract opacity by densitometry and objective optical analysis. J Cataract Refract Surg. 2008;34:1345–52.

19. Qiao L, Wan X, Cai X, et al. Comparison of ocular modulation transfer function determined by a ray-tracing aberrometer and a double-pass system in early cataract patients. Chin Med J. 2014;127:3454–8.

20. Lim SA, Hwang J, Hwang KY, Chung SH. Objective assessment of nuclear cataract: comparison of double-pass and Scheimpflug systems. J Cataract Refract Surg. 2014;40:716–21.

21. Pan AP, Wang QM, Huang F, Huang JH, Bao FJ, Yu AY. Correlation among lens opacities classification system III grading, visual function index-14, pentacam nucleus staging, and objective scatter index for cataract assessment. Am J Ophthalmol. 2015;159:241–7. e2

22. Kawamorita T, Uozato H. Modulation transfer function and pupil size in multifocal and monofocal intraocular lenses in vitro. J Cataract Refract Surg. 2005;31:2379–85.

23. Montes-Mico R, Alio JL, Munoz G, Perez-Santonja JJ, Charman WN. Postblink changes in total and corneal ocular aberrations. Ophthalmology. 2004;111:758–67.

24. Santhiago MR, Wilson SE, Netto MV, et al. Modulation transfer function and optical quality after bilateral implantation of a +3.00 D versus a +4.00 D multifocal intraocular lens. J Cataract Refract Surg. 2012;38:215–20.

25. Galliot F, Patel SR, Cochener B. Objective scatter index: working toward a new quantification of cataract? J Refract Surg. 2016;32:96–102.

26. Jiang B, Liu Y. An analysis on the equivalence of the eye to a system with aberration. Sci Sin B. 1982;25:970–80.

27. Bellucci R, Morselli S, Piers P. Comparison of wavefront aberrations and optical quality of eyes implanted with five different intraocular lenses. J Refract Surg. 2004;20:297–306.

28. Semeraro F, Romano MR, Duse S, Costagliola C. Quality of vision in patients implanted with aspherical and spherical intraocular lens: Intraindividual comparison. Indian J Ophthalmol. 2014;62:461–3.

29. Lee K, Ahn JM, Kim EK, Kim TI. Comparison of optical quality parameters and ocular aberrations after wavefront-guided laser in-situ keratomileusis versus wavefront-guided laser epithelial keratomileusis for myopia. Graefes Arch Clin Exp Ophthalmol. 2013;251:2163–9.

30. Vilaseca M, Romero MJ, Arjona M, et al. Grading nuclear, cortical and posterior subcapsular cataracts using an objective scatter index measured with a double-pass system. Br J Ophthalmol. 2012;96:1204–10.

31. Stifter E, Sacu S, Weghaupt H, et al. Reading performance depending on the type of cataract and its predictability on the visual outcome. J Cataract Refract Surg. 2004;30:1259–67.

32. Michael R, Barraquer RI, Willekens B, van Marle J, Vrensen GF. Morphology of age-related cuneiform cortical cataracts: the case for mechanical stress. Vis Res. 2008;48:626–34.

33. Swets JA. ROC analysis applied to the evaluation of medical imaging techniques. Investig Radiol. 1979;14:109–21.

34. Hajian-Tilaki K. Receiver operating characteristic (ROC) curve analysis for medical diagnostic test evaluation. Caspian J Intern Med. 2013;4:627–35.

35. Greiner M, Pfeiffer D, Smith RD. Principles and practical application of the receiver-operating characteristic analysis for diagnostic tests. Prev Vet Med. 2000;45:23–41.

36. Martinez-Roda JA, Vilaseca M, Ondategui JC, Aguirre M, Pujol J. Effects of aging on optical quality and visual function. Clin Exp Optom. 2016;99:518–25.

37. Bron AJ, Vrensen GF, Koretz J, Maraini G, Harding JJ. The ageing lens. Ophthalmologica. 2000;214:86–104.

38. Amano S, Amano Y, Yamagami S, et al. Age-related changes in corneal and ocular higher-order wavefront aberrations. Am J Ophthalmol. 2004;137:988–92.

39. Mihaltz K, Kovacs I, Weingessel B, Vecsei-Marlovits PV. Ocular Wavefront aberrations and optical quality in diabetic macular edema. Retina. 2016;36:28–36.

40. Filgueira CP, Sanchez RF, Colombo EM, Vilaseca M, Pujol J, Issolio LA. Discrimination between surgical and nonsurgical nuclear cataracts based on ROC analysis. Curr Eye Res. 2014;39:1187–93.

22

Phacoemulsification with hydrodelineation and OVD-assisted hydrodissection in posterior polar cataract

Xia Hua[1†], Yongxiao Dong[2†], Jianying Du[2], Jin Yang[3] and Xiaoyong Yuan[3*]

Abstract

Background: To evaluate the results and complications of phacoemulsification with hydrodelineation and ophthalmic viscosurgical device (OVD)-assisted hydrodissection for posterior polar cataract (PPC).

Methods: Medical records of 24 eyes from 17 patients with clinical diagnosis of PPC, who underwent phacoemulsification with hydrodelineation and OVD-assisted hydrodissection, were retrospectively reviewed.

Results: The incidence of posterior capsule rupture (PCR) was 16.67% (4/24): 2 cases occurred during epinucleus removal, and 2 cases occurred during OVD removal after the implantation of the intraocular lens into the bag. No nucleus piece or lens materials dropped into the vitreous during cataract surgery, and no obvious postoperative complications were found during follow-up. All patients had improved best-corrected visual acuity (BCVA) 1 month postoperatively.

Conclusion: OVD-assisted hydrodissection could be an effective technique in phacoemulsification to reduce the incidence of PCR and achieve satisfactory postoperative outcomes.

Keywords: Posterior polar cataract, Posterior capsule rupture, Ophthalmic viscosurgical device, Hydrodissection

Background

Posterior polar cataract (PPC) is a type of developmental cataract characterized by a white, well-defined, distinctive discoid opacity located on or in front of the central posterior capsule (PC) [1]. PPC presents a special challenge to the phaco surgeon due to its high risk of posterior capsule rupture (PCR), vitreous loss, and even nuclear drop during cataract surgery, which can occur because of extreme weakness, pre-existing dehiscence or tight adherence of opacity in the PC [2]. In general, cataract surgery, the incidence of PCR is less than 1% [2], while it is up to 36% in surgery for PPC [3–5].

During phacoemulsification, PCR occurs most often in the removal of the epinucleus [5] or the posterior polar opacity [6] for PPC cases. The recommended strategies [5–8] delay the removal of the posterior polar opacity in the epinuclear plate until complete emulsification of the whole nucleus to minimize the risk for dropping nuclear fragments and losing vitreous. In this study, we retrospectively evaluated the results of our case series of phacoemulsification with hydrodelineation, phacoemulsification of the nucleus, followed by ophthalmic viscosurgical device (OVD)-assisted hydrodissection in PPCs.

Methods

This retrospective study was approved by the ethics committee of the First People's Hospital of Xianyang, and all procedures were performed in accordance with the Declaration of Helsinki. From January 1, 2016 to December 12, 2017, patients with a clinical diagnosis of PPC based on slit lamp microscopy who underwent phacoemulsification with hydrodelineation and OVD-assisted hydrodissection were retrospectively reviewed to obtain data on the patients' demographics, preoperative and postoperative visual acuity, the integrity of the PC, and other complications during surgery.

* Correspondence: yuanxy_cn@hotmail.com

Xia Hua and Yongxiao Dong are co-first authors.

†Xia Hua and Yongxiao Dong contributed equally to this work.

[3]Tianjin Eye Hospital, Tianjin Key Lab of Ophthalmology and Visual Science, Clinical College of Ophthalmology, Tianjin Medical University, Tianjin 300020, China

Full list of author information is available at the end of the article

All surgeries were performed by the same surgeon (YD). After topical anesthesia, a 1-mm side port clear corneal incision was made, followed by injection of about 250 μl of a viscoelastic material Qisheng (Medical Sodium Hyaluronate Gel, Shanghai Qisheng Biological Agent Co., Shanghai, China), a viscous, cohesive gel with 1.5% sodium hyaluronate at a molecular weight of 2,000,000 to 2,500,000 Da, providing approximately 450,000 mPa·s at a shear rate of 0.01 Hz at 25 °C into the anterior chamber. A 2.8-mm, 3-stepped, clear corneal incision was made 90 degree to the right of the side port incision. Capsulorhexis was started by pinching the anterior capsule by the forceps, and continued with a 5.0-mm continuous curvilinear capsulorhexis (CCC), taking special care to avoiding viscoelastic escape from the incision. Only hydrodelineation was performed to separate the epinucleus and nucleus. A venture system phaco machine (Stellaris, Bausch & Lomb, Rochester, New York, USA) was set to a perimeter lower than normal at power 35%, vacuum 280 mmHg, and bottle height 70 cm. The phaco-chop technique was used. After the first division of the nucleus, we rotated the phaco tip towards one-half of the nuclear piece, followed by chopping and emulsifying in situ, avoiding any rotation of the lens pieces. Then for the

residual nucleus pieces, we left the integrated posterior epinucleus in situ. The above viscoelastic was injected carefully between PPC and PC from 3 o'clock to 9 o'clock, to lift the epinucleus with the posterior opaque and push down the PC. For large-sized PPC, bi-directional OVD-assisted hydrodissection was performed to release the synechia between PPC and PC. If the PC was judged to have integrated tentatively, routine irrigation and aspiration of the posterior epinucleus and cortex was performed by lowering the vacuum at 280 mmHg. A foldable IOL was implanted into the capsular bag.

If PCR was found during surgery, a dispersive viscoelastic (Viscoat, Alcon, Fort Worth, Texas, USA) was injected beside the OVD to see if the tear could be converted to a continuous curvilinear capsulorhexis. Vitrectomy with a high cutting rate of 800 cpm, low vacuum of 100 mmHg, and bottle height of 50 cm was then performed until the anterior chamber was free of vitreous, if necessary with viscoelastic instead of fluid irrigation, follow by IOL in the sulcus (Fig. 1).

After surgery, all the patients were given TobraDex (Alcon, Fort Worth, Texas, USA) qid. For the first week, which was tapered over the following 4 weeks. All the patients were routinely examined on the first day, first

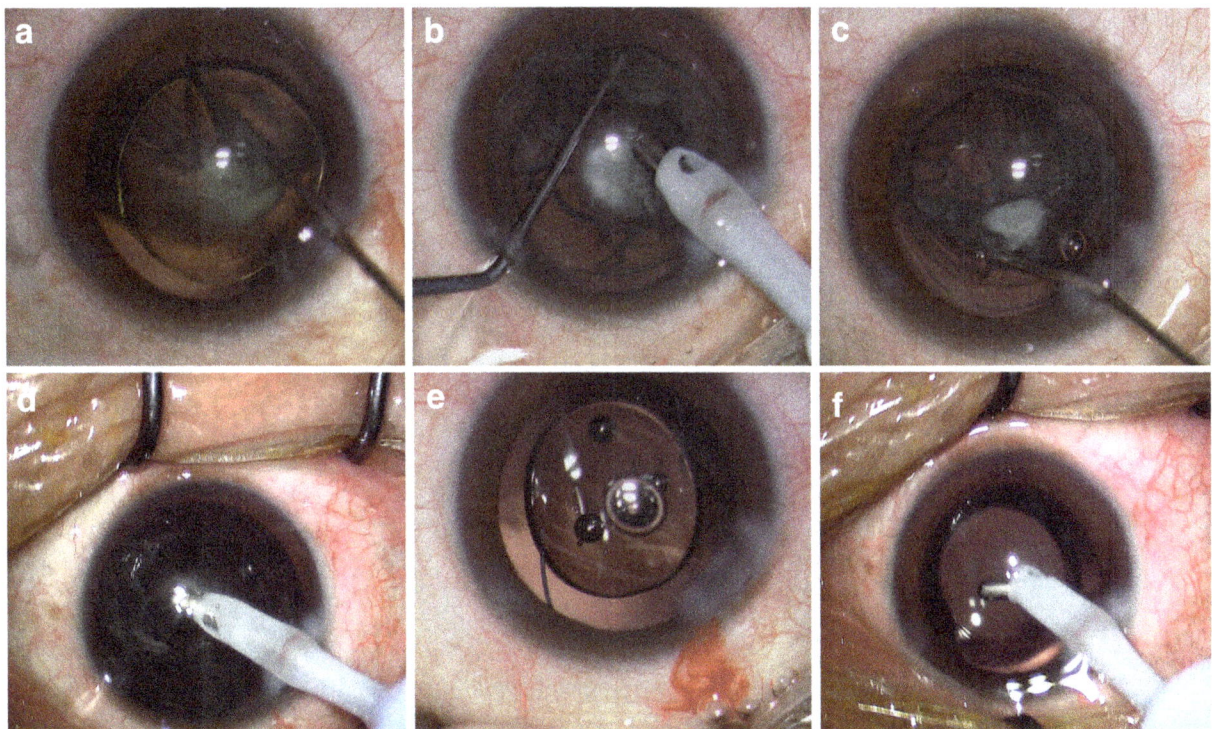

Fig. 1 a A golden ring followed hydrodelineation to separate the epinucleus and nucleus. **b** Phacoemulsification of the nucleus with the phaco-chop technique, leaving the posterior capsular cataract (PPC) with the epinucleus in situ. **c** Ophthalmic viscosurgical device (OVD)-assisted hydrodissection. The PPC was lifted with the epinucleus by injecting viscoelastic material between the PPC and the posterior capsule. **d** Irrigation/aspiration of the lifted PPC with the epinucleus. **e** A 3-piece acrylic IOL implantation into a sulcus with posterior capsular rupture. **f** A 1-piece acrylic IOL into a capsular bag with an intact posterior capsule

week, first month, and 6 months postoperatively. The data from the first month were evaluated here. And the comparisons of BCVA (logMAR) between 1 month post-operation and pre-operation were analyzed with Student's t-test. P value less than 0.05 (two tails) was considered as statistical difference.

Results
In total, 24 eyes in 17 patients with clinically diagnosed PPC were enrolled in this study (Table 1).

According to the Emery-Little classification, the nuclear sclerosis (NS) grades were II in 14 eyes, III in seven eyes, and IV in three eyes.

In all patients, CCC and hydrodelineation were performed uneventfully. The nucleus was successfully emulsified and aspirated in all cases of PPC. No PCR was noticed, and no vitreous prolapse or loss was found in this stage or before. In 22 eyes, OVD-assisted hydrodissection was successfully performed, as the OVD was injected between the capsular rim and the epinucleus. The posterior opacity was floated up and curled towards the main incision. The PC was pushed down, and a gap generated by the OVD suggested the PC was integrated at this stage. The I/A hand piece was inserted, and the epinucleus and cortex were removed by the phaco program.

In two cases, PCR was found during the OVD-assisted hydrodissection, and dense synechia was noticed between the PPC and PC. The OVD was carefully injected, and the PC was not pushed down; instead, a horizontal or an oblique rupture was noticed. A little more OVD was injected upon the PCR, followed by manual I/A of the epinucleus and residual cortex by a Simeco cannula. Of these two cases, the vitreous prolapsed in one case, and anterior vitrectomy was needed. In the other case, PPC was successfully floated up, and when automatic I/A was being performed, PCR occurred, followed by more dispersive OVD injection and manual I/A. A one-piece acrylic IOL was implanted into the bag if the PC was intact, and a three-piece acrylic IOL with PMMA haptics was inserted into the sulcus if PCR occurred. Then, OVD in the anterior and posterior chambers was removed by the I/A hand piece or Simeco canula.

After removing the OVD and before reforming the AC, two cases with acrylic IOL in the capsular bag were noticed with PCR. Therefore, some dispersive OVD was

Table 1 shows the clinical data of these patients

Demographics	
Age (years, mean ± SD)	62.12 ± 13.28
Male/female (n)	10/7
Right/left (n)	14/10
PCR	4 (16.67%)

injected upon the PCR, and the one-piece IOL was changed to the three-piece one in the sulcus.

In all patients, BCVA (logMAR) 1 month postoperation (0.15 ± 0.12) was much improved compared with pre-operation (0.58 ± 0.23) ($t = 8.23$, $p < 0.0001$). In addition, no obvious posterior segment complication was found, even in eyes with PCR. In 7 cases, minimal corneal edema and anterior chamber flare were seen on day 1 postoperation, but they had disappeared by 1 week postoperation. Temporary high IOP was found in 7 eyes, 2 of which had PCR. It was controlled by tapping some of the aqueous, and it recovered in 2 days. In 2 eyes with uneventful surgery, obvious macular degeneration was found after surgery. Both had a BCVA of 20/50, with deformation by 1 month postoperation.

Discussion
Because of the extremely thin or even defective local posterior capsule of PPC, PCR occurs at a high rate during ECCE, phaco surgery, and even femtosecond laser-assisted cataract surgery [3, 6, 9, 10]. PCR is inevitable for some cases of PPCs due to pre-existing posterior capsule defects or strong synechia between the posterior opacity and posterior capsule. Special care should be taken at all steps of cataract surgery for such cases.

In our study, all procedures started with a side port incision followed by injecting viscoelastic into the anterior chamber. We believe that the possibility of anterior chamber collapse might be lower with this approach than starting from the main incision, so this approach might be helpful for avoiding the rupture of a weak PC. Overloading viscoelastic injection should be avoided. For capsulorhexis, we preferred to use a forceps with a sharp tip, starting by pinching the anterior capsule instead of applying downward force. During the whole maneuver, it was important not to exert pressure on the incision and the operated eye; otherwise, the viscoelastic might overflow and the anterior chamber prolapse. a 5–5.5-mm capsulorhexis was performed. In our opinion, a too-large capsulorhexis is not suggested; although it can cause minimal turbulence in the capsular bag during phacoemulsification, if PCR occurs, not enough anterior capsule rim will exist to support the IOL in the sulcus [11]. Most previous studies suggested a 5.0- to 5.5-mm circular curvilinear capsulorhexis. Vasavada preferred 4.5 mm [5]. Pong and Lai suggested a 5.5- to 6.0-mm CCC for a hard nucleus [12]. Singh described an oval capsulorhexis technique with all grades of nuclear sclerosis for PPC with preexisting PCR, with good results [11]. In our cases, it was not difficult to perform the hydro process and phaco chop with a 5.5-mm-diameter anterior capsule opening, even for a moderate-hardness nucleus. Routine hydrodissection may cause a sudden fluid wave in the weak or defective PC of such cases, which should be avoided right after capsulorhexis. Many surgeons [7, 9, 13, 14] suggest only hydrodelineation at this stage for PPC. We performed conventional hydrodelineation with the cannula penetrating into the lens. As the fluid was injected from outside to inside, usually a golden ring was noticed, which indicated a successful hydrodelineation. A layer of epinucleus was in front of the PC, and the posterior polar opacity was left in situ. Then, phacoemulsification with lower vacuum and lower bottle height was started.

We selected the phaco chop technique in this case series. As the nucleus was divided into pieces, the nuclear material was emulsified in situ, without rotating with the epinuclear plane in front of PC, all of which might exert minimal stress on the capsular bag, especially the weak PC. During the process, it was important not to exert stress on the capsular bag and not to rotate the lens substance until all the nucleus was emulsified and aspirated. Another important issue was to keep the anterior chamber stable. Some viscoelastic could be injected through the side port before withdrawing the phaco tip.

Epinuclear removal might be the most dangerous and difficult part of PPC surgeries [15]. Some surgeons use a phaco tip with very low aspiration flow rate, vacuum, ultrasound power, and bottle height, to strip the epinucleus from the PC [5, 8]. In our case series, a medical sodium hyaluronate gel, Qisheng, was used as the fluid for hydrodissection at 180 degrees opposite the main incision to alleviate the epinucleus with posterior opacity from the PC. As more OVD was injected, the PC was noticed to be pushed down and the posterior opacity with the epinucleus flowed up, which was followed by the I/A tip instead of the phaco tip to remove the epinucleus gradually, and the residual cortex as well.

Posterior capsule polishing should be avoided, even the PC is intact with some opacity, because of the weak nature of such PCs [5, 6, 13]. Most PCRs in our cases were noticed during this stage, and some Viscoat was injected between the PCR plane and epinucleus. The epinucleus was then removed by manual dry aspiration with the Simcoe cannula if no or minimal vitreous was left out. Otherwise, anterior vitrectomy with a high cutting rate and low vacuum and bottle height was performed until the anterior chamber was free of vitreous. One piece of acrylic IOL was then inserted into the bag for the intact PC, or a three-piece of IOL (acrylic optical IOL with PMMA haptics) was inserted into the sulcus.

Different surgical techniques have been recommended to prevent or reduce the incidence of PCR in PPC cases. Osher et al. reported a 26% incidence of PCR during cataract surgeries with a slow motion phacoemulsification, combined with lower settings of aspiration, vacuum, and infusion pressure [6]. Using a lambda technique with dry aspiration, Lee and Lee's case series showed a PCR ratio

with 11.1% [14] . And Vasavada's group favored inside-out delineation with culmulative surgical experience, they reduced the incidence of PCR to 8% [16]. Compared with other reports of different surgical techniques for PPC, the PCR ratio in our case series is 16.67%, among which, 8.34% was found before IOL implantation, and the other 8.34% occurred after the removal of OVD in the anterior chamber.

We observed two cases of PCR when the anterior chamber collapsed after removing all the OVD. In both cases, the PC was intact after the one-piece acrylic IOL was inserted into the bag, and then, routine I/A of viscoelastic material was performed normally. After withdrawal of the I/A tip, the anterior chamber was shallowed, and then PCR was found. We believe that this kind of PC is fragile by nature and cannot endure pressure from the posterior segment and IOL as the anterior chamber disappears [9].

Only one eye did not reach satisfactory postoperative visual acuity, due to macular degeneration with uneventful cataract surgery. All other eyes had improved BCVA, whether PCR existed or not. With our technique of hydrodelineation first, then phacoemulsification of the nucleus, followed by OVD-assisted hydrodissection, the epinucleus with posterior opacity was easy to remove, and it was safe to handle the lens materials, even those with pre-existing PCR or PCR that occurred during this stage, since the chance of dropping the nucleus was minimal and leakage of vitreous was effectively pushed back.

Conclusion

In conclusion, PCR is sometimes inevitable in cases of PPC. We adopted different techniques to minimize the damages to the affected eyes. The goals of the surgery are to remove the PPC safely and to keep the integrity of the PC or reduce the chance of dropping lens materials and the loss of vitreous. Phacoemulsification with hydrodelineation and OVD hydrodissection for removal of the epinucleus was an effective treatment for PPCs.

Abbreviations
BCVA: Best-corrected visual acuity; CCC: Continuous curvilinear capsulorhexis; OVD: Ophthalmic viscosurgical device; PC: Posterior capsule; PCR: Posterior capsule rupture; PPC: Posterior polar cataract

Acknowledgements
We thank all the patients who participated in this study.

Funding
This study was financially supported by the Tianjin Research Program of Application Foundation and Advanced Technology (15JCYBJC54600, 13JCYBJC21500), and the project supported by Science & Technology Foundation for Selected Overseas Chinese Scholar, Bureau of personnel of China, Tianjin.

Authors' contributions

XH: design, data collection, analysis and interpretation of data, drafting of the manuscript. YD: case selection, data analysis and interpretation. JD: data collection, drafting of the manuscript. JY: data collection, drafting of the manuscript. XY: design, data interpretation, critical revision of the manuscript. All authors read and approved the final manuscript.

Competing interests

The authors declare that they have no competing interests.

Author details

[1]Department of Ophthalmology, the Second Hospital of Tianjin Medical University, Tianjin, China. [2]Department of Ophthalmology, the First People's Hospital of Xianyang, Shanxi 712000, China. [3]Tianjin Eye Hospital, Tianjin Key Lab of Ophthalmology and Visual Science, Clinical College of Ophthalmology, Tianjin Medical University, Tianjin 300020, China.

References

1. Vasavada AR, Raj SM, Vasavada V, Shrivastav S. Surgical approaches to posterior polar cataract: a review. Eye (Lond). 2012;26(6):761–70.
2. Osher RH, Cionni RJ. The torn posterior capsule: its intraoperative behavior, surgical management, and long-term consequences. J Cataract Refract Surg. 1990;16(4):490–4.
3. Das S, Khanna R, Mohiuddin SM, Ramamurthy B. Surgical and visual outcomes for posterior polar cataract. Br J Ophthalmol. 2008;92(11):1476–8.
4. Siatiri H, Moghimi S. Posterior polar cataract: minimizing risk of posterior capsule rupture. Eye (Lond). 2006;20(7):814–6.
5. Vasavada A, Singh R. Phacoemulsification in eyes with posterior polar cataract. J Cataract Refract Surg. 1999;25(2):238–45.
6. Osher RH, Yu BC, Koch DD. Posterior polar cataracts: a predisposition to intraoperative posterior capsular rupture. J Cataract Refract Surg. 1990;16(2):157–62.
7. Allen D, Wood C. Minimizing risk to the capsule during surgery for posterior polar cataract. J Cataract Refract Surg. 2002;28(5):742–4.
8. Fine IH, Packer M, Hoffman RS. Management of posterior polar cataract. J Cataract Refract Surg. 2003;29(1):16–9.
9. Consultation section. Cataract surgical problem. J Cataract Refract Surg. 1997;23(6):819–24.
10. Alder BD, Donaldson KE. Comparison of 2 techniques for managing posterior polar cataracts: traditional phacoemulsification versus femtosecond laser-assisted cataract surgery. J Cataract Refract Surg. 2014;40(12):2148–51.
11. Singh K, Mittal V, Kaur H. Oval capsulorhexis for phacoemulsification in posterior polar cataract with preexisting posterior capsule rupture. J Cataract Refract Surg. 2011;37(7):1183–8.
12. Pong JC, Lai JS. Managing the hard posterior polar cataract. J Cataract Refract Surg. 2008;34(4):530. author reply 530-531
13. Hayashi K, Hayashi H, Nakao F, Hayashi F. Outcomes of surgery for posterior polar cataract. J Cataract Refract Surg. 2003;29(1):45–9.
14. Lee MW, Lee YC. Phacoemulsification of posterior polar cataracts–a surgical challenge. Br J Ophthalmol. 2003;87(11):1426–7.
15. Vasavada AR, Vasavada VA. Managing the posterior polar cataract: an update. Indian J Ophthalmol. 2017;65(12):1350–8.
16. Vasavada AR, Raj SM. Inside-out delineation. J Cataract Refract Surg. 2004;30(6):1167–9.

23

Effectiveness of binocularity-stimulating treatment in children with residual amblyopia following occlusion

Haeng-Jin Lee[1,3] and Seong-Joon Kim[1,2,3*]

Abstract

Background: To evaluate the effectiveness of binocularity-stimulating treatment in children with residual amblyopia following occlusion therapy for more than 6 months.

Methods: Of patients with amblyopia caused by anisometropia and/or strabismus, patients with residual amblyopia following more than 6 months of occlusion therapy were included. Subjects underwent one of the following types of binocularity-stimulating therapy: Bangerter foil (BF), head-mounted display (HMD) game, or BF/HMD combination (BF + HMD). Factors including age, sex, types of amblyopia, visual acuity, and duration of treatment were investigated. Baseline and final (after at least 2 months of treatment) visual acuity were also compared.

Results: Twenty-two patients with a mean age of 8.7 ± 1.3 years were included. Seven patients had anisometropic amblyopia, 8 patients had strabismic amblyopia, and 7 patients had combined amblyopia. After 4.4 ± 1.8 months of treatment, logarithm of the minimum angle of resolution (logMAR) visual acuity in the amblyopic eye improved from 0.22 ± 0.20 to 0.18 ± 0.15. Five of 22 patients (22.7%) gained more than 0.2 logMAR, including 1 of 10 patients (10.0%) in the BF group, 2 of 7 patients (28.6%) in the HMD group, and 2 of 5 patients (40.0%) in the BF + HMD group. No significant differences in clinical characteristics were identified among the three groups.

Conclusions: Binocularity-stimulating therapy is somewhat beneficial in children with residual amblyopia and might be attempted when children no longer benefit from sufficient long-term period of occlusion therapy.

Keywords: Amblyopia, Residual amblyopia, Binocularity-stimulating treatment, Binocular treatment

Background

Most common treatments for amblyopia are monocular patching or penalization. By depriving the vision of sound eye, suppression of the amblyopic eye is eliminated and visual experience promote development or recovery of visual acuity of amblyopic eye. However, the response to patching usually reaches a plateau before vision in the amblyopic eye equals that of the sound eye [1–4], a condition referred to as residual amblyopia. Many amblyopes do not achieve a normal visual acuity, regardless of their patching compliance, and amblyopia often recurs after successful treatment in 25–50% of children [5–7]. In addition, older

children and adults with amblyopia are rarely treated by conventional treatment.

Recent studies have reported that abnormal binocular interactions play a key role in amblyopia [8–13]. Binocularity-stimulating therapies on amblyopia using perceptual learning or dichoptic stimulus presentation have been introduced [9, 10, 14–16]. The mechanism of dichoptic presentation is presenting a strong stimulus to the amblyopic eye and a weak stimulus to the normal sound eye. Many devices can be used for dichoptic presentation: head-mounted display (HMD) [11], liquid crystal display (LCD) shutter glasses [17], 3-dimensional (3-D) shutter glasses [18, 19], and an iPad [20–23]. Researchers have shown that this type of therapy is effective in treating childhood amblyopia, especially binocular iPad games [20, 23, 24]. However, these studies mostly examined pediatric patients with recent amblyopia diagnoses, and the effect of

* Correspondence: ophjun@snu.ac.kr
[1]Department of Ophthalmology, Seoul National University College of Medicine, Seoul, South Korea
[2]Seoul Artificial Eye Center, Seoul National University Hospital Clinical Research Institute, Seoul, South Korea
Full list of author information is available at the end of the article

binocularity-stimulation therapy on children with residual amblyopia (i.e., following patching and/or atropine therapy) has not yet been reported.

We previously developed a new software program which directly targets the binocular function using dichoptic presentation [25]. This program presents 3-D images in a virtual reality environment using a complete split screen view. The visual input to both eyes is controlled using an HMD. We evaluated the effectiveness of binocularity-stimulating treatment in children with residual amblyopia following occlusion therapy for more than 6 months using the HMD and Bangerter foil (BF).

Methods
Subjects
A medical chart review was performed on the prospectively collated subjects patients with amblyopia caused by strabismus and/or anisometropia between 2015 and 2016 at Seoul National University Hospital, South Korea. Patients with residual amblyopia following > 6 months occlusion therapy, who had good occlusion therapy compliance, and who underwent binocularity-stimulating treatment were included.

All patients underwent cycloplegic refraction at the first clinic visit to determine refractive error, which was converted to spherical equivalent values for statistical analysis (measured in diopters [D]). Myopia was defined as a negative spherical equivalent and hyperopia was defined as a positive spherical equivalent. Visual acuity was measured using a Snellen visual chart at every visit by one experienced examiner and was converted to the logarithm of the minimum angle of resolution (logMAR) for all data analyses. Ocular alignment was evaluated using the alternate prism cover test with accommodative targets for near (0.33 m) and distance (6 m) fixation. Stereoacuity was tested using the Titmus stereotest (Stereo Optical, Chicago, Illinois, USA). All values were transformed to log arcsec for the purpose of analysis.

Amblyopia was defined as an interocular difference of visual acuity between two eyes at least 0.2 LogMAR (2 lines). Types of amblyopia were divided as follows: anisometropic, strabismic, and combined. Anisometropic amblyopia was defined if there was a difference of at least 1.0D in spherical equivalent or 1.5D in astigmatism between the two eyes with no measurable strabismus. Strabismic amblyopia was defined as amblyopia in the presence of a heterotropia at distance and/or near fixation with a spherical equivalent interocular difference < 1.0D and < 1.5D interocular difference in astigmatism. The deviation is within 8 prism diopters with a history of strabismus surgery or resolution of misalignment after spectacle correction. Combined amblyopia was defined as amblyopia in the presence of both strabismus and anisometropia.

Patients with congenital or acquired ophthalmic conditions (e.g., optic nerve disease, glaucoma, media opacity, or cataract), systemic disease (e.g., neurologic disorders, developmental delays), or poor treatment compliance were excluded.

This study was approved by the Institutional Review Board of Seoul National University Hospital in South Korea and the study protocol followed the tenets of the Declaration of Helsinki. Written informed consent was obtained from the patients' parents or guardians and patients more than 7 years.

Binocularity-stimulating treatment
Patients prospectively underwent one of three randomly chosen types of binocularity-stimulating treatment. We used the randomly generated numbers using computer program. One physician who unaware of this study generated the program and sealed sequentially numbered envelopes, which were concealed from investigators. After confirming eligibility and obtaining written informed consent, one of us (H-JL or S-JK) opened a sealed envelope, and assigned the patient to the appropriated treatment. These included BF, HMD games, and combination BF/HMD game therapy and binocularity-stimulating treatment was performed for at least 2 months.

Group 1 underwent BF with 0.6-, 0.4-, and 0.2-strength BF. The BF with a similar level to the amblyopic eye was chosen and the appropriate BF was applied on the glasses of the sound eye for 6 h a day. Group 2 underwent HMD game therapy using the "Ice Cream Truck" game on an HMD for 30 min a day. This game is a casual shooting game that requires players to throw ice cream to kids running towards them. The game is presented on a split screen, which allows independent control of 3-D image contrast and intensity using the 16-level Gaussian blur method. The amblyopic eye is presented images with increased contrast and intensity, while the sound eye is presented images with decreased contrast and intensity (Fig. 1). The player has the ability to select gameplay level as normal, expert, or hard. Group 3 underwent BF/HMD game combination therapy. Patients watched a video or played the 3-D game in a virtual reality environment using HMD for 30 min a day with BF on glasses of the sound eye.

Assessment of effectiveness of binocularity-stimulating treatment
Patient age, sex, amblyopia type, visual acuity, and treatment duration were investigated. At baseline and at each follow-up visit, best-corrected visual acuity was measured in each eye. After at least 2 months of binocularity-stimulating treatment, baseline and final visual acuity were compared. We also evaluated the number of patients with a vision improvement of 2 Snellen lines (0.2 logMAR) or more after binocularity-stimulating treatment.

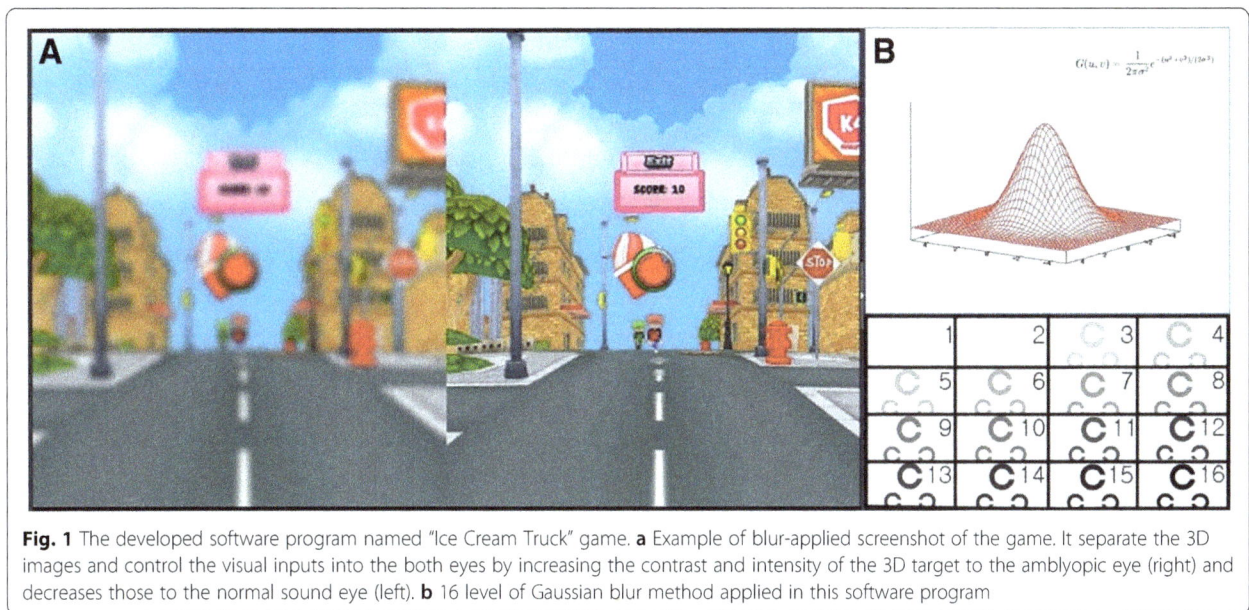

Fig. 1 The developed software program named "Ice Cream Truck" game. **a** Example of blur-applied screenshot of the game. It separate the 3D images and control the visual inputs into the both eyes by increasing the contrast and intensity of the 3D target to the amblyopic eye (right) and decreases those to the normal sound eye (left). **b** 16 level of Gaussian blur method applied in this software program

Statistical analyses

The ANOVA test and Fisher's exact test were performed using SPSS software (Version 16.0 for Windows; SPSS Science, Chicago, IL). For all tests, P-values < 0.05 were considered statistically significant. Continuous variables are reported as mean ± standard deviation.

Results

Demographic and clinical characteristics of subjects

Of total 22 patients (15 males) included, 10 patients were treated with BF, 7 patients were treated with HMD games, and 5 patients were treated with BF/HMD game combination therapy. The visual acuity at the initial visit was 0.73 ± 0.47 (range 0.2~ 1.8) LogMAR. Seven patients had anisometropic amblyopia, 8 patients had strabismic amblyopia, and 7 patients had combined amblyopia. The mean occlusion therapy duration was 2.5 ± 1.1 years (range: 0.7–4.7 years), and LogMAR visual acuity after occlusion was 0.22 ± 0.20 (range: 0.05–1.0). Occlusion therapy led to a visual gain of at least 0.2 LogMAR in 19 of 22 patients (86.4%). Mean age at the time of binocularity-stimulating treatment was 8.7 ± 1.3 years (range: 6.7–11.1 years) and mean duration of binocularity-stimulating was 4.4 ± 1.8 months (range: 2.1–8.1 months, Table 1).

Effect of binocularity-stimulating treatment on visual acuity

The visual acuity in amblyopic eye was changed from 0.22 ± 0.20 LogMAR to 0.18 ± 0.15 LogMAR after binocularity-stimulating treatment ($P = 0.252$). Of total 22 patients, there were no significantly different factors including sex, amblyopia type, and binocular treatment age, according to the types of treatment (Table 2). Five patients (22.7%) gained more than 0.2 logMAR of vision (1 of 10 patients [10%] in

Table 1 Demographic and clinical characteristics in children with residual amblyopia following occlusion for more than 6 months

	Total ($n = 22$)
Sex (male:female)	15:7
Refractive error (diopters)	
Amblyopic eye	+ 3.16 ± 4.10 (range − 5.50~ 7.50)
Fellow eye	+ 2.31 ± 2.67 (range − 2.25~ 7.75)
Laterality of amblyopic eye (right:left)	7:15
Types of amblyopia (A:S:C)	7:8:7
VA at initial visit (LogMAR)	0.73 ± 0.47 (range 0.2~ 1.8)
Duration of occlusion (years)	2.5 ± 1.1 (range 0.7~ 4.7)
VA after occlusion (LogMAR)	0.22 ± 0.20 (range 0.05~ 1.0)
Age at binocular treatment (years)	8.7 ± 1.3 (range 6.7~ 11.1)
Stereoacuities at binocular treatment (Logarcsec)	2.3 ± 0.2 (range 1.9~ 2.6)
Duration of binocular treatment (months)	4.4 ± 1.8 (range 2.1~ 8.1)
VA after binocular treatment (LogMAR)	0.18 ± 0.15 (range 0.0~ 0.5)

Continuous variables are reported as mean ± standard deviation
Abbreviations: A anisometropic, S strabismic, C combined, VA visual acuity, LogMAR logarithm of the minimum angle of resolution

Table 2 Comparison of clinical factors and visual acuity in children with residual amblyopia following occlusion for more than 6 months according to the treatment modalities

	BF (n = 10)	HMD (n = 7)	BF + HMD (n = 5)	P value
Sex (male:female)	6:4	5:2	4:1	0.852[b]
Types of amblyopia (A:S:C)	3:5:2	3:2:2	1:1:3	0.634[b]
VA at initial visit (LogMAR)	0.66 ± 0.44	0.77 ± 0.53	0.80 ± 0.58	0.844[a]
Duration of occlusion (years)	2.9 ± 1.3	2.6 ± 1.0	1.8 ± 0.5	0.215[a]
VA after occlusion (LogMAR)	0.17 ± 0.12	0.30 ± 0.32	0.21 ± 0.11	0.411[a]
Age at binocular treatment (years)	8.3 ± 1.2	8.7 ± 1.5	9.5 ± 1.4	0.289[a]
Duration of binocular treatment (months)	4.7 ± 2.4	4.2 ± 1.4	4.1 ± 1.1	0.795[a]
VA after binocular treatment (LogMAR)	0.19 ± 0.17	0.17 ± 0.07	0.17 ± 0.19	0.958[a]

Continuous variables are reported as mean ± standard deviation
Abbreviations: BF Bangerter foil, HMD Head-mounted display, A anisometropic, S strabismic, C combined, VA visual acuity, LogMAR logarithm of the minimum angle of resolution
[a]ANOVA test
[b]Fisher's exact test

the BF group, 2 of 7 patients [28.6%] in the HMD group, and 2 of 5 patients [40%] in the BF + HMD group, Fig. 2).

Discussion
Though the mainstay treatment for unilateral amblyopia has traditionally been penalization of the sound eye, there is growing interest in the role of binocular treatments. As further clinical evidence on amblyopia management is accumulated, there may be a shift from penalization and an inclination toward binocular stimulation to improve binocular interaction and promote binocularity.

Binocularity-stimulating treatments include the use of movies and video games displayed on a split screen, with some media components presented in low contrast images for the sound eye and high contrast images for the amblyopic

eye. Li et al. [26] examined the effect of watching three dichoptic movies per week for 2 weeks on 8 amblyopic patients (4 patients with anisometropic amblyopia, 1 patient with strabismic amblyopia, and 4 patients with combination amblyopia) that were 4–10 years old. Before treatment, the amblyopic eye visual acuity ranged from 0.24–1.20 LogMAR. They reported that the mean improvement in visual acuity was 2 lines. However, their study only included a small number of patients and had a short follow-up period (2 weeks).

Vedamurthy et al. [27] conducted a larger study on older patients that compared amblyopic patients who watched movies with a patch (n = 15 patients) to those who played dichoptic video games (n = 23 patients). In each treatment group, approximately half of patients had anisometropic amblyopia and half of patients had strabismic amblyopia.

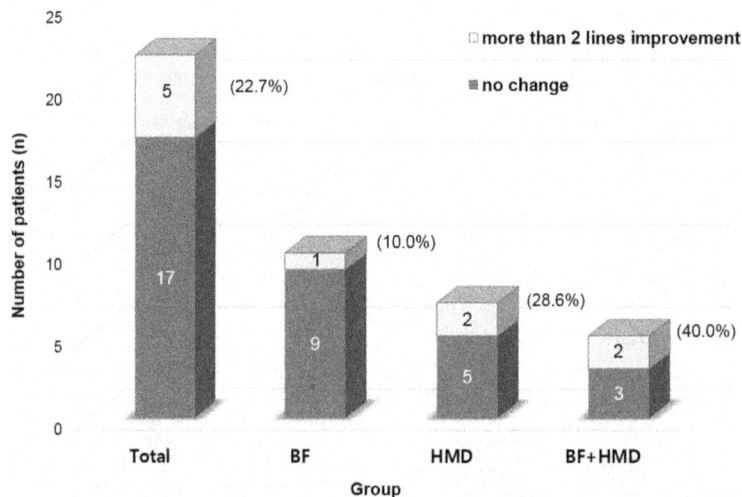

Fig. 2 Distribution and change of visual acuity in children with residual amblyopia following occlusion for more than 6 months. Five patients (22.7%) presented more than 0.2 logMAR improvement of visual acuity: 1 of 10 patients (10%) in the BF group, 2 of 7 patients (28.6%) in the HMD group, and 2 of 5 patients (40%) in the BF + HMD group

Participants were required to perform their assigned visual activities for 1.5–2 h at least 2–5 times per week for a total of 40 h. They found that the dichoptic video game group had an overall improvement in stereopsis and contrast sensitivity shortly after and 2 months after initiating the intervention.

These prior studies included patients with newly diagnosed amblyopia and treated patients with binocularity-stimulating therapies without any experience of conventional treatment (e.g., patching) [20, 23, 24, 26]. In contrast, our study included amblyopic children who had reached a treatment response plateau after a sufficiently long period of occlusion therapy (residual amblyopes). Residual amblyopia is generally considered to be an untreatable condition, and conventional therapies offer no options for further visual acuity improvements. Before binocular therapy, mean occlusion duration was 2.5 ± 1.1 years and occlusion compliance was good. Even though 86.4% of our patients gained at least 2 lines of vision with more than 6 months of patching, vision in the amblyopic eye had still not reached that of the sound eye. Therefore, different treatments were needed to further improve visual acuity.

We tried binocularity-stimulating treatment using BF and HMD games. Chen et al. [28] reported that BF can immediately reduce suppression and promote binocular summation for mid/low spatial frequencies in observers with amblyopia. In addition, we previously developed a new software program that directly targets binocular function with dichoptic presentation [25]. This program presents 3-D images in a virtual reality environment using an HMD. The system targets binocular function by presenting 3-D images on a split screen. In the virtual reality environment, image contrast and intensity can be independently adjusted for each eye and were increased in the amblyopic eye and decreased in the sound eye. Therefore, patients are forced to use both the sound and amblyopic eye to successfully play games or watch movies. In the present study, mean patient age at the time of binocular treatment was 8.7 ± 1.3 years and mean binocularity-stimulating treatment duration was 4.4 ± 1.8 months. All patients had good therapy compliance. Of the 22 patients included, 5 patients (22.7%) gained more than 0.2 logMAR of vision. Even though we only examined a small number of patients, this result could be meaningful because we only included residual amblyopes.

Our study had several limitations. First, the number of subjects was small and there was no control group which was observed without any treatment. We could not include the control subjects because of ethical issue. In addition, even if we assigned the treatment randomly by masked physician, participants and investigators were not blinded after treatment. To check the compliance and detect any complications/side effects following binocular treatment, we had to know the types of treatment. However, it would be the major limitation, so further blinded prospective research on a larger group of amblyopic children and adults is necessary to prove binocular treatment efficacy. Second, images presented by the HMD had a relatively low resolution. Therefore, display resolution improvements are needed. Investigations to determine optimum utilization in the clinic and at patient homes are also needed.

Conclusions

To the best of our knowledge, this is the first study to report results of binocularity-stimulating treatment in children with residual amblyopia. There may be some benefit of binocularity-stimulating treatments in residual amblyopic children. Therefore, binocularity-stimulating treatments should be considered in children with residual amblyopia following long-term occlusion therapy.

Abbreviations
BF: Bangerter foil; D: Diopters; HMD: Head-mounted display

Funding
This work was supported by the National Research Foundation of Korea (NRF) Grant funded by the Korean Government (MOE) (No. 2017R1D1A1B03032985).

Authors' contributions
Design of the study (SJK); Conduct of the study (HJL, SJK); Collection and management of data (HJL, SJK); Analysis and interpretation of data (HJL, SJK); Preparation, review, or approval of the manuscript (HJL, SJK). All authors read and approved the final manuscript.

Competing interests
The authors declare that they have no competing interests.

Author details
[1]Department of Ophthalmology, Seoul National University College of Medicine, Seoul, South Korea. [2]Seoul Artificial Eye Center, Seoul National University Hospital Clinical Research Institute, Seoul, South Korea. [3]Department of Ophthalmology, Seoul National University Hospital, 101 Daehak-Ro, Jongno-Gu, Seoul 110-744, Republic of Korea.

References
1. Pediatric Eye Disease Investigator Group. A randomized trial of atropine vs. patching for treatment of moderate amblyopia in children. Arch Ophthal. 2002;120(3):268–78.
2. Levartovsky S, Gottesman N, Shimshoni M, Oliver M. Factors affecting long-term results of successfully treated amblyopia: age at beginning of

treatment and age at cessation of monitoring. J Pediatr Ophthalmol Strabismus. 1992;29(4):219–23.

3. Repka MX, Cotter SA, Beck RW, Kraker RT, Birch EE, Everett DF, Hertle RW, Holmes JM, Quinn GE, Sala NA, et al. A randomized trial of atropine regimens for treatment of moderate amblyopia in children. Ophthalmol. 2004;111(11):2076–85.

4. Scott WE, Dickey CF. Stability of visual acuity in amblyopic patients after visual maturity. Graefe's Arch Clin Exp Ophthalmol. 1988;226(2):154–7.

5. Holmes JM, Beck RW, Kraker RT, Astle WF, Birch EE, Cole SR, Cotter SA, Donahue S, Everett DF, Hertle RW, et al. Risk of amblyopia recurrence after cessation of treatment. Journal of AAPOS. 2004;8(5):420–8.

6. Wallace DK, Edwards AR, Cotter SA, Beck RW, Arnold RW, Astle WF, Barnhardt CN, Birch EE, Donahue SP, Everett DF, et al. A randomized trial to evaluate 2 hours of daily patching for strabismic and anisometropic amblyopia in children. Ophthalmol. 2006;113(6):904–12.

7. Rutstein RP, Quinn GE, Lazar EL, Beck RW, Bonsall DJ, Cotter SA, Crouch ER, Holmes JM, Hoover DL, Leske DA, et al. A randomized trial comparing Bangerter filters and patching for the treatment of moderate amblyopia in children. Ophthalmol. 2010;117(5):998–1004 e1006.

8. Hess RF, Mansouri B, Thompson B. A binocular approach to treating amblyopia: antisuppression therapy. Optometry Vis Sci. 2010;87(9):697–704.

9. Hess RF, Mansouri B, Thompson B. Restoration of binocular vision in amblyopia. Strabismus. 2011;19(3):110–8.

10. Hess RF, Thompson B. New insights into amblyopia: binocular therapy and noninvasive brain stimulation. Journal of AAPOS. 2013;17(1):89–93.

11. Knox PJ, Simmers AJ, Gray LS, Cleary M. An exploratory study: prolonged periods of binocular stimulation can provide an effective treatment for childhood amblyopia. Invest Ophthalmol Vis Sci. 2012;53(2):817–24.

12. Li J, Thompson B, Deng D, Chan LY, Yu M, Hess RF. Dichoptic training enables the adult amblyopic brain to learn. Current Bio. 2013;23(8): R308–9.

13. Murphy KM, Roumeliotis G, Williams K, Beston BR, Jones DG. Binocular visual training to promote recovery from monocular deprivation. J Vis. 2015;15(1): 15.11.12.

14. Hess RF, Mansouri B, Thompson B. A new binocular approach to the treatment of amblyopia in adults well beyond the critical period of visual development. Restor Neurol Neurosci. 2010;28(6):793–802.

15. Hess RF, Thompson B, Black JM, Machara G, Zhang P, Bobier WR, Cooperstock J. An iPod treatment of amblyopia: an updated binocular approach. Optometry. 2012;83(2):87–94.

16. Li RW, Young KG, Hoenig P, Levi DM. Perceptual learning improves visual performance in juvenile amblyopia. Invest Ophthalmol Vis Sci. 2005;46(9): 3161–8.

17. Bossi M, Anderson EJ, Tailor V, Bex PJ, Greenwood JA, Dahlmann-Noor A, Dakin SC. An exploratory study of a novel home-based binocular therapy for childhood amblyopia. Investigative Ophthalmology and Visual Science. 2014;55:ARVO E-Abstract 5981.

18. Herbison N, Cobb S, Gregson R, Ash I, Eastgate R, Purdy J, Hepburn T, MacKeith D, Foss A. Interactive binocular treatment (I-BiT) for amblyopia: results of a pilot study of 3D shutter glasses system. Eye. 2013;27(9):1077–83.

19. Foss AJ, Gregson RM, MacKeith D, Herbison N, Ash IM, Cobb SV, Eastgate RM, Hepburn T, Vivian A, Moore D, et al. Evaluation and development of a novel binocular treatment (I-BiT) system using video clips and interactive games to improve vision in children with amblyopia ('lazy eye'): study protocol for a randomised controlled trial. Trials. 2013;14:145.

20. Birch EE, Li SL, Jost RM, Morale SE, De La Cruz A, Stager D Jr, Dao L, Stager DR Sr. Binocular iPad treatment for amblyopia in preschool children. J AAPOS. 2015;19(1):6–11.

21. Handa T, Ishikawa H, Shoji N, Ikeda T, Totuka S, Goseki T, Shimizu K. Modified iPad for treatment of amblyopia: a preliminary study. J AAPOS. 2015;19(6):552–4.

22. Li SL, Jost RM, Morale SE, De La Cruz A, Dao L, Stager D Jr, Birch EE. Binocular iPad treatment of amblyopia for lasting improvement of visual acuity. JAMA Ophthalmology. 2015;133(4):479–80.

23. Li SL, Jost RM, Morale SE, Stager DR, Dao L, Stager D, Birch EE. A binocular iPad treatment for amblyopic children. Eye. 2014;28(10):1246–53.

24. Kelly KR, Jost RM, Dao L, Beauchamp CL, Leffler JN, Birch EE. Binocular iPad game vs patching for treatment of amblyopia in children: a randomized clinical trial. JAMA Ophthalmology. 2016;134(12):1402–8.

25. Lee HJ, Kim S-J. Newly developed binocular treatment of amblyopia using head-mounted display. Invest Ophthalmol Vis Sci. 2016;57(12):3081–1.

26. Li SL, Reynaud A, Hess RF, Wang YZ, Jost RM, Morale SE, De La Cruz A, Dao L, Stager D Jr, Birch EE. Dichoptic movie viewing treats childhood amblyopia. J AAPOS. 2015;19(5):401–5.

27. Vedamurthy I, Nahum M, Huang SJ, Zheng F, Bayliss J, Bavelier D, Levi DM. A dichoptic custom-made action video game as a treatment for adult amblyopia. Vis Res. 2015;114:173–87.

28. Chen Z, Li J, Thompson B, Deng D, Yuan J, Chan L, Hess RF, Yu M. The effect of Bangerter filters on binocular function in observers with amblyopia. Invest Ophthalmol Vis Sci. 2015;56(1):139–49.

24

The efficacy and safety of Retcam in detecting neonatal retinal hemorrhages

Feng Chen[1], Dan Cheng[1], Jiandong Pan[1], Chongbin Huang[2], Xingxing Cai[2], Zhongxu Tian[1], Fan Lu[1] and Lijun Shen[1*]

Abstract

Background: To investigate the ability of characterizing neonatal retinal hemorrhage (RH) using RetCam in healthy newborns and the systemic effects during the procedure.

Methods: This prospective study enrolled 68 healthy newborns aged 2 to 4 days old. The RH was imaged and classified according to the location and numbers of hemorrhages. The heart rate (HR), respiration rate (RR), and oxygen saturation (OS) were recorded at 4 time points before (Phase 1, P1), during (P2 and P3) and after the examination (P4).

Results: The median exam time was 151 s. RH was present in 15 infants and 23 eyes. All 23 eyes had hemorrhage in Zone II. Grade II and III hemorrhages were present in 5 and 18 eyes, respectively. The HR increased to 168 beats per minute (bpm) in P3 and recovered to 122.5 bpm in P4. The RR increased to 38 bpm in P3 and recovered to 25 bpm in P4. The OS was reduced to 83% in P2 and recovered to 96% in P4.

Conclusions: RH in healthy newborns, mostly present in Zone II with grade II and III, can be characterized in detail by RetCam. Systemic effects during the process are mild and can be revolved spontaneously.

Keywords: Neonatal retinal hemorrhage, Digital imaging, RetCam, Fundus examination, Systemic effects

Background

With its initial detection in 1861, retinal hemorrhage (RH) in newborns has been reported frequently [1]. The incidence of neonatal RH (NRH) varies widely from 2.6 to 50.0% [2–8]. Birth-related RH is commonly bilateral, intraretinal, localized primarily to the posterior retina, and rapidly resolved without any visual deficits [1, 9, 10]. The follow-up of the development of birth-related hemorrhage may play a significant role in the process of neonatal eye examination [11]. In addition, an accurate description of retinal bleeding is extremely important given its association with abusive head trauma [1, 12]. The direct ophthalmoscope and indirect ophthalmoscope were successively used for the primary examination of the fundus of the newborns. Nevertheless, the examination results had inadequate examination range or were particularly subjective. Currently, a wide-angle fundus camera (RetCam, Clarity Medical Systems USA) allowing immediate visualization and real-time recording of fundus findings has become widely used in fundus examination and has potential in recording RH on newborns [13, 14].

To our knowledge, the systemic effects of the fundus examination in healthy newborns have not been studied. Several studies have reported on systemic effects of the screening examination on retinopathy of prematurity (ROP) in preterm infants [15–20]. The preterm infants exhibited increased blood pressure, decreased oxygen saturation, increased pulse rate [15], CRIES pain score [17], facial responses to pain [18], and salivary cortisol [19] after examination. The healthy newborns' behavior during the fundus examination may differ from the preterm infants' behavior based on the existence of different demographics. This study aimed to detect the ability of screening birth-related RH by RetCam examination and to identify any significant systemic effects during the process in healthy newborns.

* Correspondence: ljshenysg@163.com
[1]School of Optometry and Ophthalmology and Eye Hospital of Wenzhou Medical University, Number 270, West Xueyuan Road, Lucheng District, Wenzhou 325000, Zhejiang, China
Full list of author information is available at the end of the article

Methods

This study was approved by the research ethics committees at Eye Hospital of Wenzhou Medical University (Wenzhou, Zhenjiang, China), and informed parental consent was obtained before the study. This study adhered to the tenets of the Declaration of Helsinki. Consecutive 68 healthy newborns receiving neonatal RH screening examination during a two-week study period at Yueqing Maternal and Child Health Hospital (Yueqing, Zhejiang, China) were included in the study from January 2013 to February 2015. Babies with known or suspected systemic or ocular disease or congenital malformation were excluded.

The fundus examination was performed by an experienced ophthalmologist with a digital wide-angle retinal imaging device (RetCam III; Clarity Medical Systems, Pleasanton, California) within 3 days after the birth of newborns. A neonatologist was always on standby during the examination to manage the subjects' systemic condition. Every baby was offered a soother to suck during the examination unless it rejected the sucker. Pupillary dilatation was obtained with 0.5% tropicamide phenylephrine eye drops (Santen Pharmaceutical Co., Osaka, Japan) instilled twice every 5 min one hour before examination. Immediately before the eye examination, local anesthetic eye drops were administered with 0.5% proxymetacaine (Alcon Laboratories, Texas, USA). The eyelid was opened using an infant speculum (MR-0103-1, Xiehemedical, Suzhou, China). The 130 diopter camera lens was placed on the cornea after carbomer eye drops (Bausch & Lomb, Berlin, Germany) and applied onto the cornea. Both eyes of every newborn were examined, and there was an approximately 10-s pause between the time when the camera lens switched from the right eye to left eye. For each eye, 5 images were obtained that covered the posterior pole, temporal quadrant, superior quadrant, nasal quadrant and inferior quadrant, separately. By pushing the eye globe with the camera lens, the peripheral image was obtained. Fundus examination was performed in the morning between 9:00 and 12:00 AM, and the infants kept in incubators. Newborns with RH were re-examined 4 weeks later.

Hemorrhages were classified according to the location and number of the hemorrhages by two masked readers (FC and JP) after the examination [1]. Zone I encompassed one disc diameter around the optic nerve head and fovea. Zone II extended from the anterior boundary of zone I to the equator. Zone III was anterior to zone II, extending to the ora serrata. Hemorrhage grade was determined by the number of hemorrhages. One or two hemorrhages were defined as grade I, three to ten hemorrhages grade II (Fig. 1), and more than ten hemorrhages grade III (Fig. 2).

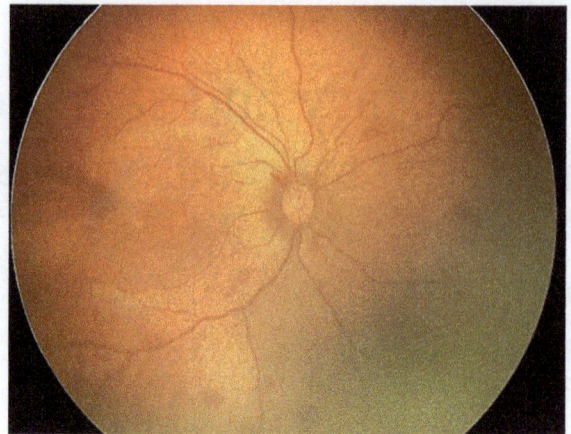

Fig. 1 Retcam photograph of a grade II retinal hemorrhage in a newborn

Heart rate (HR), respiration rate (RR) and oxygen saturation (OS) were monitored by a monitor (Mindray patient monitor, model PM-8000 Express, Shenzhen, China) during the procedure. These measurements were recorded at 4 time points before, during or after the examination. Phase 1 (P1, baseline) was at 5 min before the eye examination. Phase 2 (P2) was when the camera lens was placed on the first eye's cornea. Phase 3 (P3) was when the camera lens was switched to the second eye. Phase 4 (P4) was at 10 min after the procedure. Adverse systemic effects were monitored for during and short-term after the exam, including bradycardia (oculocardiac reflex, defined as percentage decrease in HR from baseline of ≥10%) and oxygen desaturation during examination, which was defined as a decrease in SaO2 of ≥20%.

The analyses were performed with SPSS software version 22.0 for Windows (SPSS Inc., Chicago, IL, USA).

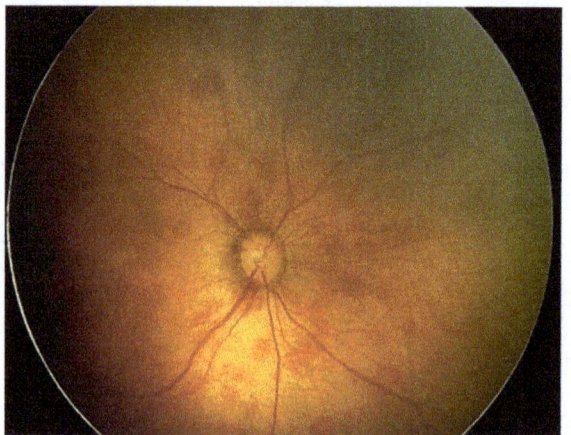

Fig. 2 Retcam photograph of a grade III retinal hemorrhage in a newborn

Given that data were not normally distributed, nonparametric statistics (2 related samples, Wilcoxon Signed Ranks Test) was performed to assess the changes in heart rate, respiration and oxygen saturation compared with baseline. The median and range was used to describe each variable. A level of $P < 0.05$ was accepted as statistically significant.

Results

Demographic features of the newborn population are provided in Table 1. The subjects included 38 males and 30 females, all of which were full-term (born at 37 weeks or older). Fifty newborns were delivered by spontaneous vaginal delivery, and eighteen were delivered by cesarean section.

The median time for each newborn's fundus examination using RetCam was 151 s (range 101–273). All hemorrhages found in 15 (22%) subjects and in 23 (17%) eyes (Table 2) were intra-retinal. Of the 15 newborns with hemorrhage, 8 (53%) had hemorrhage in both eyes, and 7 (47%) had hemorrhage in one eye. Hemorrhages were dot blot or flame shaped. Nineteen (14%) eyes had hemorrhages in Zone I, and 10 (7%) eyes had hemorrhages in zone III. All 23 eyes had hemorrhage in zone II. All the hemorrhages in this study were grade II or III, which were present in 5 (4%) and 18(13%) eyes, respectively. At the follow-up time, which was 4 weeks after birth, all the RHs disappeared completely.

At baseline, the median heart rate of the 68 newborns was 128.5 beats per minute (bpm, range 87–174). The heart rate increased to median value of 156 and 168 bpm in P2 and P3, respectively, but recovered to 122.5 bpm in P4 (Table 3, Fig. 3). Respiratory rate increased from 24 bpm in P1 to 30.5 and 38 bpm in P2 and P3, respectively, and recovered to 25 bpm in P4. Oxygen saturation levels declined from 95 to 83% during the exam and then recovered to 88% and 96% in P3 and P4, respectively.

One subject (1.5%) developed bradycardia whose heart rate declined from 112 at baseline to 62 bpm during exam and subsequently recovered to 121 bpm at 10 min after the exam. Five subjects (7%) developed oxygen desaturation during examination in this study. The median of oxygen saturation of those 5 subjects declined from 97% (range 92–99%) at baseline to 70% (range 54–76%)

Table 2 Characteristics of Retinal Hemorrhage in Healthy Newborns ($n = 136$)

	Zone			Grade		
	I	II	III	I	II	III
Eyes (n = 136, %)	19 (14%)	23 (17%)	10 (7%)	0	5 (4%)	18 (13%)

during examination but recovered to 96% (range 95–98%) in P4.

Discussion

The results of this study suggest that neonatal RH can be efficiently detected and characterized with digital imaging by RetCam. Healthy newborns have some systemic effects to RetCam examination; however, they can recover quickly after the examination. The systemic effects encompass the decrease in the heart rate and oxygen saturation.

Our study used RetCam imaging to record the morphology of RH in newborns. Previous studies have reported clinical and demographic features of infants with birth-related RH [1, 11, 21, 22]. To our knowledge, studies have rarely analyzed all the clinical grades of the hemorrhages [1, 23] in healthy newborns with RH by RetCam. RetCam imaging is an efficient tool to analyze the clinical classification of RH. The system causes minimal stress-related responses and provides rapid recording of fundus findings by images [13, 14], which may contribute to the security of neonatal screening and facilitate in clinical classification and follow-up examination. However, the incidence of the neonatal RH in this study is lower than values given in several other studies [2, 3, 5–7]. In the current study, 15 infants out of 68 didn't develop RH. One important factor may be the mode of delivery. In this study, most newborns were delivered by spontaneous vaginal delivery, and a few were delivered by cesarean section. These two delivery modes tend to cause less incidence of NRH compared with vacuum-assisted delivery. The occurrence of NRH related to delivery by vacuum extraction was 75% in Emerson's study [1] and 77.8% in Hughes' study [24]. The high incidence of hemorrhage in babies born from vacuum-assisted vaginal delivery suggests that the neonatal RH is mainly caused by the change of pressure during the birth procedure. On the other hand, the variation of the incidence of NRH appears to be due to the age of the infants examined after birth and the mode of

Table 1 Clinical Data for the Included Newborns ($n = 68$)

	Age (days)	Gestational age (weeks)	Birth weight (g)	1-minute Apgar score	5-minute Apgar score
Median	3	39.0	3300	9	10
Range	1–4	37.0–41.0	2150–4300	7–9	9–10

Table 3 Stress Responses to the Retcam Screening Examination

	P 1	P2	P 3	P 4
HR, bpm, median (range)	128.5 (87–174)	156** (78–201)	168** (62–204)	122.5 (90–156)
RR, bpm, median (range)	24 (12–53)	30.5** (18–80)	38** (16–89)	25 (11–57)
OS (%), median (range)	95% (81–100%)	83%** (54–98%)	88%** (51–100%)	96% (82–100%)

P1–4 Phase 1–4, *HR* Heart Rate, *RR* Respiratory Rate, *OS* Oxygen Saturation
**$P \leq 0.001$ compared to P1, Sign Test

delivery. The median age of the newborns at examination was 3 days old in our study, which was older than those in other studies. The birth-related neonatal RH appears to resolve quickly, and the incidence declines as time progresses. Giles et al. reported that incidence of RH was reduced from 40% at 1 h post-delivery to 20% at 72 h [25].

The systemic response in infants screened for RH with techniques of examination should be taken into account to pediatricians and ophthalmologists. Previous studies demonstrated that a comprehensive evaluation of parameters standing for systemic response have been investigated, including blood pressure, CRIES pain score, facial responses to pain, and salivary cortisol. However, it was not possible to obtain blood pressure reading during the examination without interfering with its progress. Moreover, though ROP screening is considered a painful procedure, it may be different in the examination of healthy newborns and with digital imagings. The heart rate, respiration rate and oxygen saturation, which can be monitored simultaneously during the procedure with seldom interfering are evaluated in the current study. Oculocardiac reflex and oxygen desaturation are two complications during the fundus examination on newborns or premature infants. To the best of our knowledge, no studies have investigated systemic effects in healthy newborns during the detection of neonatal RH by RetCam. In this study, oculocardiac reflex was defined as a percentage decrease in HR from baseline of $\geq 10\%$, which is similar to other studies [14, 15, 26]. Clarke et al. reported that 17 out of 54 consecutive

premature infants (31%) had oculocardiac reflex during indirect ophthalmoscopy examination [26]. The high incidence of oculocardiac reflex in their study may be associated with the method used. They depressed the sclera to detect the peripheral fundus in every infant. Mukherjee et al. reported that 8 (11.9%) in the RetCam group and 3 (8.3%) in the binocular indirect ophthalmoscopy (BIO) group developed oculocardiac reflex during ROP screening examination [14]. In their practice, a scleral depressor was used to gently rotate the globe not depress the sclera directly to obtain adequate visualization of the peripheral fundus, thus causing less oculocardiac reflex. Compared with those studies, the occurrence of oculocardiac reflex in our study is considerably reduced. One implication is that RetCam has a wider field of view than BIO, and thus globe rotation required is less than that of BIO. Another implication is that healthy newborns may behave different from premature infants during the fundus examination.

The incidence of oxygen desaturation during examination was 6% (5/80) in this study, which was similar to Laws et al.'s report [15]. The 5 subjects who developed oxygen desaturation did not suffer apneic episode, and the oxygen saturation returned to baseline levels rapidly without supplemental oxygen administration. Mehta et al. reported a much higher incidence of episodes of desaturation (9/42) in a small cohort of 12 neonates screened with BIO or RetCam [18]. They also found a greater incidence of episodes of desaturation with the RetCam and suspected that the longer time required for screening with the RetCam 120 might be a contributing

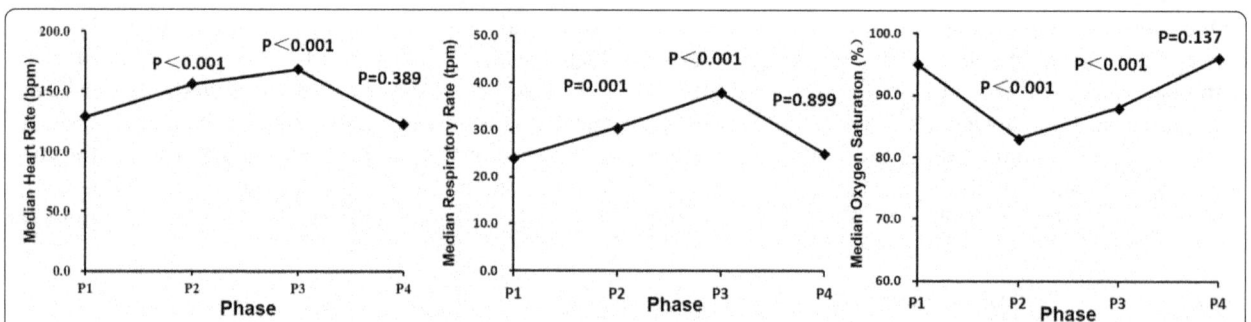

Fig. 3 Change of heart rate (HR), respiratory rate (RR) and oxygen saturation (OS) during fundus examination with Retcam. HR and RR increased, OS decreased during the exam but recovered at 10 min after the exam. Values are medians. Phase 1 (P1, baseline) was at 5 min before the eye examination. Phase 2 (P2) was when the camera lens was just placed on the cornea of the first eye. Phase 3 (P3) was when the camera lens was switched to the second eye. Phase 4 (P4) was at 10 min after the procedure.* $P < 0.05$ compared to P1

factor to the difference. Mukherjee et al. did not identify any significant difference in episodes of desaturation associated with RetCam use [14]. In our opinion, the subjects' gestational age at birth and postconceptional age at examination might account more for the occurrence of episodes of desaturation compared with the duration of the examination. In Mehta et al.'s study, the median gestational age at birth of the infants was 28 weeks, and the median postconceptional age at the first screening was 33 weeks. Younger infants may be more likely to develop oxygen desaturation during medical intervention.

Neonatal care may play an important role in the newborns' response to medical intervention. A Newborn Individualized Developmental Care and Assessment Program (NIDCAP)-based intervention has been adopted by Kleberg et al. during eye examination for ROP [19]. In that study, the NIDCAP-based intervention did not decrease pain responses but resulted in faster recovery, as measured by lower salivary cortisol. NIDCAP is an intervention program aiming at optimizing and adapting neonatal care for preterm infants. NIDCAP included individual evaluation of the infant's responses, direct support to the infant, pacing of the procedure, and modification of the environment. In the present study, we adopted some developmental care strategies that were in accordance with NIDCAP care guidelines. The examination environment was quiet and calm, and room lighting was moderate. During the examination, newborns were lying supine and wrapped with legs cocooned. A neonatologist was on standby, providing effective and individual support throughout the examination. There was a ten-second rest between the first and second eye. The above strategies seemed to minimize the newborns' systemic effects in this study.

RetCam screening have several advantages over BIO in terms of efficacy and safety in neonatal eye examination. First, the classical ophthalmoscope are subjective and leave no records, while Retcam screening has digital imaging records. Moreover, the RetCam has a wider field of view than BIO, which may has an inadequate examination rage. Therefore, the globe rotation required in the RetCam exam is less than that required for BIO. Scleral depression, which is compulsory with BIO, is not necessary with RetCam. Further, the carbomer eye drops used with RetCam will moisten the subject's cornea and avoid the sense of burning. Additionally, the level of illumination appears to be reduced with RetCam compared with BIO. Mehta et al. and Mukherjee et al. reported that the RetCam group examination time was significantly longer than that of BIO (14.5 min versus 9 min and 7.8 min versus 3.9 min, respectively) [14, 18]. In our study, the median time for each newborn's fundus examination using RetCam was 151 s (2.5 min), which was considerably reduced compared with other studies. The

difference may be partly due to the different subjects and different familiarity with the examination procedure.

The examination technique is another important factor accounting for the subject's systemic effects. Several studies have compared the impact of retinopathy of prematurity (ROP) screening examination between a digital fundus camera and conventional BIO on systemic effects [14, 18, 20].Mehta et al. found that screening with the RetCam 120 and the BIO with a speculum caused a greater change in pulse and mean blood pressure and an increase in facial responses to pain during and immediately after screening compared with the BIO without the speculum [18]. Mukherjee et al. reported that screening for ROP with a digital fundus camera was associated with a significantly reduced stress-related response compared with conventional indirect BIO [14].

The limitations of this study include the small sample size. Though neonatal eye examination has the goal of discovering serious congenital, hereditary and acquired eye diseases in the neonatal period of heathy newborns, this procedure is still optional for the families in China. Furthermore, it is understandable that parents are not sure about the necessity of the neonatal screening and worry about the security during the examination. Second, the current study included no identification of long-term side effects of examination. Future studies will include larger sample sizes and longer follow-up time to completely understand the long-term adverse effects of the exams.

The current study characterized the appearance, location and grades of neonatal RH using RetCam imaging. Transient systemic effects were presented during the screening process, and their recovery after the examination demonstrated the security of RetCam imaging. Our study indicates that RetCam is an efficient and secure screening tool in detecting birth-related RH.

Conclusions

RH in healthy newborns, mostly present in Zone II with grade II and III, can be characterized in detail by RetCam. Systemic effects during the process are mild and can be revolved spontaneously.

Abbreviations

BIO: Binocular indirect ophthalmoscopy; bpm: Beats per minute; HR: Heart rate; NIDCAP: Newborn Individualized Developmental Care and Assessment Program; OS: Oxygen saturation; RH: Retinal hemorrhage; ROP: Retinopathy of prematurity; RR: Respiration rate

Funding

This project is supported by Medical and Health Project of Zhejiang Province (2016ZDA016).

Authors' contributions

FC suggested concept of study. FL and LJS performed to conduct study. CCX and CBH measured and collected data in this study. The measurements were confirmed by DC and JDP. Analysis data and interpretation of data were performed by LJS and ZXT. FC wrote the manuscript. LJS provided a critical review of the manuscript. All authors approved the manuscript for submission.

Competing interests

The authors declare that they have no competing interests.

Author details

[1]School of Optometry and Ophthalmology and Eye Hospital of Wenzhou Medical University, Number 270, West Xueyuan Road, Lucheng District, Wenzhou 325000, Zhejiang, China. [2]Neonate Department, Yueqing Maternal and Child Health Hospital, Yueqing, China.

References

1. Emerson MV, Pieramici DJ, Stoessel KM, Berreen JP, Gariano RF. Incidence and rate of disappearance of retinal hemorrhage in newborns. Ophthalmology. 2001;108(1):36–9.
2. Bergen R, Margolis S. Retinal hemorrhages in the newborn. Ann Ophthalmol. 1976;8(1):53–6.
3. Besio R, Caballero C, Meerhoff E, Schwarcz R. Neonatal retinal hemorrhages and influence of perinatal factors. Am J Ophthalmol. 1979;87(1):74–6.
4. Van Noorden GK, Khodadoust A. Retinal hemorrhage in newborns and organic amblyopia. Arch Ophthalmol. 1973;89(2):91–3.
5. Laghmari M, Skiker H, Handor H, Mansouri B, Ouazzani Chahdi K, Lachkar R, Salhi Y, Cherkaoui O, Ouazzani Tnacheri B, Ibrahimy W, et al. Birth-related retinal hemorrhages in the newborn: incidence and relationship with maternal, obstetric and neonatal factors. Prospective study of 2,031 cases. Journal francais d'ophtalmologie. 2014;37(4):313–9.
6. Zhao Q, Zhang Y, Yang Y, Li Z, Lin Y, Liu R, Wei C, Ding X. Birth-related retinal hemorrhages in healthy full-term newborns and their relationship to maternal, obstetric, and neonatal risk factors. Graefes Arch Clin Exp Ophthalmol. 2015;253(7):1021–5.
7. Watts P, Maguire S, Kwok T, Talabani B, Mann M, Wiener J, Lawson Z, Kemp A. Newborn retinal hemorrhages: a systematic review. J AAPOS. 2013;17(1):70–8.
8. Callaway NF, Ludwig CA, Blumenkranz MS, Jones JM, Fredrick DR, Moshfeghi DM. Retinal and optic nerve hemorrhages in the newborn infant: one-year results of the newborn eye screen test study. Ophthalmology. 2016;123(5):1043–52.
9. Suzuki Y, Awaya S. Long-term observation of infants with macular hemorrhage in the neonatal period. Jpn J Ophthalmol. 1998;42(2):124–8.
10. Zwaan J, Cardenas R, O'Connor PS. Long-term outcome of neonatal macular hemorrhage. J Pediatr Ophthalmol Strabismus. 1997;34(5):286–8.
11. Li LH, Li N, Zhao JY, Fei P, Zhang GM, Mao JB, Rychwalski PJ. Findings of perinatal ocular examination performed on 3573, healthy full-term newborns. Br J Ophthalmol. 2013;97(5):588–91.
12. Adams GG, Agrawal S, Sekhri R, Peters MJ, Pierce CM. Appearance and location of retinal haemorrhages in critically ill children. Br J Ophthalmol. 2013;97(9):1138–42.
13. Wu C, Petersen RA, VanderVeen DK. RetCam imaging for retinopathy of prematurity screening. J AAPOS. 2006;10(2):107–11.
14. Mukherjee AN, Watts P, Al-Madfai H, Manoj B, Roberts D. Impact of retinopathy of prematurity screening examination on cardiorespiratory indices: a comparison of indirect ophthalmoscopy and retcam imaging. Ophthalmology. 2006;113(9):1547–52.
15. Laws DE, Morton C, Weindling M, Clark D. Systemic effects of screening for retinopathy of prematurity. Br J Ophthalmol. 1996;80(5):425–8.
16. Rush R, Rush S, Nicolau J, Chapman K, Naqvi M. Systemic manifestations in response to mydriasis and physical examination during screening for retinopathy of prematurity. Retina. 2004;24(2):242–5.
17. Belda S, Pallas CR, De la Cruz J, Tejada P. Screening for retinopathy of prematurity: is it painful? Biol Neonate. 2004;86(3):195–200.
18. Mehta M, Adams GG, Bunce C, Xing W, Hill M. Pilot study of the systemic effects of three different screening methods used for retinopathy of prematurity. Early Hum Dev. 2005;81(4):355–60.
19. Kleberg A, Warren I, Norman E, Morelius E, Berg AC, Mat-Ali E, Holm K, Fielder A, Nelson N, Hellstrom-Westas L. Lower stress responses after newborn individualized developmental care and assessment program care during eye screening examinations for retinopathy of prematurity: a randomized study. Pediatrics. 2008;121(5):e1267–78.
20. Moral-Pumarega MT, Caserio-Carbonero S, De-La-Cruz-Bertolo J, Tejada-Palacios P, Lora-Pablos D, Pallas-Alonso CR. Pain and stress assessment after retinopathy of prematurity screening examination: indirect ophthalmoscopy versus digital retinal imaging. BMC Pediatr. 2012;12:132.
21. Ju RH, Ke XY, Zhang JQ, Fu M. Outcomes of 957 preterm neonatal fundus examinations in a Guangzhou NICU through 2008 to 2011. Int J Ophthalmol. 2012;5(4):469–72.
22. Mulvihill AO, Jones P, Tandon A, Fleck BW, Minns RA. An inter-observer and intra-observer study of a classification of RetCam images of retinal haemorrhages in children. Br J Ophthalmol. 2011;95(1):99–104.
23. Studies of ocular complications of AIDS Foscarnet-Ganciclovir Cytomegalovirus Retinitis Trial: 1. Rationale, design, and methods. AIDS Clinical Trials Group (ACTG). Control Clin Trials 1992, 13(1):22–39.
24. Hughes LA, May K, Talbot JF, Parsons MA. Incidence, distribution, and duration of birth-related retinal hemorrhages: a prospective study. J AAPOS. 2006;10(2):102–6.
25. Giles CL. Retinal hemorrhages in the newborn. Am J Ophthalmol. 1960;49:1005–11.
26. Clarke WN, Hodges E, Noel LP, Roberts D, Coneys M. The oculocardiac reflex during ophthalmoscopy in premature infants. Am J Ophthalmol. 1985;99(6):649–51.

Comparison of postoperative ciliary body changes associated with the use of 23-gauge and 20-gauge system for pars plana vitrectomy

Meng-su Tang[1], Shu-qi Zhang[2] and Li-wei Ma[1]* (iD)

Abstract

Background: To compare the ciliary body changes associated with the use of 23-gauge (23G) and 20-gauge (20G) systems for pars plana vitrectomy.

Methods: A total of 60 patients (60 eyes) with idiopathic epiretinal membrane who were scheduled for surgical treatment were selected and randomly assigned to 20G group or 23G group. Time required for incision making, vitrectomy, and incision closure was compared between the two groups. Changes in ciliary body were evaluated by ultrasound microscopy (UBM). Anterior chamber inflammation was assessed with laser flare meter instrument.

Results: Incision-making time (4.5 ± 0.9 min) and incision-closure time (2.8 ± 0.7 min) in the 23G group were significantly shorter than those in the 20G group (10.1 ± 1.5 min and 11.3 ± 2.2 min, respectively). No significant intergroup difference was observed with respect to time required for vitrectomy (21.6 ± 3.3 min and 20.7 ± 3.2 min, respectively). Ciliary body thickness in the 23G group recovered back to preoperative levels after 4 weeks, as against 8 weeks in the 20G group. Postoperative ciliary body thickness in the 20G group was significantly higher than that in the 23G group ($p < 0.05$). The aqueous protein concentration in 23G group recovered back to preoperative levels after 2 weeks, as against 4 weeks in the 20G group. Postoperative aqueous protein concentration in the 20G group was significantly higher than that in the 23G group ($p < 0.05$).

Conclusions: The use of 23G system was associated with significantly milder injury to the ciliary body as compared to that associated with the use of 20G system.

Keywords: Pars plana vitrectomy, Ciliary body, Idiopathic epiretinal membrane, 23-gauge system

Background

Technological advancements in vitreoretinal surgery have made it possible to treat certain diseases which were hitherto considered untreatable. Pioneered by Machemer in the early 1970s, the pars plana vitrectomy technique has evolved into an increasingly advanced minimally-invasive treatment modality. Introduced for the first time by Claus

Eckardt in 2005, the 23-gauge (23G) transconjunctival vitrectomy technique is commonly used by vitreoretinal surgeons in daily practice. The advantages of use of 23G system include a smaller incision, milder inflammatory response, and more rapid recovery [1–5]. However, use of 23G system may lead to low intraocular pressure, choroidal detachment, and incisional vitreous incarceration in the short term after the procedure [6–8].

Pars plana vitrectomy is a safe procedure used to manage vitreoretinal disease. However, it could also alter the anterior segment morphology and increase the risk of early postoperative complications such as transient

* Correspondence: lwma@cmu.edu.cn
[1]Department of Ophthalmology, the Fourth Affiliated Hospital of China Medical University, No. 11 Xinhua Road, Heping District, Shenyang 110004, Liaoning Province, China
Full list of author information is available at the end of the article

decrease in depth of anterior chamber, angle narrowing, persistent hypotony, and supraciliary effusion [9–11]. The underlying retinal microangiopathy increases the risk of postoperative inflammation, uveal congestion, and changes of the ciliary body in patients with vitreoretinal disease; these changes may be severe in some cases. However, clinical evidence pertaining to post-vitrectomy changes of the ciliary body in such patients is not well documented.

Ultrasound biomicroscopy has been used to monitor postoperative incision healing after use of 20G and 25G vitrectomy systems, [12–15] by serial measurements of the thickness of the ciliary body. In addition, laser flare meter provides a non-invasive means for quantitative monitoring of blood-aqueous barrier function, through laser reflection of the anterior pupil area to indicate the aqueous protein concentration; the technique allows for evaluation of ciliary body wound healing from another aspect [16–18]. In this study, changes of ciliary body thickness and aqueous protein concentration before and after operation were studied to explore the impact on 23G and 20G vitrectomy.

Methods
Objects
A total of 60 patients (60 eyes) with idiopathic epiretinal membrane, who underwent surgical treatment at our hospital during January 2016 and February 2017 were selected. The patients included 22 men and 38 women (age range, 39 to 60 years). The subjects were randomly assigned to 23G group or 20G group using a random number table. No statistical difference was observed on age and gender distribution between two groups. Patients in the 23G group received 23G minimally invasive vitrectomy and those in the 20G group received 20G traditional standard three-channel vitrectomy. Written informed consent was obtained from all patients prior to their enrolment. The study was approved by the institutional ethics committee. The clinical study registration number was ChiCTR-INR-17011082.

Inclusion criteria: (1) idiopathic epiretinal membrane diagnosed based on optical coherence tomography and fundus fluorescein angiography; (2) best corrected visual acuity ≤0.3; (3) diopter between ±3.0 D.

Exclusion criteria: (1) history of eye surgery; (2) glaucoma, familial glaucoma history, or intraocular hypertension; (3) uveitis; (4) severe lenticular opacity requiring cataract extraction; (5) need for intraocular tamponade, such as silicone oil or gas; (6) patients with diabetes, hypertension, and autoimmune conditions, such as rheumatoid arthritis, systemic lupus erythematosus, and multiple sclerosis.

Operation method
All patients were operated under general or local anesthesia by the same surgeon (L.M.). Vitrectomy machine system

(ACCURUS, ALCON) was used for 23-gauge vitrectomy and 20-gauge vitrectomy. In the 23G group, the conjunctiva was pushed laterally using a pressure plate. Subsequently, two-step tunnel-like transconjuctival incisions were made using a sharp 23G blade at a 20–30° angle parallel to the limbus facilitating insertion of the trocars. After vitrectomy, the trocars were removed and the sclerotomies were covered by the conjunctiva.

In the 20G group, the conjunctiva was opened in a nasal triangle and a temporal quadrangle 1 mm from the limbus followed by scleral incisions 3.5–4 mm behind the limbus without electrocoagulation. After vitrectomy, the sclerotomies and conjunctiva were closed with vicryl 8.0 sutures. In both groups, a thorough vitrectomy was performed with the goal of removing vitreous. Time required for incision-making, vitrectomy, and - incision-closure was recorded for all patients.

All patients were administered topical levofloxacin 6 times per day and atropine ophthalmic gel 2 times per day from 3 days before the operation. After the operation, the subjects received topical tobramycin dexamethasone 4 times per day and atropine ophthalmic gel 2 times per day. The tobramycin dexamethasone was tapered off over 4 weeks and changed to pranoprofen 4 times per day for another 4 weeks. Atropine ophthalmic gel was stopped after 2 weeks.

Postoperative observation
The evaluation of ciliary body by ultrasound microscopy (UBM) (ODM-3000, Tianjin Meda Medical Technology Co., Ltd.) was performed by the same technician. The ciliary body thickness at three incisions was measured to obtain the mean value. Each measurement was repeated three times to calculate the mean value. Ethylene oxide was used to sterilize the eye cup and absolute alcohol was adopted to wipe the UBM probe. Anterior chamber inflammation was detected by laser flare meter(FM600, Kowa) to measure the aqueous protein concentration. Each measurement was repeated three times to calculate the mean value. All subjects were assessed with UBM and laser flare meter preoperatively, on postoperative day 1, week 1, week 2, and week 4. UBM examination was performed again at the postoperative week 8.

Statistical analysis
All data analyses were performed with SPSS 19.0 software(IBM Corporation, NY). The ciliary body thickness and aqueous protein concentration before and after the operation were compared by two-way ANOVA. Ciliary body thickness, aqueous protein concentration, and operation time of the two groups were compared by t test. $p < 0.05$ was considered statistically significant.

Results

General information
The baseline demographic data of the two groups were listed in Table 1. The lens was not exceed C1N1P0 according to LOCSII classification.

Complications
Eight patients in the 23G group and six patients in the 20G group developed punctate hemorrhage in the macular area. The bleeding was self-absorbed without laser or electrocoagulation intervention. The lens was retained in all patients, and no intraocular tamponade was used at the end of surgery. Six patients in the 23G group experienced mild choroidal detachment on the first day after operation, which recovered in one week. However, none of the patients in the 20G group experienced choroidal detachment. Fifteen patients in the 23G group and two patients in the 20G group had low intraocular pressure on the first postoperative day and recovered in one week. Vitreous incarceration was observed in 3(10%, 23G) and 0(0%, 20G) eyes on the first postoperative day. None of the patients developed postoperative endophthalmitis.

Time for surgery
The 23G group exhibited significantly shorter time for incision-making (4.5 ± 0.9 min) and incision-closure (2.8 ± 0.7 min) as compared to that in the 20G group (10.1 ± 1.5 min and 11.3 ± 2.2 min), respectively ($t = 17.771$, $p < 0.05$; $t = 19.868$, $p < 0.05$). No statistically significant intergroup difference was observed with respect to time for vitrectomy (21.6 ± 3.3 min vs. 20.7 ± 3.2 min, $t = 1.038$, $p > 0.05$).

Measurement of ciliary body thickness
As shown in Fig. 1a, no significant intergroup difference was observed with respect to preoperative ciliary body thickness ($t = 0.064$, $p > 0.05$). A significant increase in ciliary body thickness was observed postoperatively in both groups ($F = 263.83$, $p < 0.05$). Ciliary body thickness in the 23G group recovered to preoperative levels after 4 weeks as against 8 weeks in the 20G group.

Table 1 Patient demographic data

	23G	20G
Cases(eye)	30	30
Mean age	52	51
Age range	39—60	41—60
Male	10	12
Female	20	18
preoperative ciliary body thickness (mm)	0.25 ± 0.02	0.25 ± 0.02
preoperative aqueous protein concentration (pc/ms)	6.7 ± 1.6	6.9 ± 1.4

Postoperative ciliary body thickness in the 20G group was significantly higher than that in the 23G group ($F = 18.913$, $p < 0.05$). The measurement method of ciliary body thickness was exhibited in Fig. 2.

Measurement of aqueous protein concentration
As shown in Fig. 1b, no significant intergroup difference was observed with respect to preoperative aqueous protein concentration ($t = 0.592$, $p > 0.05$). A significant increase in aqueous protein concentration was observed postoperatively in both groups ($F = 117.246$, $p < 0.05$). Aqueous protein concentration in the 23G group recovered to preoperative levels in 2 weeks as against 4 weeks in the 20G group. Aqueous protein concentration in the 20G group was significantly higher than that in the 23G group ($F = 7.775$, $p < 0.05$).

Discussion
Minimal-invasive procedures are the tendency of modern ocular surgery. According to many previous studies, sutureless vitrectomy has its benefits and risks. The sutureless vitrectomy system shortens the operation time to some extent, thus providing quicker recovery time. However, low intraocular pressure and ciliary body detachment may appear in the early stage of postoperative period [19–21].

In our study, small-incision vitrectomy(23G) was associated with shorter operation time and faster postoperative recovery. This mirrors the results of previous studies [19–21]. 23G system with the wider cutter opening and much closer to the cutter head can not only increase the cutting rate, but also reduce the unnecessary disturbances to the retina which makes up its lower efficiency due to the thinner pipe. This is proven by the result of our study that the vitrectomy time was no significant difference in 20G and 23G groups. Due to the shorter incision-making and incision-closure time, the total operation time was much shorter in 23G group..

Previous studies mainly focused on ciliary body detachment and vitreous incarceration. However, it is less investigated about the impact of the two systems on the thickness of ciliary body. In this study, we focused on the quantative change of ciliary body at the incision site. In addition, all the patients retained the lens, which helped avoid thermal damage caused by phacoemulsification. Furthermore, no silicone oil or gas tamponade were used in these cases, which avoids the impact of intraocular tamponade on the ciliary body. The ciliary body changes were mainly caused by the two different vitrectomy systems. The results of this study indicated postoperative increase in thickness of the ciliary body in both the groups; however, the amplitude of increase in the 23G group was significantly lower than that in the 20G group. Additionally, the ciliary body thickness

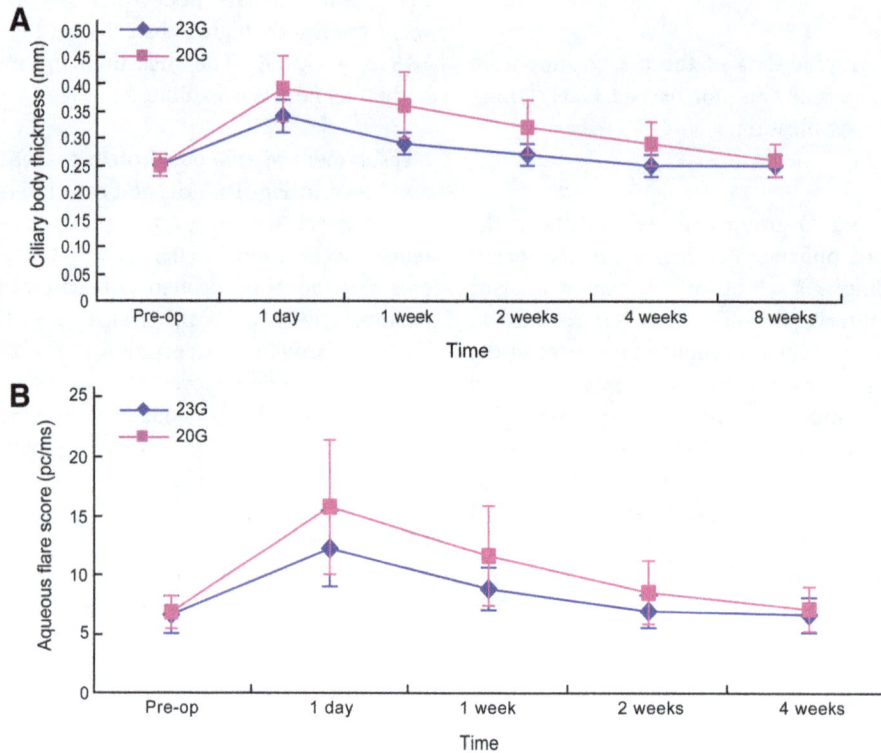

Fig. 1 Postoperative changes of ciliary body thickness and aqueous flare score. **a**, ciliary body thickness. **b**, aqueous flare score

recovered to the preoperative level after two weeks in 23G group, as compared to 4 weeks in the 20G group, which suggests that 23G vitrectomy system caused lesser damage to the ciliary body. This is attributable to several factors. Firstly, compared with the traditional 20G system, 23G vitrectomy system enters the eye through the trocar fixed on pars plana of the ciliary body, without direct contact with the sclera and the ciliary body. The trocar helped avoid the direct contact of surgical instruments with the ciliary body. The lesser friction of the surgical instruments minimized the mechanical damage to the ciliary body. Secondly, the presence of a part of the trocar in the eye effectively reduces intraoperative vitreous spillover and the

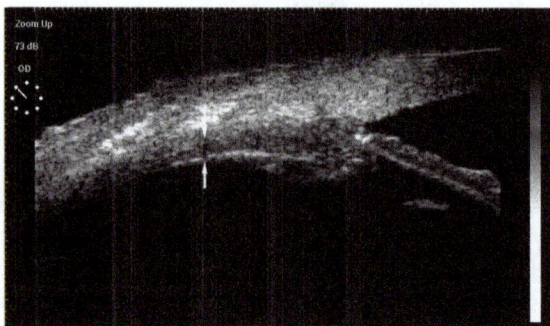

Fig. 2 Ciliary body thickness in 20 G group at 4 weeks after surgery detected by UBM (arrow)

traction effect of the ciliary body in the vicinity of the incision site. In the 20G group, 4 patients, who were found that part of the pigment epithelium of ciliary body was brought out together with the spilled vitreous, experienced a particularly high degree of postoperative increase in ciliary body thickness. Thirdly, a conjunctival oblique incision (two-step method) was applied in 23G group, which was subject to automatic closure and required no suture. On the contrary, incisions in the 20G group were closed by absorbent suture. Granulomatous inflammation during degradation of the suture may affect the repair of the ciliary body, and prolong the time required for recovery of ciliary body. Though previous studies did not involve direct observation of ciliary body damage after pars plana vitrectomy, several studies indicate that unsutured vitrectomy is associated with lesser postoperative inflammation and shorter recovery time, which is consistent with our results [22, 23].

The blood-aquoeus barrier function is disturbed after trauma or surgery. The operation-induced blood-aquoeus barrier dysfunction may be related to mechanical damage and thermal injury.. None of the patients in this study received retinal photocoagulation treatment or cataract phacoemulsification, which helped exclude the impact of thermal injury. Blood-aquoeus barrier dysfunction may be mainly caused by mechanical damage in the anterior uvea. We employed laser flare meter to measure aquoeus

Comparison of postoperative ciliary body changes associated with the use of 23-gauge...

169

protein concentration in order to assess the degree of damage to the blood-aqueous barrier function. Smaller incisions for cataract surgery have been shown to attenuate damage to the blood-aqueous barrier function as compared to larger incisions [24, 25]. In this study, postoperative aqueous protein concentrations were increased to varying degrees in both the groups, which indicates that all patients suffered from blood-aqueous barrier function damage because of mechanical injury. However, the increasement of aqueous protein concentration in the 23G group was significantly smaller than that in the 20G group, which suggests that mechanical injury to the ciliary body in the 23G group was lesser than that in the 20G group. In addition, the time required for aqueous protein concentration recovery was 2 weeks in the 23G group and 4 weeks in the 20G group, which further demonstrates that 23G vitrectomy system was relatively less invasive.

Besides the benefits of sutureless vitrectomy discussed above, there still some risks of it are worth of attention. The incidence of hypotony and choroidal detachment in the 23G group was significantly higher than that in the 20G group, which was associated with intraoperative fluid filler and postoperative incision leakage [26, 27]. According to our results, the higher incidence of hypotony and choroidal detachment in 23G group mostly happened in the early postoperative stage, and this transient phenomenon can be restored in about 1 week. While the thickness of ciliary body recovered in 4 weeks in 23G group compared with 8 weeks in 20G group, the transient postoperative hypotony and choroidal detachment did not affect the recovery of ciliary body's morphology and function. Theoretically, sutureless surgical procedures are associated with a higher risk of endophthalmitis. However, no case of endophthalmitis occurred in our study, although the number of patients is too small to draw any definitive conclusions in this respect.

Conclusions

In summary, compared with the 20G vitrectomy system, the 23G vitrectomy system apparently reduced the total operation time owing to faster incision-making and closure. The use of the 23G system was associated with significantly less damage to the ciliary body as compared to the use of 20G system.

Abbreviation
UBM: Ultrasound microscopy

Acknowledgements
Ming-yu Shi and Fan Zhang contributed equally to this work.

Funding
This study was not supported by any research grants.

Authors' contributions
Meng-su Tang analyzed the data and wrote the manuscript. Shu-qi Zhang analyzed the data and wrote the manuscript. Li-wei Ma designed the study, analyzed and interpreted the patient data, and was a major contributor in writing the manuscript. All authors read and approved the final manuscript.

Competing interests
The authors declare that they have no competing interests.

Author details
[1]Department of Ophthalmology, the Fourth Affiliated Hospital of China Medical University, No. 11 Xinhua Road, Heping District, Shenyang 110004, Liaoning Province, China. [2]Department of Ophthalmology, the 463 Hospital of the Chinese People's Liberation Army, Shenyang 110021, Liaoning Province, China.

References
1. Karadag R, Gunes B, Demiorok A. Trocar-assisted intrascleral sutureless fixation of a dislocated three-piece sulcus intraocular lens. Arq Bras Oftalmol. 2017;80(6):393–5.
2. Gurelik G, Sul S, Kilic G, Ozsaygili C. A modified foveal advancement technique in the treatment of persistent large macular holes. Ophthalmic Surg Lasers Imaging Retina. 2017;48(10):793–8.
3. Bajgai P, Tigari B, Singh R. Outcomes of 23- and 25-gauge transconjunctival sutureless vitrectomies for dislocated intraocular lenses. Int Ophthalmol. 2017.
4. Hsu CM, Chen SC, Wu TT, Sheu SJ. Outcomes of 23-gauge transconjunctival sutureless vitrectomy for acute postoperative endophthalmitis. J Chin Med Assoc. 2017;80(8):503–7.
5. Dehghani A, Rezaei L, Tavallali A, Dastborhan Z. Upper eyelid silicone oil migration after Sutureless 23-gauge vitrectomy. Advanced biomedical research. 2017;26:58.
6. Kucuk E, Yilmaz U, Zor KR, Kalayci D, Sarikatipoglu H. Risk factors for suture requirement and early hypotony in 23-gauge vitrectomy for complex vitreoretinal diseases. Int Ophthalmol. 2017;37(4):989–94.
7. Xu H, Lutrin D, Wu Z. Outcomes of 23-gauge pars plana vitrectomy combined with phacoemulsification and capsulotomy without intraocular lens implantation in rhegmatogenous retinal detachment associated with choroidal detachment. Medicine. 2017;96(34):e7869.
8. Takashina H, Watanabe A, Mitooka K, Tsuneoka H. Examination of self-sealing Sclerotomy for Vitrectomized eye under gas tamponade in 23-gauge Transconjunctival Sutureless vitrectomy. Semin Ophthalmol. 2016; 31(3):210–4.
9. Chen WL, Yang CM, Chen YF, Yang CH, Shau WY, Huang JS, Ho TC, Chen MS, Hung PT. Ciliary detachment after pars plana vitrectomy: an ultrasound biomicroscopic study. Retina. 2002;22(1):53–8.
10. Hikichi T, Ohnishi M, Hasegawa T. Transient shallow anterior chamber induced by supraciliary fluid after vitreous surgery. Am J Ophthalmol. 1997; 124(5):696–8.
11. Minamoto A, Nakano KE, Tanimoto S, Mizote H, Takeda Y. Ultrasound biomicroscopy in the diagnosis of persistent hypotony after vitrectomy. Am J Ophthalmol. 1997;123(5):711–3.
12. Ghomi Z, Ghassemi F. Changes in anterior segment parameters following pars Plana vitrectomy measured by ultrasound biomicroscopy (UBM). Medical hypothesis, discovery and innovation in ophthalmology. 2017;6(1):14–8.
13. Benitez-Herreros J, Lopez-Guajardo L, Camara-Gonzalez C, Perez-Crespo A, Silva-Mato A, Alvaro-Meca A, Teus MA. Evaluation of conjunctival bleb detection after vitrectomy by ultrasound biomicroscopy, optical coherence tomography and direct visualization. Curr Eye Res. 2014;39(4):390–4.
14. Lopez-Guajardo L, Vleming-Pinilla E, Pareja-Esteban J, Teus-Guezala MA. Ultrasound biomicroscopy study of direct and oblique 25-gauge vitrectomy sclerotomies. Am J Ophthalmol. 2007;143(5):881–3.
15. Rizzo S, Genovesi-Ebert F, Vento A, Miniaci S, Cresti F, Palla M. Modified incision in 25-gauge vitrectomy in the creation of a tunneled airtight sclerotomy: an ultrabiomicroscopic study. Graefe's archive for clinical and experimental ophthalmology = Albrecht von Graefes Archiv fur klinische und experimentelle Ophthalmologie. 2007;245(9):1281–8.

16. X.B. Gao, X.L. Zhang, G. Chen, X.K. Huang, X.J. Zhong, M.K. Lin, J Ge, [The blood-aqueous barrier changes after laser peripheral iridotomy or surgery peripheral iridectomy], [Zhonghua yan ke za zhi] Chinese journal of ophthalmology 2011;47(10): 876–880.

17. Sawa M. Laser flare-cell photometer: principle and significance in clinical and basic ophthalmology. Jpn J Ophthalmol. 2017;61(1):21–42.

18. Bernasconi O, Papadia M, Herbort CP. Sensitivity of laser flare photometry compared to slit-lamp cell evaluation in monitoring anterior chamber inflammation in uveitis. Int Ophthalmol. 2010;30(5):495–500.

19. Ho J, Grabowska A, Ugarte M, Muqit MM. A comparison of 23-gauge and 20-gauge vitrectomy for proliferative sickle cell retinopathy - clinical outcomes and surgical management. Eye (Lond). 2018;22.

20. Kim IG, Lee SJ, Park JM. Comparison of the 20-gauge conventional vitrectomy technique with the 23-gauge releasable suture vitrectomy technique. Korean J Ophthalmol. 2013;27(1):12–8.

21. Yokota R, Inoue M, Itoh Y, Rii T, Hirota K, Hirakata A. Comparison of microinsicion vitrectomy and conventional 20-gauge vitrectomy for severe proliferative diabetic retinopathy. Jpn J Ophthalmol. 2015;59(5):288–94.

22. Romero P, Salvat M, Almena M, Baget M, Mendez I. Experience with 25-gauge transconjunctival vitrectomy compared to a 20-gauge system. Analysis of 132 cases. J Fr Ophtalmol. 2006;29(9):1025–32.

23. Chen E. 25-Gauge transconjunctival sutureless vitrectomy. Curr Opin Ophthalmol. 2007;18(3):188–93.

24. Miyake K, Masuda K, Shirato S, Oshika T, Eguchi K, Hoshi H, Majima Y, Kimura W, Hayashi F. Comparison of diclofenac and fluorometholone in preventing cystoid macular edema after small incision cataract surgery: a multicentered prospective trial. Jpn J Ophthalmol. 2000;44(1):58–67.

25. Laplace O, Goldschild M, De Saint Jean M, Guepratte N, Baudouin C. Evaluation by laser flare meter of the inflammatory response after cataract surgery. J Fr Ophtalmol. 1998;21(4):265–9.

26. Tahiri Joutei Hassani R, El Sanharawi M, Adam R, Monin C, Dupont-Monod S, Baudouin C. Influence of sutureless 23-gauge sclerotomy architecture on postoperative intraocular pressure decrease: results of a multivariate analysis. Graefe's Arch Clin Exp Ophthalmol. 2013;251(5):1285–92.

27. Ho LY, Garretson BR, Ranchod TM, Balasubramaniam M, Ruby AJ, Capone A Jr, Drenser KA, Williams GA, Hassan TS. Study of intraocular pressure after 23-gauge and 25-gauge pars plana vitrectomy randomized to fluid versus air fill. Retina. 2011;31(6):1109–17.

26

Retinal vascular flow and choroidal thickness in eyes with early age-related macular degeneration with reticular pseudodrusen

So Min Ahn[1], Suk Yeon Lee[1], Soon-Young Hwang[2], Seong-Woo Kim[1], Jaeryung Oh[1] and Cheolmin Yun[1]* ⓘ

Abstract

Background: To investigate the characteristics of retinal vessels and retinal thickness in eyes with early age-related macular degeneration (AMD) with or without reticular pseudodrusen.

Methods: We retrospectively evaluated the clinical history and optical coherence tomography (OCT) and OCT angiography images of consecutive patients with early AMD. We calculated the retinal vessel densities of the superficial and deep capillary plexus with the ImageJ software (National Institutes of Health, Bethesda, MD, USA) and investigated the relationship with mean retinal thickness and subfoveal choroidal thickness.

Results: We included 135 early AMD eyes and classified 60 of them into a reticular pseudodrusen group and 75 into a non-reticular pseudodrusen group. The vascular densities of the superficial and deep capillary plexus in the reticular pseudodrusen group (32.35% ± 3.67 and 26.71% ± 2.88%) were not different from those of the non-reticular pseudodrusen group (33.18% ± 2.2% and % 27.43 ± 1.79%; $P = 0.546$ and $P = 0.318$, respectively). The retinal thickness of the reticular pseudodrusen group (287.31 μm ± 24.36 μm) did not differ from that of the non-reticular pseudodrusen group (294.27 μm ± 20.71 μm; $P = 0.493$), while subfoveal choroidal thickness in the reticular pseudodrusen group (158. 13 μm ± 42.53 μm) was lower than that in the non-reticular pseudodrusen group (237.89 μm ± 60.94 μm; $P < 0.001$). Multivariate analysis revealed that lower vascular density of the superficial capillary plexus and subfoveal choroidal thickness were associated with retinal thinning in reticular pseudodrusen group ($P = 0.003$ and $P = 0.036$) and older age was associated with retinal thickness in the non-reticular pseudodrusen group ($P = 0.005$).

Conclusions: Retinal thinning in early AMD patients with reticular pseudodrusen was accompanied by choroidal and retinal vascular loss, which suggests a possible linkage of retinal thinning with vascular alterations.

Keywords: Early age-related macular degeneration, Reticular pseudodrusen, Retinal atrophy, Optical coherence tomography angiography

Background

Age-related macular degeneration (AMD) is a leading cause of legal blindness and its pathogenesis remains insufficiently understood [1]. Drusen are recognized as a hallmark in eyes with AMD and are considered to be risk factors for late AMD including neovascular AMD and geographic atrophy [1, 2]. However, with the development of ocular imaging techniques, an additional different phenotype, reticular pseudodrusen, has been identified and reported on. Reticular pseudodrusen, which was proposed by Mimoun et al., appears as a yellowish interlacing network on fundus examination and the appearance of subretinal drusenoid deposit located above the retinal pigment epithelium on optical coherence tomography (OCT) has been suggested to be associated with the development of late AMD [3–5].

Geographic atrophy is an advanced stage of late AMD characterized by the loss of the outer retina, retinal

* Correspondence: yuncheolmin@gmail.com
[1]Department of Ophthalmology, Korea University College of Medicine, 123, Jeokgeum-ro, Danwon-gu, Ansan-si, Gyeonggi-do, Seoul, South Korea
Full list of author information is available at the end of the article

pigment epithelium, and underlying choriocapillaris [6]. Retinal atrophy in early AMD has been suggested to develop in retina-overlying drusen and these areas may subsequently progress to geographic atrophy [6–8]. However, recently, several studies have reported the distinct clinical features of retinal atrophy found in eyes with drusen versus in those with reticular pseudodrusen [6–11]. Eyes with geographic atrophy tend to have a higher prevalence of reticular pseudodrusen and their presence has been suggested to be associated with the progression of early AMD to geographic atrophy rather than to neovascular AMD [6, 12–15].

To date, the pathogenesis of reticular pseudodrusen is still not clear, but various imaging and histologic studies note that these eyes may have choroidal perfusion problems and suggest the existence of a possible association between such and a vascular basis [14, 16–20]. Recently, several studies performed involving OCT angiography (OCTA) revealed that early AMD eyes had significant retinal vascular alterations and that retinal vascular loss might be associated with retinal thinning in eyes with reticular pseudodrusen [21–23]. However, previous studies didn't consider the effects of choroidal thickness as well as various factors including age, gender, and the presence of drusen that may affect the retinal thickness [24–28]. Because the choroid is composed of vessels and capillaries, choroidal thickness may represent the choroidal circulation and thinner choroid may be a marker of a damaged choroidal circulation which have insufficient blood flow to the choroid [29]. Several previous studies noted that abnormal choroidal circulation may be involved in the development of AMD [30, 31]. Therefore, in this study, we investigated the retinal vascular densities of the superficial capillary plexus and deep capillary plexus in early AMD with or without reticular pseudodrusen and their association with retinal thickness, considering choroidal thickness.

Methods

This study was approved by the institutional review board of Korea University Medical Center in Seoul, Korea. All data collection and analysis efforts were conducted in accordance with the tenets of the Declaration of Helsinki.

We reviewed the medical records of early AMD patients who visited the clinic at Korea University Medical Center between June 2016 and January 2018 retrospectively. We defined early AMD cases as those eyes that demonstrated an early or intermediate stage of AMD according to the classifications of the Age-Related Eye Disease Study [32]. Presentations of late AMD included both neovascular AMD and geographic atrophy. All patients received comprehensive ophthalmic examinations including wide-field fundus photography, autofluorescence, and spectral domain OCT (SD-OCT) (Cirrus

HD-OCT 5000; Carl Zeiss Meditec, Dublin, CA, USA.) and OCTA. We also collected information about systemic diseases, hypertension, and diabetes. We excluded any cases with a history of vitreoretinal surgery, vitreoretinal disease including diabetic retinopathy, epiretinal membrane, retinal vein occlusion, bilateral neovascular AMD, geographic atrophy, uveitis, and/or high myopia (axial length greater than 26.0 mm). In cases of bilateral early AMD patients, the right eye was chosen for analysis.

The reticular pseudodrusen area was defined as yellow interlacing network lesions ranging from 125 μm to 250 μm based on fundus examination and color fundus photography [18, 33]. The reticular lesions were identified on SD-OCT and defined when five or more hyperreflective triangular lesions or mounds are present above the retinal pigment epithelium in at least one of the B-scans in all images of the macular cube scans [34, 35]. Two independent observers (S.A. and C.Y.) classified AMD status and confirmed the existence of reticular pseudodrusen in each participant. In cases of disagreement, both observers reviewed the cases again and a final decision was made jointly. Data on the area of drusen under the retinal pigment epithelium in 3-mm- and 5-mm-diameter areas centered on the fovea were collected using advanced retinal pigment epithelium analysis using SD-OCT software [36]. The area provided by the software does not include the area of reticular pseudodrusen over the retinal pigment epithelium. The drusen area and volume were transformed to the square root value for statistical analysis [37].

The OCT device generated a volume scan with a 512×128 scan pattern and a line scan centered on the fovea with enhanced depth imaging protocol. Retinal thickness at the fovea and at four sectors of the 3 mm inner circle (i.e., the superior, nasal, inferior, and temporal) in the Early Treatment of the Diabetic Retinopathy Study chart were collected. Both observers (C.Y. and S.A.) reviewed all OCT B-scan images of volume scan and manually corrected segmentation errors together with assistance from the built-in OCT software in cases with segmentation errors.

Choroidal thickness was measured manually at the fovea using the line scan and a caliper tool integrated into the OCT software. The length was measured from the RPE to the inner surface of the sclera perpendicularly. Two retinal specialists (C.Y. and S.A.) performed independent measurements and the mean of the two measurements was used in the analysis.

The OCT device uses an 840 nm wavelength and an 68,000 A-scans/second speed with an OCT microangiography complex algorithm. The OCTA examination employed a 3 mm × 3 mm volume scan pattern centered on the fovea. We exported the en-face OCTA images of superficial capillary plexus and deep capillary plexus from the software. The superficial capillary plexus was segmented from the internal limiting membrane to the bottom of the inner nuclear layer, while the deep capillary plexus was segmented from the internal aspect of the inner nuclear layer to below the outer plexiform layer [38]. Each of the images were automatically segmented and both observers examined the segmentation errors. If segmentation errors are present, the observers corrected it together. We calculated the vascular density in the superficial capillary plexus and deep capillary plexus using the ImageJ software (version 1.49; National Institutes of Health, Bethesda, MD, USA) [39]. Initially, the en-face OCTA image was imported in the software. Then, the eight-bit image was processed with the command path Adjust > Auto local threshold with Otsu method > Process > Binary > Make binary > Edit > Selection > Create selection > Measure. Using the total number of pixels with vessels, the vascular densities of the superficial capillary plexus and deep capillary plexus were calculated as a ratio of the occupied area by vessels in the 3×3 area (number of pixels in the vessel area / number of pixels in total area $\times 100$). The foveal avascular zone area of the superficial capillary plexus and deep capillary plexus was measured manually using the ImageJ software by two observers (C.Y. and S.A.). The mean foveal avascular zone area of the superficial capillary plexus and the deep capillary plexus was then calculated from the mean values obtained by the two observers and used in the analysis.

For image analysis, poor quality images (those with a signal strength of less than 7), OCTA images with motion artifacts extending over more than two lines, and those with vessel-duplication artifacts were excluded.

The normal distribution of continuous variables was determined with a Kolomogorov–Smirnov test. A comparison of variables between the two groups was performed with an independent t-test or Mann–Whitney U test for continuous variables and a chi-squared test for the categorical variables. To adjust for the differences of age between the two groups, the analysis of covariance (ANCOVA) test was applied. Pearson's correlation or Spearman's rank test was used to analyze the relationship between continuous variables. Simple linear regression was used to analyze the relationship of various parameters and the RT. Based on the results of simple linear regression, we included variables with statistical significance for the multiple linear regression and determined significant factors with backward elimination. Inter-observer reliability was assessed with an intraclass correlation coefficient. Statistical analysis was performed with the SPSS software (version 20.0 for Windows; IBM Corporation, Armonk, NY, USA). P-values < 0.05 were considered to be statistically significant. In cases of comparisons, because there were multiple comparisons for outcome parameters between two groups, we used an adjusted P-value with the Bonferroni correction.

Results

The reticular pseudodrusen group and non- reticular pseudodrusen group included 60 eyes and 75 eyes, respectively. The mean age (years) of the patients in the reticular pseudodrusen group was greater than that of those in the non- reticular pseudodrusen group ($P = 0.001$). The gender, history of hypertension, diabetes, and mean axial length were not different between the two groups (Table 1). The mean subfoveal choroidal thicknesses of the two groups were different ($P < 0.001$) and the square root of the 5 mm drusen area of the reticular pseudodrusen group was greater than that of the non- reticular pseudodrusen group ($P = 0.045$). Conversely, the mean retinal thickness and square root of the 3 mm drusen area were not different between the two groups ($P = 0.075$ and $P = 0.071$). After adjustment for age, the square root of the 5 mm drusen area was not different between the two groups ($P = 0.434$) (Table 2). In each group, 16 patients in the reticular pseudodrusen group and 24 patients in the non-reticular pseudodrusen group had late AMD in one eye.

The mean foveal avascular zone areas of the superficial capillary plexus and deep capillary plexus of the reticular pseudodrusen group were not different from those of the non- reticular pseudodrusen group ($P = 0.734$ and $P = 0.594$). The mean vascular densities of the superficial capillary plexus and deep capillary plexus of the reticular pseudodrusen group also did not show differences in comparison with those of the non- reticular pseudodrusen group ($P = 0.106$ and $P = 0.089$) (Table 3).

In the reticular pseudodrusen group, the mean retinal thickness was associated with age, subfoveal choroidal thickness, square root of the 5 mm drusen area, and vessel density of the superficial capillary plexus and deep capillary plexus (Fig. 1 and Table 4). In the non- reticular pseudodrusen group, the mean retinal thickness was associated with age, subfoveal choroidal thickness, and the square root of the 5 mm drusen area (Fig. 1 and Table 5). In multivariate analysis, a thinner subfoveal choroidal thickness and a lower vessel density of the superficial capillary plexus were associated with lower retinal thickness in the reticular pseudodrusen group (Table 6), while older age was associated with lower retinal thickness in the non- reticular pseudodrusen group. Representative cases are presented in Fig. 2.

We assessed the interobserver reproducibility for the subfoveal choroidal thickness and foveal avascular zone area of the superficial capillary plexus and deep capillary plexus with an intraclass correlation coefficient. The intraclass correlation coefficient was 0.895 [95% confidence interval (CI): 0.852–0.925] for subfoveal choroidal thickness; 0.931 (95% CI: 0.903–0.951) for the foveal avascular zone of the superficial capillary plexus; and 0.861 (95% CI: 0.804–0.901) for the foveal avascular zone of the deep capillary plexus, respectively.

Table 1 Comparison of baseline characteristics between early AMD patients with and without reticular pseudodrusen

	Reticular pseudodrusen group (n = 60)	Non-reticular pseudodrusen group (n = 75)	P-value
Age (years)	74.77 ± 8.70	68.76 ± 10.97	0.001*
Gender (male:female)	14:46	26:49	0.152[†]
Hypertension, n (%)	28 (46.7%)	36 (48.0%)	0.728*
Diabetes, n (%)	17 (28.3%)	22 (29.3%)	0.899*
Axial length (mm)	23.38 ± 1.23	23.11 ± 1.01	0.223*

*Independent t-test
[†]Chi-square test

Discussion

Recently, several studies have suggested that vascular alterations are involved in the pathogenesis of AMD [1, 6, 7, 22, 23, 30, 31]. Diminished vascular flow in the retina and choroid has been considered as a factor associated with AMD development and progression [30, 31]. In the current study, the mean vascular density of the superficial and deep capillary plexus were not different between in the reticular pseudodrusen group versus in the non-reticular pseudodrusen group after adjustment for age. In the reticular pseudodrusen group, thinner choroidal thickness and lower retinal vascular density were associated with retinal thinning, while age was associated with retinal thickness in the non-reticular pseudodrusen group.

Previous studies have suggested that eyes with early AMD demonstrate significant changes in retinal vascular flow and that such was more pronounced in eyes with reticular pseudodrusen [21–23]. Toto et al. reported the occurrence of retinal vascular impairment and associated retinal damage in patients with early AMD [21, 22]. However, because they did not consider the presence of reticular pseudodrusen, the impact of reticular pseudodrusen on vascular flow was not suggested. More recently, Cicinelli et al. investigated the retinal vessels according to the presence of reticular pseudodrusen on OCTA and suggested that retinal vascular loss is present in early AMD patients and that these features are more pronounced in eyes with reticular pseudodrusen [23].

These reports suggested that retinal thickness is reduced with changes in retinal vascular loss. However, retinal thickness has been reported to be affected by various factors including age, gender, spherical equivalent, and drusen [8, 27, 28, 40, 41]. In addition, alterations in choroidal thickness are accompanied by retinal vascular changes in early AMD patients [21]. However, these previous studies did not consider these factors in the context of association with retinal thickness. Therefore, we included these factors in the analysis in the present study. The results of our study are similar to those from previous studies. However, we found additional factors that might be associated with retinal thickness in eyes with early AMD in addition to the retinal vascular changes.

In this study, in spite of the similarity of retinal thickness and vascular densities of superficial and deep capillary plexus, different associations of retinal thickness and vascular density were observed between the two groups. This suggests that development of retinal thinning in early AMD eyes may have different features of retinal vasculature according to the presence of reticular pseudodrusen. Previous studies suggested that ocular perfusion is decreased in several ocular diseases and correlated with the degree of the severity or damage of neural retina [26, 42, 43]. Retinal thickness has a correlation with the retinal vascular perfusion and the decreased retinal vascular flow might reflect the status of damaged retina [44]. Drusen-related retinal atrophy

Table 2 Comparison of baseline optical coherence tomographic characteristics between early AMD patients with and without reticular pseudodrusen

	Reticular pseudodrusen group (n = 60)	Non-reticular pseudodrusen group (n = 75)	P-value*	Age-adjusted P-value[†]
Mean retinal thickness (μm)	287.31 ± 24.36	294.27 ± 20.71	0.075	0.493
Subfoveal choroidal thickness (μm)	158.13 ± 42.53	237.89 ± 60.94	< 0.001	< 0.001
3 mm drusen area (mm²)**	0.50 ± 0.74	0.37 ± 0.73	0.308	0.929
5 mm drusen area (mm²)**	0.80 ± 1.07	0.55 ± 1.02	0.182	0.764
Square root of 3 mm drusen area	0.50 ± 0.51	0.33 ± 0.51	0.071	0.519
Square root of 5 mm drusen area	0.65 ± 0.62	0.44 ± 0.61	0.045	0.434

*Independent t-test, P-value < 0.005 (0.05/10) was considered to be statistically significant with the Bonferroni correction
[†]ANCOVA test, P-value < 0.005 (0.05/10) was considered to be statistically significant with the Bonferroni correction
**Drusen area under the retinal pigment epithelium

Table 3 Comparison of angiographic features between early AMD patients with and without reticular pseudodrusen

	Reticular pseudodrusen group (n = 60)	Non-reticular pseudodrusen group (n = 75)	P-value*	Age-adjusted P-value[†]
Superficial capillary plexus				
Foveal avascular zone area (mm²)	0.34 ± 0.11	0.34 ± 0.13	0.734	0.553
Vascular density (%)	32.35 ± 3.67	33.18 ± 2.22	0.106	0.615
Deep capillary plexus				
Foveal avascular zone area (mm²)	1.28 ± 3.78	1.31 ± 3.80	0.594	0.322
Vascular density (%)	26.71 ± 2.88	27.43 ± 1.79	0.089	0.352

*Independent t-test, P-value < 0.005 (0.05/10) was considered to be statistically significant with the Bonferroni correction
[†]ANCOVA test, P-value < 0.005 (0.05/10) was considered to be statistically significant with the Bonferroni correction

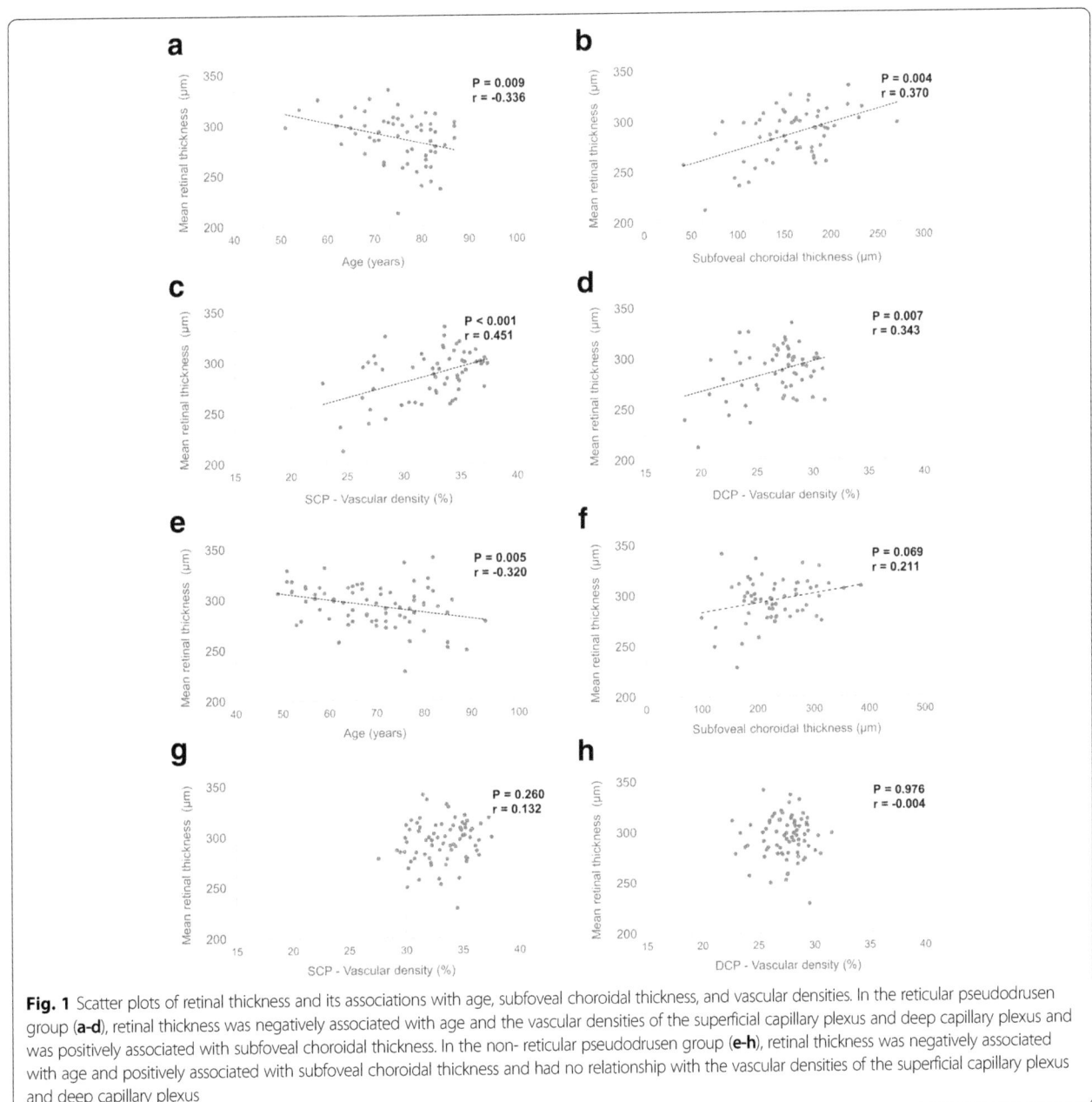

Fig. 1 Scatter plots of retinal thickness and its associations with age, subfoveal choroidal thickness, and vascular densities. In the reticular pseudodrusen group (**a-d**), retinal thickness was negatively associated with age and the vascular densities of the superficial capillary plexus and deep capillary plexus and was positively associated with subfoveal choroidal thickness. In the non- reticular pseudodrusen group (**e-h**), retinal thickness was negatively associated with age and positively associated with subfoveal choroidal thickness and had no relationship with the vascular densities of the superficial capillary plexus and deep capillary plexus

Table 4 Univariate analysis for estimating factors associated with mean retinal thickness in the reticular pseudodrusen group

Variables	ß	Standard error	P-value*
Age (years)	−1.020	0.376	0.009
Gender (female)	11.510	7.344	0.122
Hypertension	−5.331	6.336	0.404
Diabetes	5.888	6.995	0.403
Axial length (mm)	−3.353	3.036	0.275
Subfoveal choroidal thickness (μm)	0.212	0.070	0.004
Square root of the 3 mm drusen area[†]	−10.090	6.160	0.107
Square root of the 5 mm drusen area[†]	−8.991	5.049	0.080
Foveal avascular zone area of superficial capillary plexus (mm^2)	−26.571	28.805	0.360
Foveal avascular zone area of deep capillary plexus (mm^2)	4.938	8.437	0.561
Vessel density of superficial capillary plexus (%)	2.995	0.778	< 0.001
Vessel density of deep capillary plexus (%)	2.900	1.044	0.007

*Simple linear regression
[†]Drusen area under the retinal pigment epithelium

usually develops on the area overlying the drusen and after drusen regression [7]. It is confined to areas affected by the drusen and thus, the retinal degenerative changes are focal rather than overall and the changes may not induce whole macular changes. Thus, retinal thickness measurements might not reflect the whole retinal change in the non- reticular pseudodrusen group in this study. However, in eyes with reticular pseudodrusen, diffuse changes in retinal thickness which were associated with retinal and choroidal vascular changes were noted. Because the reticular pseudodrusen group had similar drusen characteristics to those of the non- reticular pseudodrusen group, there might be another factor that may affect the retinal changes. Previous studies suggested that the eyes with reticular pseudodrusen are under diffuse choroidal changes and the etiology of

which was suggested to be a vascular problem by comparison with eyes without pseudodrusen [14, 16, 23, 45–47]. In addition, the characteristics of retinal atrophy in eyes with AMD were reported to be different between eyes with and without reticular pseudodrusen, and the eyes with reticular pseudodrusen have a tendency to have diffuse and multilobular retinal atrophy [48]. In conjunction with previous reports and our study, diffuse changes in retina and choroid are present in eyes with reticular pseudodrusen compared to those without reticular pseudodrusen, and this might be associated with retinal thinning on a vascular basis.

In the non-reticular pseudodrusen group, lower retinal thickness was associated with older age, a larger area of drusen, and a thinner subfoveal choroidal thickness. Because the square root of drusen area and subfoveal

Table 5 Univariate analysis for estimating factors associated with mean retinal thickness in the non- reticular pseudodrusen group

Variables	ß	Standard error	P-value*
Age (years)	−0.622	0.215	0.005
Gender (female)	−2.716	5.049	0.592
Hypertension	−6.025	4.767	0.210
Diabetes	−5.711	5.246	0.280
Axial length (mm)	4.010	2.813	0.160
Subfoveal choroidal thickness (μm)	0.072	0.039	0.069
Square root of 3 mm drusen area[†]	−7.404	3.255	0.118
Square root of 5 mm drusen area[†]	−6.723	2.321	0.089
Foveal avascular zone area of superficial capillary plexus (mm^2)	−14.296	19.013	0.455
Foveal avascular zone area of deep capillary plexus (mm^2)	−0.161	6.393	0.980
Vessel density of superficial capillary plexus (%)	1.229	1.084	0.260
Vessel density of deep capillary plexus (%)	−0.041	1.354	0.976

*Simple linear regression
[†]Drusen area under the retinal pigment epithelium

Table 6 Multivariate analysis for estimating factors associated with mean retinal thickness in the reticular pseudodrusen group

Variables	ß	Standard error	P value*
Vessel density of superficial capillary plexus (%)	2.475	0.792	0.003
Subfoveal choroidal thickness (μm)	0.147	0.068	0.036

*Multiple linear regression

choroidal thickness had a relationship with age in this study, their effects on retinal thickness became attenuated with multivariate analysis (See Additional file 1). Usually, it has been suggested that the amount of drusen increase over time in early AMD eyes and that the choroid undergoes atrophy with advancements in age [25, 37]. Thus, even though various factors were associated with retinal thinning in the non- reticular pseudodrusen group, retinal thickness in early AMD eyes without reticular pseudodrusen might be predominantly influenced by aging. However, in the reticular pseudodrusen group, there might be other mechanisms that affect retinal thickness. Several investigators including individuals from our group previously reported about decreased choroidal thickness in early AMD eyes with reticular pseudodrusen when they were compared with early AMD eyes without reticular pseudodrusen [26, 45–47]. In addition to the finding of decreased choroidal thickness, we also suggested that the progression of choroidal atrophy is more prominent in eyes with reticular pseudodrusen and hypothesized that eyes with reticular pseudodrusen have an altered choroid that cannot compensate for changes in perfusion pressure appropriately, and that this might be associated with the prominent choroidal atrophy seen in eyes with reticular pseudodrusen [26]. Because the choroid

supplies blood to the outer retina, changes in the choroid might therefore affect retinal status. The different features between the two groups in our study supports previous theories that have suggested that early AMD eyes with reticular pseudodrusen might be distinctly different from early AMD eyes without reticular pseudodrusen [7, 10, 17, 48–52].

We can suggest two possibilities with respect to the results of this study. First, the eyes with reticular pseudodrusen under chronic choroidal insufficiency might contribute to retinal atrophy [11, 20, 53]. It is well-known that retinal atrophy is common in eyes with reticular pseudodrusen [9, 11]. Decreased metabolic demand associated with outer retinal atrophy might induce secondary decreased retinal vascular flow and this means that choroidal changes might also contribute to secondary retinal change. Second, eyes with reticular pseudodrusen may be co-morbid for choroidal insufficiency and retinal vascular dysregulation. The regulation of blood flow to the retina and the choroid is quite different: while retinal flow vasculature employs autoregulation, choroidal flow employs autonomic regulation [42–44]. Although the exact mechanism of autoregulation of the retinal blood flow is unclear, several studies have shown that retinal blood flow

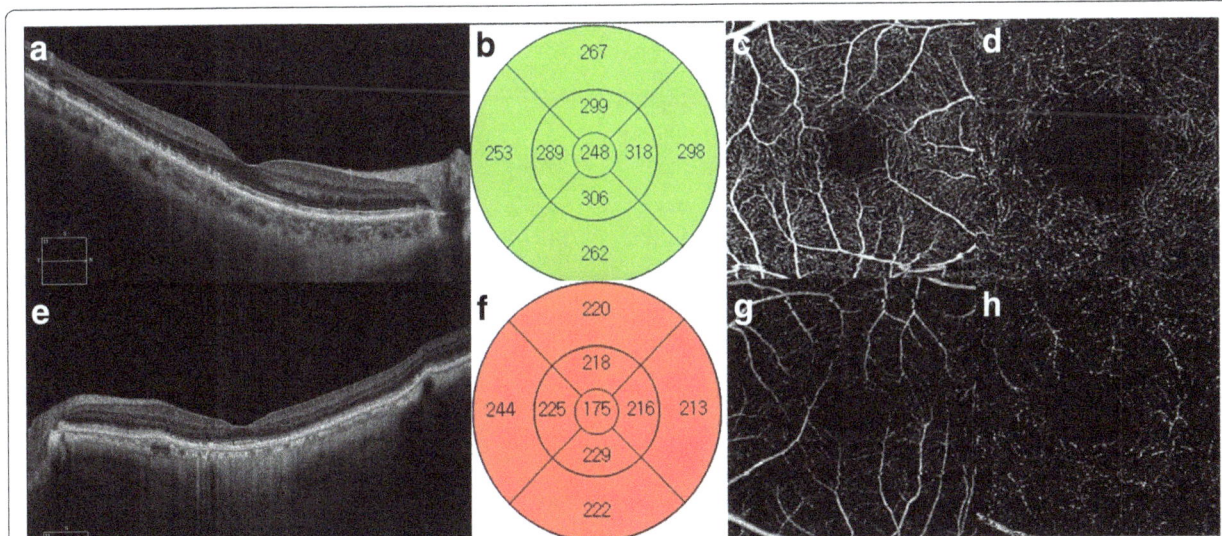

Fig. 2 Representative cases of patients with early AMD and reticular pseudodrusen. OCT and OCTA images of a 71-year-old female patient (**a-d**) and a 75-year-old male patient (**e-h**) with early AMD and reticular pseudodrusen. **a** Line scan shows multiple subretinal drusenoid deposits with 193 μm subfoveal choroidal thickness. **b** ETDRS grid shows normal range retinal thickness. **c** and **d** OCTA shows relatively preserved superficial capillary plexuses and deep capillary plexuses. **e** Line scan shows multiple subretinal drusenoid deposits with 65 μm subfoveal choroidal thickness. **f** ETDRS grid shows decreased retinal thickness. **g** and **h** OCTA shows relatively decreased vascular densities of the superficial capillary plexus and deep capillary plexus

responds to changes in ocular perfusion pressure and attempts to maintain a constant blood flow [42–44]. However, previous research has also reported that retinal vascular reactivity might decrease with age [42–44]. We hypothesized that eyes with reticular pseudodrusen may have a limited compliance with changes in ocular perfusion pressure both in choroid and retinal vessels, while the choroid and retinal vessels in early AMD eyes without reticular pseudodrusen might compensate better for changes in ocular perfusion pressure [26]. The contribution of decreased retinal vascular density independently with the choroidal thickness in this study might support this possibility. The etiology of reticular macular disease is controversial, but there are some findings that support the existence of a vascular basis with the alteration of choroid and choriocapillaris blood flow [14, 16, 54]. Smith et al. previously reported about the relationship between various systemic diseases that may affect systemic circulatory status and reticular macular disease [13, 16, 18]. They suggested a hypothesis that the impairment of blood flow is involved in the pathogenesis of reticular macular disease [14, 16, 54]. Retinal vascular changes including generalized narrowing of arteriole and venule has been recently reported to be associated with cardiovascular disease [55, 56]. In addition to the suggestions of previous investigations, the results of our study may give rise to a suspicion about the role of vascular origin in retinal atrophy in eyes with reticular pseudodrusen.

This study has several limitations. First, it has a retrospective design and includes a limited number of cases. There might be selection bias due to hospital-based sampling. Second, we diagnosed and classified patients into two groups based only on fundus examination and OCT. Other multimodal imaging options including infrared imaging might improve the diagnostic rate, even though reticular pseudodrusen can be detected with higher sensitivity and specificity only with OCT [34]. Third, because reticular pseudodrusen patients have characteristics associated with older age, which also have been reported in previous epidemiologic studies, we had to adjust the age with the statistical method [13, 35, 53]. Fourth, because of the limited scan area of OCTA, we investigated only in 3 mm × 3 mm area. Fifth, because we used SD-OCT with limited resolution on choriocapillaris, we could not investigate the OCTA images of choriocapillaris [57, 58].

In conclusion, patients with early AMD with reticular pseudodrusen showed retinal thinning accompanied by choroidal and retinal vascular loss, while patients without reticular pseudodrusen did not. This provides a suggestion that progression of retinal thinning in eyes

with reticular pseudodrusen may be occur a vascular basis.

Abbreviations
AMD: Age-related macular degeneration; OCT: Optical coherence tomography; OCTA: Optical coherence tomography angiography; SD-OCT: Spectral domain optical coherence tomography

Funding
This research was supported by grants from Korea University (K1723451). However, the funding organization had no role in the design or conduct of this research.

Authors' contributions
Study design (CY); study conduct (SA, CY); data collection (SA, SL); data analysis and interpretation (SA, SH, CY); and preparation, review, and approval of the manuscript (SA, SL, SH, SK, JO, CY). CY contributed the manuscript as a corresponding author. All authors read and approved the final manuscript.

Competing interests
J. Oh is a consultant of Topcon Corporation. The remaining authors declare that they have no competing interests.

Author details
[1]Department of Ophthalmology, Korea University College of Medicine, 123, Jeokgeum-ro, Danwon-gu, Ansan-si, Gyeonggi-do, Seoul, South Korea.
[2]Department of Biostatistics, Korea University College of Medicine, Seoul, South Korea.

References
1. Lim LS, Mitchell P, Seddon JM, Holz FG, Wong TY. Age-related macular degeneration. Lancet (London, England). 2012;379:1728–38.
2. Schaal KB, Rosenfeld PJ, Gregori G, Yehoshua Z, Feuer WJ. Anatomic clinical trial endpoints for nonexudative age-related macular degeneration. Ophthalmology. 2016;123:1060–79.
3. Mimoun G, Soubrane G, Coscas G. Macular druse. Journal francais d'ophtalmologie. 1990;13:511–30.
4. Finger RP, Wu Z, Luu CD, Kearney F, Ayton LN, Lucci LM, et al. Reticular pseudodrusen: a risk factor for geographic atrophy in fellow eyes of individuals with unilateral choroidal neovascularization. Ophthalmology. 2014;121:1252–6.
5. Hogg RE, Silva R, Staurenghi G, Murphy G, Santos AR, Rosina C, et al. Clinical characteristics of reticular pseudodrusen in the fellow eye of patients with unilateral neovascular age-related macular degeneration. Ophthalmology. 2014;121:1748–55.
6. Fleckenstein M, Mitchell P, Freund KB, Sadda S, Holz FG, Brittain C, et al. The progression of geographic atrophy secondary to age-related macular degeneration. Ophthalmology. 2018;125:369–90.
7. Klein ML, Ferris FL 3rd, Armstrong J, Hwang TS, Chew EY, Bressler SB, et al. Retinal precursors and the development of geographic atrophy in age-related macular degeneration. Ophthalmology. 2008;115:1026–31.
8. Schuman SG, Koreishi AF, Farsiu S, Jung SH, Izatt JA, Toth CA. Photoreceptor layer thinning over drusen in eyes with age-related macular degeneration imaged in vivo with spectral-domain optical coherence tomography. Ophthalmology. 2009;116:488–96. e482
9. Hamel CP, Meunier I, Arndt C, Ben Salah S, Lopez S, Bazalgette C, et al. Extensive macular atrophy with pseudodrusen-like appearance: a new clinical entity. Am J Ophthalmol. 2009;147:609–20.
10. Mones J, Biarnes M. Geographic atrophy phenotype identification by cluster analysis. Br J Ophthal. 2018;102:388–92.
11. Spaide RF. Outer retinal atrophy after regression of subretinal drusenoid deposits as a newly recognized form of late age-related macular degeneration. Retina. 2013;33:1800–8.

12. Finger RP, Chong E, McGuinness MB, Robman LD, Aung KZ, Giles G, et al. Reticular pseudodrusen and their association with age-related macular degeneration: the Melbourne collaborative cohort study. Ophthalmology. 2016;123:599–608.

13. Klein R, Meuer SM, Knudtson MD, Iyengar SK, Klein BE. The epidemiology of retinal reticular drusen. Am J Ophthalmol. 2008;145:317–26.

14. Pumariega NM, Smith RT, Sohrab MA, Letien V, Souied EH. A prospective study of reticular macular disease. Ophthalmology. 2011;118:1619–25.

15. Zhou Q, Daniel E, Maguire MG, Grunwald JE, Martin ER, Martin DF, et al. Pseudodrusen and incidence of late age-related macular degeneration in fellow eyes in the comparison of age-related macular degeneration treatments trials. Ophthalmology. 2016;123:1530–40.

16. M AM, Marsiglia M, M DL, Pumariega N, Bearelly S, Smith RT. Is reticular macular disease a choriocapillaris perfusion problem? Med Hypothesis Discov Innov Ophthalmol. 2012;1:37–41.

17. Querques G, Querques L, Martinelli D, Massamba N, Coscas G, Soubrane G, et al. Pathologic insights from integrated imaging of reticular pseudodrusen in age-related macular degeneration. Retina. 2011;31:518–26.

18. Smith RT, Sohrab MA, Busuioc M, Barile G. Reticular macular disease. Am J Ophthalmol. 2009;148:733–43. e732

19. Zweifel SA, Spaide RF, Curcio CA, Malek G, Imamura Y. Reticular pseudodrusen are subretinal drusenoid deposits. Ophthalmology. 2010;117: 303–12. e301.

20. Alten F, Heiduschka P, Clemens CR, Eter N. Exploring choriocapillaris under reticular pseudodrusen using OCT-angiography. Graefes Arch Clin Exp Ophthalmol. 2016;254:2165–73.

21. Toto L, Borrelli E, Di Antonio L, Carpineto P, Mastropasqua R. Retinal vascular plexuses' changes in dry age-related macular degeneration, evaluated by means of optical coherence tomography angiography. Retina. 2016;36: 1566–72.

22. Toto L, Borrelli E, Mastropasqua R, Di Antonio L, Doronzo E, Carpineto P, et al. Association between outer retinal alterations and microvascular changes in intermediate stage age-related macular degeneration: an optical coherence tomography angiography study. Br J Ophthalmol. 2017;101:774–9.

23. Cicinelli MV, Rabiolo A, Sacconi R, Lamanna F, Querques L, Bandello F, et al. Retinal vascular alterations in reticular pseudodrusen with and without outer retinal atrophy assessed by optical coherence tomography angiography. Br J Ophthalmol. 2018;

24. Lee JY, Lee DH, Lee JY, Yoon YH. Correlation between subfoveal choroidal thickness and the severity or progression of nonexudative age-related macular degeneration. Invest Ophthalmol Vis Sci. 2013;54:7812–8.

25. Spaide RF. Age-related choroidal atrophy. Am J Ophthalmol. 2009;147: 801–10.

26. Yun C, Ahn J, Kim M, Hwang SY, Kim SW, Oh J. Ocular perfusion pressure and choroidal thickness in early age-related macular degeneration patients with reticular pseudodrusen. Invest Ophthalmol Vis Sci. 2016;57:6604–9.

27. Myers CE, Klein BE, Meuer SM, Swift MK, Chandler CS, Huang Y, et al. Retinal thickness measured by spectral-domain optical coherence tomography in eyes without retinal abnormalities: the beaver dam eye study. Am J Ophthalmol. 2015;159:445–56. e441

28. Song WK, Lee SC, Lee ES, Kim CY, Kim SS. Macular thickness variations with sex, age, and axial length in healthy subjects: a spectral domain-optical coherence tomography study. Invest Ophthalmol Vis Sci. 2010;51:3913–8.

29. Ardeljan D, Chan CC. Aging is not a disease: distinguishing age-related macular degeneration from aging. Prog Retin Eye Res. 2013;37:68–89.

30. Coleman DJ, Silverman RH, Rondeau MJ, Lloyd HO, Khanifar AA, Chan RV. Age-related macular degeneration: choroidal ischaemia? Br J Ophthalmol. 2013;97:1020–3.

31. McLeod DS, Grebe R, Bhutto I, Merges C, Baba T, Lutty GA. Relationship between RPE and choriocapillaris in age-related macular degeneration. Invest Ophthalmol Vis Sci. 2009;50:4982–91.

32. Age-Related Eye Disease Study Research G: A randomized, placebo-controlled, clinical trial of high-dose supplementation with vitamins C and E, beta carotene, and zinc for age-related macular degeneration and vision loss: AREDS report no. 8. Arch Ophthalmol 2001;119:1417–1436.

33. Arnold JJ, Sarks SH, Killingsworth MC, Sarks JP. Reticular pseudodrusen. A risk factor in age-related maculopathy. Retina. 1995;15:183–91.

34. Ueda-Arakawa N, Ooto S, Tsujikawa A, Yamashiro K, Oishi A, Yoshimura N. Sensitivity and specificity of detecting reticular pseudodrusen in multimodal imaging in Japanese patients. Retina. 2013;33:490–7.

35. Zweifel SA, Imamura Y, Spaide TC, Fujiwara T, Spaide RF. Prevalence and significance of subretinal drusenoid deposits (reticular pseudodrusen) in age-related macular degeneration. Ophthalmology. 2010;117:1775–81.

36. Gregori G, Wang F, Rosenfeld PJ, Yehoshua Z, Gregori NZ, Lujan BJ, et al. Spectral domain optical coherence tomography imaging of drusen in nonexudative age-related macular degeneration. Ophthalmology. 2011;118:1373–9.

37. Yehoshua Z, Wang F, Rosenfeld PJ, Penha FM, Feuer WJ, Gregori G. Natural history of drusen morphology in age-related macular degeneration using spectral domain optical coherence tomography. Ophthalmology. 2011;118: 2434–41.

38. Spaide RF, Curcio CA. Evaluation of segmentation of the superficial and deep vascular layers of the retina by optical coherence tomography angiography instruments in normal eyes. JAMA Ophthalmol. 2017;135:259–62.

39. Al-Sheikh M, Phasukkijwatana N, Dolz-Marco R, Rahimi M, Iafe NA, Freund KB, et al. Quantitative OCT angiography of the retinal microvasculature and the choriocapillaris in myopic eyes. Invest Ophthalmol Vis Sci. 2017;58:2063–9.

40. Duan XR, Liang YB, Friedman DS, Sun LP, Wong TY, Tao QS, et al. Normal macular thickness measurements using optical coherence tomography in healthy eyes of adult Chinese persons: the Handan eye study. Ophthalmology. 2010;117:1585–94.

41. Gupta P, Sidhartha E, Tham YC, Chua DK, Liao J, Cheng CY, et al. Determinants of macular thickness using spectral domain optical coherence tomography in healthy eyes: the Singapore Chinese eye study. Invest Ophthalmol Vis Sci. 2013;54:7968–76.

42. Costa VP, Harris A, Anderson D, Stodtmeister R, Cremasco F, Kergoat H, et al. Ocular perfusion pressure in glaucoma. Acta Ophthalmol. 2014;92:e252–66.

43. Falsini B, Anselmi GM, Marangoni D, D'Esposito F, Fadda A, Di Renzo A, et al. Subfoveal choroidal blood flow and central retinal function in retinitis pigmentosa. Invest Ophthalmol Vis Sci. 2011;52:1064–9.

44. Yu J, Gu R, Zong Y, Xu H, Wang X, Sun X, et al. Relationship between retinal perfusion and retinal thickness in healthy subjects: an optical coherence tomography angiography study. Invest Ophthalmol Vis Sci. 2016;57:204–10.

45. Garg A, Oll M, Yzer S, Barile GR, Merriam JC, Tsang SH, et al. Reticular pseudodrusen in early age-related macular degeneration are associated with choroidal thinning. Invest Ophthalmol Vis Sci. 2013;54:7075–81.

46. Haas P, Esmaeelpour M, Ansari-Shahrezaei S, Drexler W, Binder S. Choroidal thickness in patients with reticular pseudodrusen using 3D 1060-nm OCT maps. Invest Ophthalmol Vis Sci. 2014;55:2674–81.

47. Querques G, Querques L, Forte R, Massamba N, Coscas F, Souied EH. Choroidal changes associated with reticular pseudodrusen. Invest Ophthalmol Vis Sci. 2012;53:1258–63.

48. Xu L, Blonska AM, Pumariega NM, Bearelly S, Sohrab MA, Hageman GS, et al. Reticular macular disease is associated with multilobular geographic atrophy in age-related macular degeneration. Retina. 2013;33:1850–62.

49. Curcio CA, Presley JB, Malek G, Medeiros NE, Avery DV, Kruth HS. Esterified and unesterified cholesterol in drusen and basal deposits of eyes with age-related maculopathy. Exp Eye Res. 2005;81:731–41.

50. Mrejen S, Sato T, Curcio CA, Spaide RF. Assessing the cone photoreceptor mosaic in eyes with pseudodrusen and soft drusen in vivo using adaptive optics imaging. Ophthalmology. 2014;121:545–51.

51. Oak AS, Messinger JD, Curcio CA. Subretinal drusenoid deposits: further characterization by lipid histochemistry. Retina. 2014;34:825–6.

52. Querques G, Massamba N, Srour M, Boulanger E, Georges A, Souied EH. Impact of reticular pseudodrusen on macular function. Retina. 2014;34:321–9.

53. Querques G. Reticular pseudodrusen: a common pathogenic mechanism affecting the choroid-bruch's membrane complex and retinal pigment epithelium for different retinal and macular diseases. Invest Ophthalmol Vis Sci. 2015;56:5914–5.

54. Cymerman RM, Skolnick AH, Cole WJ, Nabati C, Curcio CA, Smith RT. Coronary artery disease and reticular macular disease, a subphenotype of early age-related macular degeneration. Curr Eye Res. 2016;41:1482–8.

55. Mitchell P, Wang JJ, Wong TY, Smith W, Klein R, Leeder SR. Retinal microvascular signs and risk of stroke and stroke mortality. Neurology. 2005; 65:1005–9.

56. Wang JJ, Liew G, Wong TY, Smith W, Klein R, Leeder SR, et al. Retinal vascular calibre and the risk of coronary heart disease-related death. Heart. 2006;92:1583–7.

27

Comparison of different settings for yellow subthreshold laser treatment in diabetic macular edema

Jay Chhablani[1*], Rayan Alshareef[2], David Ta Kim[3], Raja Narayanan[1], Abhilash Goud[1] and Annie Mathai[1]

Abstract

Background: To assess the safety and efficacy of two subthreshold parameters (5 and 15% duty cycle (DC)) compared to standard ETDRS (early treatment of diabetic retinopathy study) continuous wave (CW) laser.

Methods: In this prospective randomized study, 30 eyes from 20 patients with non-center involving macular edema were randomized into 3 different groups: 5% DC, 15% DC and CW navigated modified ETDRS laser treatment. Titration in subthreshold groups was performed with 30% of the threshold power, decided with microsecond pulses. CW laser was titrated to a barely visible burn. All patients underwent microperimetry, thickness measurements and visual acuity examinations at baseline, 6 weeks and 12 weeks post treatment.

Results: At three months follow up, retinal sensitivity was significantly reduced in the CW group by − 2.2 dB whereas in both subthreshold groups, retinal sensitivity increased by 2.4 dB for 5% and 1.9 dB for 15% DC with no significant difference. Retinal volume (mm^3) decreased in both subthreshold groups by 0.08 ± 0.3 and 0.12 ± 0.11 in 5 and 15% DC group respectively. Whereas the CW group showed volume increase of 0.55 ± 0.92 ($p = 0.02$ and 0.01 for 5 and 15% DC groups). Visual acuity remained stable in all 3 groups (− 0.7 letter in 5% DC; 2.11 letters in 15% DC and 0.88 in CW with no significant difference).

Conclusion: Subthreshold microsecond laser was shown to be safe and effective with both 5 and 15% DC as compared to conventional photocoagulation with ETDRS parameters. The 15% DC setting trended to achieve better anatomical, visual and functional outcomes.

Keywords: Subthreshold laser, Microsecond, Micropulse, Diabetic macular edema, Microperimetry, Laser photocoagulation

Background

After various randomized and non-randomized clinical trials, anti- vascular endothelial growth factor (VEGF) therapy has become a gold standard in management of diabetic macular edema [1–5]. However, in the RISE and RIDE trials, the Phase 3 trials for ranibizumab in diabetic macular edema, 13.9% of patients receiving monthly intravitreal injections of ranibizumab showed no gain of letters compared to baseline at 24 months [3]. Frequent visits with frequent injections, causes a major economic burden

for these patients. In a study from Wallick et al., patients with diabetic macular edema were found to have, on average, 25.5 annual days with a health care related visit [6]. In a Canadian study published in 2014 by Gonder et al., the mean 6-month DME-related cost was $2092 per patient [7]. The present day cost is likely higher since the study considered that 70% of patients were injected with bevacizumab and the rest with ranibizumab. Thus, there is a constant need for a therapy with long term efficacy for this visually debilitating disease.

Laser photocoagulation was proposed as treatment of choice for diabetic macular edema after ETDRS (Early Treatment of Diabetic Retinopathy Study) [8], much before the anti-VEGF era. Maintenance rather than the

* Correspondence: jay.chhablani@gmail.com
[1]Smt. Kanuri Santhamma Retina Vitreous Centre, L.V.Prasad Eye Institute, Kallam Anji Reddy Campus Banjara Hills, Hyderabad 500034, India
Full list of author information is available at the end of the article

vision improvement along with the loss of contrast sensitivity, poor color vision, accidental foveal damage and expansion of macular scars were the primary complication of laser photocoagulation, which brought the laser photocoagulation in the back seat. However, in recent past with improved technology, subthreshold laser photocoagulation has got more interest and shown to be effective in various macular diseases such as diabetic macular edema [9–13], CSCR (central serous chorioretinopathy) [14–16], and venous occlusions [17].

Laser parameters were standardized after ETDRS study for diabetic macular edema [15]. Unlike conventional laser photocoagulation, there is no standard parameters have been proposed for subthreshold laser. In the literature, there is a lot of variability for subthreshold laser settings in terms of titration, duty cycle (ranging from 5 to 15% duty cycle (DC)), laser power and pulse duration.

This study aims to assess the safety and efficacy of two of the most frequently used subthreshold parameters (5 and 15% DC) when compared to standard ETDRS threshold laser.

Methods

This prospective randomized double-masked pilot study was performed at L V Prasad eye institute, Hyderabad. The study was approved by the institutional review committee and adhered to the tenets of the Declaration of Helsinki. All participants gave written informed consent before enrollment in the study. The Hyderabad Eye Research Foundation, India, supported this study. Patients were recruited from January 2012 through February 2013 at LV Prasad Eye Institute, Hyderabad, India.

Patient eligibility

Inclusion criteria: Eyes with naive non-center involving macular edema (central subfield thickness less than 350 μm) with visual acuity 20/30 or better. The key exclusion criteria were: (1) Dense lens opacity impeding the visualization or laser photocoagulation; (2) Previous macular laser photocoagulation in the study eye; (3) Use of intraocular or periocular corticosteroids in the study eye within the previous 3 months; (4) Previous treatment with anti-VEGF drugs in the study eye.

Study design

Subjects were randomized into 3 different groups. Groups A and B received navigated microsecond laser treatments at 5% DC (100 μs on time) and 15% DC (300 μs on time), respectively. Group C received a continuous wave (CW) navigated ETDRS threshold laser treatment with visible endpoints. In situation when both eyes of the patient were eligible, each eye was randomized as per the randomization. Patient and the visual acuity assessor were masked.

Color fundus photograph

Color fundus photographs of the optic disc, macula, and temporal retina (30°) were captured with a mydriatic camera (Zeiss FF450, Carl Zeiss Meditec, Jena, Germany).

Fundus fluorescein angiography (FFA)

FFA was performed using fluorescein sodium 20% and imaging on Navilas® system (OD-OS GmbH, Teltow, Germany) to determine the site of leakage at baseline, and at three months from baseline.

Spectral Domain Optical Coherence Tomography (SD-OCT):

Cirrus HD-OCT (Carl Zeiss Meditec, Inc., Dublin, CA.) was used to obtain SD-OCT scans. Scanning protocol included HD5 line raster, HD single line raster, enhanced depth imaging, and macular cube. Central retinal thickness (CRT) (1 mm central retinal thickness area as described in the Early Treatment Diabetics Retinopathy Study (ETDRS) fields) was determined automatically and analyzed by OCT software, by generating images using the Macular Cube 512×128 scan over 6×6 mm area, the cube being composed of 128 horizontal examination lines of 512 A-scans each.

Microperimetry (MAIA ™, Centervue, Padova, Italy)

Microperimetry was performed using the microperimeter (MAIA ™, Centervue, Padova, Italy) after dilation of pupils. Goldmann III stimuli and a 4–2–1 staircase strategy with a test grid with 37 stimulus locations covering an area of 10 degrees was applied. Fixation was tracked using built-in fixation target. The stimuli were projected on a white background with black illumination set to 1.27 cd/m2 and a stimulus presentation time of 200 milliseconds. Mean differential light sensitivity in decibels (dB) of all test locations was analyzed for the study. Three fixation classes were defined: stable, relatively unstable, unstable. Stable if more than 75% of the fixation points were inside the 2 degree diameter circle; relatively unstable if less than 75% were inside the 2 degree diameter circle, but more than 75% inside the 4 degree diameter circle; and unstable if less than 75% of the fixation sites were inside the 4 degree diameter circle. A change in sensitivity of 1 dB or more, a change in stability of fixation, or both was considered significant.

All patients underwent microperimetry, thickness measurements and visual acuity examinations at baseline, 6 weeks and 12 weeks post treatment.

Laser photocoagulation

Subthreshold laser used was 577 nm navigated laser using Navilas® system (OD-OS GmbH, Teltow, Germany), however, conventional laser was 532 nm using PASCAL® (OptiMedica) system. Both subthreshold laser groups (A and B) were treated with confluent grids to cover areas of

Table 1 Baseline Characteristics of study groups

	Group A (5% DC)	Group B (15% DC)	Group C (CW)
Number of eyes	10	10	10
Mean duration of diabetes (years)	6.5 ± 1.3	7.1 ± 1.1	6.3 ± 2.1
Mean age (years)	58 ± 6.6	59 ± 6	57 ± 10.6
Lens status	Clear (5), NS1(2), NS2 (3)	Clear (5), NS1(4), NS2 (1)	Clear (4), NS1(4), NS2 (2)
Mean BCVA (ETDRS letters)	76 ± 10	80 ± 5	80 ± 7
Mean CMT (microns)	258 ± 28	255 ± 58	248 ± 37
Retinal Sensitivity (dB)	19 ± 5	22 ± 4	23 ± 4

BCVA Best corrected visual acuity
CMT Central Macular Thickness

diffuse edema whereas the threshold laser group was treated with mETDRS modified grids. Fluorescein angiography was used to identify and target leaking microaneurysms, which were targeted directly using navigated laser in all groups.

Titration and settings: Titration in subthreshold groups (5 and 15% DC group) was performed with microsecond pulses to a barely visible burn, after which power was reduced to 30% to reliably achieve subthreshold effects. CW laser was titrated to a barely visible burn. Spot size and envelop pulse durations was set to 100 μm and 100 ms for each group.

Study visits

Patients were followed at week 6 and week 12 after the baseline visit. Comprehensive examination including microperimetry and SD-OCT were performed at all visits, however, FFA was performed at baseline and at week 12.

Outcome measures

Primary outcome measures included change in retinal sensitivity at week 12 compared to baseline. Secondary outcome measures included change in CMT, BCVA, retinal volume on SD-OCT macular thickness map.

Statistical analysis

Intention to treat analysis was performed. The changes compared to baseline, in retinal sensitivity, BCVA, CMT, and retinal volume, at 6 weeks and 12 weeks, were analyzed with Kruskal-Wallis-Test. P-value of < 0.05 was considered as statistically significant.

Results

Thirty eyes of 20 patients with a mean age of 57 ± 8.7 years were enrolled in the study with 10 eyes in each group. Sixteen were males and four were females. At presentation, lens status was clear in 14 eyes; grade 1 nuclear sclerosis 10 and grade 2 nuclear sclerosis in 6 eyes. Baseline clinical characteristics of the groups are shown in Table 1. There was no significant difference between the groups for BCVA, CMT and retinal sensitivity.

The laser parameter used for each group is listed in Table 2. The number of spots applied was significantly lower in group C (CW) as CW laser for modified grid was one burn width apart unlike subthreshold group where confluent laser applications were performed. Representative cases are shown as Figs. 1, 2, and 3. As expected the adjusted laser power values were significantly higher in the 5%DC group as compared to 15%DC and CW. This can be attributed to the titration paradigm as the power has to be increased in order to obtain a barely visible burn to compensate the fact of a chopped microsecond pulsing laser beam. Nevertheless, the fluence in both subthreshold groups is comparable and represents about 30% of the threshold energy obtained with CW lasers.

No complications were reported in any of the groups except in one eye of the 15% DC group, the evidence of the microsecond laser was detected at three months

Table 2 Laser parameter characteristics among different groups

	Group A (5% DC)	Group B (15% DC)	Group C (CW)
Number of spots applied	435 ± 282	335 ± 313	128 ± 112
Fluence applied mJ/mm²	144.4 ± 28.8	167.8 ± 28.7	488.2 ± 142.4
Power range used in mW (range)	424 ± 92.8 (220–500)	168 ± 42.9 (130–280)	87.3 ± 37.2 (50–180)

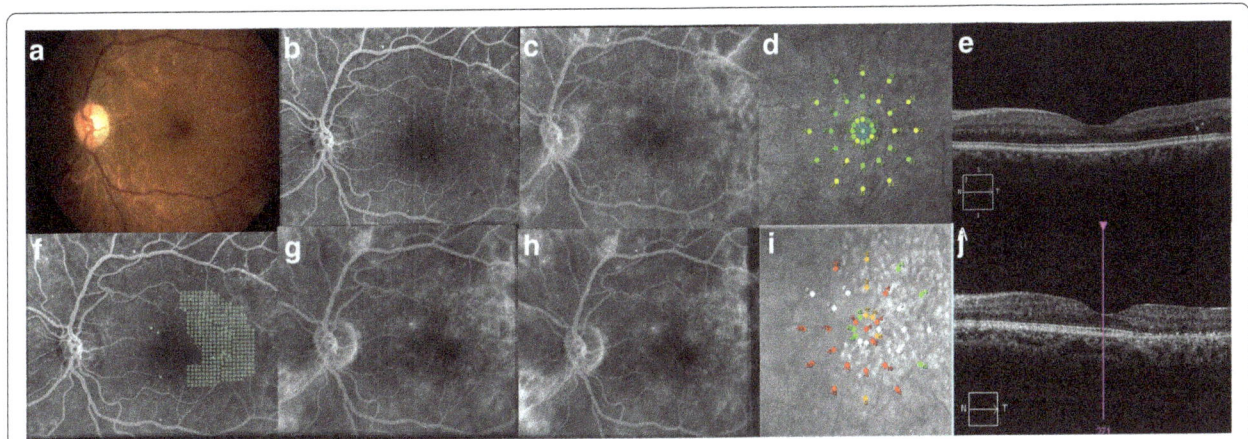

Fig. 1 Continuous wave laser photocoagulation: Color fundus photograph (**a**) shows signs of extrafoveal macular edema with few microaneurysms in early phase of fluorescein angiogrpahy (FA) (**b**) with late leakage in late phase (**c**). Microperimetry map (**d**) shows retinal sensitivity map at baseline. Spectral domain optical coherence tomography (SD-OCT) (**e**) shows normal foveal contour with minimal extrafoveal edema. Laser planning map (**f**) on NAVILAS® device with continuous wave with 60mw power, 100 msec pulse duration, and single burn width apart. At three months follow up FA early and late phases show decrease in overall leakage along with laser scars (**g** and **h**). Microperimetry shows decrease in retinal sensitivity (**i**). SD-OCT shows normal foveal contour with outer retinal damage due to laser scars

follow up on fluorescein angiography. This patient was therefore excluded from further evaluation.

Outcome measures
Changes in primary and secondary outcome measures are shown as Table 3.

Retinal sensitivity outcome
At three months, the retinal sensitivity was slightly reduced in the CW group by − 0.3 dB whereas in both subthreshold groups, retinal sensitivity increased by

0.9 dB for 5% and 1.7 dB for 15% DC ($p = 0.6$ and 0.2 as compared to threshold group) from baseline.

Visual acuity outcome
Best corrected visual acuity remained stable during the follow up period in all 3 groups with no significant difference among the groups (0.7 letter losses in 5% DC; 1.9 letters gain in 15% DC and 0.5 letters gain in CW, respectively). As indicated in Fig. 4 the 15% DC group demonstrated an improvement ($p = 0.04$). Change in BCVA is shown as Fig. 4.

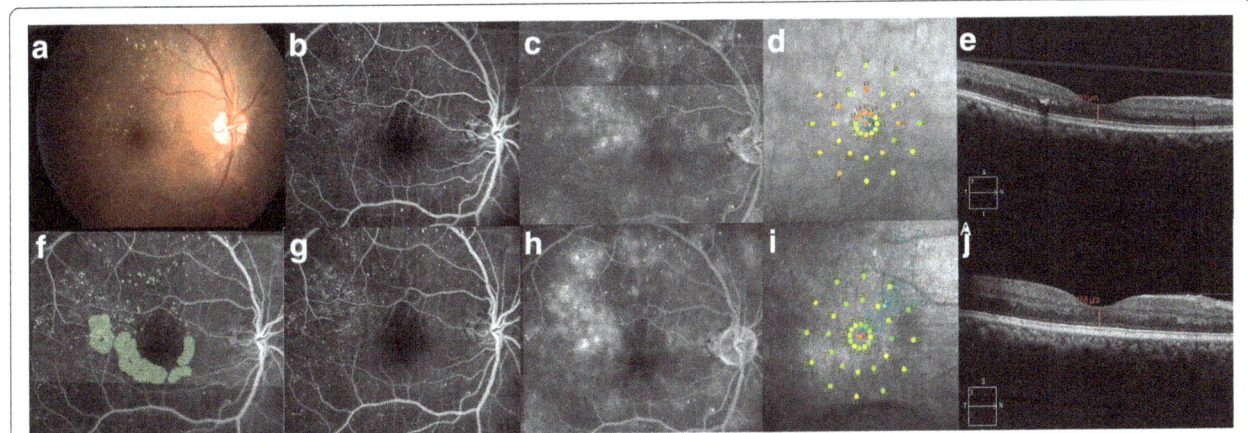

Fig. 2 Subthreshold 5% duty cycle laser photocoagulation: Color fundus photograph (**a**) shows signs of extrafoveal macular edema with few microaneurysms in early phase of fluorescein angiogrpahy (FA) (**b**) with late leakage in late phase (**c**). Microperimetry map (**d**) shows retinal sensitivity map at baseline. Spectral domain optical coherence tomography (SD-OCT) (**e**) shows normal foveal contour with minimal extrafoveal edema. Laser planning map (**f**) on NAVILAS® device with 5%DC with 400mw power, 100 msec pulse duration, and confluent burns. At three months follow up, FA early and late phases show almost same leakage, compared to baseline without any visible laser scars (**g** and **h**). Microperimetry shows improvement in retinal sensitivity (**i**). SD-OCT shows normal foveal contour without any outer retinal damage

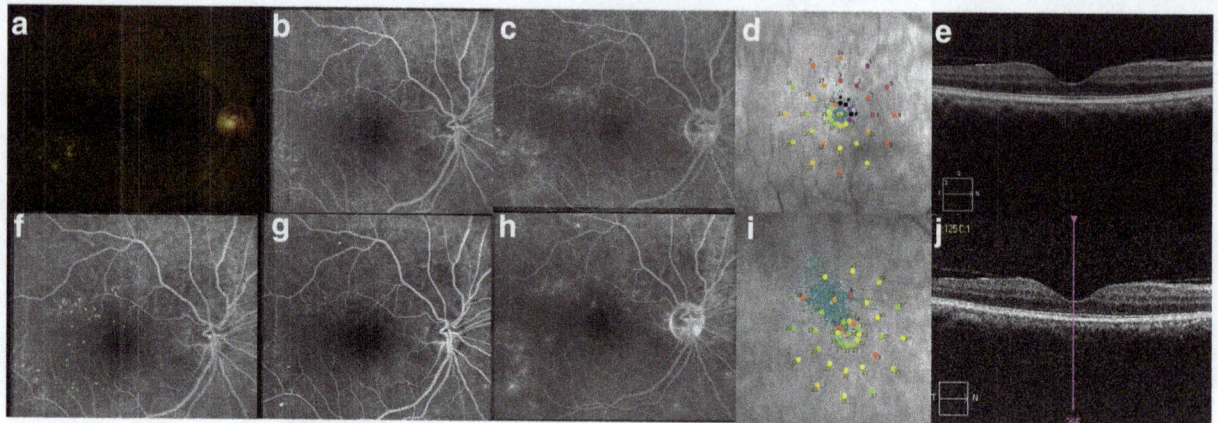

Fig. 3 Subthreshold 15% duty cycle laser photocoagulation: Color fundus photograph (**a**) shows signs of extrafoveal macular edema with few microaneurysms in early phase of fluorescein angiogrpahy (FA) (**b**) with late leakage in late phase (**c**). Microperimetry map (**d**) shows retinal sensitivity map at baseline. Spectral domain optical coherence tomography (SD-OCT) (**e**) shows normal foveal contour. Laser planning map (**f**) on NAVILAS® device with 15%DC with 240mw power, 100 msec pulse duration, and single burn width apart. At three months follow up, FA early and late phase shows almost same leakage, compared to baseline without any visible laser scars (**g** and **h**). Microperimetry shows improvement in retinal sensitivity (**i**). SD-OCT shows normal foveal contour without any outer retinal damage

Anatomical outcome

Retinal volume and central retinal thickness remained stable at three months follow up, with a slight trend toward decreasing in both subthreshold groups with 0.08 ± 0.3 in 5% DC group and 0.12 ± 0.11 in 15% DC group. Whereas, CW group represented a slight volume increase of 0.55 ± 0.92 ($p = 0.02$ and 0.01 for 5 and 15% DC groups as compared to threshold group). The same applies to the CRT where a positive development of reduced CRT can be noted as compared to an increase in CRT in the CW group (See Fig. 5).

Discussion

Subthreshold microsecond laser is a novel, tissue-sparing approach to treat diabetic macular edema. Unlike with conventional focal laser, there is no standard protocol for laser settings for subthreshold treatments. Tables 4 and 5 shows an overview of studies on subthreshold laser (including 810 nm and 577 nm) and the myriad of parameters used in diabetic macular edema [9–12, 18–

26]. Vujosevic et al. compared yellow with infrared subthreshold laser in 26 and 27 eyes respectively, and found no differences in central retinal thickness, macular volume, foveal choroidal thickness, and best-corrected visual acuity [23]. Our study shows that the subthreshold microsecond laser was safe and effective with both 5 and 15% DC following careful titration as compared to CW laser. In trend, 15% DC setting seems to achieve highest ETDRS letter gain and largest decrease in volume.

Lavinsky et al. did a detailed analysis of retinal structures changes under certain fluence reductions and concluded that 30% of threshold energy does not create any tissue defects [27, 28]. Our parameters cannot be compared directly as Lavinsky et al. used CW mode with 7-10 ms pulse durations. However, considering that shortening the pulse duration results in lesser damage, we performed subthreshold microsecond laser with 30% of threshold laser power and found it to be successful. Therefore, these settings can be considered as safe and effective with microsecond laser.

Table 3 Change in outcome measures at week 12

Parameters	CW	5%	15%
Retinal sensitivity (dB)	-2.2 ± 2.4	$+2.4 \pm 6.04(p*=0.3)$	$+1.9 \pm 4.1(p*=0.2)$ Compared to 5% ($p = 0.8$)
ETDRS letters loss/gain	0.9 ± 2.5	$-0.7 \pm 7.7(p*=0.6)$	2.11 ± 2.5 ($p*=0.3$) Compared to 5% ($p = 0.3$)
Central Retinal Thickness (microns)	12.3 ± 41.2	-12.4 ± 36.6 ($p*=0.2$)	$0.6 \pm 21.3(p*=0.5)$ Compared to 5% ($p = 0.4$)
Retinal volume (mm^3)	$+0.55 \pm 0.92$	-0.08 ± 0.3 ($p*=0.02$)	-0.12 ± 0.11 ($p*=0.01$) Compared to 5% ($p = 0.4$)

ETDRS Early Treatment Of Diabetic Retinopathy Study
* = Compared to CW (conventional) threshold laser

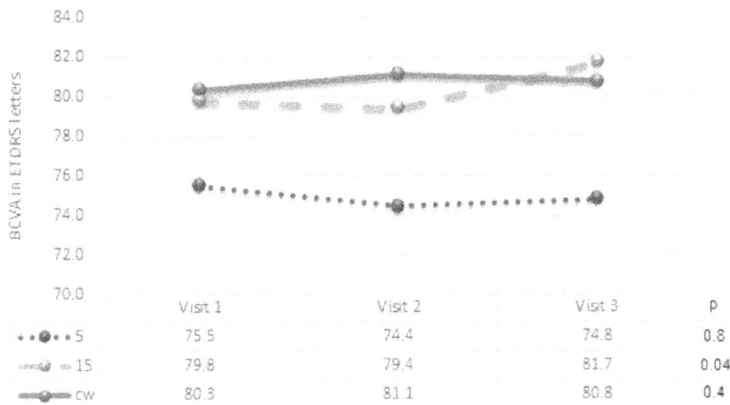

Fig. 4 Change in best-corrected visual acuity (BCVA) during study visits

	Visit 1	Visit 2	Visit 3	p
5	75.5	74.4	74.8	0.8
15	79.8	79.4	81.7	0.04
CW	80.3	81.1	80.8	0.4

One of the challenges with micropulse is the invisibility of laser applications, which makes it difficult to follow up the patients and re-treatment. NAVILAS® provides an additional advantage over other micropulse laser systems is that it provides the reports with treated area along with laser parameters. Application of confluent laser marks could be challenging using conventional slit lamp laser systems due to eye movement and the unavailability of eye tracking. NAVILAS® provides a computerized laser planning and eye tracking during laser application which is accurate and beneficial for subthreshold laser as the laser spots are not visible. Two studies have shown that use of the NAVILAS® results in higher accuracy of targets for photocoagulation compared to the conventional method without the navigating system [29–31]. However, previous reports suggest subthreshold laser application in the "whole posterior pole" which doesn't require the information about the previously performed subthreshold laser applications. [32, 33]

Luttrull et al. showed increased burn risk for 810 nm subthreshold laser with more than 5%DC. [34] This risk increases with decreasing wavelength, which may have been the reason for visible burn in one out 10 eyes with 15%DC. This needs further clarification in terms of safety with larger sample size including 5%DC group. However, this study supports the safety of subthreshold laser over the CW laser.

Limitations of our study include small sample size in each group and short follow up. Our study did not scientifically analyze microaneurysm closure rate. However, this is the first study, which compares effect of different duty cycle subthreshold dosage with standard ETDRS laser dosage in diabetic macular edema. However, less number of subthreshold laser applications over a limited area of DME may be the reason for suboptimal response. Due to ethical issues, we did not include center-involving edema, which may have responded differently due to more severity and further loss of retinal sensitivity, and may have influenced the outcome measures.

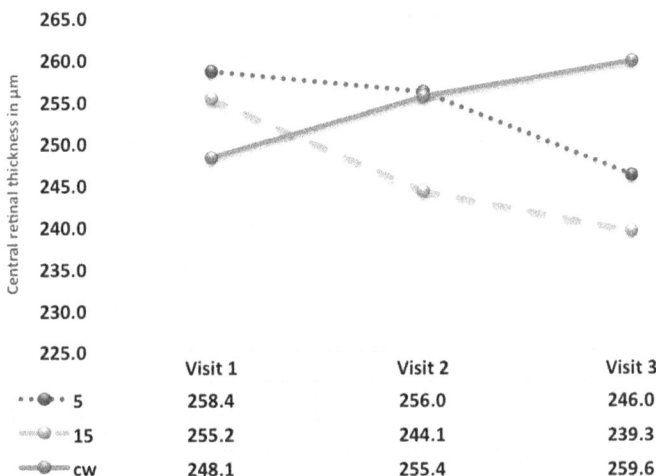

	Visit 1	Visit 2	Visit 3
5	258.4	256.0	246.0
15	255.2	244.1	239.3
cw	248.1	255.4	259.6

Fig. 5 Change in central retinal thickness during study visits

Table 4 Overview on parameters used in 810 nm subthreshold laser treatments

	Wavelength (nm)	Spot size (um)	Duration (ms)	Duty Cycle	Power definition method
Laursen et al. [9]	810	125	100	5%	50% of barely visible burn
Figueira et al. [10]	810	125	300	30%	200% of barely visible burn
Lavinsky et al. [11]	810	125	300	15%	120% of barely visible burn
Vujosevic et al. [12]	810	125	200	5%	750 mW
Luttrull et al. [19]	810	125	300	5%	750 mW
Sivaprasad et al. [20]	810	125	200	5%	100% of a barely visible burn (unless more than 1200 mW in which case duty cycle was increased to 10%)
Othman et al. [21]	810	75–125	300	15%	100% barely visible burn
Inagaki et al. [22]	810	200	200	15%	200% barely visible burn

Table 5 Overview on parameters used in yellow (577 nm) subthreshold treatments

Author	Spot Size	ms	DC	Power	Fluence mmJ/mm²	Power definition method
Kwon et al. [24]	100	20	15%	140	54	Titration in cw; starting at 100 mW upwards until barely visible burn; after switch to μp power remains immediately below test burn
Vujosevic et al. [23]	100	200	5%	250	318	Fixed power setting
Yadav et al. [25]	100	200	10%	70–200	340	Titration burn in cw, until mild retinal whitening; then μs mode and Half power
Inagaki et al. [22]	200	200	15%	204	197	Test burn in cw mode with 100 ms and 200 μm; then switch to 15% DC and doubling the power which is 60% of threshold energy
Pei-pei et al. [30]	60	10	100%	32,4 J/cm²	324	50% of power, no switch of Pulse duration

Conclusion

In conclusion, our pilot study reports the subthreshold laser with 15% DC appears to be more efficacious to reduce the retinal thickness and improve the retinal sensitivity, however, safety needs further evaluation on larger studies. Further studies are warranted to evaluate subthreshold laser in center-involving diabetic macular edema with or without anti-VEGF therapy. Subthreshold laser could be considered as cheap treatment option and finally a retinal restorative therapy without any structural and functional damage.

Abbreviations

BCVA: Best Corrected Visual Acuity; CMT: Central Macular Thickness; CRT: Central Retinal Thickness; CSCR: Central Serous Chorioretinopathy; CW: Continuous Wave; DC: Duty Cycle; DME: Diabetic Macular Edema; ETDRS: Early Treatment Diabetic Retinopathy Study; FFA: Fundus Fluorescence Angiography; SD-OCT: Spectral Domain Ocular Coherence Tomography; VEGF: Vascular Endothelial Growth Factor

Author's contributions

Conception and design: JC, RN,AM; Data collection: JC, RN, AG, AM. Analysis and interpretation: JC, RA, DTK; writing the article: JC, RA, DTK. Critical Revision of the article: JC, RA, DTK, RN, AG, AM. Final approval of the article: JC, RA, DTK, RN, AG, AM.

Competing interests

Jay Chhablani is a member of the editorial board.

Author details

[1]Smt. Kanuri Santhamma Retina Vitreous Centre, L.V.Prasad Eye Institute, Kallam Anji Reddy Campus Banjara Hills, Hyderabad 500034, India. [2]Department of Ophthalmology, McGill University, Montreal, Quebec, Canada. [3]Department of Surgery, Division of Ophthalmology, Faculty of Medicine and Health Sciences, Université de Sherbrooke, Sherbrooke, Quebec, Canada.

References

1. Michaelides M, Kaines A, Hamilton RD, Fraser-Bell S, Rajendram R, Quhill F, Boos CJ, Xing W, Egan C, Peto T. A prospective randomized trial of intravitreal bevacizumab or laser therapy in the management of diabetic macular edema (BOLT study):12-month data: report 2. Ophthalmology. 2010;117(6):1078–1086. e1072.
2. Arevalo JF, Sanchez JG, Fromow-Guerra J, Wu L, Berrocal MH, Farah ME, Cardillo J, Rodríguez FJ. Group P-ACRS: comparison of two doses of primary intravitreal bevacizumab (Avastin) for diffuse diabetic macular edema: results from the pan-American collaborative retina study group (PACORES) at 12-month follow-up. Graefes Arch Clin Exp Ophthalmol. 2009;247(6):735–43.
3. Brown DM, Nguyen QD, Marcus DM, Boyer DS, Patel S, Feiner L, Schlottmann PG, Rundle AC, Zhang J, Rubio RG. Long-term outcomes of ranibizumab therapy for diabetic macular edema: the 36-month results from two phase III trials: RISE and RIDE. Ophthalmology. 2013;120(10):2013–22.
4. Brown DM, Schmidt-Erfurth U, Do DV, Holz FG, Boyer DS, Midena E, Heier JS, Terasaki H, Kaiser PK, Marcus DM. Intravitreal aflibercept for diabetic macular edema: 100-week results from the VISTA and VIVID studies. Ophthalmology. 2015;122(10):2044–52.
5. Network DRCR. Aflibercept, bevacizumab, or ranibizumab for diabetic macular edema. N Engl J Med. 2015;2015(372):1193–203.

6. Wallick CJ, Hansen RN, Campbell J, Kiss S, Kowalski JW, Sullivan SD. Comorbidity and health care resource use among commercially insured non-elderly patients with diabetic macular edema. Ophthalmic Surg Lasers Imaging Retina. 2015;46(7):744–51.

7. Gonder JR, Walker VM, Barbeau M, Zaour N, Zachau BH, Hartje JR, Li R. Costs and quality of life in diabetic macular edema: Canadian burden of diabetic macular edema observational study (C-REALITY). J Ophthalmol. 2014;2014:939315.

8. Photocoagulation for diabetic macular edema. Early treatment diabetic retinopathy study report number 1. Early treatment diabetic retinopathy study research group. Archives of ophthalmology (Chicago, Ill : 1960). 1985;103(12):1796–806.

9. Laursen M, Moeller F, Sander B, Sjoelie A. Subthreshold micropulse diode laser treatment in diabetic macular oedema. Br J Ophthalmol. 2004;88(9):1173–9.

10. Figueira J, Khan J, Nunes S, Sivaprasad S, Rosa A, de Abreu JF, Cunha-Vaz JG, Chong N. Prospective randomised controlled trial comparing sub-threshold micropulse diode laser photocoagulation and conventional green laser for clinically significant diabetic macular oedema. Br J Ophthalmol. 2009;93(10):1341–4.

11. Lavinsky D, Cardillo JA, Melo LA, Dare A, Farah ME, Belfort R. Randomized clinical trial evaluating mETDRS versus normal or high-density micropulse photocoagulation for diabetic macular edema. Invest Ophthalmol Vis Sci. 2011;52(7):4314–23.

12. Vujosevic S, Bottega E, Casciano M, Pilotto E, Convento E, Midena E. Microperimetry and fundus autofluorescence in diabetic macular edema: subthreshold micropulse diode laser versus modified early treatment diabetic retinopathy study laser photocoagulation. Retina. 2010;30(6):908–16.

13. Venkatesh P, Ramanjulu R, Azad R, Vohra R, Garg S. Subthreshold micropulse diode laser and double frequency neodymium: YAG laser in treatment of diabetic macular edema: a prospective, randomized study using multifocal electroretinography. Photomed Laser Surg. 2011;29(11):727–33.

14. Koss M, Beger I, Koch F. Subthreshold diode laser micropulse photocoagulation versus intravitreal injections of bevacizumab in the treatment of central serous chorioretinopathy. Eye. 2012;26(2):307–14.

15. Roisman L, Magalhães FP, Lavinsky D, Moraes N, Hirai FE, Cardillo JA, Farah ME. Micropulse diode laser treatment for chronic central serous chorioretinopathy: a randomized pilot trial. Ophthalmic Surg Lasers Imaging Retina. 2013;44(5):465–70.

16. Chen S-N, Hwang J-F, Tseng L-F, Lin C-J. Subthreshold diode micropulse photocoagulation for the treatment of chronic central serous chorioretinopathy with juxtafoveal leakage. Ophthalmology. 2008; 115(12):2229–34.

17. Parodi MB, Spasse S, Iacono P, Di Stefano G, Canziani T, Ravalico G. Subthreshold grid laser treatment of macular edema secondary to branch retinal vein occlusion with micropulse infrared (810 nanometer) diode laser. Ophthalmology. 2006;113(12):2237–42.

18. Luttrull JK, Musch DC, Mainster MA. Subthreshold diode micropulse photocoagulation for the treatment of clinically significant diabetic macular oedema. Br J Ophthalmol. 2005;89(1):74–80.

19. Sivaprasad S, Sandhu R, Tandon A, Sayed-Ahmed K, McHugh DA. Subthreshold micropulse diode laser photocoagulation for clinically significant diabetic macular oedema: a three-year follow up. Clin Exp Ophthalmol. 2007;35(7):640–4.

20. Othman IS, Eissa SA, Kotb MS, Sadek SH. Subthreshold diode-laser micropulse photocoagulation as a primary and secondary line of treatment in management of diabetic macular edema. Clin Ophthalmol (Auckland, NZ). 2014;8:653.

21. Inagaki K, Ohkoshi K, Ohde S, Deshpande GA, Ebihara N, Murakami A. Comparative efficacy of pure yellow (577-nm) and 810-nm subthreshold micropulse laser photocoagulation combined with yellow (561–577-nm) direct photocoagulation for diabetic macular edema. Jpn J Ophthalmol. 2015;59(1):21–8.

22. Kwon YH, Lee DK, Kwon OW. The short-term efficacy of subthreshold micropulse yellow (577-nm) laser photocoagulation for diabetic macular edema. Korean J Ophthalmol. 2014;28(5):379–85.

23. Vujosevic S, Martini F, Longhin E, Convento E, Cavarzeran F, Midena E. Subthreshold micropulse yellow laser versus subthreshold micropulse infrared laser in center-involving diabetic macular edema: morphologic and functional safety. Retina. 2015;35(8):1594–603.

24. Yadav N, Jayadev C, Mohan A, Vijayan P, Battu R, Dabir S, Shetty B, Shetty R. Subthreshold micropulse yellow laser (577 nm) in chronic central serous chorioretinopathy: safety profile and treatment outcome. Eye. 2015;29(2):258–65.

25. Pei-Pei W, Shi-Zhou H, Zhen T, Lin L, Ying L, Jiexiong O, Wen-Bo Z, Chen-Jin J. Randomised clinical trial evaluating best-corrected visual acuity and central macular thickness after 532-nm subthreshold laser grid photocoagulation treatment in diabetic macular oedema. Eye. 2015;29(3):313–22.

26. Group ETDRSR. Treatment techniques and clinical guidelines for photocoagulation of diabetic macular edema: early treatment diabetic retinopathy study report number 2. Ophthalmology. 1987;94(7):761–74.

27. Lavinsky D, Sramek C, Wang J, Huie P, Dalal R, Mandel Y, Palanker D. Subvisible retinal laser therapy: titration algorithm and tissue response. Retina. 2014;34(1):87–97.

28. Lavinsky D, Palanker D. Nondamaging photothermal therapy for the retina: initial clinical experience with chronic central serous retinopathy. Retina. 2015;35(2):213–22.

29. Muqit MM, Denniss J, Nourrit V, Marcellino GR, Henson DB, Schiessl I, Stanga PE. Spatial and spectral imaging of retinal laser photocoagulation burns. Invest Ophthalmol Vis Sci. 2011;52(2):994–1002.

30. Kozak I, Oster SF, Cortes MA, Dowell D, Hartmann K, Kim JS, Freeman WR. Clinical evaluation and treatment accuracy in diabetic macular edema using navigated laser photocoagulator NAVILAS. Ophthalmology. 2011;118(6):1119–24.

31. Kernt M, Cheuteu RE, Cserhati S, Seidensticker F, Liegl RG, Lang J, Haritoglou C, Kampik A, Ulbig MW, Neubauer AS. Pain and accuracy of focal laser treatment for diabetic macular edema using a retinal navigated laser (Navilas®). Clin Ophthalmol (Auckland NZ). 2012;6:289.

32. Luttrull J, Musch D, Mainster M. Subthreshold diode micropulse photocoagulation for the treatment of clinically significant diabetic macular oedema. Br J Ophthalmol. 2005;89(1):74–80.

33. Luttrull JK, Dorin G. Subthreshold diode micropulse laser photocoagulation (SDM) as invisible retinal phototherapy for diabetic macular edema: a review. Curr Diabetes Rev. 2012;8(4):274–84.

34. Luttrull JK, Sramek C, Palanker D, Spink CJ, Musch DC. Long-term safety, high-resolution imaging, and tissue temperature modeling of subvisible diode micropulse photocoagulation for retinovascular macular edema. Retina. 2012;32(2):375–86.

28

Risk factors of presenile nuclear cataract in health screening study

Seung Wan Nam[1], Dong Hui Lim[1,2,4*], Kyu Yeon Cho[1], Hye Seung Kim[3], Kyunga Kim[3] and Tae-Young Chung[1,4*]

Abstract

Background: To identify risk factors for the development of presenile nuclear cataract in health screening test.

Methods: The cross sectional study included a total of 532 eyes of 266 participants aged 30 to 49 years of Samsung Medical Center from February 2013 to April 2015. Presence of nuclear cataract was defined when the log MAR visual acuity with correction was greater than or equal to 0.2 and one or more of the following were met: Pentacam Nuclear Staging (PNS) grading score $\geq$ 1, average value of nuclear density $\geq$ 15%, maximum value of nuclear density $\geq$ 30%. Possible risk factors were obtained from blood tests and questionnaires of a health screening test of Samsung Medical Center. Association between nuclear cataract and risk factors was investigated using univariate and multivariate logistic regression analysis by generalized estimating equation (GEE) models.

Results: Five factors were significantly associated with presenile nuclear cataract: current smoking [odds ratio (OR) = 2.80, 95% confidence interval (CI), 1.10–7.12, $p = 0.0310$], non-exercise and high amount of daily physical exercise (OR = 3.99, 95% CI, 1.27–12.52, $p = 0.0178$; OR = 2.92, 95% CI, 1.38–6.22, $p = 0.0053$), asthma (OR = 8.93, 95% CI, 1.12–71.15, $p = 0.0386$), tuberculosis (OR = 4.28, 95% CI, 1.36–13.50, $p = 0.0131$), and higher total iron binding capacity (OR = 1.01, 95% CI, 1.00–1.02, $p = 0.0059$).

Conclusions: Presenile nuclear cataract is related to current smoking, non-exercise or high amount of physical exercise, asthma, tuberculosis, and iron deficiency status. The association of non-exercise group and presenile nuclear cataract seems to be related to co-morbidity. Patients with asthma, tuberculosis, or iron deficiency anemia are recommended to receive frequent ophthalmic examination to detect cataract.

Keywords: Presenile cataract, Health screening test, Scheimpflug image, Smoking, Exercise

Background

Cataract, caused by degenerative changes in the lens, is a major cause of blindness globally, and often occurs after 50 years of age [1]. The Lens Opacification Classification System III (LOCS), the most commonly used grading system for evaluating cataract, grades cataract by nuclear color and opacity, cortical opacity, and posterior subcapsular opacity [2].

Pentacam Nucleus Staging (PNS) using Pentacam Scheimpflug (Oculus, Wetzlar, Germany) [3] images is a quantitative method of measuring nuclear cataract that provides average and maximal lens density [4]. In the previous study, we suggested that Pentacam imaging system is effective in screening cataract patients and has

the potential to be applied in health examination [4]. The correlation between PNS and LOCS III has been revealed in many studies [5–7], especially in nuclear cataract [8]. PNS detects early nuclear cataract and quantitatively analyzes nuclear cataract [6].

Presenile cataract refers to onset before the age of 50 years [9]. According to a previous study, posterior subcapsular cataract related with atopy is the most common type of cataract in presenile age [9]. However, early diagnosis of other types of cataract including nucleosclerosis in presenile age is important to make a clinical decision of cataract surgery and prevent progression of cataract. Unlike senile nuclear cataract, the risk factors of presenile nuclear cataract is well not known.

The purpose of the present study is to detect and reveal the risk factors of presenile nuclear cataract diagnosed by Pentacam image in the health screening test.

* Correspondence: ldhlse@gmail.com; tychung@skku.ac.kr
[1]Department of Ophthalmology, Samsung Medical Center, Sungkyunkwan University School of Medicine, Seoul, South Korea
Full list of author information is available at the end of the article

Methods

The study population included 4605 consecutive participants undergoing screening cataract using Pentacam Schiempflug imaging as part of routine health check-up examinations at the Center for Health Promotion of Samsung Medical Center in Seoul, Korea from February 2013 to April 2015. Of these, 532 eyes of 266 participants aged 30 to 49 years were included. All participants had no history of ocular trauma, laser treatments, or ocular surgeries. Participants diagnosed with any ocular disease except age-related cataract were excluded. If a participant had more than one Scheimpflug image during the study period, only the last Scheimpflug image was included.

The Institutional Review Board of Samsung Medical Center (Seoul, Korea) approved the study protocol (IRB File Number: 2015–06-050). The Institutional Review Board of Samsung Medical Center exempted the requirement for informed consent because the study was based on retrospective analyses of de-identified existing administrative and clinical data.

Health screening examination

Over 1200 predictor variables were obtained by health screening examination. According to previous reports [10–16], 42 of these predictors known to be associated with cataract were selected for the analysis: age [14], sex [17], history of smoking [18], alcohol consumption [19], physical exercise [20], diabetes [21], asthma [22, 23], tuberculosis [24], hypertension [25], dyslipidemia [26], medication use such as statin [27] or aspirin [28] as reported by a self-questionnaire, height, weight, body mass index (BMI, kg/m^2) [29], waist circumference, and blood tests including markers of diabetes, dyslipidemia, inflammation [30], dehydration [31], iron deficiency [32], and viral infection [33, 34].

Daily exercise duration was categorized into 3 subgroups. According to 2013 AHA/ACC guideline [35], 40-min exercise per day was suggested to affect blood pressure and cholesterol. Therefore, we divided low and high amount of daily exercise duration by 40 min. Blood tests including white blood cell count, red blood cell count, platelet count, sodium, potassium, fasting glucose, hemoglobin A1c, total cholesterol, triglycerides, high-density lipoprotein (HDL) cholesterol, low-density lipoprotein (LDL) cholesterol, hemoglobin, and total iron binding capacity (TIBC) were performed. Blood samples were collected after at least 10 h of fasting. The Department of Laboratory Medicine and Genetics at Samsung Medical Center has participated in several proficiency testing programs operated by the Korean Association of Quality Assurance for Clinical Laboratory, the Asian Network of Clinical Laboratory Standardization and Harmonization, and the College of American Pathologists.

Pentacam nuclear staging

Quantitative lens density was measured with Pentacam device, as in the previous report [4]. All images were obtained using the same device and consistent environment after equipment calibration. Participants without pupil dilation placed their chins on a chin rest. The Scheimpflug image of each eye was manually focused and centered. Built-in densitometry software automatically measured PNS measurements (Fig. 1). To increase the reliability of the data, Scheimpflug images of the medical examination included in the study were verified by the ophthalmologist, and ophthalmologist confirmed that PNS measurements were obtained at the nucleus position of lens. The grading scores from 0 to 5, and the average and maximum value of nuclear density from 0 to 100% were recorded.

Presence of nuclear cataract was defined by corrected visual acuity and PNS measurements. According to our previous criteria [4], presenile nuclear cataract was diagnosed when the log MAR visual acuity with correction was greater than or equal to 0.2 [4] and one or more of the following were met: PNS grading score ≥ 1, average value of nuclear density $\geq 15\%$, maximum value of nuclear density $\geq 30\%$.

Statistical analysis

Between-group differences (normal group vs. presenile nuclear cataract group) were evaluated using Wilcoxon test for continuous variables, chi-squared test for categorical variables, and Fisher's exact test for analysis of factors with small counts of ≤ 5. To identify risk factors for presenile nuclear cataract, generalized estimation equation (GEE) models were constructed by considering paired eyed data. In the first step, univariate GEE was performed to identify possible prognostic factors. In the second step, multivariate GEE was performed using variables with p values less than 0.2 on univariate GEE to refine the predictive model. All statistical tests were two-tailed and performed with $p < 0.2$ considered statistically significant in univariate analysis, and $p < 0.05$ considered statistically significant in multivariate analysis. Distributions for continuous variables are expressed as means $\pm$ standard deviations (SDs). Statistical analysis was performed using SAS version 9.4 (SAS Institute, Cary, NC).

Results
Descriptive characteristics

A total of 532 eyes of 266 participants were included in this study. Seventy-four eyes (13.91%) were diagnosed with presenile nuclear cataract by PNS. The age of subjects was 45.12 ± 3.78 years (range, 31–49), and 183 participants (68.80%) of the total analyzed population were men. The log MAR visual acuity with correction

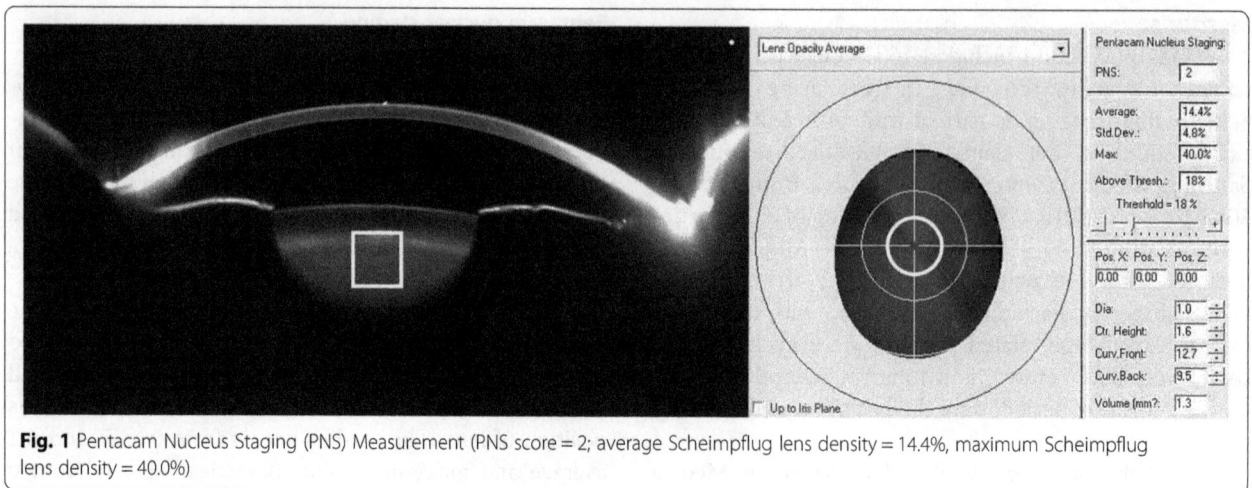

Fig. 1 Pentacam Nucleus Staging (PNS) Measurement (PNS score = 2; average Scheimpflug lens density = 14.4%, maximum Scheimpflug lens density = 40.0%)

was 0.07 ± 0.17, and PNS measurements were as follows; PNS score = 0.52 ± 0.54, average Scheimpflug lens density = 10.72 ± 1.55%, maximum Scheimpflug lens density = 38.05 ± 16.22%.

Descriptive characteristics and between-group differences were analyzed in Table 1. 32.24% of participants were current smokers; 2.44% of participants reported daily alcohol intake; 9.72% of participants performed no physical exercise, 14.66% of participants had hypertension, 6.02% of participants had diabetes, 16.92% of participants had dyslipidemia, 1.88% of participants had asthma, 4.14% of participants had tuberculosis, and 4.14% of participants showed hepatitis B virus (HBV) seropositivity.

Univariate analysis

The univariate GEE analysis for each factor is reported in Additional file 1: Table S1. Variables with a p value less than 0.2 on univariate GEE were considered possible risk factors for presenile nuclear cataract. Compared to normal group, presenile nuclear cataract group showed higher proportion of current smokers (odds ratio (OR) = 1.72, 95% confidence interval (CI), 0.97–3.08, $p = 0.0656$), younger age at starting smoking (OR = 0.90, 95% CI, 0.80–1.01, $p = 0.0791$), longer smoking duration (OR = 1.04, 95% CI, 0.99–1.09, $p = 0.1636$), smoked over 30 cigarettes per day (OR = 2.13, 95% CI, 0.67–6.79, $p = 0.1998$), no physical exercise and a high amount of physical exercise (OR = 2.45, 95% CI, 1.08–5.58, $p = 0.0322$; OR = 1.97, 95% CI, 1.10–3.52, $p = 0.0223$), taller (OR = 1.02, 95% CI, 0.99–1.05, $p = 0.1520$), asthma (OR = 4.87, 95% CI, 0.99–23.84, $p = 0.0510$), tuberculosis (OR = 3.30, 95% CI, 1.09–9.97, $p = 0.0341$), lower hemoglobin A1c (OR = 0.71, 95% CI, 0.45–1.13, $p = 0.1509$), lower glucose level (OR = 0.99, 95% CI, 0.97–1.00, $p = 0.1015$), higher TIBC (OR = 1.00, 95% CI, 1.00–1.01, $p = 0.0533$), and higher HBV seropositivity (OR = 2.82, 95% CI, 0.91–8.74, $p = 0.0729$).

The association with presenile nuclear cataract was not significantly different with age (OR = 0.97, 95% CI, 0.91–1.04, $p = 0.3422$) and sex (OR = 1.24, 95% CI, 0.73–2.10, $p = 0.4223$). Other descriptive characteristics were comparable between normal and presenile nuclear cataract groups. There was no significant association between presenile nuclear cataract and other modifiable lifestyle-related risk factors, such as alcohol consumption, weight, BMI, and waist-hip ratio (WHR, $p > 0.2$). Cholesterol profile including total cholesterol, HDL, LDL, and triglyceride did not show a significant association with nuclear cataract ($p > 0.2$).

Multivariate analysis

The results of multivariate GEE analysis adjusted for variables with a p value less than 0.2 on univariate analysis are reported in Table 2. Data regarding smoking, alcohol consumption, and physical exercise were collected using various survey questions. Variables in these questionnaire items were then adjusted by considering clinical and statistical significance. Smoking status, alcohol consumption frequency, and daily physical exercise duration were analyzed.

The multivariate model identified current smoker (OR = 2.80, 95% CI, 1.10–7.12, $p = 0.0310$), non-exercise and high amount of physical exercise (OR = 3.99, 95% CI, 1.27–12.52, $p = 0.0178$; OR = 2.92, 95% CI, 1.38–6.22, $p = 0.0053$), asthma (OR = 8.93, 95% CI, 1.12–71.15, $p = 0.0386$), tuberculosis (OR = 4.28, 95% CI, 1.36–13.50, $p = 0.0131$), and higher TIBC (OR = 1.01, 95% CI, 1.00–1.02, $p = 0.0059$) as predictive of presenile nuclear cataract. Alcohol consumption frequency, height, hemoglobin A1c, and HBV seropositivity did not show significant associations with nuclear cataract ($p > 0.05$).

Table 1 Demographic characteristics and between-group analysis of participants

	Total (n = 266)	Normal (n = 192)	Presenile nuclear cataract (n = 74)[d]	p value
Age (years)	45.12 ± 3.78 (N = 266)	45.26 ± 3.65 (N = 192)	44.76 ± 4.12 (N = 74)	0.471[a]
Sex, male	183/266 (68.8%)	136/192 (72.18%)	47/74 (63.51%)	0.248[b]
Smoking status				0.306[b]
Never	116/245 (47.35%)	86/174 (49.43%)	30/71 (42.25%)	
Former (quit ≥1 year ago)	50/245 (20.41%)	37/174 (21.26%)	13/71 (18.31%)	
Current	79/245 (32.24%)	51/174 (29.31%)	28/71 (39.44%)	
Age at starting smoking (years)	20.11 ± 3.99 (N = 131)	20.45 ± 4.09 (N = 92)	19.33 ± 3.69 (N = 39)	0.210[a]
Smoking duration (years)	21.30 ± 7.81 (N = 121)	20.93 ± 7.88 (N = 85)	22.17 ± 7.70 (N = 36)	0.448[a]
Smoking cigarettes per day				0.366[a]
≤ 10 cigarettes	38/126 (30.16%)	29/88 (32.95%)	9/38 (23.68%)	
11–20 cigarettes	48/126 (38.10%)	34/88 (38.64%)	14/38 (36.84%)	
21–30 cigarettes	33/126 (26.19%)	22/88 (25.00%)	11/38 (28.95%)	
≥ 30 cigarettes	7/126 (5.56%)	3/88 (3.41%)	4/38 (10.53%)	
Alcohol consumption status				0.456[b]
Never	53/261 (20.31%)	36/188 (19.15%)	17/73 (23.29%)	
Ever	208/261 (79.69%)	152/188 (80.85%)	56/73 (76.71%)	
Alcohol consumption duration (years)	23.07 ± 7.07 (N = 192)	23.04 ± 7.20 (N = 141)	23.14 ± 6.78 (N = 51)	0.734[a]
Alcohol consumption frequency				0.532[c]
≤ 1 day/month	24/205 (11.71%)	16/149 (10.74%)	8/56 (14.29%)	
2–3 days/month	63/205 (30.73%)	46/149 (30.87%)	17/56 (30.36%)	
1–2 days/week	63/205 (30.73%)	49/149 (32.89%)	14/56 (25.00%)	
3–4 days/week	41/205 (20.00%)	29/149 (19.46%)	12/56 (21.43%)	
5–6 days/week	9/205 (4.39%)	7/149 (4.70%)	2/56 (3.57%)	
Everyday	5/205 (2.44%)	2/149 (1.34%)	3/56 (5.36%)	
Alcohol consumption amount (Units/time)				0.940[b]
1~2	56/203 (27.59%)	39/147 (26.53%)	17/56 (30.36%)	
3~6	48/203 (23.65%)	36/147 (24.49%)	12/56 (21.43%)	
7~13	76/203 (37.44%)	55/147 (37.41%)	21/56 (37.50%)	
≥ 14	23/203 (11.33%)	17/147 (11.56%)	6/56 (10.71%)	
Physical exercise degree, n (%)				0.558[b]
Almost absent	26/253 (10.28%)	20/182 (10.99%)	6/71 (8.45%)	
Mild	67/253 (26.48%)	47/182 (25.82%)	20/71 (28.17%)	
Moderate	134/253 (52.96%)	99/182 (54.40%)	35/71 (49.30%)	
Vigorous	26/253 (10.28%)	16/182 (8.79%)	10/71 (14.08%)	
Physical exercise frequency, n (%)				0.324[b]
None	27/245 (11.02%)	18/178 (10.11%)	9/67 (13.43%)	
1–2 days/week	99/245 (40.41%)	75/178 (42.13%)	24/67 (35.82%)	
3–4 days/week	79/245 (32.24%)	60/178 (33.71%)	19/67 (28.36%)	
≥ 5 days/week	40/245 (16.33%)	25/178 (14.04%)	15/67 (22.39%)	
Daily exercise duration, n (%)				0.065[b]
Low amounts (1–40 min/day)	105/247 (42.51%)	83/178 (46.63%)	22/69 (31.88%)	
None	24/247 (9.72%)	14/178 (7.87%)	10/69 (14.49%)	
High amounts (≥41 min/day)	118/247 (47.77%)	81/178 (45.51%)	37/69 (53.62%)	

Table 1 Demographic characteristics and between-group analysis of participants (Continued)

	Total (n = 266)	Normal (n = 192)	Presenile nuclear cataract (n = 74)[d]	p value
Height (cm)	169.66 ± 8.55 (N = 266)	169.35 ± 8.39 (N = 192)	170.45 ± 8.98 (N = 74)	0.349[a]
Weight (kg)	72.50 ± 16.27 (N = 266)	72.34 ± 16.43 (N = 192)	72.92 ± 15.96 (N = 74)	0.793[a]
BMI (kg/m^2)	24.98 ± 4.23 (N = 266)	25.01 ± 4.29 (N = 192)	24.90 ± 4.12 (N = 74)	0.923[a]
WHR	0.91 ± 0.07 (N = 266)	0.91 ± 0.07 (N = 192)	0.92 ± 0.08 (N = 74)	0.586[a]
Hypertension, n (%)	39/266 (14.66%)	30/192 (15.63%)	9/74 (12.16%)	0.474[b]
Diabetes, n (%)	16/266 (6.02%)	14/192 (7.29%)	2/74 (2.70%)	0.249[c]
Dyslipidemia, n (%)	45/266 (16.92%)	31/192 (16.15%)	14/74 (18.92%)	0.589[b]
Asthma, n (%)	5/266 (1.88%)	2/192 (1.04%)	3/74 (4.05%)	0.133[b]
Tuberculosis, n (%)	11/266 (4.14%)	5/192 (2.60%)	6/74 (8.11%)	0.078[b]
Thyroid disease, n (%)	8/266 (3.01%)	7/192 (3.65%)	1/74 (1.35%)	0.450[c]
HbA1c (%)	5.58 ± 0.68 (N = 256)	5.62 ± 0.77 (N = 183)	5.48 ± 0.36 (N = 73)	0.511[a]
Glucose (mg/dL)	95.89 ± 21.91 (N = 266)	97.48 ± 24.71 (N = 192)	91.74 ± 11.00 (N = 74)	0.058[a]
Cholesterol (mg/dL)	197.09 ± 35.88 (N = 266)	198.67 ± 35.65 (N = 192)	192.99 ± 36.41 (N = 74)	0.257[a]
HDL cholesterol (mg/dL)	58.65 ± 17.79 (N = 265)	57.92 ± 15.41 (N = 191)	60.53 ± 22.84 (N = 74)	0.578[a]
LDL cholesterol (mg/dL)	125.69 ± 32.18 (N = 265)	127.09 ± 31.64 (N = 191)	122.07 ± 33.49 (N = 74)	0.312[a]
Triglyceride (mg/dL)	126.50 ± 127.86 (N = 265)	133.31 ± 143.60 (N = 191)	108.92 ± 70.87 (N = 74)	0.097[a]
WBC (/mm^3)	5763.8 ± 1761.3 (N = 266)	5906.8 ± 1872.3 (N = 192)	5392.7 ± 1377.2 (N = 74)	0.074[a]
CRP (mg/dL)	0.20 ± 0.51 (N = 247)	0.18 ± 0.41 (N = 177)	0.24 ± 0.72 (N = 70)	0.235[a]
Sodium (mmol/L)	141.66 ± 1.83 (N = 245)	141.63 ± 1.87 (N = 176)	141.74 ± 1.75 (N = 69)	0.734[a]
Potassium (mmol/L)	4.24 ± 0.31 (N = 245)	4.24 ± 0.33 (N = 176)	4.23 ± 0.26 (N = 69)	0.966[a]
Hemoglobin (g/dL)	14.73 ± 1.79 (N = 266)	14.78 ± 1.75 (N = 192)	14.60 ± 1.91 (N = 74)	0.476[a]
TIBC (μg/dL)	324.66 ± 44.73 (N = 245)	321.31 ± 44.96 (N = 176)	333.20 ± 43.28 (N = 69)	0.040[a]
HBV seropositive, n (%)	11/266 (4.14%)	6/192 (3.13%)	5/74 (6.76%)	0.186[a]
HCV seropositive, n (%)	3/266 (1.13%)	2/192 (1.04%)	1/74 (1.35%)	1.000[a]
Medication history of aspirin	17/266 (6.39%)	13/192 (6.77%)	4/74 (5.41%)	0.787[b]
Medication history of statin	20/266 (7.52%)	17/192 (8.85%)	3/74 (4.05%)	0.183[b]
Medication history of nutritional supplements	39/266 (14.66%)	30/192 (15.63%)	9/74 (12.16%)	0.474[b]

[a]Wilcoxon rank sum test, [b]Chi-squared test, [c]Fisher's exact test
[d]If at least one eye was diagnosed as presenile nuclear cataract, it was considered a presenile nuclear cataract patient
Examples of physical exercise degree: almost absent (walking for less than 10 min), mild (walking, golf, housework), moderate (bicycle, fast walking, tennis, swimming, hiking), vigorous (aerobics, jogging, soccer)
Alcohol consumption units: 10 g of alcohol
BMI body mass index, WHR waist-hip ratio, HbA1c hemoglobin A1c, HDL high-density lipoprotein, LDL low-density lipoprotein, CRP C-reactive protein, TIBC total iron binding capacity, HBV hepatitis B virus, HCV hepatitis C virus
Values are either absolute values or mean ± standard deviation values

Discussion

Detection of early nuclear cataract is important in clinical and preventive medicine [36]. Relatively high incidence of presenile nuclear cataract (13.91%) in the current study indicates that health screening exams are important in early diagnosis of presenile nuclear cataract. Pentacam detects early nuclear cataract and quantitatively measures the severity of nuclear cataract [6]. Health screening data allows a large sample size and less biased selection of participants without significant ophthalmologic problems as the normal population. Therefore, risk factors for presenile nuclear cataract were identified using Pentacam and a health screening test in this study.

In the present study, current smokers showed a higher risk than never smokers (OR = 2.80, 95% CI, 1.10–7.12, p = 0.0310), consistent with previous reports [18, 37]. Ye et al. reported that smoking is a significant risk factor for nuclear cataract [18]. Copper, cadmium, and lead concentrations in crystalline lenses were higher in cataract patients, and this could be related with smoking [38]. In the present study, early smoking age, smoking duration, and heavy smoking (≥ 30 cigarettes/day) showed significant effects on univariate analysis (p < 0.2) and could also affect formation of nuclear cataract. Therefore, smoking prevention and cessation are important in preventing formation of nuclear cataract.

Table 2 Risk factors for presenile nuclear cataract, as estimated from univariable and multivariable generalized estimation equation

Risk factors	Univariate analysis		Multivariate analysis	
	OR (95% CI)	p value	OR (95% CI)	p value
Smoking status		0.1894		0.1296
Never	Reference		Reference	
Former (quit ≥1 year ago)	1.04 (0.51–2.12)	0.9206	1.83 (0.74–4.51)	0.1882
Current	1.72 (0.97–3.08)	0.0656	2.80 (1.10–7.12)	0.0310
Alcohol consumption frequency		0.7793		0.9150
≤1 day/month	Reference		Reference	
2–3 days/month	1.04 (0.44–2.46)	0.9381	1.43 (0.42–4.85)	0.5662
1–2 days/week	0.91 (0.37–2.23)	0.8367	0.83 (0.26–2.61)	0.7505
3–4 days/week	1.34 (0.52–3.43)	0.5409	1.00 (0.27–3.73)	0.9951
5–6 days/week	0.64 (0.14–2.97)	0.5691	0.81 (0.13–4.95)	0.8205
Everyday	2.20 (0.64–7.49)	0.2087	1.00 (0.24–4.20)	0.9970
Daily exercise duration, n (%)		0.0295		0.0107
Low amounts (1-40 min/day)	Reference		Reference	
None	2.45 (1.08–5.58)	0.0322	3.99 (1.27–12.52)	0.0178
High amounts (≥41 min/day)	1.97 (1.10–3.52)	0.0223	2.92 (1.38–6.22)	0.0053
Height (cm)	1.02 (0.99–1.05)	0.1520	1.04 (1.00–1.10)	0.0808
Asthma	4.87 (0.99–23.84)	0.0510	8.93 (1.12–71.15)	0.0386
Tuberculosis	3.30 (1.09–9.97)	0.0341	4.28 (1.36–13.50)	0.0131
HbA1c (%)	0.71 (0.45–1.13)	0.1509	0.70 (0.38–1.28)	0.2508
TIBC (μg/dL)	1.01 (1.00–1.01)	0.0533	1.01 (1.00–1.02)	0.0059
HBV seropositive	2.82 (0.91–8.74)	0.0729	2.98 (0.82–10.89)	0.0979

OR odds ratio, CI confidence interval, HbA1c hemoglobin A1c, TIBC total iron binding capacity, HBV hepatitis B virus

In the current study, daily physical exercise duration and presenile nuclear cataract showed a U-shaped relationship. Participants with low amount of exercise (1–40 min/day) showed the lowest nuclear cataract formation. Participants that were non-exerciser (OR = 3.99, 95% CI, 1.27–12.52, p = 0.0178) or who had a high amount (≥41 min/day) of exercise (OR = 2.92, 95% CI, 1.38–6.22, p = 0.0053) showed more nuclear cataract formation. Non-exercise group showed larger proportion co-morbidity than any amount of exercise group such as stroke history (4.2% vs 2.2%) in this study. Therefore, we should consider the possibility that co-morbidity has affected cataract formation [39]. Zheng et al. reported that Leisure time inactivity (< 1 h/day) was associated with increased risk of cataract [20]. However, they did not perform sub-group analysis of non-exerciser and any amount of exercise group, especially less than an hour daily. High amounts of physical exercise group showed variable incidence of presenile nuclear cataract in previous study [40]. High amounts of physical exercise group could create more free radicals [41] and could be exposed high amount of ultraviolet radiation during outdoor activity. However, high amounts of physical exercise also reduce glucose levels and are correlated to

a healthy life style. Therefore, to eliminate the effect of these confounding variables for physical exercise, further study is required.

Asthma was a significant risk factor for presenile nuclear cataract in this study (OR = 8.93, 95% CI, 1.12–71.15, p = 0.0386). Asthma patients may receive systemic steroid treatments, which likely explain the higher incidence of cataract [22]. However, because the current study used health screening data, only a small number of participants with asthma were included in the study. Also, information on steroid treatment history was not recorded. Additional study is necessary to reveal the relationship between asthma and nuclear cataract formation.

Tuberculosis is also a significant risk factor of presenile nuclear cataract in this study (OR = 4.28, 95% CI, 1.36–13.50, p = 0.0131). The possible mechanism of cataract formation with tuberculosis was suggested in a previous report [24]. The mechanism is likely complicated and includes direct and indirect biological effects of tuberculosis, steroid treatments, toxicity of anti-tuberculosis treatments, and low socioeconomic status [24]. Also, only a small number of participants with tuberculosis were included, and the confidence interval was wide because this study is based on health screening. Further study is needed to reveal the relationship of tuberculosis and nuclear cataract formation.

Higher TIBC level is related to iron deficiency [42]. Iron deficiency is related to cataract [43], and iron supplementation may reduce oxidative stress [44]. In the current study, higher TIBC was a significant risk factor for cataract (OR = 1.01, 95% CI, 1.00–1.02, $p = 0.0059$).

Age is a strong risk factor for nuclear cataract [14]. However, in this study, age was not significantly related to nuclear cataract. Most previous studies regarding nuclear cataract did not include presenile age under 50 or did not analyze the association with age due to low incidence of presenile nuclear cataract. Klein et al. included participants 43 to 83 years old and showed nuclear cataract prevalence of 12.4% in the 43 to 54 years old age group. However, they did not perform subgroup analysis of this group in the Beaver Dam Eye Study [45]. Foster et al. included participants 40 to 81 years old and showed a significant association between age and nuclear cataract (OR = 5.6, 95% CI. 4.6–6.8, $p < 0.001$), but they did not perform subgroup analysis of this group in the Tanjong Pagar Survey [46]. Therefore, there is currently insufficient evidence for age as a risk factor of nuclear cataract in the presenile age group. Another explanation for the lack of association with age is sampling bias of the current study. Patients with severe cataract in older age received early cataract surgery and were excluded from this study.

Alcohol showed conflicting results with cataract in a previous study [47]. In the current study, alcohol did not show any association with nuclear cataract formation in status, duration, amount, or frequency. Alcohol could be a confounder of age, diet, smoking, and socioeconomic status. Prospective study is necessary to reveal the effect of alcohol on presenile nuclear cataract. In the current study, blood glucose and hemoglobin A1c level did not show relationships with nuclear cataract formation. Although diabetes is an important risk factor for cataract, diabetes shows conflicting results in nuclear type [48]. Furthermore, data from the health screening test causes selection bias from the healthy user effect. Participants who received health screening may have a healthy life style and low possibility of diabetes.

There were several studies about risk factors of age-related cataract. According to Taizhou Eye Study, age-related cataract is related with older age, increased outdoor activity, lower education level, female, no outdoor eye protection, low high-density lipoprotein, high low-density lipoprotein, high myopia, and increased pickled food intake [49]. In Los Angeles Latino Eye Study, older age, smoking, and myopia were related with age-related cataract. These studies included senile age group and used slit lamp examination for qualitative cataract grading [50]. In our study, smoking and amount of physical exercise were related with presenile nuclear cataract. We revealed relationship of smoking and nuclear cataract with detailed smoking questionnaire, and U-shaped relationship of daily physical exercise duration and nuclear cataract. High incidence of presenile nuclear cataract in high amounts of exercise group might not only be related with free radical, but also ultraviolet radiation while outdoor activity. Unfortunately, the questionnaires used in this study did not distinguish between indoor and outdoor activity. In addition, high incidence of presenile nuclear cataract in non-exercise group might be related with co-morbidity such as stroke [39].

Our study has several strengths, including its large sample size and detailed information on a number of potential risk factors for presenile nuclear cataract. Previously, few studies have investigated risk factors for presenile nuclear cataract because of relatively low incidence of this disease and absence of control data in the clinical setting. However, Pentacam method provides objective measurements to evaluate cataracts, especially in health examination. Our study has a large sample size and accurate detailed information for both cases and controls, providing helpful results that current smoking, asthma, tuberculosis, and iron deficiency status are risk factors for presenile nuclear cataract. In addition, the non-exerciser and high amount of daily physical exercise duration is risk factors for presenile nuclear cataract.

However, the current study is limited by its cross sectional nature using health screening data. In a cross-sectional study, the temporal relationship cannot be clearly defined, and it is difficult to establish causal inferences. There may also have been selection bias and healthy user bias. Also, confounding variables could not be perfectly excluded. Information on socioeconomic status, occupation, and residence area, which could be related to cataract formation, was not obtained. In addition, without pupil dilation, the accuracy of PNS score might be reduced. However, non-dilated PNS score could be a good screening tool for presenile nuclear cataract in general health examination setting which pupil dilatation is difficult.

Conclusion

Presenile nuclear cataract is also related to current smoking, non-exercise and high amounts of physical exercise, asthma, tuberculosis, and iron deficiency status. Patients with asthma, tuberculosis, and iron deficiency anemia who complain of visual discomfort should receive frequent ophthalmic examinations to detect cataract and other eye problems.

Acknowledgments
The authors would like to thank Kyunga Kim, PhD and Hye Seung Kim, MS from the Statistics and Data Center, Samsung Medical Center for their contributions to statistical analysis in this article.

Authors' contributions
SW Nam contributed to the manuscript as the first authors. DH Lim and T-Y Chung contributed to the manuscript as corresponding authors. SW Nam and DH Lim designed the study. DH Lim and T-Y Chung provided the required clinical data. SW Nam, KY Cho, HS Kim and K Kim analyzed the clinical data. SW Nam, DH Lim, and T-Y Chung reviewed the design, reviewed the results and wrote/reviewed the final paper. All authors read and approved the final manuscript.

Competing interests
None of the authors have financial or proprietary interests (such as personal or professional relationships, affiliations, knowledge or beliefs) in any of the materials or methods mentioned in this study. The authors declare that they have no competing interests.

Author details
[1]Department of Ophthalmology, Samsung Medical Center, Sungkyunkwan University School of Medicine, Seoul, South Korea. [2]Department of Preventive Medicine, Graduate School, The Catholic University of Korea, Seoul, South Korea. [3]Biostatistics and Clinical Epidemiology Center, Research Institute for Future Medicine, Samsung Medical Center, Seoul, South Korea. [4]Department of Ophthalmology, Samsung Medical Center, #81 Irwon-ro, Gangnam-gu, Seoul 06351, South Korea.

References
1. Thylefors B. The World Health Organization's programme for the prevention of blindness. Int Ophthalmol. 1990;14(3):211–9.
2. Chylack LT Jr, Wolfe JK, Singer DM, Leske MC, Bullimore MA, Bailey IL, Friend J, McCarthy D, Wu SY. The Lens opacities classification system III. The longitudinal study of cataract study group. Arch Ophthalmol (Chicago, Ill: 1960). 1993;111(6):831–6.
3. Datiles MB 3rd, Magno BV, Freidlin V. Study of nuclear cataract progression using the National eye Institute Scheimpflug system. Br J Ophthalmol. 1995;79(6):527–34.
4. Lim DH, Kim TH, Chung ES, Chung TY. Measurement of lens density using Scheimpflug imaging system as a screening test in the field of health examination for age-related cataract. Br J Ophthalmol. 2015;99(2):184–91.
5. Grewal DS, Brar GS, Grewal SP. Correlation of nuclear cataract lens density using Scheimpflug images with Lens opacities classification system III and visual function. Ophthalmology. 2009;116(8):1436–43.
6. Pan AP, Wang QM, Huang F, Huang JH, Bao FJ, Yu AY. Correlation among lens opacities classification system III grading, visual function index-14, pentacam nucleus staging, and objective scatter index for cataract assessment. Am J Ophthalmol. 2015;159(2):241–247.e242.
7. Pei X, Bao Y, Chen Y, Li X. Correlation of lens density measured using the Pentacam Scheimpflug system with the Lens opacities classification system III grading score and visual acuity in age-related nuclear cataract. Br J Ophthalmol. 2008;92(11):1471–5.
8. Magalhaes FP, Costa EF, Cariello AJ, Rodrigues EB, Hofling-Lima AL. Comparative analysis of the nuclear lens opalescence by the Lens opacities classification system III with nuclear density values provided by oculus Pentacam: a cross-section study using Pentacam nucleus staging software. Arq Bras Oftalmol. 2011;74(2):110–3.
9. Praveen MR, Shah GD, Vasavada AR, Mehta PG, Gilbert C, Bhagat G. A study to explore the risk factors for the early onset of cataract in India. Eye (Lond). 2010;24(4):686–94.
10. Chang JR, Koo E, Agron E, Hallak J, Clemons T, Azar D, Sperduto RD, Ferris FL 3rd, Chew EY. Risk factors associated with incident cataracts and cataract surgery in the age-related eye disease study (AREDS): AREDS report number 32. Ophthalmology. 2011;118(11):2113–9.
11. Karppi J, Laukkanen JA, Kurl S. Plasma lutein and zeaxanthin and the risk of age-related nuclear cataract among the elderly Finnish population. Br J Nutr. 2012;108(1):148–54.
12. Mukesh BN, Le A, Dimitrov PN, Ahmed S, Taylor HR, McCarty CA. Development of cataract and associated risk factors: the visual impairment project. Arch Ophthalmol (Chicago, Ill : 1960). 2006;124(1):79–85.
13. Richter GM, Choudhury F, Torres M, Azen SP, Varma R. Risk factors for incident cortical, nuclear, posterior subcapsular, and mixed lens opacities: the Los Angeles Latino eye study. Ophthalmology. 2012;119(10):2040–7.
14. Rim TH, Kim MH, Kim WC, Kim TI, Kim EK. Cataract subtype risk factors identified from the Korea National Health and nutrition examination survey 2008-2010. BMC Ophthalmol. 2014;14:4.
15. Tang Y, Ji Y, Ye X, Wang X, Cai L, Xu J, Lu Y. The Association of Outdoor Activity and age-Related Cataract in a rural population of Taizhou eye study: phase 1 report. PLoS One. 2015;10(8):e0135870.
16. Wei L, Liang G, Cai C, Lv J. Association of vitamin C with the risk of age-related cataract: a meta-analysis. Acta Ophthalmol. 2016;94(3):e170–6.
17. Chatziralli IP, Sergentanis TN, Peponis VG, Papazisis LE, Moschos MM. Risk factors for poor vision-related quality of life among cataract patients. Evaluation of baseline data. Graefes Arch Clin Exp Ophthalmol. 2013;251(3):783–9.
18. Ye J, He J, Wang C, Wu H, Shi X, Zhang H, Xie J, Lee SY. Smoking and risk of age-related cataract: a meta-analysis. Invest Ophthalmol Vis Sci. 2012;53(7):3885–95.
19. Gong Y, Feng K, Yan N, Xu Y, Pan CW. Different amounts of alcohol consumption and cataract: a meta-analysis. Optom Vis Sci. 2015;92(4):471–9.
20. Zheng Selin J, Orsini N, Ejdervik Lindblad B, Wolk A. Long-term physical activity and risk of age-related cataract: a population-based prospective study of male and female cohorts. Ophthalmology. 2015;122(2):274–80.
21. Machan CM, Hrynchak PK, Irving EL. Age-related cataract is associated with type 2 diabetes and statin use. Optom Vis Sci. 2012;89(8):1165–71.
22. Sweeney J, Patterson CC, Menzies-Gow A, Niven RM, Mansur AH, Bucknall C, Chaudhuri R, Price D, Brightling CE, Heaney LG. Comorbidity in severe asthma requiring systemic corticosteroid therapy: cross-sectional data from the optimum patient care research database and the British thoracic difficult asthma registry. Thorax. 2016;71(4):339–46.
23. Park SJ, Lee JH. Cataract and Cataract Surgery: Nationwide Prevalence and Clinical Determinants. J Korean Med Sci. 2016;31(6):963–71.
24. Hsia NY, Ho YH, Shen TC, Lin CL, Huang KY, Chen CH, Tu CY, Shih CM, Hsu WH, Sung FC. Risk of cataract for people with tuberculosis: results from a population-based cohort study. Int J Tuberc Lung Dis. 2015;19(3):305–11.
25. Yu X, Lyu D, Dong X, He J, Yao K. Hypertension and risk of cataract: a meta-analysis. PLoS One. 2014;9(12):e114012.
26. Hiller R, Sperduto RD, Reed GF, D'Agostino RB, Wilson PW. Serum lipids and age-related lens opacities: a longitudinal investigation: the Framingham studies. Ophthalmology. 2003;110(3):578–83.
27. Dobrzynski JM, Kostis JB. Statins and cataracts--a visual insight. Curr Atheroscler Rep. 2015;17(2):477.
28. Christen WG, Manson JE, Glynn RJ, Ajani UA, Schaumberg DA, Sperduto RD, Buring JE, Hennekens CH. Low-dose aspirin and risk of cataract and subtypes in a randomized trial of U.S. physicians. Ophthalmic Epidemiol. 1998;5(3):133–42.
29. Mahdi AM, Rabiu M, Gilbert C, Sivasubramaniam S, Murthy GV, Ezelum C, Entekume G. Prevalence and risk factors for lens opacities in Nigeria: results of the national blindness and low vision survey. Invest Ophthalmol Vis Sci. 2014;55(4):2642–51.
30. Boey PY, Tay WT, Lamoureux E, Tai ES, Mitchell P, Wang JJ, Saw SM, Wong TY. C-reactive protein and age-related macular degeneration and cataract: the Singapore malay eye study. Invest Ophthalmol Vis Sci. 2010;51(4):1880–5.
31. Taylor HR. Epidemiology of age-related cataract. Eye (Lond). 1999;13(Pt 3b):445–8.
32. Schoenfeld ER, Leske MC, Wu SY. Recent epidemiologic studies on nutrition and cataract in India, Italy and the United States. J Am Coll Nutr. 1993;12(5):521–6.
33. Kushnir VN, Slepova OS, Zaitseva NS, Titarenko ZD, Dumbrava VA, Vovk EM. Viral hepatitis B as a factor in the etiology of cataracts in adults and children. Vestn oftalmol. 1996;112(1):46–50.
34. Rasmussen LD, Kessel L, Molander LD, Pedersen C, Gerstoft J, Kronborg G, Obel N. Risk of cataract surgery in HIV-infected individuals: a Danish Nationwide population-based cohort study. Clin Infect Dis. 2011;53(11):1156–63.

35. Eckel RH, Jakicic JM, Ard JD, de Jesus JM, Houston Miller N, Hubbard VS, Lee IM, Lichtenstein AH, Loria CM, Millen BE, et al. 2013 AHA/ACC guideline on lifestyle management to reduce cardiovascular risk: a report of the American College of Cardiology/American Heart Association task force on practice guidelines. Circulation. 2014;129(25 Suppl 2):S76–99.

36. McGinty SJ, Truscott RJ. Presbyopia: the first stage of nuclear cataract? Ophthalmic Res. 2006;38(3):137–48.

37. Lindblad BE, Hakansson N, Wolk A. Smoking cessation and the risk of cataract: a prospective cohort study of cataract extraction among men. JAMA ophthalmology. 2014;132(3):253–7.

38. Racz P, Erdohelyi A. Cadmium, lead and copper concentrations in normal and senile cataractous human lenses. Ophthalmic Res. 1988;20(1):10–3.

39. Chen Y-C, Liu L, Peng L-N, Lin M-H, Liu C-L, Chen L-K, Chen T-J, Hwang S-J. Cataract surgery utilization after acute stroke: a nationwide cohort study. J Clin Gerontol Geriatr. 2013;4(1):7–11.

40. Williams PT. Prospective epidemiological cohort study of reduced risk for incident cataract with vigorous physical activity and cardiorespiratory fitness during a 7-year follow-up. Invest Ophthalmol Vis Sci. 2009;50(1):95–100.

41. Sachs-Olsen C, Berntsen S, Lodrup Carlsen KC, Anderssen SA, Mowinckel P, Carlsen KH. Time spent in vigorous physical activity is associated with increased exhaled nitric oxide in non-asthmatic adolescents. Clin Respir J. 2013;7(1):64–73.

42. Lopez A, Cacoub P, Macdougall IC, Peyrin-Biroulet L. Iron deficiency anaemia. Lancet (London, England). 2016;387(10021):907–16.

43. Tarwadi KV, Chiplonkar SA, Agte V. Dietary and nutritional biomarkers of lens degeneration, oxidative stress and micronutrient inadequacies in Indian cataract patients. Clin Nutr. 2008;27(3):464–72.

44. Kurtoglu E, Ugur A, Baltaci AK, Undar L. Effect of iron supplementation on oxidative stress and antioxidant status in iron-deficiency anemia. Biol Trace Elem Res. 2003;96(1–3):117–23.

45. Klein BE, Klein R, Lee KE, Gangnon RE. Incidence of age-related cataract over a 15-year interval the beaver dam eye study. Ophthalmology. 2008;115(3):477–82.

46. Foster PJ, Wong TY, Machin D, Johnson GJ, Seah SK. Risk factors for nuclear, cortical and posterior subcapsular cataracts in the Chinese population of Singapore: the Tanjong Pagar survey. Br J Ophthalmol. 2003;87(9):1112–20.

47. Hiratsuka Y, Ono K, Murakami A. Alcohol use and cataract. Curr Drug Abuse Rev. 2009;2(3):226–9.

48. Li L, Wan XH, Zhao GH. Meta-analysis of the risk of cataract in type 2 diabetes. BMC Ophthalmol. 2014;14:94.

49. Tang Y, Wang X, Wang J, Jin L, Huang W, Luo Y, Lu Y: Risk factors of age-related cataract in a Chinese adult population: the Taizhou eye study. 2017.

50. Richter GM, Torres M, Choudhury F, Azen SP, Varma R. Risk factors for cortical, nuclear, posterior subcapsular, and mixed lens opacities: the Los Angeles Latino eye study. Ophthalmology. 2012;119(3):547–54.

29

Assessing amblyopia treatment using multifocal visual evoked potentials

Junwon Jang and Sungeun E. Kyung[*]

Abstract

Background: To evaluate the effect of occlusion treatment for anisometropic amblyopia using multifocal visual evoked potentials (mfVEPs).

Methods: The patients for this study comprised 19 patients (mean age 6.05 ± 1.65 years) with anisometropic amblyopia underwent mfVEP analysis using the RETIscan® system before and after occlusion treatment. After dividing the area into six ring areas and four quadrants, we analyzed the amplitudes and latencies of the mfVEPs.

Results: The amplitudes of ring 1 (central field) in amblyopic eyes after treatment were significantly higher than those in the other rings ($p = 0.001$). The mfVEP amplitudes in each of the six rings between amblyopic eyes and fellow eyes at diagnosis and after occlusion treatment showed no significant differences. In quadrant 1 the amplitudes of the amblyopic eyes and fellow eyes were significantly different at the time of diagnosis ($p = 0.005$), whereas after occlusion treatment there was no significant difference ($p = 0.888$). The amplitudes for each of the six rings at diagnosis and after occlusion treatment in amblyopic eyes versus fellow eyes showed no significant difference. There were also no differences in the amplitudes in each of the four quadrants at the time of diagnosis and after occlusion treatment in amblyopic eyes versus fellow eyes. No significant difference was found in the comparison of latency values in each of the six rings or in each of the four quadrants at diagnosis and after occlusion treatment in amblyopic eyes versus their fellow eyes.

Conclusions: The amplitudes of quadrant 1 in amblyopic eyes compared with those of the fellow eyes at diagnosis were increased after occlusion treatment. Changes of the difference between amblyopic eyes and fellow eyes in quadrant 1 after occlusion treatment could be a useful, objective method for monitoring improvement in visual acuity.

Keywords: mfVEP (multifocal visual evoked potential), Anisometropia, Amblyopia, Amplitude, Latency

Background

Amblyopia is a developmental loss of visual sensitivity caused by experiencing discordant binocular images early in life. It specifically refers to a decrease in best-corrected visual acuity in an eye with no organic pathology [1]. Amblyopia is commonly associated with visual deprivation, anisometropia, and strabismus. Anisometropic amblyopia is a decrease in the best-corrected visual acuity in one eye that results from considerably different refractive errors in the patient's eyes. The eye that provides a more blurred image to the retina, and subsequently the brain, develops amblyopia [2].

Most anisometropic amblyopia patients in therapy are children due to the urgency of the critical development window, and occlusion (i.e. patching, atropinization) of the fellow eye is the usual tratment.[2] Also, treatments including refractive correction, and atropine eye drops to the fellow eye have been shown to improve the vision of the amblyopic eye [3].

Because most of the patients are children, it has been necessary to develop objective methods in addition to measuring visual acuity to monitor vision after treatment with occlusion. Visual evoked potentials are commonly used for this purpose. Conventional visual evoked potentials testing in all types of amblyopia yields abnormal results [4, 5].

Relative to the normal eye, the decrease of visual acuity and contrast sensitivity in the amblyopic eye is far

* Correspondence: Kseeye@hanmail.net
Department of ophthalmology, University of Dankook, Dankook University Hospital, 359 Manghang-Ro, Dongnam-Gu, Cheonan-City, Chungchungnam-Do, South Korea

more significant in the fovea than at the periphery of the visual field [6, 7]. Standard visual evoked potentials do not provide topographic information in the retino-cortical pathway, limiting information about topographic differences in processing. This information might be overcome by employing a multifocal stimulation technique. Multifocal visual evoked potentials are used to investigate pathological or functional changes in the visual system, and specifically as a diagnostic tool for optic neuritis, glaucoma, amblyopia and ischemic optic neuropathy [8–11]. For recording multifocal visual evoked potentials, adjacent locations in the visual field are stimulated simultaneously with temporally uncorrelated stimuli. Individual responses in the visual field are extracted using cross-correlation methods [12].

In the present study, we evaluated the effect of occlusion treatment of unilateral anisometropic amblyopia using the multifocal visual evoked potentials technique. The purpose of our study is to validate the use of the multifocal visual evoked potentials in amblyopia management.

Methods

Patients

A retrospective chart review of patients diagnosed with unilateral anisometropic amblyopia, who performed multifocal visual evoked potentials at the university medical center from March 2013 to May 2015, was conducted. This study has been granted an exemption from Dankook university ethics approval and it was conducted according to the tenets of the Declaration of Helsinki. The patients for this study comprised 19 patients (mean age 6.05 ± 1.65 years) with anisometropic amblyopia who underwent multifocal visual evoked potentials testing at Dankook University at the time of diagnosis and again after occlusion treatment. The recording was usually carried out between 10 AM and 3 PM. Amblyopia was diagnosed on the basis of a clear history after the age of 4 to < 12 years. A difference of at least one diopter of anisometropia and a difference of two Snellen lines were required at diagnosis. None had either unsteady foveal or eccentric fixation. The best-corrected visual acuity was measured in each eye using Snellen chart or Tumbling E chart. Protocol-specified follow-up visits for occlusion were conducted 6 weeks after spectacle correction. Patients were prescribed two continuous hours of daily patching with spectacle correction until the difference in the best-corrected visual acuity between the eyes must be less than two lines. We followed them for average 12 months (6 months -18 months).

Inclusion criteria for unilateral anisometropic amblyopes were as follows: clear cornea and lens, no ocular pathology and no oculomotor disorders such as strabismus or nystagmus. The difference in the best-corrected visual acuity between the eyes must be less than two lines in the amblyopic eyes after occlusion treatment were included. Two patients with poor attendance (unexplained missing visits or no documented follow up) or poor compliance (failure of spectacle correction or 2 h occlusion) were excluded. Follow-up examination was performed after at least 6 months. Patient information is given in Table 1. Institutional review board approval was not required for this study.

Multifocal visual evoked potential test procedure and analysis

The multifocal visual evoked potentials test was conducted using the RETIscan® system (Roland, Brandenburg, Germany). The distance to the 21-in. color cathode ray tube monitor was 30 cm, which corresponded to a total angular subtense of 60°. The stimulus was comprised of 60 checkerboard sections, most effective among all the check sizes, each containing eight white and eight black alternating squares [13]. Luminance of the white squares was 200 cd/m², and that of the black squares was < 1 cd/m2, producing a Michelson contrast of 99%. Background luminance of the screen was maintained at the maximal level of 200 cd/m². The visual stimuli were generated on a computer screen with a refresh rate of 50 Hz, and the pattern of reversals for each quadrant followed a pseudo-random sequence.

Gold cup electrodes were placed on the occipital scalp using electroencephalography paste to minimize impedance below 5KΩ. These electrode placements were based on the four-channel recording of Klistorner and Graham [14]. This modified, four-channel recording is currently the most widely used technique for recording multifocal visual evoked potentials. Two active electrodes were placed along the vertical midline 4 cm above the inion and 3 cm below the inion. Two more active electrodes were placed 4 cm on either side of the inion. A forehead electrode placed at the glabella served as the reference electrode and an earlobe electrode served as the ground electrode.

To measure the amplitude of responses, a signal to noise ratio (SNR) was calculated across the interval from 0 to 500 msec by specifying signal window (0 to 200 msec) and a "noise-only" window (300 to 500 msec). The amplification gain was ±100 μV. The low- and high-frequency cutoffs were set at 1 and 30 Hz, respectively. The signals were bandpass-filtered at 50 and 100 Hz, respectively. The same stimuli were administered to all subjects with the same electrode positions to obtain the multifocal visual evoked potentials responses. The extracted waveforms were analyzed via the best visual evoked potentials response method. The best visual evoked potentials response method is the

Table 1 Demographic characteristics of the participants

Case	Sex	Refractive error(D)		BCVA[a] (At diagnosis)		BCVA (After treatment)	
		Amblyopic eye	Fellow eye	Amblyopic eye	Fellow eye	Amblyopic eye	Fellow eye
1	M	sph + 5.5	sph + 0.75	20/30	20/20	20/20	20/20
2	M	sph + 2.5,cyl + 1.5	sph + 1.5	20/30	20/15	20/20	20/15
3	M	sph + 4.5, cvl + 2.0	sph + 3.5, cyl + 1.5	20/40	20/25	20/20	20/20
4	F	sph + 0.5, cyl − 3.5	sph + 0.25, cyl − 2.0	20/25	20/15	20/20	20/15
5	F	sph + 4.0	sph + 0.5	20/30	20/20	20/20	20/20
6	M	sph + 5.5	sph + 0.25	20/30	20/20	20/20	20/20
7	F	sph + 3.0, cyl −1.0	sph + 1.0	20/30	20/20	20/20	20/20
8	F	sph + 2.0, cyl-4.5	sph + 0.5	20/30	20/15	20/20	20/15
9	F	sph + 5.0, cyl + 1.0	sph + 3.0, cyl + 1.0	20/30	20/20	20/20	20/15
10	F	sph + 1.5, cyl −2.5	sph + 1.0	20/30	20/20	20/20	20/20
11	F	sph + 4.5, cyl-6.0	sph + 0.5	20/100	20/15	20/20	20/15
12	F	sph + 1.0, cyl + 1.5	sph + 1.25	20/40	20/20	20/20	20/20
13	F	sph + 6.0	sph + 2.0	20/30	20/20	20/20	20/20
14	F	sph −1.75	sph −0.5	20/30	20/20	20/20	20/20
15	M	sph + 4.5	sph + 1.0	20/40	20/15	20/20	20/15
16	M	sph + 3.75	sph + 2.75	20/70	20/20	20/20	20/20
17	F	sph + 3.0, cyl −4.0	sph + 2.25	20/30	20/15	20/20	20/15
18	M	sph + 2.0	sph + 0.25	20/50	20/20	20/20	20/20
19	M	sph + 7.0	sph + 5.0	20/50	20/20	20/20	20/20

[a]BCVA = Best corrected visual acuity
D: Diopter

custom-designed program of RETIscan which selecting the waveform of maximal amplitude among various waveforms recorded in each channel [15].

Before amblyopia treatment, the patients were tested with their manifest refractive correction. They were instructed to maintain their fixation on the center of the stimulus. The non-tested eye was patched. Two runs were completed for each eye in a right–left–right–left sequence, always beginning with the right eye. The averaged data from the two trials were analyzed. During recording, the position of the stimulated eye was monitored constantly by the examiner via the camera display provided in the RETIscan. Recording segments contaminated by fixation loss, unsteady fixation or external noises were discarded.

In a field divided into 60 areas, we analyzed the mean amplitudes and the mean latencies of each topographical region from two trials, with six ring-shaped areas and four quadrants. The six rings were divided by their distance from the foveal center: ring 1, 0–5°; ring 2, 5°–10°; ring 3, 10°–20°; ring 4, 20°–30°; ring 5, 30°–45°; ring 6, 45°–60 (Fig. 1). The four quadrants were also divided according to the horizontal meridian and the vertical midline: quadrant 1, superior and temporal (right); quadrant 2, inferior and temporal (right); quadrant 3, inferior and nasal (left); quadrant 4, superior and nasal (left) (Fig. 1).

After amblyopia treatment the multifocal visual evoked potentials testing was repeated (see additional file 1).

Statistical analysis

All statistics were calculated using SPSS version 18.0 software (SPSS Inc., Chicago, IL, USA). The Friedman test was performed to identify any significant differences among the six rings and four quadrants in the amblyopic eyes at the time of diagnosis and after occlusion treatment. The Wilcoxon sign rank test was performed to identify any significant differences for each ring and each quadrant between the time of diagnosis and after occlusion treatment, as well as between the amblyopic and fellow eyes. A value of $p < 0.05$ was considered to indicate statistical significance.

Results

The 19 patient cohort showed significant visual acuity changes from the pre-treatment baseline tests. The mean visual acuity change was from 0.27 ± 0.15 to 0 ± 0 in logMAR (Table 1).

Amplitude

The multifocal visual evoked potentials waveforms were classified and sorted according to the loci and eccentricities of their stimuli. In amblyopic eyes, the mean values

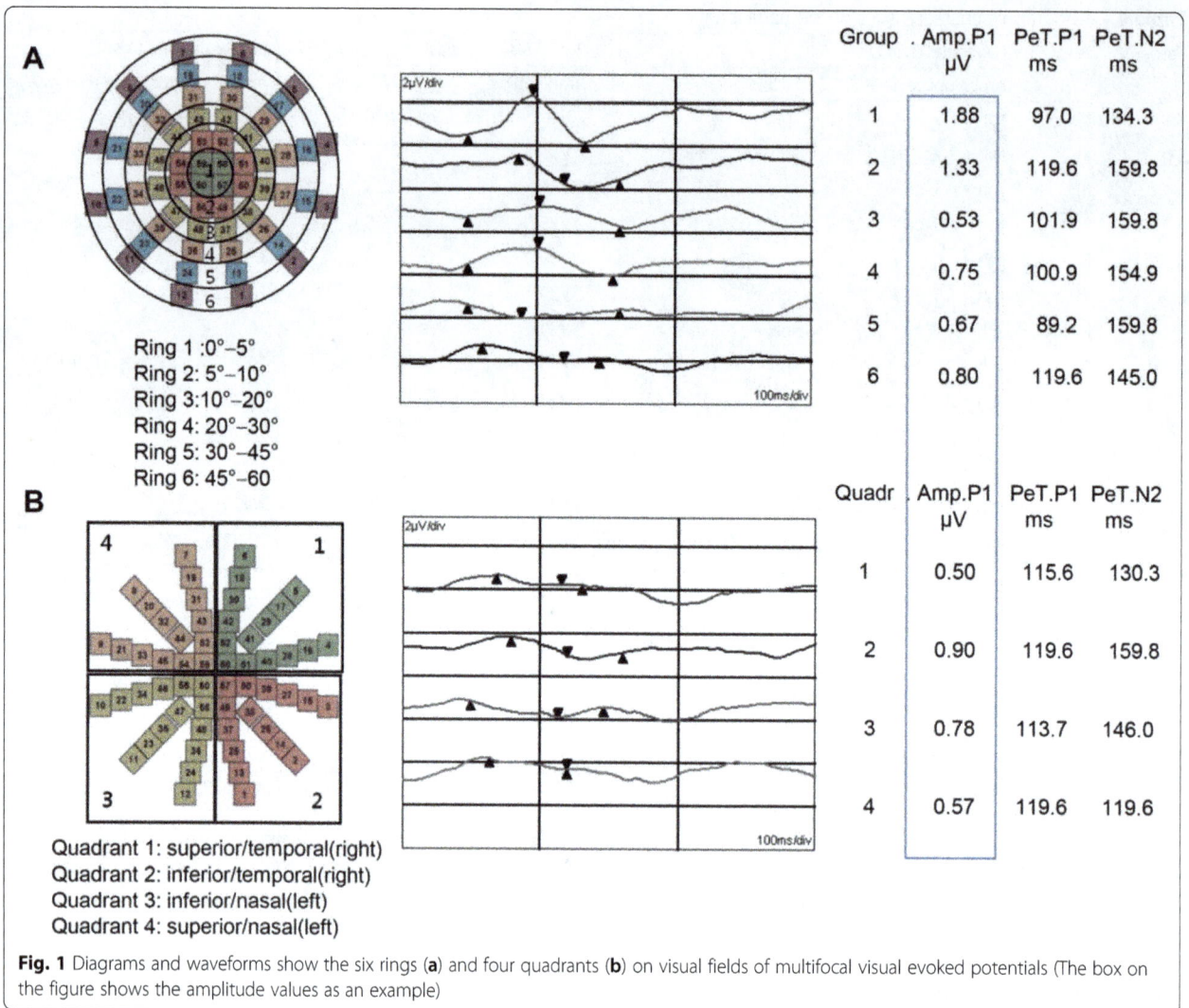

A

Ring 1 :0°–5°
Ring 2: 5°–10°
Ring 3:10°–20°
Ring 4: 20°–30°
Ring 5: 30°–45°
Ring 6: 45°–60

Group	Amp.P1 µV	PeT.P1 ms	PeT.N2 ms
1	1.88	97.0	134.3
2	1.33	119.6	159.8
3	0.53	101.9	159.8
4	0.75	100.9	154.9
5	0.67	89.2	159.8
6	0.80	119.6	145.0

B

Quadrant 1: superior/temporal(right)
Quadrant 2: inferior/temporal(right)
Quadrant 3: inferior/nasal(left)
Quadrant 4: superior/nasal(left)

Quadr	Amp.P1 µV	PeT.P1 ms	PeT.N2 ms
1	0.50	115.6	130.3
2	0.90	119.6	159.8
3	0.78	113.7	146.0
4	0.57	119.6	119.6

Fig. 1 Diagrams and waveforms show the six rings (**a**) and four quadrants (**b**) on visual fields of multifocal visual evoked potentials (The box on the figure shows the amplitude values as an example)

of the each topographical rings did not differ significantly from each other at diagnosis ($p = 0.391$, Friedman test). After treatment, however, the value of ring 1 (central field) was significantly higher than those of the other rings ($p = 0.001$, Friedman test) (Fig. 2). The amplitudes in each rings at the time of diagnosis and after treatment in amblyopic eyes were shown in Fig. 3.

The comparison of multifocal visual evoked potentials amplitudes between amblyopic eyes and fellow eyes in the six rings at the time of diagnosis showed no significant difference (Wilcoxon sign rank test) (Fig. 3). Comparison of the amplitudes of the six rings between amblyopic eyes and fellow eyes after treatment also showed no significant difference (Wilcoxon sign rank test) (Fig. 3).

The difference in the amplitudes in each of the six rings at the time of diagnosis and after treatment in amblyopic eyes and fellow eyes did not differ significantly (Wilcoxon sign rank test) (Fig. 3).

The multifocal visual evoked potentials waveforms were also classified by four quadrants, divided by horizontal and vertical midlines, and then analyzed. The quadrant 1 values for the amblyopic versus fellow eyes were significantly different at the time of diagnosis ($p = 0.005$, Wilcoxon sign rank test) (Fig. 4), whereas after treatment there was no significant difference ($p = 0.888$, Wilcoxon sign rank test) (Fig. 4).

The difference in the amplitudes in the quadrants at diagnosis and after treatment in amblyopic eyes and fellow eyes also showed no significant difference (Wilcoxon sign rank test) (Fig. 4).

Latency

The comparison of latency values in each of the six rings at the time of diagnosis and after treatment in amblyopic and fellow eyes showed no significant differences (Table 2). The comparison of latencies for the six rings

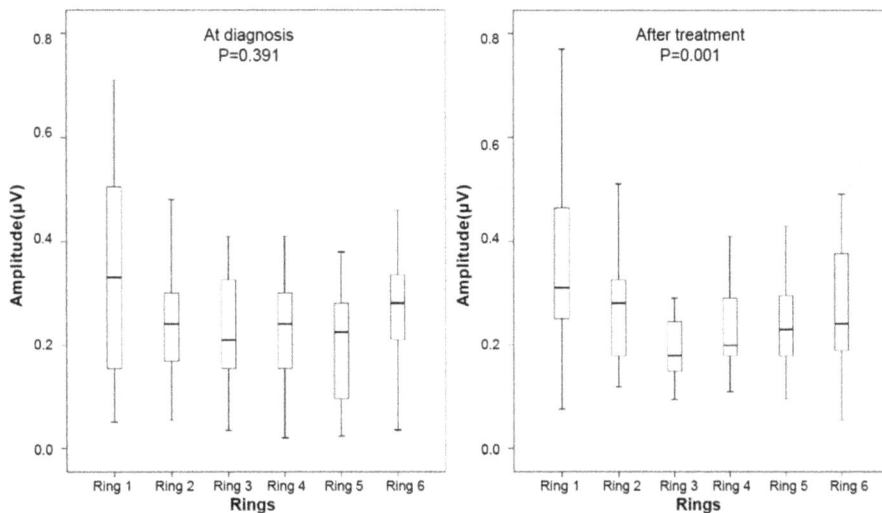

Fig. 2 Box plots of data show the mean amplitude of multifocal visual evoked potentials in rings at diagnosis and after occlusion treatment of amblyopia. In amblyopic eyes, the values of the rings did not differ significantly at the time of diagnosis ($p = 0.391$, Friedman test). After treatment, however, the value in ring 1 (central field) was significantly higher ($p = 0.001$, Friedman test) than that of the other rings (Wilcoxon test): rings 1 vs. 2 ($p = 0.042$); rings 1 vs. 3 ($p = 0.003$); rings 1 vs. 4 ($p = 0.006$), rings 1 vs. 5 ($p = 0.004$); rings 1 vs. 6 ($p = 6$ 0.033)

in amblyopic eyes and fellow eyes at diagnosis and after treatment showed no significant differences (Table 2).

The comparison of latencies for each of the four quadrants between the time of diagnosis and after treatment in amblyopic eyes and fellow eyes showed no significant differences (Table 3). The comparison of latencies for the four quadrants between amblyopic eyes and fellow eyes at diagnosis and after treatment also showed no significant differences (Table 3).

Discussion

Jeon et al. [16] reported that visual acuity quantification using absolute value of amplitude in pattern visual evoked potentials was useful in confirming subjective visual acuity. They found that the relationship between amplitude and logMAR acuity was linear. We also evaluated the correlation between visual acuity (logMAR) and amplitude or latency in multifocal visual evoked potentials. We found no significant relationship between visual acuity and amplitude or latency (linear regression: $P = 0.271$, 0.276, respectively). There were great variations of responses in mfVEP obtained from ring 1 in normal eye. Baseler et al. [8] suggested that the clinical utility of the mfVEP is limited because of the variation of responses obtained from identical locations in normal individuals. And Graham et al. and Hood et al. [17] suggested interocular comparison of mfVEP. Therefore we evaluated the effect of occlusion treatment of unilateral anisometropic amblyopia by correlating the differences in visual acuity before and after treatment in amblyopic eyes, and the difference between the two eyes to the equivalent difference in mfVEP parameters.

Kim et al. [18] reported that the multifocal visual evoked potentials were significantly greater in ring 1 than in the other five rings in normal adult controls. In a recent study, Jeon et al. [19] demonstrated, using multifocal visual evoked potentials, that the amplitudes of ring 1 of the anisometropic amblyopic eyes were not significantly different from those of the other rings before treatment. After occlusion treatment, however, the amplitude of ring 1 in the amblyopic eyes exhibited a significantly greater changes than the other rings, suggesting that increased VA in amblyopic eyes are associated with improved visual function in the central field. In our study, the amplitudes in ring 1 of the amblyopic eyes were significantly greater after treatment than those of the other rings. This finding is consistent with the results of Yu et al. [20] who demonstrated that visual acuity as more severely impaired in the foveal area than in the periphery of amblyopic eyes. A possible explanation for this phenomenon is that the center of the visual field, which vision is the clearest region and it demands an accurately focused image for development, whereas the periphery of the visual field is less clear region and it requires a less accurately focused image.

The most prominent deficit in amblyopia is in spatial vision, as measured by either Snellen acuity or grating acuity. The amblyopes also show decreased contrast sensitivity and visual discrimination ability. The same ranges of characteristics were revealed by experimentally created amblyopia in the macaque monkeys [21]. It has been suggested that anisometropic and strabismic amblyopia do not originate from a common pathophysiological process. The high spatial

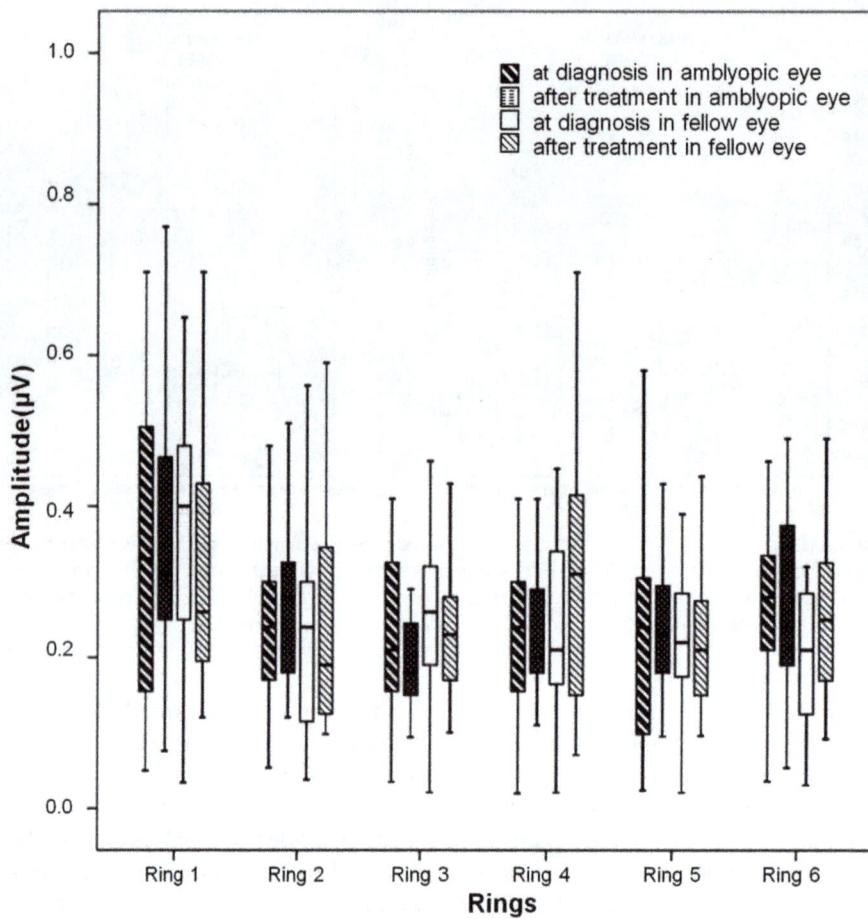

Fig. 3 Comparison of multifocal visual evoked potential) (mfVEP) amplitudes for amblyopic eyes and fellow eyes in the six rings at the time of diagnosis and after occlusion treatment. There were no significant differences among the rings. Values are presented as mean ± SD (ms). *P* value derived from t-test for the comparison P: between amblyopic eyes and fellow eyes at the time of diagnosis *P:between amblyopic eyes and fellow eyes after treatment. **P: between at the time of diagnosis and after treatment in amblyopic eye ***P:between at the time of diagnosis and after treatment in fellow eye

frequency (low temporal frequency) losses are inferred to represent parvocellular pathway deficits and lower spatial frequency (higher temporal frequency) losses are inferred to represent magnocellular pathway deficits. They have hypothesized that the distinction between the two types of amblyopia depends on the severity of magnocellular or parvocellular visual

pathway defects [22]. We also think anisometropic and strabismic amblyopia might have similar neural anomalies even though they have different etiologies (chronic unilateral blur vs chronic unilateral suppression). The results would depend on the severity of magnocellular or parvocellular visual pathway defects than types of amblyopia.

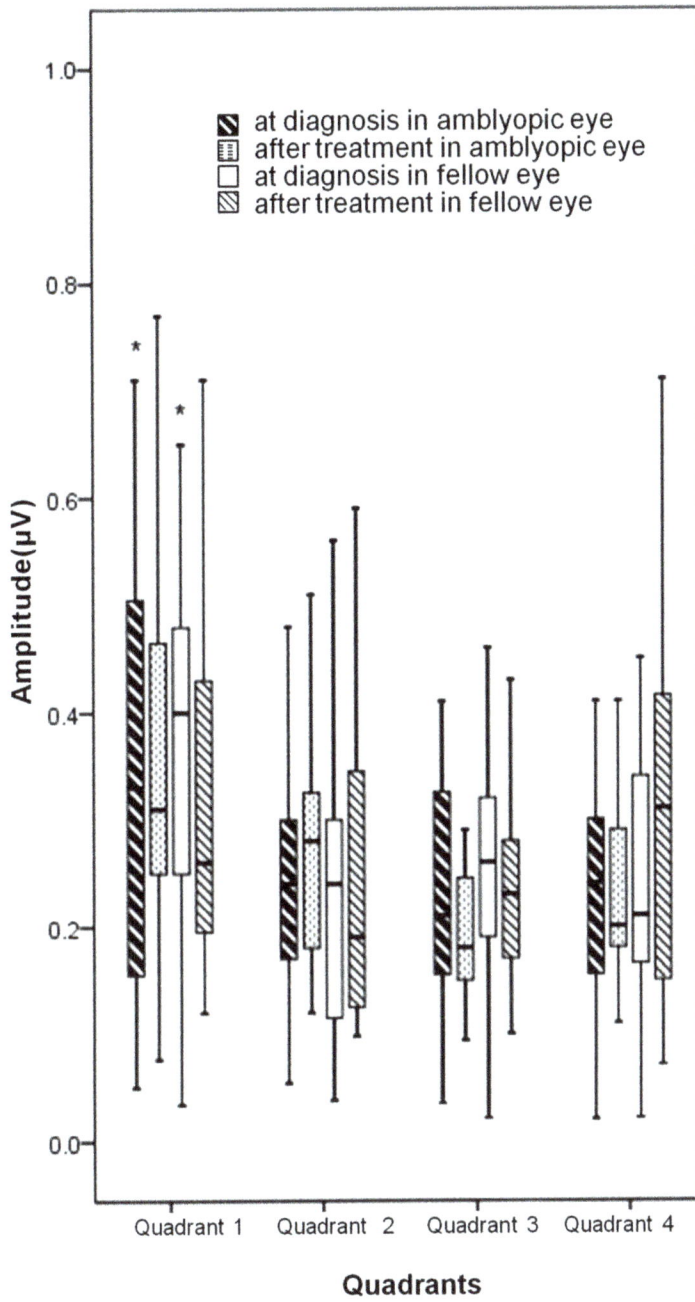

Fig. 4 (See legend on next page.)

Area	Amblyopic eye		Fellow eye		P value			
	At diagnosis	After treatment	At diagnosis	After treatment				
Quadrant 1	0.19±0.83	0.26±0.15	0.28±0.16	0.25±0.98	P=0.005	*P=0.888	**P=0.087	***P=0.267
Quadrant 2	0.34±0.17	0.36±0.16	0.33±0.21	0.36±0.16	P=0.810	*P=0.601	**P=0.747	***P=0.375
Quadrant 3	0.40±0.28	0.39±0.18	0.40±0.22	0.39±0.18	P=0.984	*P=0.763	**P=0.983	***P=0.888
Quadrant 4	0.25±0.16	0.23±0.12	0.24±0.14	0.23±0.12	P=0.546	*P=0.469	**P=0.384	***P=0.687

(See figure on previous page.)

Fig. 4 Comparison of multifocal visual evoked potentials (mfVEP) amplitudes for amblyopic eyes and fellow eyes in the four quadrants of the visual field at the time of diagnosis and after occlusion treatment. The values of quadrant 1 between amblyopic eyes and fellow eyes only show statistically significant differences at the time of diagnosis ($p = 0.005$) but not after treatment ($p = 0.888$). *quadrant 1 at diagnosis in amblyopic eyes and fellow eyes: statistically significant difference, $p = 0.005$. Values are presented as mean ± SD (ms). P value derived from t-test for the comparison P: between amblyopic eyes and fellow eyes at the time of diagnosis *P:between amblyopic eyes and fellow eyes after treatment. **P: between at the time of diagnosis and after treatment in amblyopic eye ***P:between at the time of diagnosis and after treatment in fellow eye.

Shan et al. [23] suggested that anisometropic amblyopia is primarily associated with an abnormal parvocellular visual system, rather than an abnormal magnocellular visual system. Parvocellular pathways tend to reflect the visual function of the fovea and account for the relatively greater defects observed in central visual function than is seen with peripheral visual function in amblyopic individuals [24]. Therefore, in this study, a significant change of amplitude in the central field in the amblyopic eye after treatment might reflect improvement of the abnormal parvocellular visual system function.

Another study showed a significant response latency difference between the amblyopic and normal eyes which the responses in the central region of the visual field (rings 1 and 2) had a longer latency in amblyopic eyes than normal eyes [25]. Most of the patients showed severe degree of anisometopia (6/60–6/9). In our study, however, the comparison of the latencies in each of the six rings and each of the four quadrants showed no significant difference between the amblyopic eyes and fellow eyes. This discrepancy may be due to the mild degree of anisometropia seen in our cases (20/100 in one patient, Table 1) or lack of optimization in the process not using multiple stimuli in our study.

A number of studies have examined the associations among the degree of anisometropia, baseline visual acuity, and final visual acuity in patients with anisometropic amblyopia [25]. Kutschke et al. [26] reported that the degree of anisometropia is not related to the baseline visual acuity but, rather, to the final visual acuity of amblyopic eye. In this study, we compared amplitude and latency values of each of six rings and four quadrants of amblyopic eyes versus fellow eyes after treatment. In quadrant 1, the amplitudes were significantly lower in amblyopic eyes than in fellow eyes at the time of diagnosis. After treatment, however, this parameter was no longer significantly different. These statistical changes in quadrant 1 may reflect the improvement in visual acuity (i.e., final visual acuity).

We evaluated the effect of occlusion treatment on amblyopia using multifocal visual evoked potentials to compare anisometropic amblyopic eyes and fellow eyes. There was no significant difference between the amplitudes for each ring in anisometropic amblyopic eyes and fellow eyes at the time of diagnosis and after treatment. The values for quadrant 1 in amblyopic eyes were significantly lower than those of fellow eyes at the time of diagnosis but showed no significant differences after treatment, suggesting that in quadrant 1 the amblyopic eyes improved from the pre-treatment baseline ($p = 0.087$). The occlusion treatment and the plasticity caused quadrant 1 in the amblyopic eyes to become similar to those of their fellow eyes. The fibers from the macula occupy the temporal portion. This papillomacular bundle is highly sensitive to visual function, and quadrant 1 is included in the superotemporal area [27]. There have been a report that the

Table 2 Comparison of latency values in each of the six rings in amblyopic and fellow eyes

Area	Amblyopic eye		Fellow eye		P value			
	At diagnosis	After treatment	At diagnosis	After treatment				
Ring 1	141.2 ± 20.8	147.3 ± 16.9	147.1 ± 17.5	136.2 ± 25.2	$P = 0.221$	*$P = 0.155$	**$P = 0.46$	***$P = 0.12$
Ring 2	144.0 ± 19.9	145.3 ± 13.3	142.9 ± 15.5	141.6 ± 19.0	$P = 0.906$	*$P = 0.755$	**$P = 0.81$	***$P = 0.72$
Ring 3	138.0 ± 20.5	144.3 ± 15.2	143.0 ± 17.1	140.8 ± 17.2	$P = 0.334$	*$P = 0.384$	**$P = 0.56$	***$P = 0.98$
Ring 4	141.7 ± 21.5	141.9 ± 16.3	137.6 ± 20.0	146.3 ± 17.5	$P = 0.244$	*$P = 0.407$	**$P = 0.84$	***$P = 0.22$
Ring 5	140.7 ± 16.6	145.6 ± 16.5	141.1 ± 19.3	139.5 ± 18.8	$P = 0.950$	*$P = 0.187$	**$P = 0.31$	***$P = 0.55$
Ring 6	144.1 ± 19.6	150.5 ± 13.0	135.4 ± 18.2	142.5 ± 19.9	$P = 0.214$	*$P = 0.080$	**$P = 0.25$	***$P = 0.18$
	† $P = 0.84$	† $P = 0.48$	† $P = 0.30$	† $P = 0.65$				

Values are presented as mean ± SD (ms)

P value derived from t-test for the comparison

P: between amblyopic eyes and fellow eyes at the time of diagnosis

*P:between amblyopic eyes and fellow eyes after treatment

**P: between at the time of diagnosis and after treatment in amblyopic eye

***P:between at the time of diagnosis and after treatment in fellow eye

†P value derived from t-test for the comparison between rings

Table 3 Comparison of latencies for each of the four quadrants in amblyopic eyes and fellow eyes

Area	Amblyopic eye		Fellow eye		P value			
	At diagnosis	After treatment	At diagnosis	After treatment				
Quadrant 1	132.6 ± 21.3	141.4 ± 23.6	138.7 ± 22.4	141.8 ± 17.2	$P = 0.35$	$*P = 0.95$	$**P = 0.22$	$***P = 0.63$
Quadrant 2	141.5 ± 20.7	137.8 ± 24.2	135.3 ± 18.5	132.1 ± 24.1	$P = 0.22$	$*P = 0.33$	$**P = 0.53$	$***P = 0.63$
Quadrant 3	139.8 ± 19.4	142.2 ± 18.0	134.8 ± 20.0	140.1 ± 18.2	$P = 0.40$	$*P = 0.68$	$**P = 0.68$	$***P = 0.41$
Quadrant 4	142.9 ± 23.7	139.7 ± 23.8	134.9 ± 21.1	138.4 ± 22.1	$P = 0.12$	$*P = 0.85$	$**P = 0.62$	$***P = 0.50$
	$^\dagger P = 0.16$	$^\dagger P = 0.66$	$^\dagger P = 0.77$	$^\dagger P = 0.20$				

Values are presented as mean ± SD (ms)
P value derived from t-test for the comparison
P: between amblyopic eyes and fellow eyes at the time of diagnosis
*P:between amblyopic eyes and fellow eyes after treatment
**P: between at the time of diagnosis and after treatment in amblyopic eye
***P:between at the time of diagnosis and after treatment in fellow eye
†P value derived from t-test for the comparison between rings

amplitudes in the multifocal visual evoked potentials (RETIscan® system, Roland, Brandenburg, Germany) were larger in the inferior field than superior field. [18] The subtle difference in quadrant 2 (inferotemporal) may not be reflected to the relatively large amplitude in the inferior field. Therefore, in our study, the quadrant 2 did not show treatment effect like quadrant 1, even though it is also included in the papillomacular bundle.

It has been reported that the change in amplitude on the central field (ring 1) in amblyopic eyes could be a useful, objective monitoring method for observing the improvement in VA [16]. However, the multifocal visual evoked potentials results might prove to have low reproducibility among tests and individuals [28]. Large-amplitude noise can be analyzed as the neural response if the electrical responses are too small. Therefore, it could be a better method for monitoring the effect of amblyopic treatment with quadrant 1 because it (superotemporal region) is a larger area than that of ring 1. Comparisons using the values of quadrant 1, rather than those of ring 1, in patients whose visual acuity was improved after treatment will help quantify the amplitude changes even when considering the fixation unreliability of multifocal visual evoked potentials. Our study also confirmed the larger changes in the central responses than the peripheral responses with less severely impaired eye.

There were some limitations to our study. First, because of the relatively small number of patients, we could not analyze amplitude changes based on the degree of anisometropia. Second, because the test might have a learning curve and patient compliance could differ according to age, additional studies of correlations among age, follow-up period, and total numbers of tests are needed. The interpretation of results must also take the effects of unstable fixation during measurements into consideration. The fixation stability is crucial for good VEP results, and it may be more useful in cooperative children. The usefulness of mfVEP in pre-verbal children should be evaluated by further study. Third, we did not take into consideration on the effect with stimulus size, and we use only the 16 checks/segments. Recording responses to more than one check size, to make sure the optimal response in the amblyopia is not obtained [13, 28]. Therefore, no significant difference is found for any of the latency comparisons. (Tables 2,3) It must be considered with caution in this study.

The standard method of visual acuity assessment in cooperative children is a standard letter acuity tests, and these tests are subjective tests. Clinicians have difficulty confirming objective visual acuity whether it is in the course of visual and cognitive development. We also need objective method to evaluate the level of underlying organic dysfunction in patients with non-organic overlay superimposed upon real dysfunction. Therefore mfVEP can be used as an objective VA test in cooperative children with amblyopia treatment and malingering even though it takes a longer time. In the present study, we focused on multifocal visual evoked potentials amplitude, which could be considered a useful, objective measurement to replace visual acuity testing. Comparing the results of the multifocal visual evoked potentials recordings of amblyopic eyes with those of fellow eyes can be an effective method for verifying an abnormality.

Conclusion

In conclusion, the multifocal visual evoked potentials have the advantage that it produces a topographical measure of damage compared with standard visual evoked potentials. Using multifocal visual evoked potentials, we found changes of smaller dysfunctional areas in anisometropic amblyopia after treatment using hundreds of stimulations presented in the same amount of time. Changes in the differences between amblyopic eyes and fellow eyes in quadrant 1 could be a useful, objective method for monitoring improvements in visual acuity even when taking fixation reliability into consideration.

Abbreviations

BCVA: Best corrected visual acuity; D: Diopter; mfVEP: (multifocal visual evoked potential); VA: Visual acuity

Funding

The present research was conducted by the fund of Dankook University in Cheonan city, South Korea in 2016.

Authors' contributions

KS designed and coordinated the study, and wrote the article. JJ performed the statistical analysis and interpreted the data. KS analyzed and interpreted the data. KS approved final manuscript. All authors read and approved the final manuscript.

Competing interests

The authors declare that they have no competing interests

References

1. von Noorden GK. Mechanism of amblyopia. Doc Ophthalmol. 1977;34:93–6.
2. Sen DK. Anisometropic amblyopia. J Pediatr Ophthalmol Strabismus. 1980; 17:180–4.
3. Repka MX, Kraker RT, Holmes JM, et al. Atropine vs patching for treatment of moderate amblyopia: follow-up at 15 years of age of a randomized clinical trial. JAMA Ophthalmol. 2014;132(7):799–805.
4. Sokol S. Abnormal evoked potentials in amblyopia. Br J Ophthalmol. 1983; 67:310–4.
5. Davis ET, Bass SJ, Sherman J. Flash visual evoked potential (VEP) in amblyopia and optic nerve disease. Optom Vis Sci. 1995;72:612–8.
6. Kirschen DG, Flom MC. Visual acuity at different retinal loci of eccentrically fixating functional amblyopia. Am J Optom Physiol Optic. 1978;55:144–50.
7. Levi DM, Klein SA, Aitsebaomo AP. Detection and discrimination of the direction of the motion in central and peripheral vision of normal and amblyopic observers. Vis Res. 1984;24:789–800.
8. Hood DC, Zhang X, Greenstein VC, et al. An interocular comparison of the multifocal VEP: a possible technique for detecting local damage to the optic nerve. Invest Ophthalmol Vis Sci. 2000;41:1580–7.
9. Graham SL, Klistorner AI, Grigg JR, Billson FA. Objective VEP perimetry in glaucoma: asymmetry analysis to identify early deficits. J Glaucoma. 2000;9:10–9.
10. Hood DC, Odel JG, Zhang X. Tracking the recovery of local optic nerve function after optic neuritis: a multifocal VEP study. Invest Ophthalmol Vis Sci. 2000;41:4032–8.
11. Pérez-Rico C, García-Romo E, Gros-Otero J, et al. Evaluation of visual function and retinal structure in adult amblyopes. Optom Vis Sci. 2015;92:375–83.
12. Fortune B, Hood DC. Comparison of conventional and multifocal VEPs. Invest Ophthalmol Vis Sci. 2003;44:1364–75.
13. Balachandran C, Klistorner AI, Graham SL. Effect of stimulus check size on multifocal visual evoked potential. Doc Ophthalmol. 2003;106:183–8.
14. Klistorner A, Graham SL. Objective perimetry in glaucoma. Ophthalmology. 2000;107:2283–99.
15. Park SM, Park SH, Chang JH, Ohn YH. Study for analysis of the multifocal visual evoked potential. Korean J Ophthalmol. 2011;25(5):334–40.
16. Jeon JH, Ph SY, Kyung SE. Assessment of visual disability using visual evoked potentials. BMC Ophthalmol. 2012;12:36.
17. Baseler HA, Sutter EE, Klein SA, Carney T. The topography of visual evoked response properties across the visual field. Electroencephlogr Clin Neurophysiol. 1994;90:65–81.
18. Kim DH, Park SH, Ohn YH. Multifocal visual evoked potential in normal subjects. J Korean Ophthalmol Soc. 2010;51:532–41.
19. Jeon JH, Kyung SE. The change of multifocal visual evoked potential in unilateral Anisometropic amblyopia before and after occlusion treatment. J Korean Ophthalmol. 2012;53:1851–6.
20. Yu M, Brown B, Edwards MH. Investigation of multifocal visual evoked potentials in anisometropic and esotropic amblyopes. Invest Ophthalmol Vis Sci. 1998;39: 2033–40.
21. Kiorpes L, Movshon JA. Amblyopia: a developmental disorder of the central visual pathways. Cold Spring Harb Symp Quant Biol. 1996;61:39–48.
22. von Noorden GK. Amblyopia: a multidisciplinary approach. Proctor lecture Invest Ophthalmol Vis Sci. 1985;26:1704–16.
23. Shan Y, Moster ML, Roemer RA, et al. Abnormal function of the parvocellular visual cells in amblyopia. J Pediatr Ophthalmol Strabismus. 2000;37:73–8.
24. Donahue SP. The relationship between anisometropia, patient age and the development of amblyopia. Trans Am Ophthalmol Soc. 2005;103:313–6.
25. Barrett BT, Bradley A, Candy TR. The relationship between anisometropia and amblyopia. Prog Retin Eye Res. 2013;36:120–58.
26. Kutschke PJ, Scott WE, Keech RV. Anisometropic amblyopia. Ophthalmology. 1991;98:258–63.
27. Honjo M, Omodaka K, Ishizaki T, et al. Retinal thickness and the structure/ function relationship in the eyes of older adults with Glaucoma. PLoS One. 2015;10:e0141293.
28. Wenner Y, Heinrich SP, Beisse C, Fuchs A, Bach M. Visual evoked potential-based acuity assessment: overestimation in amblyopia. Doc Ophthalmol. 2014;128:191–200.

30

Phospholipase Cγ2 is critical for Ca^{2+} flux and cytokine production in anti-fungal innate immunity of human corneal epithelial cells

Xudong Peng[1], Guiqiu Zhao[1*], Jing Lin[1], Jianqiu Qu[1], Yingxue Zhang[2] and Cui Li[1]

Abstract

Background: Fungal keratitis (FK) is a sight-threatening disease, accounting for a significant portion with its complex presentation, suboptimal efficacy of the existing therapies and uncontrollable excessive innate inflammation. Phospholipase C-γ2 (PLCγ2) is a non-receptor tyrosine kinase that plays an important role at the early period of innate immunity. This study aimed to identify the role of PLCγ2 in Dectin-1-mediated Ca^{2+} Flux and its effect on the expression of proinflammatory mediators at the exposure to *Aspergillus fumigatus* (*A. fumigatus*) hyphae antigens in human corneal epithelial cells (HCECs).

Methods: The HCECs were preincubated with or without different inhibitors respectively before *A. fumigatus* hyphae stimulation. Intracellular calcium flux in HCECs and levels of PLCγ2 and spleen-tyrosine kinase (Syk) were detected by fluorescence imaging and Western Blotting. The expression of proinflammatory mediators was determined by reverse transcriptase polymerase chain reaction (RT-PCR) and enzyme-linked immunosorbent assay (ELISA).

Results: We demonstrated that an intracellular Ca^{2+} flux in HCECs was triggered by *A. fumigatus* hyphae and could be reduced by pre-treatment with PLCγ2-inhibitor U73122. *A. fumigatus* hyphae induced PLCγ2 phosphorylation was regulated by Dectin-1 via Syk. Furthermore, PLCγ2-deficient HCECs showed a drastic impairment in the Ca^{2+} signaling and the secretion of IL-6, CXCL1 and TNF-α.

Conclusions: PLCγ2 plays a critical role for Ca^{2+} Flux in HCECs stimulated by *A. fumigatus* hyphae. Syk acts upstream of PLCγ2 in the Dectin-1 signaling pathway. The expressions of proinflammatory mediators induced by *A. fumigatus* are regulated by the activation of Dectin-1-mediated PLCγ2 signaling pathway in HCECs.

Keywords: PLCγ, Dectin-1, Ca^{2+}, Innate immunity, Corneal epithelium, *Aspergillus fumigatus*

Background

FK is a sight threatening disorder associated with multiple risk factors, such as ocular surface disease, extended wear contact lenses, and traumatic ocular surface accidents [1], presenting a therapeutic challenge due to the lack of effective antifungal agents and uncontrollable excessive innate inflammation. Innate immunity is an important defence against microbial infections in cornea.

However, excessive innate inflammatory response could damage normal corneal epithelial cells whilst slowing down the pathological progress of FK [2].

On one hand, cytoplasmic Ca^{2+} flux has been demonstrated to play an important role in innate immune response. In airway epithelia, cytoplasmic Ca^{2+} regulates *P. aeruginosa*- or *flagellin*- activated innate immune responses [3]. Additionally, cytoplasmic Ca^{2+} flux promotes macrophage to recognize carbohydrate structures on pathogenic fungi via C-type lectin receptors (CLRs) [4–7]. In lymphocytes, cytoplasmic Ca^{2+} flux is one of the hallmarks of B cell receptor (BCR) signaling [8, 9], in

---
* Correspondence: zhaoguiqiu_good@126.com
[1]Department of Ophthalmology, The Affiliated Hospital of Qingdao University, NO. 16 Jiangsu Road, Qingdao 266003, Shandong Province, China
Full list of author information is available at the end of the article

which the enzymatic activity of PLCγ2 is enssential for the induction of Ca^{2+} flux [10]. PLCγ2 is a non-receptor tyrosine kinase, playing an important role at the early period of innate immunity. It is documented that PLCγ2 is the key component in Dectin-2 signaling pathway, mediating anti-fungal innate immune responses in macrophages [11]. However, there is little evidence showing the relationship between PLCγ2 and the induction of Ca^{2+} flux in human corneal epithelial cells (HCECs) [12].

On the other hand, pattern-recognition receptors (PRRs) exert the regulatory role in innate immune response [2, 13]. At the early period of fungal infection, the innate immune system recognizes pathogen associated molecular pattern (PAMP) of pathogenic microorganism using PRRs, such as C-type lectin receptors (CLRs), Toll-like receptors (TLRs) and NOD-like receptors (NLRs) [14–17]. Dectin-1 is a CLR that can identify β-glucan of fungal cytoderm, mediating a variety of fungal innate immune responses and triggers signal transduction via its cytoplasmic hemi-ITAM [18]. The phosphorylated ITAM-like motif of Dectin-1 could directly recruit Syk, which subsequently signals downstream to activate mitogen-activated protein kinases (MAPKs) and nuclear factor κB (NF-κB). Additionally, Syk plays a significant role in Dectin-1 mediated signaling pathway as an antigen-receptor-like manner in magrophages [19, 20]. However, the function of Syk in the Dectin-1 signal pathway in HCECs is still unclear. Recently, we reported that Dectin-1 induced cytoplasmic Ca^{2+} flux upon A. fumigatus infection in HCECs [21], suggesting a potential relationship between PLCγ2 and Dectin-1, as well as cytoplasmic Ca^{2+} flux.

In this study, we demonstrated that the participation of Dectin-1 regulated the expression of PLCγ2 via Syk upon the treatment of A. fumigatus in HCECs. Moreover, PLCγ2 is the critical phospholipases in the process of Dectin-1-mediated Ca^{2+} flux and the secretion of pro-inflammatory mediators (IL-6, CXCL1 and TNF-α) in HCECs.

Methods
Materials and reagents
RNAiso Plus and RT-PCR kits were from TaKaRa (Dalian, China). RIPA (radioimmunopreci- pitation assay) was from Solarbio (Beijing, China). The BCA Protein Assay Kit, polyvinylidene difluoride (PVDF) membranes, confining liquid and enhanced chemiluminescence (ECL) kit were from Beyotime Biotechnology (Shanghai, China). The following reagents were purchased: PLCγ2 inhibitor-U73122 (MilliporeSigma, MO, USA), syk inhibitor-Piceatannol(Selleck, Texas, USA)and Dectin-1 inhibitor-Laminarin (MilliporeSigma, MO, USA). Antibodies used for confocal microscope were from AAT Bioquest (California, USA). Antibodies used for Western

blot were from Cell Signaling(Danvers, MA): anti-PLCγ2, anti-phospho-PLCγ2 (Tyr759), anti-Syk, anti-phospho-Syk.

The preparation of A. fumigatus suspension
A.fumigatus standard strain (CPCC 3.0772) was cultured in Sabouroud liquid culture at 37 °C 200 rpm for 2–3 days, and then the harvested mycelia of Aspergillus fumigatus was washed twice by sterile phosphate buffere saline (PBS) and sterilized by 70% ethanol at 4 °C for 12 h. The density of the fungal mycelia was read in a blood cell counting board and reached the final concentrations of 1×10^8 colony-forming units per 1 ml. The inactived A. fumigatus mycelia was stored at – 20 °C [22, 23].

Cell culture
HCECs were kindly offered by Ocular Surface Laboratory of Xia Men Eye Center and grown in DMEM/F12 with 6.4% Fetal bovine serum (FBS), 7.52 ng/ml Insulin, 7.52 µg/ml Epidermal Growth Factor (EGF), 100u/ml penicillin G and 100µg/ml streptomycin sulfate in a humidified 5% CO2 incubator at 37 °C. The medium was replaced every 2 days before experiments. HCECs suspensions of 1×10^5/ml were seeded onto 12- or 6-well tissue culture plates and when 90 % of the cells were attaehed, the medium was replaced.

HCECs stimulation assay
HCECs untreated were set as controls, anothers were added with A. fumigatus hyphea (5×10^6/ml). Or HCECs were treated with 0.3 mg/ml laminarin, 5 µmol PLCγ2 inhibitor (U73122) or 10 µmol syk inhibitor (Piceatannol) for 30 min prior to A. fumigatus hyphae antigens stimulation in order to block Dectin-1, PLCγ2 and syk. After 15 min or 8 h' incubation, HCECs were harvested to detect the protein and mRNA expression by western blot and RT-PCR.

Calcium imaging
For analysis of cytoplasmic calcium, HCECs which seeded on the glass-bottom culture dishes (NEST) were labeled with Fluo-3 AM (5 µM;AAT Bioquest) for 60 min.To block PLCγ2, Fluo-3-loaded HCECs were preincubated with U73122 for 30 min at room temperature. After resting for 30 min, cells were stimulated with A. fumigatus hyphea(5×10^6/ml) and cytoplasmic calcium was monitored on a Leica TCS SPE confocal microscope in real time for 6–8 min. The images were acquired using Leica LAS software before and after A. fumigatus hyphea were added for each condition. The fluoresecence intensity were measured using Image J software [21].

Western blot

Cells were lysed in RIPA buffer for 1 h, and then were centrifuged. After estimation of protein content, addition of SDS sample buffer, and boiling, total protein was separated on 10% acrylamide SDS-PAGE and transferred onto a polyvinylidene difluoride membrane. The membranes were blocked with 5% BSA liquid, and then were incubated with a monoclonal antibody to human β-actin, and a monoclonal antibody to human Primary antibody at 4 °C overnight. After washed in PBST for three times, the membranes were incubated with corresponding peroxidase-conjugated secondary antibodies at 37 °C for 1 h. Then the blots.

were developed using chemiluminescence (ECL; Thermo Scientific).

Real-time PCR

RNAiso plus reagent were used to extract total RNA from samples according to the manufacturer's protocol, and the RNA was quantified by sprctrophotometry. The first strand cDNA was synthesized by RT from total RNA. The Real-Time PCR was performed in a Mx3005PTM system (Stratagene) with 20ul reaction volume containing 2ul of cDNA. cDNA was amplified by PCR using primers shown below. β-actin was used as the endogenous control. The thermocycler parameters were 95 °C for 30s, followed by 40 cycles of 95 °C for 5 s and 60 °C for 30s. A melting curve was used to confirm the specificity of the PCR products following each reaction. The ΔΔCT method was used for quantization of target gene.

products of stimulated and unstimulated group. Data are expressed as fold of increase in mRNA expressio. Each experiment was performed in triplicate. The double-stranded probes used are as follow: The following primers were used (5′-3′): AAGCCAGAGCTGTG CAGATGAGTA(forward) and TGTCCTGCAGCCAC TGGTTC(reverse) for Human-IL-6; AGGGAATTC ACCCCAAGAAC(forward) and CACCAGTGAGCTTC CTCCTC(reverse) for Human-CXCL1; TGCTTGTTC CTCAGCCTCTT(forward) and CAGAGGGCTGATTA GAGAGAGGT(reverse) for Human-TNF-α; TGGCACC CAGCACAATGAA(forward) and CTAAGTCATAGTC CGCCTAGAAGCA (reverse) for Human-β-actin as housekeeping gene.

Enzyme-linked immunosorbent assay

According to the manufacturer's protocol Enzyme-linked Immunosorbent Assay, Double-sandwich ELISA for human IL-6, CXCL1and TNF-α was performed, to detect the concentration of IL-6, CXCL1and TNF-α protein in conditioned media and culture cell lysates from different treatments. Absorbance was read at 450 nm with a reference wavelength of 570 nm by a VERSAmax microplate reader (Molecular Devices, Sunnyvale, CA) [21].

Statistical analysis

All data were presented as mean ± SD from independent experiments. The data were analyzed using SPSS19.0 statistical package. One-way ANOVA test was used to make comparison among three or more groups, and LSD was used to identify between each two groups. $P < 0.05$ was considered statistically significant and data are shown as mean ± SEM.

Results

A. fumigatus induces cytokines production in a time- and dose-dependent manner

To investigate A. fumigatus hyphae-induced IL-6, CXCL1 and TNF-α mRNA expression and protein secretion, hyphae-treated cells and supernatants were analyzed by RT-PCR and ELISA. The assys were performed over a period of 16 h and 36 h, with cells being exposed to 5×10^5, 5×10^6 and 5×10^7/ml of hyphae, respectively. The level of IL-6, CXCL1 and TNF-α mRNA expression was elevated and peaked at 8 h (5×10^6/ml), then returned to decrease after hyphae stimulation, as shown in Fig. 1a-c. The maximal protein production was recorded at 24 h (5×10^6/ml) (Fig. 1d-f). The data demonstrated that IL-6, CXCL1 and TNF-α mRNA expression and protein secretion were induced by hyphae in a time- and dose-dependent manner in HCECs.

PLCγ2 could be activated by A. fumigatus and induced by the engagement of Dectin-1 in HCECs

We stimulated HCECs with A. fumigatus hyphae, and the data showed that the stimulation led to the activation of PLCγ2 as indicated by their phosphorylation status. The phosphorylation of PLCγ2 was significantly increased after A. fumigatus hyphae infection with a time-dependent manner, and peaked at 15 min, whereas no significant difference was seen in total PLCγ2 protein (Fig. 2a). But we wondered whether the engagement of Dectin-1 could increase the activition of PLCγ2 in HCECs. To address this question, we preincubated HCECs with the Dectin-1 inhibitor laminarin before the stimulation of hyphae and data showed that this prior treatment could decrease the expression of p-PLCγ2 (Fig. 2b). Thus, it proved that the engagement of Dectin-1 played an important role in the activation of PLCγ2 with the stimulaton of hyphae in HCECs.

PLCγ2 plays a role in the stimulation of Ca²⁺ flux induced by A. fumigates

To confirm whether PLCγ2 could induce Ca²⁺ flux in the infected HCECs, we preincubated the cells with U73122, the inhibitor of PLCγ2, prior to A. fumigatus hyphae treatment. As shown in Fig. 3, the Ca²⁺ flux elicited by treatment of hyphae in HCECs could be

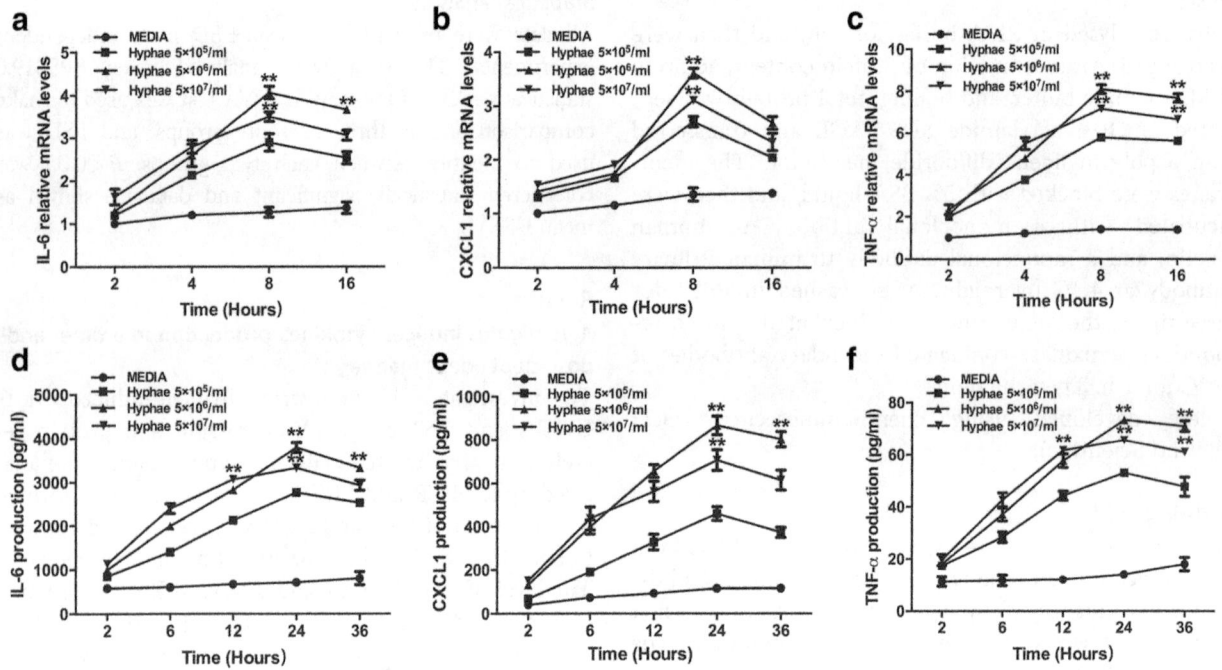

Fig. 1 The effect of hyphae on mRNA and protein expression of IL-6, CXCL1 and TNF-α. **a-c** The RNA from HCECs treated with different concentrations of *A. fumigatus* hyphae ($5 \times 10^5, 5 \times 10^6$ and 5×10^7 /ml) were harvested and tested by RT-PCR. **d-f** Cells were stimulated with *A. fumigatus* hyphae at 37 °C. The supernatants were collected and assayed by ELISA. The data represented the mean ± SEM of three separate experiments. **$p < 0.001$

inhibited by U73122, which suggested that PLCγ2 played an important role in triggering Ca^{2+} signaling in HCECs.

Syk is important for Dectin-1-induced PLCγ2 activation

To investigate the stimulatory effects on Syk with the *A. fumigatus* hyphae, the HCECs were incubated with the *A. fumigatus* hyphae (5×10^6/mL) for 5, 15, 30 and 45 min, tested by western blotting. As shown in Fig. 4a, the findings indicated the phosphorylation of Syk was activated at 30 min by *A. fumigatus* hyphae stimulation in HCECs. We indicated that Dectin-1 was critical in the activation of Syk, because the inhibition of Dectin-1 abrogated hyphae-induced phosphorylation of Syk (Fig. 4b). To assess if the tyrosine kinase is important for

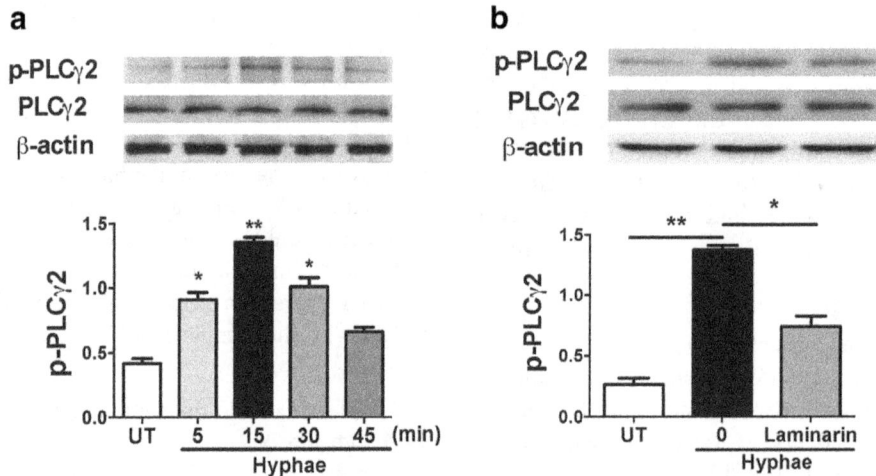

Fig. 2 Engagement of Dectin-1 activates PLCγ2 in HCECs. **a** HCECs were treated with 5×10^6/ml *A. fumigates hyphae* for various times as indicated their activation status determined by Western Blot. **b** HCECs were preincubated for 30 min with Dectin-1 inhibitor Laminarin, followed by the treatment of *hyphae* for 15 min. The activation of PLCγ was assayed by Western Blot. Data shown are representative of more than three independent sets of experiments. *$p < 0.05$, **$p < 0.001$

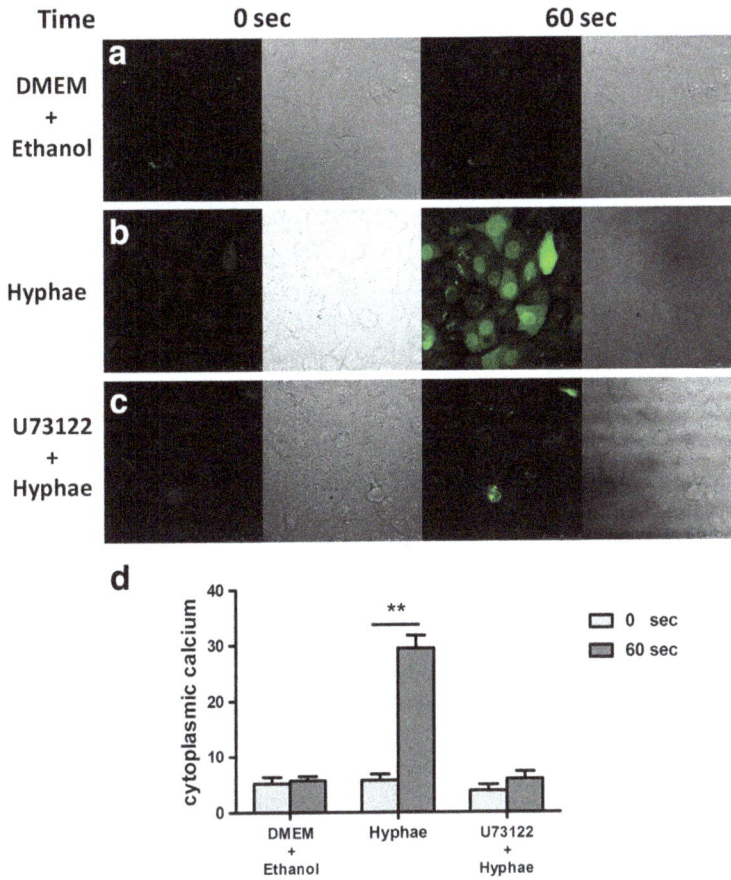

Fig. 3 PLCγ2 plays an important role for the elicitation of Ca^{2+} flux in HCECs. **a-c** HCECs were loaded with Fluo-3 and treated with DMEM in the presence of Ethanol, 5×10^6/ml *A. fumigates hyphae* or 5×10^6/ml *A. fumigates hyphae* in the presence of 1μMol/L inhibitor of PLCγ2-U73122. Confocal images of HCECs showed cytoplasmic calcium expression (green stain). **d** The corresponding results of fluoresecence intensity were measured by Image J software. Data are representative of more than three independent sets of experiments. Magnifications 400X. **$p < 0.001$

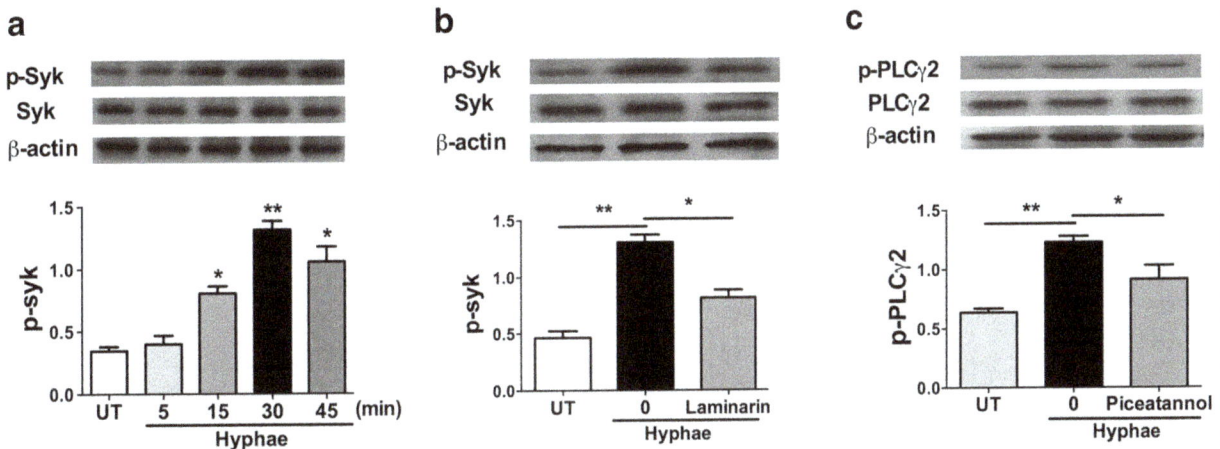

Fig. 4 Syk Plays a crucial role for the activation of Dectin-1-induced PLCγ2 in HCECs. **a** The phosphorylation of Syk was activated after *A. fumigatus* hyphae stimulation in HCECs. The activation status was measured by Western Blot at 5, 15, 30 and 45 min. **b, c** HCECs were preincubated for 30 min with Dectin-1 inhibitor Laminarin or syk inhibitor Piceatannol, followed by treatment with hyphae for 30 or 15 min. The activation of syk or PLCγ was assayed by Western Blot. Results shown are mean ± SD of three independent experiments. *$p < 0.05$, **$p < 0.001$

Dectin-1-induced activation of PLCγ2, we pretreated HCECs with the Syk inhibitor Piceatannol(10 μM) for 30 min followed the stimulation of hyphae. Then we examined the phosphorylation status of PLCγ2. As shown in Fig. 4c, hyphae-stimulated phosphorylation of PLCγ2 was markedly reduced when Syk was inhibited by its specific inhibitor Piceatannol in HCECs. Consistent with the finding that Syk play important role in Dectin-1 signaling, our results further suggested that Syk acted upstream of PLCγ2 in the Dectin-1 signaling pathway as their activities are crucial for the activation of PLCγ2.

PLCγ2 is essential for the up-regulation of cytokine production in HCECs

To determine whether PLCγ2 can regulate cytokine secretion upon *A. fumigatus* hyphae stimulation in HCECs, RT-PCR and ELISA were used to detect the expression of cytokine at 8 and 24 h. As seen in Fig. 5a-c, relative mRNA levels of IL-6, CXCL1 and TNF-α was significantly reduced with the pretreatment of U73122 compared with untreated controls. Protein analysis confirmed the mRNA data, with significant reduction between U73122 treated groups and controls (Fig. 5b-d). It suggested that PLCγ2 signaling critically regulated these cytokines in antifungal immunity.

Discussion

FK is a blinding infection of the corneas, accounting for a significant portion in all keratitis. However, the pathogenesis of FK and the underlying molecular mechanisms are still unclear [24]. In the development of FK, innate immune response against *A. fumigatus* plays a crucial role in controlling microbial infection with the participation of inflammatory mediators [19]. In this study, we demonstrated that Dectin-1 mediated PLCγ2 signaling plays a critical role in *A. fumigatus* hyphae induced innate immune response in HCECs, and Syk acts as an upstream mediator in the Dectin-1 PLCγ2 signaling pathway. Above all, we showed that *A. fumigatus* hyphae significantly upregulated the expression of inflammatory factors IL-6, CXCL1 and TNF-α in HCECs. These fungi-induced cytokines resist fungal infection and promote the infiltration of inflammatory cells to remove pathogens.

In addition, our results suggested that PLCγ2 plays an important role in the stimulation of Ca²⁺ flux induced by *A. fumigates* in HCECs, which is consistent with that the enzymatic activity of PLCγ2 is required for the induction of Ca²⁺ flux in B cells [10]. Cytoplasmic Ca²⁺ flux is the hallmark of B cell receptor (BCR) signaling pathway, in which the engagement of PRRs is essential for the elicitation of Ca²⁺ flux in lymphocytes [9]. It is in

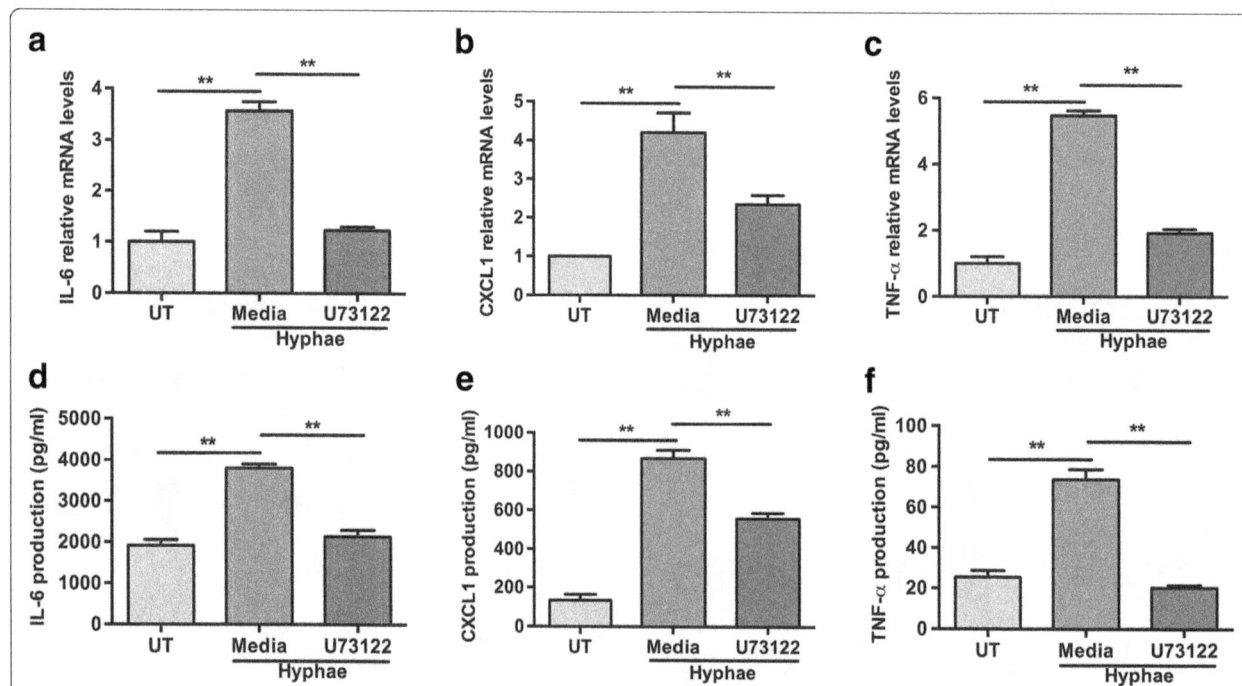

Fig. 5 *A. fumigatus*-induced expression of inflammatory cytokines was regulated by PLCγ2 in HCECs. Cells were pre-treated with indicated concentrations of U73122 for 30 min prior to stimulation with 5 × 10⁶/ ml *A. fumigatus* hyphae. **a-c** mRNAs levels of IL-6, CXCL1 and TNF-α were reduced significantly after U73122 treatment. **d-f** Protein levels of these cytokines were also significantly reduced with the treatment of U73122. The data represented the mean ± SEM of three separate experiments. **P < 0.001

the agreement with our previous study that the innate PRRs such as Dectin-1 could elicit intracellular Ca^{2+} flux [21]. It is also consistent with the importance of PLCγ2 for intracellular Ca^{2+} flux with the engagement of Dectin-1in DCs [25]. Recently, Lu et al. showed that the maintaince of intracellular Ca^{2+} homeostasis was involved in the potential mechanisms of hypoxia-induced inflammation and apoptosis in microglia BV2 cells [26]. Besides functioning in BCR signaling, PLCγ2 also plays an critical role in the innate immune system as a key component of the downstream signaling pathway for many receptors in response to fungal infection [11]. A previous study has shown that PLCγ2 functions downstream of Dectin-2 in response to the stimulation by the hyphal form of *Candida albicans* (*C. albicans*), an opportunistic pathogenic fungus [11]. In addition, they found that PLCγ2-deficient mice are defective in clearing *C. albicans* infection in vivo [11]. In this study, our findings showed that the lack of Dectin-1 impaired the phosphorylation of PLCγ2 in response to the infection with *A. fumigatus*, suggesting that Dectin-1 mediated the activation of PLCγ2 in the infected HCECs. Taken together, our data suggested that the intracellular Ca^{2+} mobilization, as a mechanism of cellular signaling in HCECs, is elicited by Dectin-1-mediated PLCγ2 signaling pathway.

Moreover, Dectin-1 is one of C-type lectin receptors (CLRs), functioning as PRRs to sense fungal infection. However, Dectin-1 induced PLCγ2 signaling pathway remains largely unknown. Here we explored how PLCγ2 was activated by determining which upstream kinase is required for its activation in the Dectin-1 signal transduction pathway. Recent studies demonstrated that Syk played critical roles in Dectin-1 signaling in macrophages [19, 20]. While in HCECs, we indicated that Syk was identified as a critical component downstream of Dectin-1 signaling, because the inhibition of Dectin-1 abrogated hyphae-induced activation of Syk. During BCR signaling, Syk is important for PLCγ2 activation and Ca^{2+} flux in B cells [27, 28]. Consistent with the results of BCR signaling, we found that the hyphae-stimulated phosphorylation of PLCγ2 was markedly reduced after Syk inhibition by its specific inhibitor Piceatannol in HCECs. Taken together, these findings demonstrated that Syk plays a critical role in Dectin-1-induced PLCγ2 signaling pathways, governing antifungal innate immune responses in HCECs.

Futhermore, it is reported that the lack of PLCγ2 impaired cytokine production in response to infection with *C. albicans* in PLCγ2-deficient macrophages [11]. Its deficiency resulted in the defective activation of NF-κB and MAPK and in a significantly reduced production of reactive oxygen species (ROS) following fungal challenge [11]. In our study, inflammatory mediators (IL-6, CXCL1 and TNF-α) stimulated by *A. fumigatus* hyphae were markedly blocked by PLCγ2 inhibitor in HCECs, suggesting that Dectin-1-mediated PLCγ2 signaling pathway is involved in the innate immune response of HCECs against *A. fumigatus* hyphae. PLCγ2 activation is essential to the expression of inflammatory mediators. These findings demonstrated that inflammatory cytokines and chemokines production could be upregulated through activation of Dectin-1-mediated PLCγ2 after *A. fumigatus* hyphae stimulation.

Last, but not least, it is increasingly acknowledged that C-type lectins act critically in the regulation of initiating and sustaining immune response against various pathogens. Therefore, the elucidation of the signaling of these CLRs would make a major impact on our understanding of host defense and microbial spread in the epithelium cells. For example, Dectin-1 is important for host recognition of β-glucan structure that exists in cell wall of *aspergillus*, *yeast*, *candida*, *penicillium* and other fungus [29–32]. Our current study demonstrated that PLCγ2 in Dectin-1 signal transduction could provide new targets for therapeutic intervention to enhance or suppress the host response.

Conclusions

In conclusion, our findings demonstrate that PLCγ2 plays a critical role for Ca^{2+} Flux in HCECs stimulated by *A. fumigatus* hyphae. Syk acts upstream of PLCγ2 in the Dectin-1 signaling pathway. The expressions of proinflammatory mediators induced by *A. fumigatus* are regulated by the activation of Dectin-1-mediated PLCγ2 signaling pathway in HCECs. The further study of PLCγ2 pathway will provide new targets for the prevention and therapeutic intervention of fungal infection.

Abbreviations

A. fumigatus: Aspergillus fumigatus; BCR: B cell receptor; *C. albicans*: *Candida albicans*; CLR: C-type lectin receptor; EGF: Epidermal Growth Factor; ELISA: Enzyme-linked immunosorbent assay; FBS: Fetal bovine serum; FK: Fungal keratitis; HCECs: Human corneal epithelial cells; MAPKs: Mitogen-activated protein kinases; NF-κB: Nuclear factor κB; PAMP: Pathogen associated molecular pattern; PBS: Phosphate buffere saline; PLCγ2: Phospholipase C-γ2; PRRs: Pattern-recognition receptors; RT-PCR: Reverse transcriptase polymerase chain reaction; Syk: Spleen-tyrosine kinase

Funding

This study was supported by the National Natural Science Foundation of China (No. 81470609; No. 81170825), Youth Project of Natural Science Foundation of Shandong Province (ZR2013HQ007) and Key Project of Natural Science Foundation of Shandong Province (ZR2012FZ001).

Authors' contributions

All of the authors contributed substantially to this study. Conceived and designed the Experiments: GZ JL and XP. Performed the experiments: XP JL CL JQ and YZ. Analyzed the data: JQ YZ and CL. Contributed reagents/

materials/analysis tools: JQ and CL. Wrote the paper: XP GZ and YZ. All authors read and approved the final manuscript.

Competing interests

The authors declare that they have no competing interests.

Author details

[1]Department of Ophthalmology, The Affiliated Hospital of Qingdao University, NO. 16 Jiangsu Road, Qingdao 266003, Shandong Province, China. [2]Department of Biochemistry, Immunology and Microbiology, Wayne State University School of Medicine, 540 E. Canfield Avenue, Detroit, MI 48201, USA.

References

1. Mascarenhas J, Lalitha P, Prajna NV, Srinivasan M, Das M, D'Silva SS, Oldenburg CE, Borkar DS, Esterberg EJ, Lietman TM, et al. Acanthamoeba, fungal, and bacterial keratitis: a comparison of risk factors and clinical features. Am J Ophthalmol. 2014;157(1):56–62.
2. Li C, Zhao G, Che C, Lin J, Li N, Hu L, Jiang N, Liu Y. The role of LOX-1 in innate immunity to aspergillus fumigatus in corneal epithelial cells. Invest Ophthalmol Vis Sci. 2015;56(6):3593–603.
3. Fu Z, Bettega K, Carroll S, Buchholz KR, Machen TE. Role of Ca2+ in responses of airway epithelia to Pseudomonas aeruginosa, flagellin, ATP, and thapsigargin. Am J Physiol Lung Cell Mol Physiol. 2007;292(1):L353–64.
4. Rabes A, Zimmermann S, Reppe K, Lang R, Seeberger PH, Suttorp N, Witzenrath M, Lepenies B, Opitz B. The C-type lectin receptor Mincle binds to Streptococcus pneumoniae but plays a limited role in the anti-pneumococcal innate immune response. PLoS One. 2015;10(2):e0117022.
5. Schoenen H, Bodendorfer B, Hitchens K, Manzanero S, Werninghaus K, Nimmerjahn F, Agger EM, Stenger S, Andersen P, Ruland J, et al. Cutting edge: Mincle is essential for recognition and adjuvanticity of the mycobacterial cord factor and its synthetic analog trehalose-dibehenate. J Immunol. 2010;184(6):2756–60.
6. Bugarcic A, Hitchens K, Beckhouse AG, Wells CA, Ashman RB, Blanchard H. Human and mouse macrophage-inducible C-type lectin (Mincle) bind Candida albicans. Glycobiology. 2008;18(9):679–85.
7. Yamasaki S, Matsumoto M, Takeuchi O, Matsuzawa T, Ishikawa E, Sakuma M, Tateno H, Uno J, Hirabayashi J, Mikami Y, et al. C-type lectin Mincle is an activating receptor for pathogenic fungus, Malassezia. Proc Natl Acad Sci U S A. 2009;106(6):1897–902.
8. Weiss A, Irving BA, Tan LK, Koretzky GA. Signal transduction by the T cell antigen receptor. Semin Immunol. 1991;3(5):313–24.
9. Cambier JC, Pleiman CM, Clark MR. Signal transduction by the B cell antigen receptor and its coreceptors. Annu Rev Immunol. 1994;12:457–86.
10. Kurosaki T, Maeda A, Ishiai M, Hashimoto A, Inabe K, Takata M. Regulation of the phospholipase C-gamma2 pathway in B cells. Immunol Rev. 2000;176:19–29.
11. Gorjestani S, Yu M, Tang B, Zhang D, Wang D, Lin X. Phospholipase Cgamma2 (PLCgamma2) is key component in Dectin-2 signaling pathway, mediating anti-fungal innate immune responses. J Biol Chem. 2011;286(51):43651–9.
12. Landreville S, Coulombe S, Carrier P, Gelb MH, Guerin SL, Salesse C. Expression of phospholipases A2 and C in human corneal epithelial cells. Invest Ophthalmol Vis Sci. 2004;45(11):3997–4003.
13. Opitz B, van Laak V, Eitel J, Suttorp N. Innate immune recognition in infectious and noninfectious diseases of the lung. Am J Respir Crit Care Med. 2010;181(12):1294–309.
14. Zhao J, Wu XY. Aspergillus fumigatus antigens activate immortalized human corneal epithelial cells via toll-like receptors 2 and 4. Curr Eye Res. 2008;33(5):447–54.
15. Leal SM Jr, Cowden S, Hsia YC, Ghannoum MA, Momany M, Pearlman E. Distinct roles for Dectin-1 and TLR4 in the pathogenesis of aspergillus fumigatus keratitis. PLoS Pathog. 2010;6:e1000976.
16. Xu ZJ, Zhao GQ, Wang Q, Che CY, Jiang N, Hu LT. Xu Q: nucleotide oligomerization domain 2 contributes to the innate immune response in THCE cells stimulated by aspergillus fumigatus conidia. Int J Ophthalmol. 2012;5(4):409–14.
17. Feriotti C, Loures FV, Frank de Araujo E, da Costa TA, Calich VL. Mannosyl-recognizing receptors induce an M1-like phenotype in macrophages of susceptible mice but an M2-like phenotype in mice resistant to a fungal infection. PLoS One. 2013;8(1):e54845.
18. Xu S, Huo J, Gunawan M, Su IH, Lam KP. Activated dectin-1 localizes to lipid raft microdomains for signaling and activation of phagocytosis and cytokine production in dendritic cells. J Biol Chem. 2009;284(33):22005–11.
19. Rogers NC, Slack EC, Edwards AD, Nolte MA, Schulz O, Schweighoffer E, Williams DL, Gordon S, Tybulewicz VL, Brown GD, et al. Syk-dependent cytokine induction by Dectin-1 reveals a novel pattern recognition pathway for C type lectins. Immunity. 2005;22(4):507–17.
20. Underhill DM, Rossnagle E, Lowell CA, Simmons RM. Dectin-1 activates Syk tyrosine kinase in a dynamic subset of macrophages for reactive oxygen production. Blood. 2005;106(7):2543–50.
21. Peng XD, Zhao GQ, Lin J, Jiang N, Xu Q, Zhu CC, Qu JQ, Cong L, Li H. Fungus induces the release of IL-8 in human corneal epithelial cells, via Dectin-1-mediated protein kinase C pathways. Int J Ophthalmol. 2015;8(3):441–7.
22. Jie Z, Wu XY, Yu FS. Activation of toll-like receptors 2 and 4 in aspergillus fumigatus keratitis. Innate immunity. 2009;15(3):155–68.
23. Gantner BN, Simmons RM, Canavera SJ, Akira S, Underhill DM. Collaborative induction of inflammatory responses by dectin-1 and toll-like receptor 2. J Exp Med. 2003;197(9):1107–17.
24. Li D, Dong B, Tong Z, Wang Q, Liu W, Wang Y, Liu W, Chen J, Xu L, Chen L, et al. MBL-mediated opsonophagocytosis of Candida albicans by human neutrophils is coupled with intracellular Dectin-1-triggered ROS production. PLoS One. 2012;7(12):e50589.
25. Xu S, Huo J, Lee KG, Kurosaki T, Lam KP. Phospholipase Cgamma2 is critical for Dectin-1-mediated Ca2+ flux and cytokine production in dendritic cells. J Biol Chem. 2009;284(11):7038–46.
26. Lu Y, Gu Y, Ding X, Wang J, Chen J, Miao C. Intracellular Ca2+ homeostasis and JAK1/STAT3 pathway are involved in the protective effect of propofol on BV2 microglia against hypoxia-induced inflammation and apoptosis. PLoS One. 2017;12(5):e0178098.
27. DeFranco AL. The complexity of signaling pathways activated by the BCR. Curr Opin Immunol. 1997;9(3):296–308.
28. Kurosaki T. Genetic analysis of B cell antigen receptor signaling. Annu Rev Immunol. 1999;17:555–92.
29. Robinson MJ, Sancho D, Slack EC, LeibundGut-Landmann S, Reis e Sousa C. Myeloid C-type lectins in innate immunity. Nat Immunol. 2006;7(12):1258–65.
30. Brown GD. Dectin-1: a signalling non-TLR pattern-recognition receptor. Nat Rev Immunol. 2006;6(1):33–43.
31. Yadav M, Schorey JS. The beta-glucan receptor dectin-1 functions together with TLR2 to mediate macrophage activation by mycobacteria. Blood. 2006;108(9):3168–75.
32. Rothfuchs AG, Bafica A, Feng CG, Egen JG, Williams DL, Brown GD, Sher A. Dectin-1 interaction with Mycobacterium tuberculosis leads to enhanced IL-12p40 production by splenic dendritic cells. J Immunol. 2007;179(6):3463–71.

31

Changes in corneal endothelial cells after trabeculectomy and EX-PRESS shunt: 2-year follow-up

Saki Omatsu, Kazuyuki Hirooka[*], Eri Nitta and Kaori Ukegawa

Abstract

Background: To compare trabeculectomy and EX-PRESS device implantation procedures for treating glaucoma and evaluate changes in corneal endothelial cell density (CECD).

Methods: This study prospectively evaluated changes in the CECD in 60 eyes of 60 patients who underwent trabeculectomy and 50 eyes of 45 patients who underwent EX-PRESS device implantation. Baseline patient data recorded included age at surgery, sex, type of glaucoma medications, and lens status. Using a noncontact specular microscope, corneal specular microscopy was performed preoperatively at the central cornea and then at 6, 12, 18 and 24 months after surgery. CECD before and after surgery was compared using a paired t-test.

Results: There was a significant decrease in the IOP and number of antiglaucoma medications in both groups after the surgery. The mean CECD in the trabeculectomy group was 2505 ± 280 cells/mm^2 at baseline, while it was 2398 ± 274 cells/mm^2 ($P < 0.001$), 2349 ± 323 cells/mm^2 ($P < 0.001$), 2293 ± 325 cells/mm^2 ($P < 0.001$), and 2277 ± 385 cells/mm^2 ($P = 0.003$) at 6, 12, 18, and 24 months, respectively. However, the CECD in the EX-PRESS group was 2377 ± 389 cells/mm^2 at baseline, while it was 2267 ± 409 cells/mm^2 ($P = 0.007$), 2292 ± 452 cells/mm^2 ($P = 0.043$), 2379 ± 375 cells/mm^2 ($P = 0.318$), and 2317 ± 449 cells/mm^2 ($P = 0.274$) at 6, 12, 18, and 24 months, respectively.

Conclusions: As compared to trabeculectomy, EX-PRESS device implantation appears to be a safer procedure with regard to the endothelial cell loss risk.

Keywords: Trabeculectomy, EX-PRESS, Corneal endothelial cell density, Intraocular pressure

Background

The aim of glaucoma treatments is to slow disease progression while preserving visual functions without changing the patient's quality of life. In general, these treatments are primarily designed to lower the intraocular pressure (IOP), with first approaches utilizing medical therapies with antiglaucomatous drugs. When maximal tolerable medical therapy is not able to sufficiently lower the IOP, patients are treated using trabeculectomy in order to prevent optic nerve damage or visual field deterioration. Although trabeculectomies are commonly used, the procedure is not without risk. Thus, the EX-PRESS drainage device (Alcon Laboratories, Fort Worth, TX) was designed and created as a safer alternative for controlling the IOP [1]. This device,

which consists of a nonvalved stainless steel tube, is inserted under a partial-thickness scleral flap and serves as a connection between the anterior chamber and the subconjunctival space.

In young adults, the corneal endothelial cell density (CECD) is approximately 3000 cells/mm^2. However, due to aging, the mean CECD value is reduced by $0.5 \pm 0.6\%$ every year [2]. This loss can be accelerated by several risk factors that include, surgery, argon laser iridotomy, and even glaucoma itself [3–9]. Although it has been previously shown that trabeculectomy can damage corneal endothelial cells [10–13], no changes have been observed in the CECD at either 1 or 3 months after EX-PRESS implantation surgery [12]. In contrast, Ishida et al. reported finding significant decreases in the CECD at 24 months after EX-PRESS implantation [14]. Even so, it should be noted that this previous study did not

* Correspondence: kazuyk@med.kagawa-u.ac.jp
Department of Ophthalmology, Kagawa University Faculty of Medicine, 1750-1 Ikenobe, Miki, Kagawa 761-0793, Japan

compare eyes undergoing implantation to a control group of eyes undergoing trabeculectomy.

The purpose of this study was to evaluate the long-term changes in corneal endothelial cells that occurred for up to 1 year after undergoing trabeculectomy and EX-PRESS shunt surgeries for the treatment of glaucoma.

Methods

This observational study examined eyes undergoing treatments between April 2014 and May 2016 with either the EX-PRESS glaucoma filtration device or trabeculectomy. Trabeculectomies were performed in more than 200 eyes during the study observation period. Eyes selected for inclusion in the study were age and gender matched with the eyes from the EX-PRESS group. Written informed consent for participation in the study was obtained from participants. All procedures and follow-ups took place at the Kagawa University Hospital, Kagawa, Japan. When treatments included both eyes, data from the first eye operated on in the patient was selected and used for the study. The Institutional Review Board of the Kagawa University Faculty of Medicine approved this study protocol. In addition to the standard consent for surgery, all subjects provided written informed consent prior to their enrollment and taking part in the research study.

To be included in the study, patients were required to be older than 20 years of age, and have preoperative uncontrolled IOP despite being administered the maximum tolerated medical therapy. Exclusion criteria included having any significant ocular diseases or history in the operated eye (other than glaucoma or cataract), or exhibiting any other corneal epithelial or stromal disorders that could potentially cause issues during the specular microscopy. The study also excluded patients who did not provide specific reasons on why they were unable to complete the entire 1-year follow-up.

A noncontact specular microscope with an autofocus device, the Tomey EM-3000 (Tomey Corporation, Nagoya, Japan), was used for all observations. All measurements of the endothelial cell count were carried out at the center of the cornea, with the incorporated screen on the device used to visualize the endothelium. The device automatically measured the CECD, with cell density recorded as the number of cells per square millimeter. CECD measurements were obtained prior to and at 6 and 12 months after the surgery. Thereafter, all subsequent measurements were performed every 6 months.

Patients who had a history of vitreous surgery or severe vision loss of their fellow eye underwent the EX-PRESS glaucoma filtration device procedure, with all of the surgeries performed by one surgeon (KH). After administration of retrobulbar anesthesia with lidocaine 2%, all eyes were prepared and draped. In the first step of the procedure, after placing a corneal traction suture (5–0 silk suture), the surgeon dissected a fornix-based conjunctival flap, and then created a one-half thickness scleral flap (approximately 3.5×3.5 mm). Mitomycin C (MMC) was applied to the sclera over the proposed scleral flap site. Subsequently, after positioning 6 to 8 sponges containing 0.04% MMC solution in the subconjunctival space, the sponges were maintained in place for 3 to 5 min. Once the sponges were removed, the area was copiously irrigated using 250 ml of physiologic saline. After removing a block of clear cornea and trabecular meshwork tissue at the edge of the corneoscleral bed, peripheral iridectomy was performed, followed by suturing of the scleral flap using 6 to 7 monofilament 10–0 nylon sutures. Sutures were adjusted to ensure that a small amount of leakage could be observed around the scleral flap margin without causing any shallowing of the anterior chamber.

In the EX-PRESS group, a 26G needle was used to enter the anterior chamber slightly posterior to the blue-gray zone under the scleral flap, and the EX-PRESS (model P50) shunt was introduced into the anterior chamber through the needle track. Suturing of the scleral flap was performed using 2 to 4 monofilament 10–0 nylon sutures, while closure of the conjunctiva used 10–0 nylon sutures at the edges of the incision. For the conjunctiva, one or more of the horizontal mattress sutures were placed centrally. Once the anterior chamber was reformed by using a balanced salt solution, the wound was then checked for leaks. After instillation of a corticosteroid/antibiotic ointment, a sterile eye patch and shield was placed over the eye.

The procedure for the trabeculectomy group used a fornix-based, superior, one site approach, with the cataract surgery (phacoemulsification and intraocular lens insertion) combined with the trabeculectomy. The phacoemulsification procedure in the EX-PRESS group was performed via a 2.4 mm temporal clear cornea incision. After making the incision, the intraocular lens was then placed into the capsular bag. All patients were administered a topical corticosteroid (four times daily) and an antibiotic during the following 8 to 12 weeks after the surgery. If the filtration was judged to be too low by the surgeon or the IOP was too high to meet the target pressure, patients underwent suture lysis with an argon laser under topical anesthesia.

All statistical analyses were performed using SPSS version 19.0 (IBM, New York, NY). CECD and IOP were compared before and after surgery using paired t-tests. A P value less than 0.05 was considered to be statistically significant. Data are presented as the mean ± standard deviation.

Results

Table 1 summarizes the patient characteristics. No significant differences were observed for the patient age, gender, and lens status between the trabeculectomy and EX-PRESS shunt groups. The number of combined cataract surgeries

Table 1 Baseline patient characteristics of the trabeculectomy and EX-PRESS groups

	Trabeculectomy	EX-PRESS	P value
Mean Age (years)	63.7 ± 9.5	63.1 ± 12.3	0.85[a]
Gender (M/F)	31/33	30/20	0.22[b]
Diagnosis			
POAG	24	30	
NTG	24	12	
SG	11	8	
EG	5		
Lens status			0.06[b]
Phakia	47	28	
Pseudophakia	17	22	

M male, F female, POAG primary open-angle glaucoma, NTG normal-tension glaucoma, SG secondary glaucoma, EG exfoliation glaucoma
[a]independent t-test
[b]χ^2 test

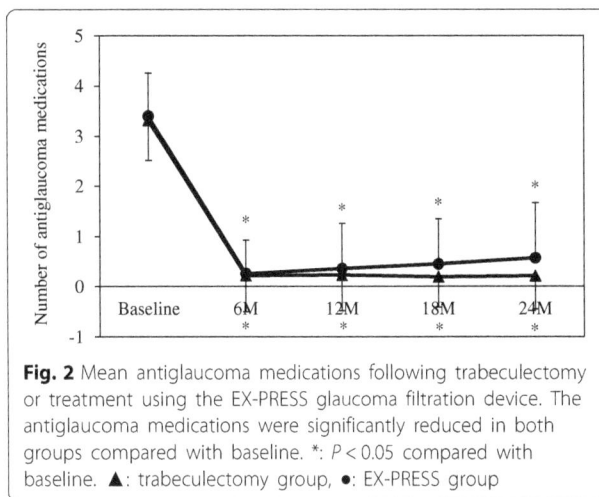

Fig. 2 Mean antiglaucoma medications following trabeculectomy or treatment using the EX-PRESS glaucoma filtration device. The antiglaucoma medications were significantly reduced in both groups compared with baseline. *: $P < 0.05$ compared with baseline. ▲: trabeculectomy group, ●: EX-PRESS group

performed in the trabeculectomy and EX-PRESS shunt groups were 29 and 22, respectively ($P = 0.72$).

Significant decreases in the IOP and in the number of antiglaucoma medications were observed after the surgery in both procedures (Figs. 1 and 2). The mean IOP in the trabeculectomy group was 18.3 ± 8.7 mmHg at baseline, while it was 9.8 ± 3.6 mmHg, 10.9 ± 4.3 mmHg, 10.9 ± 4.3 mmHg, and 11.2 ± 4.8 mmHg at 6, 12, 18, and 24 months, respectively. The IOP in the EX-PRESS group was 17.7 ± 5.6 mmHg at baseline, while it was 11.4 ± 4.3 mmHg, 12.4 ± 3.9 mmHg, 11.8 ± 3.3 mmHg and 13.1 ± 4.8 mmHg at 6, 12, 18, and 24 months, respectively.

Table 2 shows the trends of the CECD over the course of the study between the two groups. The mean CECD in the trabeculectomy group was 2505 ± 280 cells/mm^2 at baseline, while it was 2398 ± 275 cells/mm^2, 2349 ± 323 cells/mm^2, 2293 ± 325 cells/mm^2, and 2277 ± 385 cells/mm^2 at 6, 12, 18, and 24 months, respectively. The

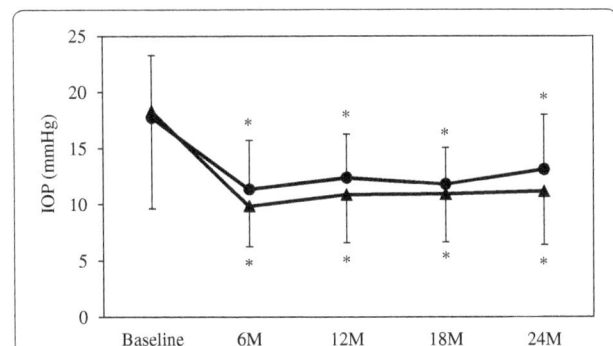

Fig. 1 Mean intraocular pressure following trabeculectomy or treatment using the EX-PRESS glaucoma filtration device. The intraocular pressure was significantly reduced in both groups compared with baseline. *: $P < 0.05$ compared with baseline. ▲: trabeculectomy group, ●: EX-PRESS group

CECD in the EX-PRESS group was 2377 ± 389 cells/mm^2 at baseline, while it was 2267 ± 409 cells/mm^2, 2292 ± 452 cells/mm^2, 2379 ± 375 cells/mm^2, and 2317 ± 449 cells/mm^2 at 6, 12, 18, and 24 months, respectively. In the trabeculectomy group, there was a significant reduction in the IOP from the baseline observed for all of the study visits. For the CECDs, however, at month 18 in the EX-PRESS group, there were no longer significant differences from the baseline noted for the density.

Table 3 shows the pre- and postoperative CECD with or without cataract surgery. While there was a significant difference from baseline for the CECD at each of the study visits in the trabeculectomy group, the CECD in the EX-PRESS combined cataract surgery group at 12 months no longer exhibited any significant difference from the baseline. Furthermore, in the patients undergoing only the EX-PRESS procedure, the CECD did not exhibit any significant difference from baseline at any of the study visits.

Discussion

To ensure maintenance of the corneal integrity and transparency, the corneal endothelium is essential [15]. Aging, surgery, and trauma have been reported by several studies to be able to reduce the CECD [2, 4, 12–14]. Our current study showed that while there were no changes in the CECD after the EX-PRESS implantation, there were significant decreases observed in the CECD after the trabeculectomies.

Several studies that have investigated trabeculectomies reported finding a reduction in the postoperative CECD after the procedure [10, 11, 16]. While several possible mechanisms for the reductions in CECD after trabeculectomy have been proposed, the exact mechanism responsible for the endothelial cell loss after trabeculectomy has yet to be fully clarified and is most likely multifactorial. Although it has been shown that MMC has a toxic effect on the corneal endothelium [17], other trabeculectomy

Table 2 Endothelial cell count before and after trabeculectomy and EX-PRESS

	Trabeculectomy (cells/mm^2)	EX-PRESS (cells/mm^2)
Baseline	2505 ± 280	2377 ± 389
6 months	2398 ± 275	2267 ± 409
P value	< 0.001	0.007
12 months	2349 ± 323	2292 ± 452
P value	< 0.001	0.043
18 months	2293 ± 325	2379 ± 375
P value	< 0.001	0.32
24 months	2277 ± 385	2317 ± 449
P value	0.003	0.27

studies have reported finding a decrease in CECD without the use of MMC [16]. Therefore, this indicates that other factors might be contributing to the observed endothelial damage. Our study also showed that were no changes in the CECD after 18 months or 24 months in the EX-PRESS shunt implantation cases that were administered MMC during surgery. Therefore, our current results indirectly support the possibility that other factors might contribute to the endothelial damage.

This study also showed that there were changes in the CECD after 6 months or 12 months in the EX-PRESS shunt implantation cases. Since there was no effect on the CECD after the EX-PRESS shunt implantation without cataract surgery, this suggests that the cataract surgery may be responsible for these changes. Casini et al. also found that there were no changes in the CECD at 1 or 3 months after the EX-PRESS shunt implantation surgery [12]. In contrast, Ishida et al. showed that there was a significant decreased in the CECD at 24 months after the EX-PRESS shunt implantation [14]. The authors speculated that the reason for the differences seen in these studies is that the decreases in the CECD are only observed after a specific length of time. In the current study, however, during the initial 24 months after the EX-PRESS

shunt implantation, we did not observe any decreases of CECD, with these changes occurring at 24 months after the implantation.

Although there were no changes in the CECD at 18 months or 24 months after the EX-PRESS shunt implantation, we did observe significant decreases at 6 or 12 months after the implantation. This suggests that the observed recovery of the CECD might be the result of cellular migration from the peripheral cornea.

Suturing of the scleral flap was performed using 6 to 7 10–0 nylon sutures in the trabeculectomy group and 2 to 4 10–0 nylon sutures in the EX-PRESS group. The physical properties of the apertures that connect the anterior chamber to the sub-scleral space are not same in the two procedures. Since the aqueous flow through EX-PRESS is probably different from the flow through sclerectomy of the trabeculectomy, the numbers of sutures were difference between the two techniques.

There were several limitations for our current study. First, it is possible that the area of the cornea examined might not have been the same at each of the visits. Second, the number of patients included in this study was quite small. Third, there was only a short follow-up period, which might not have been long enough to observe the changes. Furthermore, the EX-PRESS shunt consists of a stainless steel tube, and after insertion under a partial-thickness scleral flap, it provides a connection to the anterior chamber. Therefore, long-term follow-ups of patients will need to be performed in order to verify the effect of the EX-PRESS implantation on CECD. In addition, it should also be noted that we have combined data from several types of glaucoma, which could be an issue, as the pathogenesis could vary in each of the different types. There was a bias in the selection of patients. Patients who had a history of vitreous surgery or severe vision loss of their fellow eye underwent the EX-PRESS glaucoma filtration device procedure. As a result, the above limitations could potentially limit the general applicability of the current results. Additional studies that perform evaluations of the long-term

Table 3 Endothelial cell count before and afyer trabeculectomy and EX-PRESS with or without cataract surgery

	Trabeculectomy (cells/mm^2)		EX-PRESS (cells/mm^2)	
	Combined cataract surgery	Trabeculectomy alone	Combined cataract surgery	EX-PRESS alone
Baseline	2539 ± 264 (n = 29)	2462 ± 281 (n = 35)	2512 ± 329 (n = 22)	2279 ± 415 (n = 28)
6 months	2429 ± 286 (n = 29)	2387 ± 253 (n = 35)	2309 ± 410 (n = 21)	2236 ± 413 (n = 27)
P value	< 0.001	0.018	0.034	0.11
12 months	2373 ± 344 (n = 29)	2338 ± 288 (n = 35)	2399 ± 333 (n = 19)	2216 ± 512 (n = 27)
P value	< 0.001	0.014	0.10	0.25
18 months	2344 ± 256 (n = 26)	2225 ± 393 (n = 27)	2429 ± 319 (n = 15)	2339 ± 419 (n = 19)
P value	< 0.001	0.008	0.29	0.81
24 months	2218 ± 393 (n = 10)	2272 ± 398 (n = 15)	2379 ± 416 (n = 8)	2284 ± 477 (n = 15)
P value	0.016	0.071	0.20	0.92

effect of glaucoma surgery on CECD will need to be undertaken in the future.

Conclusions

In conclusion, our comparison of the EX-PRESS shunt implantation and trabeculectomy procedures showed there were no effects on the corneal endothelial cells until at least 24 months after the initial surgery. These findings suggest the benefit of using this procedure in patients who have a lower CECD prior to the surgery.

Abbreviations
CECD: Corneal endothelial cell density; IOP: Intraocular pressure; MMC: Mitomycin C

Acknowledgements
The authors thank FORTE for the professional service that edited our manuscript.

Funding
This work was supported by a Grant-in-Aid for Scientific Research from the Ministry of Education, Culture, Sports, Science, and Technology of Japan (26462689).

Authors' contributions
KH suggested concept of study. SO, KH, KU and EN performed to conduct study. SO.
measured and collected data in this study. The measurements were confirmed by KH. Analysis data and interpretation of data were performed by KH. KH wrote the manuscript. All authors provided a critical review of the manuscript. All authors approved the manuscript for submission.

Competing interests
The authors declare that they have no competing interests.

References
1. Mariotti C, Dahan E, Nicolai M, Levitz L, Bouee S. Long-term outcomes and risk factors for failure with the EX-press glaucoma drainage device. Eye. 2014;28:1–8.
2. Laule A, Cable MK, Hoffman CE, Hanna C. Endothelial cell population changes of human cornea during life. Arch Ophthalmol. 1978;96:2031–5.
3. Friberg TR, Doran DL, Lazenby FL. The effect of vitreous and retinal surgery on corneal endothelial cell density. Ophthalmology. 1984;91:1166–9.
4. Bourne RR, Minassian DC, Dart JK, Rosen P, Kaushal S, Wingate N. Effect of cataract surgery on the corneal endothelium: modern phacoemulsification compared with extracapsular cataract surgery. Ophthalmology. 2004;111:679–85.
5. Pollack IP. Current concepts in laser iridotomy. Int Ophthalmol Clin. 1984;24: 153–80.
6. Schwartz AL, Martin NF, Weber PA. Corneal decompensation after argon laser iridectomy. Arch Ophthalmol. 1988;106:1572–4.
7. Hong C, Kitazawa Y, Tanishima T. Influence of argon laser treatment of glaucoma on corneal endothelium. Jpn J Ophthalmol. 1983;27:567–74.
8. Wilhelmus KR. Corneal edema following argon laser iridotomy. Ophthalmic Surg. 1992;23:533–7.
9. Gagnon MM, Boisjoly HM, Brunette I, Charest M, Amyot M. Corneal endothelial cell density in glaucoma. Cornea. 1997;16:314–8.
10. Storr-Paulsen T, Norregaard JC, Ahmed A, Storr-Paulsen A. Corneal endothelial cell loss after mitomycin C-augmented trabeculectomy. J Glaucoma. 2008;17:654–7.
11. Pastor SA, Williams R, Hetherington J, Hoskins HD, Goodman D. Corneal endothelial cell loss following trabeculectomy with mitomycin C. J Glaucoma. 1993;2:112–3.
12. Casini G, Loiudice P, Pellegrini M, Sframeli AT, Martinelli P, Passani A, Nardi M. Trabeculectomy versus EX-PRESS shunt versus Ahmed valve implant: short-term effects of corneal endothelial cells. Am J Ophthalmol. 2015;160: 1185–90.
13. Kim MS, Kim KN, Kim C. Changes in corneal endothelial cells after Ahmed glaucoma valve implantation and trabeculectomy: 1-year follow-up. Korean J Ophthalmol. 2016;30:416–25.
14. Ishida K, Moroto N, Murata K, Yamamoto T. Effect of glaucoma implant surgery on intraocular pressure reduction, flare count, anterior chamber depth, and corneal endothelium in primary open-angle glaucoma. Jpn J Ophthalmol. 2017;61:334–46.
15. Mishima S. Clinical investigations on the corneal endothelium. Ophthalmology. 1982;89:525–30.
16. Arnavielle S, Lafontaine PO, Bidot S, Creuzot-Garcher C, D'Athis P, Bron AM. Corneal endothelial cell changes after trabeculectomy and deep sclerectomy. J Glaucoma. 2007;16:324–8.
17. Dreyer EB, Chaturvedi N, Zurakowski D. Effect of mitomycin C and fluorouracil-supplemented trabeculectomis on the anterior segment. Arch Ophthalmol. 1995;113:578–80.

32

Corneal densitometry in high myopia

Jing Dong[1†], Yaqin Zhang[2†], Haining Zhang[2], Zhijie Jia[2], Suhua Zhang[2], Bin Sun[2], Yongqing Han[3] and Xiaogang Wang[2*]

Abstract

Background: To investigate corneal densitometry values obtained using Scheimpflug tomography in normal and highly myopic (HM) eyes and to assess the differences in densitometry values between them.

Methods: Highly myopic and normal corneas were examined using the Pentacam Scheimpflug imaging system. Corneal densitometry was automatically performed over a 12-mm diameter area, which was divided on the basis of annular concentric zones (0–2 mm, 2–6 mm, 6–10 mm, 10–12 mm, total diameter) and depth (anterior layer: inner 120 μm; center layer: from 120 μm to the last 60 μm; posterior layer: last 60 μm; total corneal thickness).

Results: A total of 100 normal and 100 HM eyes were enrolled in this study. Upon total corneal thickness densitometry, the HM group was found to have significantly lower values compared with the normal group in 4 annuli, including the 2 mm central zone, 2-6 mm zone, 6–10 mm zone, and 0–12 mm total diameter. Upon anterior layer densitometry, the HM group demonstrated statistically lower values in the 2-6 mm and 6–10 mm zones. Upon densitometry of the central and posterior layers, the HM group was found to have lower values in all annuli.

Conclusions: The densitometry map reveals that light backscatter was lower in most portions of the HM cornea than in the normal cornea.

Keywords: Corneal densitometry, High myopia, Scheimpflug, Normal

Background

High myopia (HM) is characterized by a refractive error greater than – 6.0 diopters. The prevalence of HM is approximately 2.7% worldwide, whereas the prevalence in young Chinese individuals is about 20% [1, 2]. With HM being the fourth leading cause of blindness, 70% of HM eyes have the chance to progress to sight-threatening pathologic retinal impairments, including retinal detachment, retinal degeneration, choroidal neovascularization, and choroidal degeneration [3]. Changes in corneal-related parameters in HM eyes, such as corneal curvature, corneal thickness, and endothelial density, are still under debate [4–7].Previous study of biomechanical properties of cornea demonstrated that corneal hysteresis was significantly lower in HM, which may indicate that some aspects of corneal biomechanical properties such as elasticity, viscosity, hydration, stiffness may be compromised in HM eyes [8].

As a relatively new imaging method, Scheimpflug photography can provide a quantification assessment of light scattering and help assess corneal infiltrates [9]. PentacamHR, a noninvasive, rapid, and reproducible optical system (Oculus GMbH, Wetzlar, Germany), can be used to assess the ocular anterior segment from the anterior corneal surface to the posterior lens surface for corneal topography, corneal pachymetry, anterior chamber depth analysis, and lens clarity analysis [10]. The ability of Pentacam to measure corneal transparency changes objectively and noninvasively may help monitor corneal disease progression and even improve corresponding management.

Corneal densitometry, as an indicator for corneal health, has many applications in corneal diagnosis, such as the diagnosis of bacterial keratitis, keratoconus, pseudoexfoliation syndrome, Fuchs endothelial dystrophy, and rheumatoid arthritis, etc. [11–15] The use of this technique to assess corneal transparency in HM patients has not been reported before, and this technique may provide some useful information when assessing the corneal clarity of HM eyes. The aim of this study was to

* Correspondence: movie6521@163.com
†Jing Dong and Yaqin Zhang contributed equally to this work.
2Department of Ophthalmology, Shanxi Eye Hospital, No. 100 Fudong Street, Taiyuan 030002, Shanxi, People's Republic of China
Full list of author information is available at the end of the article

perform corneal densitometry of normal and HM corneas, to investigate the imaging capabilities of Pentacam in patients with HM and the potential differences in corneal densitometry values between normal and HM eyes.

Methods

This study was performed at the Shanxi Eye Hospital (Taiyuan, Shanxi, China). The research protocols were approved by the institutional review boards of Shanxi Eye Hospital and were carried out in accordance with the tenets of the Declaration of Helsinki. Written informed consent was obtained from each patient.

Subjects

We chose Han Chinese subjects to eliminate the possible influences of differences in ethnic groups. The participants with normal and HM eyes were chosen from the Ophthalmic Clinic Center at the Shanxi Eye Hospital. The inclusion criteria for the normal participants were as follows: best-corrected visual acuity (BCVA) of ≥16/20, a refractive error < 5 diopter (D) spheres and IOLMaster axial length (AL) less than 25 mm, normal slit-lamp and fundoscopy results, intraocular pressure (IOP) < 21 mmHg, and no history of ocular or systemic corticosteroid use. The inclusion criteria for the participants with HM were as follows: BCVA ≥20/40, spherical refractive error more negative than − 6 diopters, IOLMaster axial length longer than 25 mm, and central fixation sufficiently stable for image capture. Participants with keratoconus; previous corneal lesions; prior surgery of the cornea; severe cataracts; glaucoma; posterior abnormalities, such as choroidal neovascularization, retinoschisis, retinal detachment, or macular holes; and missing data were excluded.

Data acquisition

Corneal densitometry was performed using the rotating Scheimpflug anterior segment analyzer (Pentacam HR, Oculus GMbH, Wetzlar, Germany). The participant was asked to place his/her chin on the chin rest and press his/her forehead against the forehead strap. The participant's eye was aligned to the visual axis with a central fixation target. After proper alignment and blinking a few times, the automatic release mode, with 25 single Scheimpflug images, was started for each eye. Only cases with acceptable image quality were included in the final analysis. A single trained operator performed all examinations. All parameters were automatically calculated by the Pentacam software (Version 1.20r36).

An internal standard corneal densitometry analysis software measures the backscattered light over a 12-mm diameter corneal area (Fig. 1). Zonal corneal densitometry values were automatically measured in 4 concentric annular zones centered at the apex of the cornea (0–2 mm, 2–6 mm, 6–10 mm, 10–12 mm, total diameter) and by depth (anterior layer: inner 120 μm; center layer: from 120 μm to the last 60 μm; posterior layer: last 60 μm; total corneal thickness; Fig. 2).

Statistical analysis

Statistical analysis was performed using SPSS ver. 13.0. The statistical significance of the intergroup differences in age and axial length was evaluated using the independent sample t-test. The Mann-Whitney U test was used to assess the differences in corneal densitometry values between the two groups. Corneal densitometry values and age were correlated using Pearson's bivariate regression. The significance level for all of the tests was set at 5%.

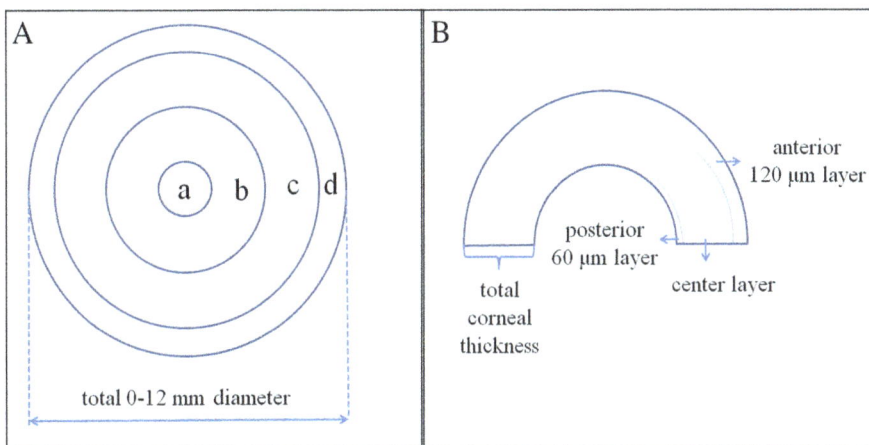

Fig. 1 Schematic diagram of standard corneal densitometry analysis using Pentacam. Panel A: densitometry analysis of concentric annular zones centered at the corneal apex (a: 0–2 mm, b: 2–6 mm, c: 6–10 mm, d: 10–12 mm); Panel B corneal densitometry analysis based on different depths (anterior layer: inner 120 μm; center layer: from 120 μm to the last 60 μm; posterior layer: last 60 μm; total corneal thickness)

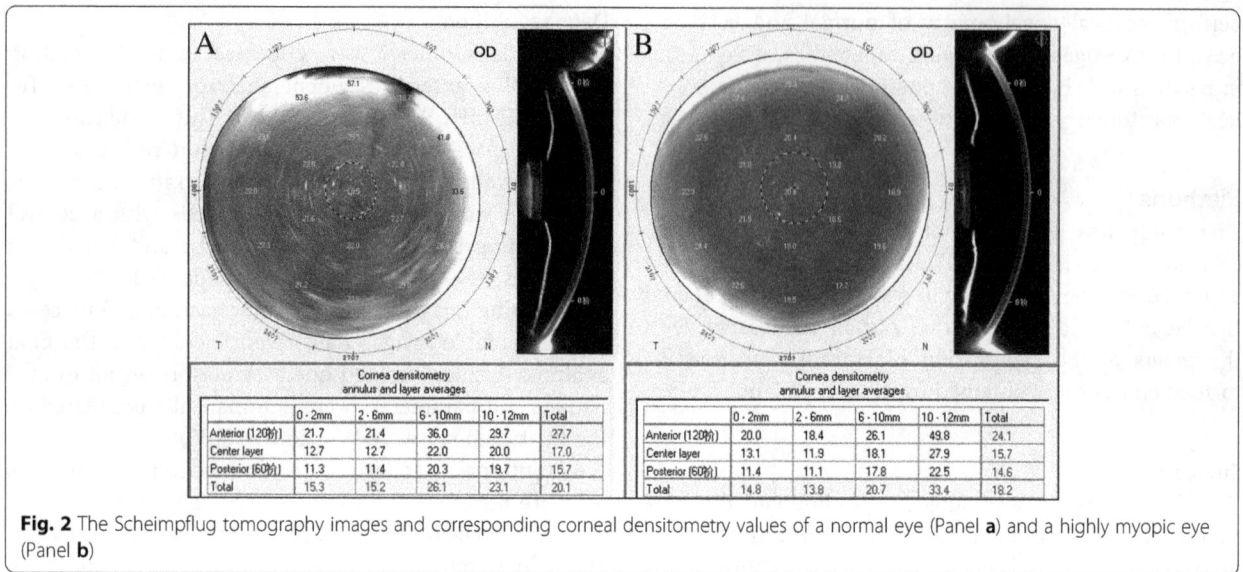

Fig. 2 The Scheimpflug tomography images and corresponding corneal densitometry values of a normal eye (Panel **a**) and a highly myopic eye (Panel **b**)

Results

A total of 200 participants were included in the study: 100 participants with normal corneas and 100 participants with HM corneas. There were 44 female and 56 male participants in the normal group and 42 female and 58 male participants in the HM group. No significant sex differences were found between the two groups ($P = 0.435$). The mean age in the normal group was 65 ± 10 years (range, 20–87 years), which was not significantly higher than that in the HM group 62 ± 13 years (range, 18–92 years; $P = 0.086$). The AL in the normal group was 23.08 ± 0.79 mm (range, 21.76–24.83 mm), which was statistically shorter than that in the HM group, that is, 28.79 ± 2.52 mm (range, 25.03–35.12 mm; $P < 0.001$).

Total corneal light backscatter was significantly lower in the HM group (HM = 18.9 ± 4.4, normal = 20.3 ± 4.3, $P = 0.008$) than in the normal group. Considering the densitometry values for the total corneal thickness, which was separated by concentric annular zones around the apex, the corneal light backscatter in the first 3 annuli (center to 2 mm, 2–6 mm diameter, and 6–10 mm diameter) was statistically lower in the HM group than in the normal group (HM = 14.7 ± 1.5, normal = 15.2 ± 1.6, $P = 0.028$; HM = 14.1 ± 2.1, normal = 15.4 ± 3.9, $P = 0.001$; HM = 22.1 ± 8.8, normal = 25.2 ± 8.0, $P = 0.002$, respectively). However, no significant difference was found in the 10–12 mm diameter annular zone between the two groups ($P = 0.203$).

When the cornea was divided into 3 layers, densitometry of the anterior layer of the concentric annular zones in the first 3 annuli and the total 0–12 mm diameter revealed the same tendency of a lower backscatter in the central cornea in the HM group. However, the anterior layer densitometry values of the 10–12 mm annular zone were higher in the HM group than in the normal group (HM = 46.4 ± 14.2, normal = 41.1 ± 13.5, $P = 0.004$). Upon densitometry of the central and posterior layers, all concentric annular zones were found to have a lower light backscatter in the HM group than in the normal group. These results are summarized in Fig. 3 and Table 1.

The densitometry values of the total corneal thickness were significantly correlated with age in both the normal and HM group ($r = 0.540$, $P < 0.001$; $r = 0.711$, $P < 0.001$). Moreover, the densitometry values of the anterior layer, center layer, and posterior layer were all correlated well with age in both groups (normal: $r = 0.504$, $r = 0.520$, $r = 0.570$; HM: $r = 0.678$, $r = 0.721$, $r = 0.747$; all $P < 0.001$). Central corneal thickness was positively correlated with total corneal densitometry values in HM group ($r = 0.198, P = 0.048$) but not in the normal group ($r = 0.135$, $P = 0.181$). No significant correlation was found between AL, mean keratometry and total corneal densitometry values in both groups (all $P > 0.05$).

Discussion

In previous studies, HM eyes were reported to have different cornea-related parameters, such as corneal curvature, corneal thickness, corneal endothelial density, corneal hysteresis, and corneal resistance factor, compared with normal eyes [4, 5, 8, 16–19]. Clinical analysis of corneal light backscatter played an important role in the evaluation of the corneal status and in monitoring the progression of some corneal diseases [11–15]. In our study, we found a decrease in light backscatter in the central cornea (10 mm in diameter) and total diameter in the HM group. A lower densitometry in the central cornea was also seen in the anterior, center, and posterior layers.

As demonstrated in a previous study, corneal densitometry provides useful information about corneal

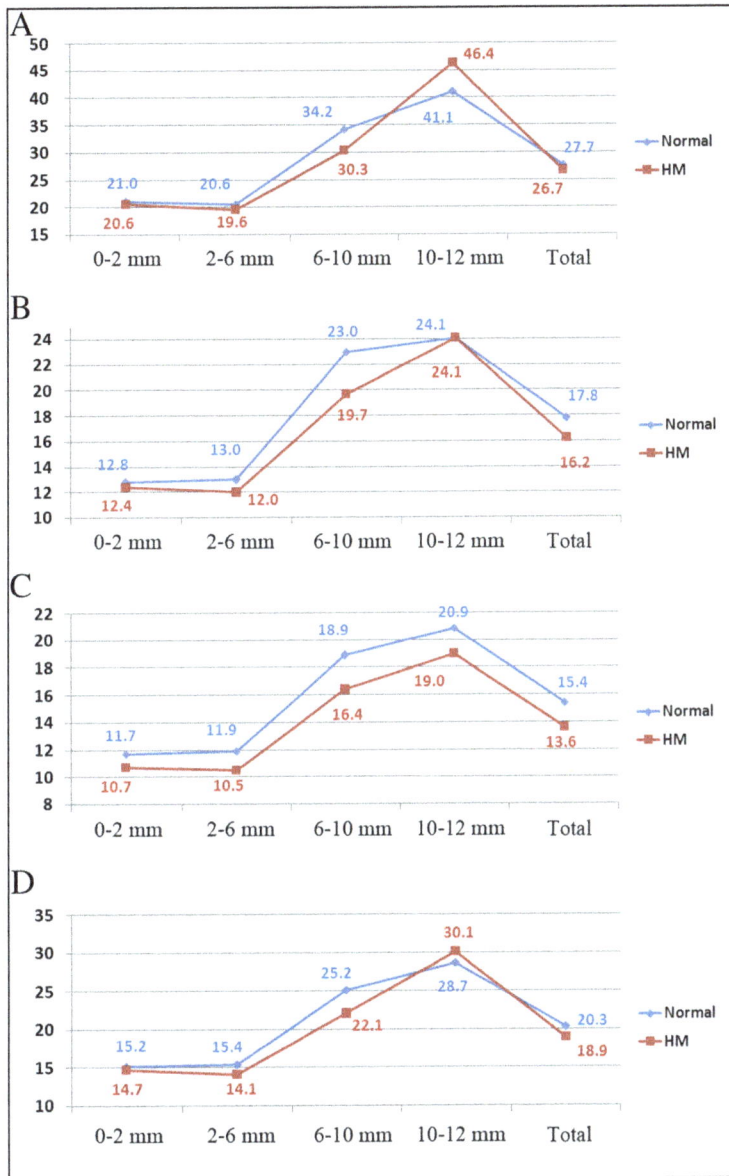

Fig. 3 Mean densitometry values of the anterior layer (panel **a**), center layer (panel **b**), posterior layer (panel **c**), and total corneal thickness (panel **d**) in the normal and HM groups. HM = high myopia; Total = total 0–12 mm diameter

clarity [14]. In a normal cornea, the anterior superficial epithelium, stromal, and the posterior corneal endothelium contribute to the total corneal densitometry value. In the HM group, decreased corneal densitometry values were found for both the total corneal thickness and the 3 seperated layers. This changing tendency may be attributed to several factors: 1) Corneal biomechanical property changes in HM. The study by Shen et al. showed that corneal hysteresis (CH) was significantly lower in HM corneas [8]. CH is a parameter related to momentary deformation of the cornea. In the current study, participants with HM corneas had lower corneal densitometry values. However, corneal damage could

not be proven. We hypothesize that lower densitometry values, as well as lower CH, indicate that some biomechanical properties of the cornea have been altered. 2) Corneal endothelial cell density changes in low and moderate myopic eyes. Delshad et al. demonstrated that the more myopic eyes tend to have a lower endothelial cell density and cell hexagonality [16]. As endothelial cells are a part of the light scattering corneal tissue, the lower endothelial cell density may result in lower corneal densitometry values. Our present study showed significantly lower corneal densitometry values for the posterior layer in HM eyes, which confirms the corneal endothelial cell density changes. 3) Potential changes in

Table 1 Corneal densitometry values of the normal and highly myopic groups

	Normal Group (n = 100)	HM Group (n = 100)	Difference	P*
Anterior 120 μm				
0–2 mm	21.0 ± 2.7	20.6 ± 2.2	0.4 ± 0.3	0.474
2–6 mm	20.6 ± 3.3	19.6 ± 2.9	1.1 ± 0.4	**0.017**
6–10 mm	34.2 ± 11.6	30.3 ± 13.4	3.9 ± 1.8	**0.004**
10–12 mm	41.1 ± 13.5	46.4 ± 14.2	− 5.3 ± 2.0	**0.004**
Total 0–12 mm	27.7 ± 6.1	26.7 ± 6.3	1.0 ± 0.9	0.143
Center layer				
0–2 mm	12.8 ± 1.2	12.4 ± 0.9	0.4 ± 0.1	**0.030**
2–6 mm	13.0 ± 2.2	12.0 ± 1.7	1.0 ± 0.3	**< 0.001**
6–10 mm	23.0 ± 8.0	19.7 ± 8.3	3.3 ± 1.2	**0.001**
10–12 mm	24.1 ± 7.1	24.1 ± 6.6	0 ± 1.0	0.823
Total 0–12 mm	17.8 ± 4.2	16.2 ± 3.9	1.6 ± 0.6	**0.002**
Posterior 60 μm				
0–2 mm	11.7 ± 1.9	10.7 ± 1.4	1.1 ± 0.2	**< 0.001**
2–6 mm	11.9 ± 2.3	10.5 ± 1.5	1.4 ± 0.3	**< 0.001**
6–10 mm	18.9 ± 4.9	16.4 ± 5.3	2.5 ± 0.7	**< 0.001**
10–12 mm	20.9 ± 5.5	19.0 ± 5.2	1.9 ± 0.8	**0.009**
Total 0–12 mm	15.4 ± 3.0	13.6 ± 2.8	1.7 ± 0.4	**< 0.001**
Total corneal thickness				
0–2 mm	15.2 ± 1.6	14.7 ± 1.5	0.5 ± 0.2	**0.028**
2–6 mm	15.4 ± 3.9	14.1 ± 2.1	1.3 ± 0.4	**0.001**
6–10 mm	25.2 ± 8.0	22.1 ± 8.8	3.1 ± 1.2	**0.002**
10–12 mm	28.7 ± 7.9	30.1 ± 8.0	−1.4 ± 1.1	0.203
Total 0–12 mm	20.3 ± 4.3	18.9 ± 4.4	1.4 ± 0.6	**0.008**

HM high myopia; * Mann-Whitney u test for statistical analysis; numbers in bold are statistically significant results

the structures inside the cornea, such as nerves, cell nuclei, the spacing of the corneal fibrils, size of the collagen fibrils, the extracellular matrix surrounding the collagen fibrils, and corneal hydration. Previous research has demonstrated that changes in the above-mentioned corneal structures play an important role in corneal transparency [20–22]. Therefore, our findings on the lower corneal densitometry values in HM eyes may be correlated with these structural changes. However, more cellular and histological studies are needed to prove these potential changes in HM corneas.

In the periphery (10–12 mm diameter), either no significant difference was found between the two groups or higher corneal densitometry values were found in the HM group than in the control group. Because of the low repeatability and reproducibility of peripheral densitometry measurements reported a previous normative study, this result has to be interpreted with caution in clinical practice [23]. Moreover, the white-to-white distance variation, which may lead to the inclusion of some proportion of the limbus and sclera in automatic corneal densitometry analysis, could mistakenly cause higher

corneal densitometry values [13]. A recent study demonstrated that corneal densitometry values increased with age in Spanish patients [24]. Our study confirmed this correlation.

Similar to a previous study, neither mean keratometry readings nor central corneal thickness was correlated with total corneal densitometry values in the normal group in this study [24]. However, the positive correlation between central corneal thickness and total corneal densitometry values was found in the HM group. This may be attributed to the relatively less endothelial cell density with myopic increasing, which has been demonstrated in a previous study [16].

A previous study has shown that participants of different races, even different subpopulations in the same race, may have different cornea-related parameters [25]. The current study involved a limited number of eyes and only included Chinese participants; therefore the results cannot be directly generalized to different ethnic backgrounds. Despite the above-mentioned limitation, this prospective study to investigate the corneal densitometry values in HM eyes provides useful information for clinical practice.

Conclusions

In conclusion, the Scheimpflug densitometry map revealed that light backscatter was lower in most portions of a HM cornea than in the normal cornea. Moreover, age was positively correlated with the total corneal densitometry values in both groups. Therefore, corneal densitometry may play a valuable role in characterizing HM corneas.

Abbreviations
AL: Axial length; BCVA: Best-corrected visual acuity; CH: Corneal hysteresis; D: Diopter; HM: High myopia; IOP: Intraocular pressure

Funding
This work was supported by the National Natural Science Foundation of China under Grant No. 81501544.

Authors' contributions
XGW: conception, design, data acquisition, analysis, drafting, critical revision. JD: conception design, data acquisition, drafting, critical revision. BS, SHZ, HNZ, YQZ ZJJ, YQH: conception, analysis, critical revision. All authors: final approval of the manuscript.

Competing interests
The authors declare that they have no competing interest.

Author details
[1]Department of Ophthalmology, The First Hospital of Shanxi Medical University, Taiyuan 030001, Shanxi, People's Republic of China. [2]Department of Ophthalmology, Shanxi Eye Hospital, No. 100 Fudong Street, Taiyuan 030002, Shanxi, People's Republic of China. [3]Department of Ophthalmology, Affiliated Hospital of Inner Mongolia University for the Nationalities, Tongliao 028007, Inner Mongolia, People's Republic of China.

References
1. Holden BA, Fricke TR, Wilson DA, et al. Global prevalence of myopia and high myopia and temporal trends from 2000 through 2050. Ophthalmology. 2016;123(5):1036–42.
2. Lin LL, Shih YF, Hsiao CK, et al. Epidemiologic study of the prevalence and severity of myopia among schoolchildren in Taiwan in 2000. J Formos Med Assoc. 2001;100(10):684–91.
3. Grossniklaus HE, Green WR. Pathologic findings in pathologic myopia. Retina. 1992;12(2):127–33.
4. Chang SW, Tsai IL, Hu FR, et al. The cornea in young myopic adults. Br J Ophthalmol. 2001;85(8):916–20.
5. Wang X, Dong J, Wu Q. Corneal thickness, epithelial thickness and axial length differences in normal and high myopia. BMC Ophthalmol. 2015;15:49.
6. Fam HB, How AC, Baskaran M, et al. Central corneal thickness and its relationship to myopia in Chinese adults. Br J Ophthalmol. 2006;90(12):1451–3.
7. Cho P, Lam C. Factors affecting the central corneal thickness of Hong Kong-Chinese. Curr Eye Res. 1999;18(5):368–74.
8. Shen M, Fan F, Xue A, et al. Biomechanical properties of the cornea in high myopia. Vis Res. 2008;48(21):2167–71.
9. Wegener A, Laser-Junga H. Photography of the anterior eye segment according to Scheimpflug's principle: options and limitations - a review. Clin Exp Ophthalmol. 2009;37(1):144–54.
10. Cho YK, Chang HS, La TY, et al. Anterior segment parameters using Pentacam and prediction of corneal endothelial cell loss after cataract surgery. Korean J Ophthalmol. 2010;24(5):284–90.
11. Anayol MA, Bostanci B, Sekeroglu MA, et al. Assessment of corneal densitometry in rheumatoid arthritis patients. Turk J Ophthalmol. 2017;47(3):125–9.
12. Chu HY, Hsiao CH, Chen PY, et al. Corneal backscatters as an objective index for assessing Fuchs' endothelial corneal dystrophy: a pilot study. J Ophthalmol. 2017;2017:8747013.
13. Lopes B, Ramos I, Ambrosio R Jr. Corneal densitometry in keratoconus. Cornea. 2014;33(12):1282–6.
14. Otri AM, Fares U, Al-Aqaba MA, Dua HS. Corneal densitometry as an indicator of corneal health. Ophthalmology. 2012;119(3):501–8.
15. Sekeroglu MA, Anayol MA, Gulec M, et al. Corneal densitometry: a new technique for objective assessment of corneal clarity in Pseudoexfoliation syndrome. J Glaucoma. 2016;25(9):775–9.
16. Delshad S, Chun JM. Corneal endothelial cell density and morphology in low and moderate myopic Chinese eyes. Int J Ophthalmol. 2013;6(4):467–70.
17. Scheiman M, Gwiazda J, Zhang Q, et al. Longitudinal changes in corneal curvature and its relationship to axial length in the correction of myopia evaluation trial (COMET) cohort. J Optom. 2016;9(1):13–21.
18. Tong L, Saw SM, Siak JK, et al. Corneal thickness determination and correlates in Singaporean schoolchildren. Invest Ophthalmol Vis Sci. 2004;45(11):4004–9.
19. Pedersen L, Hjortdal J, Ehlers N. Central corneal thickness in high myopia. Acta Ophthalmol Scand. 2005;83(5):539–42.
20. O'Donnell C, Wolffsohn JS. Grading of corneal transparency. Cont Lens Anterior Eye. 2004;27(4):161–70.
21. Daxer A, Misof K, Grabner B, et al. Collagen fibrils in the human corneal stroma: structure and aging. Invest Ophthalmol Vis Sci. 1998;39(3):644–8.
22. Maurice DM. The structure and transparency of the cornea. J Physiol. 1957;136(2):263–86.
23. Ni Dhubhghaill S, Rozema JJ, Jongenelen S, et al. Normative values for corneal densitometry analysis by Scheimpflug optical assessment. Invest Ophthalmol Vis Sci. 2014;55(1):162–8.
24. Garzon N, Poyales F, Illarramendi I, et al. Corneal densitometry and its correlation with age, pachymetry, corneal curvature, and refraction. Int Ophthalmol. 2017;37(6):1263–8.
25. Aghaian E, Choe JE, Lin S, Stamper RL. Central corneal thickness of Caucasians, Chinese, Hispanics, Filipinos, African Americans, and Japanese in a glaucoma clinic. Ophthalmology. 2004;111(12):2211–9.

33

Central corneal thickness in a Jordanian population and its association with different types of Glaucoma: cross-sectional study

Sana' Muhsen[1], Feras Alkhalaileh[2], Mohammad Hamdan[2] and Saif Aldeen AlRyalat[3*] (iD)

Abstract

Background: Central corneal thickness (CCT) has long been implicated to affect glaucoma predisposition. Several reports have identified that thinner CCT is a risk factor for open-angle glaucoma, and that CCT can be very variable between different ethnic groups. In this study, we aim to identify the relation between CCT and different glaucoma parameters in different types of glaucoma in an Arabian ethnicity.

Methods: We classified our participants into four main groups: primary open-angle glaucoma (POAG), primary angle-closure glaucoma (PACG), pseudoexfoliative glaucoma (PXFG), and a control group. We obtained demographics, intraocular pressure (IOP), cup to disc ratio (CDR), visual field mean deviation (MD) and pattern standard deviation (PSD), CCT, and retinal nerve fiber layer (RNFL) thickness for each participant.

Results: We included A total of 119 eyes with glaucoma, including POAG (54 eyes), PXFG (31 eyes) and PACG (34 eyes), we also included 57 control eyes. We found that PACG eyes have the thinnest CCT. Mean measurements of CCT for our groups were: 538.31 μm (SD = 36.30) in eyes with POAG, 544.45 μm (SD = 28.57) in eyes with PXFG, 506.91 μm (SD = 34.55) in eyes with PACG and 549.63 μm (SD = 42.9) in the control group. We found that CCT is significantly correlated with CDR ($p = 0.012$, $r = -0.231$), MD ($p < 0.001$, $r = 0.327$), and RNFL thickness ($p = .007$, $r = .283$).

Conclusion: In Arabian ethnicity, PACG patients have the thinnest CCT compared to other types of glaucoma, namely POAG and PXFG. We demonstrated that glaucomatous eyes with thinner corneas will probably have more advanced glaucomatous optic neuropathy. Our results emphasize the importance of taking ethnicity into account upon glaucoma management.

Keywords: Glaucoma, Central corneal thickness, Ethnicity

Background

Glaucoma is the second leading cause of blindness in the world, after cataracts, and is the leading cause of blindness among African-Americans [1]. It is generally classified into open-angle and closed-angle glaucoma, and both can be either primary or secondary. It is estimated that the number of people with primary open-angle glaucoma (POAG) worldwide will reach 58.6 million by 2020, while 21 million will be affected by primary angle-closure glaucoma (PACG)

* Correspondence: saifryalat@yahoo.com
[3]Department of Ophthalmology, University of Jordan Hospital, The University of Jordan, Amman 11942, Jordan
Full list of author information is available at the end of the article

[1]. Of those, 5.9 and 5.3 million will be blind from irreversible optic nerve damage associated with POAG and PACG, respectively [1]. This means that early detection and identification of risk factors are key elements in controlling the disease and preventing its progression. Secondary open-angle glaucoma is another entity with diverse types, but Pseudoexfoliation glaucoma (PXFG) is currently the leading cause of secondary open-angle glaucoma with a prevalence reaching 40% in patients over the age of 80 [2], and is highly dependent on race and ethnicity [3].

Evidence in the recent literature has shown the importance of central corneal thickness (CCT) in relation to several ocular conditions. Most notably, thinner CCT has been identified as a risk factor for open-angle glaucoma [4]. Goldmann and Schmidt discussed the association between the corneal thickness and the intra-ocular pressure (IOP) in their publication in 1957 [5]. Fourteen years later, Hansen and Ehlers demonstrated the presence of a positive linear correlation between CCT and IOP [6]. More recently, a meta-analysis of worldwide CCT literature proposed a correction factor of 2.5 mmHg for each 50 μm change in CCT [7].

CCT can be very variable between different ethnic groups, as shown in studies comparing mean CCT in both normal and glaucomatous eyes between Caucasian, Hispanic, African American, and Asians, where the thinnest corneas being more prevalent among African American ethnicity [8, 9]. Other studies also showed significant variation in CCT between ethnic sub-groups, as in a study that included different Asian populations; Chinese, Japanese, Korean, Filipino, Pacific Islander, and South Asian, and showed that the thinnest corneas are found in South Asian populations [10]. Moreover, several studies have shown that CCT varies among individuals with different types of glaucoma (POAG, PACG, and PXFG) and normal eyes, as in Bechmann et al. study that showed thinner corneas in patients with PXFG and POAG compared with patients with PACG and normal eyes [11]. In Jordanian population; an Arabian, Middle-eastern ethnicity, previous studies showed that glaucoma is one of the leading causes of blindness [12], and at the same time, the level of knowledge about glaucoma among Jordanians is poor (around 75% have either no or low level of knowledge) compared to other parts of the world [13], leading to delayed diagnosis of this silent disease. Ophthalmologists in Jordan usually depend on studies that were done on other ethnicities upon treating their glaucoma patients, due to lack of studies on the characteristics of glaucoma among Jordanians. Given the importance of early detection of risk factors of glaucoma, and as corneal thickness is one of the main risk factors for glaucoma and is the one associated with ethnicity, we aim to assess the corneal thickness in different types of glaucoma and in normal controls in a Jordanian population. We further aim to explore the relationship between CCT and the severity of glaucomatous optic neuropathy in different types of glaucoma.

Methods

Participants

This is a cross-sectional observational study that was conducted on subjects visiting the glaucoma clinics in 2 centers in Jordan between November 2015 and May 2017. We obtained ethical approval from the Institutional Review Board (IRB) and all patients were consented and approved to participate in this study.

This study was conducted in accordance with the Declaration of Helsinki latest update (2013). We included both patients with glaucoma and age-gender matching controls. Glaucoma patients were classified into three types of glaucoma: POAG, PACG, and PXFG. A diagnosis of POAG or PACG was made based on IOP, gonioscopy and both characteristic visual field (VF) defects (nasal step, arcuate scotoma, and paracentral defect), and optic nerve changes (enlarged cup to disc ratio (CDR), localized notch, and disc hemorrhage) in at least 1 eye as well as Ocular Coherence tomography (OCT) showing thinning of Retinal Nerve Fiber Layer (RNFL). For PXFG, pupils were dilated and exfoliation was checked and recorded as present or absent. PXFG was defined as an open-angle glaucoma with concomitant exfoliation material observed at pupillary border or anterior lens capsule with dilated pupil that is associated with glaucomatous optic neuropathy, as defined earlier.

To be included in this study the patients had to have all of the following inclusion criteria:

– Adult patients (age more than 18 years).
– A diagnosis of POAG, PACG or PXFG in at least 1 eye.
– A reliable VF examination taken within 3 months of the pachymetry. Reading had to be available for both eyes.

If the subject had any of the following exclusion criteria he/she was exempted from the study:

– Glaucoma types other than the aforementioned three types.
– Corneal pathology or surgery that might influence pachymetry.
– Underwent a cataract surgery.
– Patients with systemic diseases that might result in VF changes.
– Keratoconus.
– Contact lens use.
– Corneal dystrophy.

For controls, we included them from general ophthalmology clinics with matching gender and age (±2 years), and with a corneal topography of acceptable quality. We adopted the following exclusion criteria:

– Being a first or a second degree relative of any of our included patients.
– Keratoconus or other corneal disease
– History of Glaucoma or clinical signs of glaucoma
– History of corneal or intraocular surgery or trauma

We ran a power analysis to calculate the minimum sample size required for our study, the sample size was calculated based on the following assumptions: Effect size based on previous studies (see discussion) = 0.59; power = 80%; and two-sided alpha level = 0.05. The required total sample size was 90.

Parameters measured

Diagnosis of glaucoma and classification was confirmed by the attending ophthalmologist based on IOP measurements, gonioscopy, optic nerve changes, visual field defects and OCT RNFL thinning as stated before. We also asked included patients about their demographic data including age, gender, and ethnicity, as well as their previous ocular and medical history.

We measured the IOP using a Goldmann applanation tonometer, where our consultant ophthalmologist performed three measurements for each participant, and the average value was calculated. IOP readings included in the analysis were of patients treated with one or more antiglaucoma eye drops. Gonioscopy was done using a 4-mirror Sussman lens to classify angles into open or closed and to illicit signs of PXFG. A detailed anterior segment examination by slit lamp was performed to rule out corneal pathology that would exclude the patients from the study and also to help detect pseudoexfoliation. Optic nerve assessment including cup-to-disc ratio (CDR) using indirect biomicroscopy and a super field lens were performed by the consultant ophthalmologist.

We measured CCT via Oculus Pentacam HR for both glaucoma patients and controls. The Pentacam HR is a high-resolution rotating Scheimpflug camera system for anterior segment analysis. It provides crisp images of cornea, iris and lens. An ophthalmic technician performed the imaging during daytime (from 9:00 am to 4:00 pm). We then analyzed the Pentacam printouts to rule out any corneal pathologies, such as keratoconus, that would exclude patients from our study and to determine the central corneal thickness at the apex.

Other parameters were assessed for glaucoma patients only. Visual Field assessment was performed using Oculus Centerfield analyzer with a screening 24-2 Threshold strategy. RNFL thickness measurement was performed using Optovue RTVue Optical Coherence Tomography OCT, which generates high-resolution, cross-sectional (3D) images of the retina, optic disc and anterior segment.

Statistical analysis

We used SPSS 21.0 (Chicago, USA) in our statistical analysis. We first described our sample population and eyes included via descriptive statistics including numbers (percentages) and mean (+\- standard deviation SD).

We used logistic regression with generalized estimating equation to analyze effect of gender on type of glaucoma developed and eyes included. We used Independent sample t-test to study differences in general parameters and both the gender and the eye involved. To account for the within-subject effect, we used one-way repeated measure univariate analysis to study the relation between type of glaucoma and general parameters, followed by post-hoc analysis using Tukey analysis. We used Pearson's correlation to study the correlation between age and the other parameters. We also performed Spearman's test, after controlling for gender, to confirm association results. We finally adopted a model building strategy for a regression analysis to find predictors of visual field mean deviation (MD), where we corrected for age and gender. We inspected our data visually using boxplots and histograms, and we used Levene's test to check for homogeneity of variance. We also used Mauchly's test for sphericity to apply univariate analysis. We used a threshold of 0.05 for p value to indicate statistical significance.

Results

We included a total of 68 Jordanian patients in this study, with a mean age of 65.9 years (SD = 8.9). There were 42 (62%) men and 26 (38%) women. From the sample included, 119 eyes met our inclusion criteria and were included in our study, they were 61 (51.3%) right eyes and 58 (48.7%) left eyes (51 bilateral and 17 unilateral eyes). Eyes with glaucoma were categorized according to type of glaucoma into: POAG (54 eyes), PXFG (31 eyes) and PACG (34 eyes), as shown in (Table 1). We also included 29 control participants with a mean age of 55 years. They were 14 men and 15 women and a total of 57 eyes.

Upon analyzing the correlation between gender discrepancy and type of glaucoma developed, we found a significant difference ($p < 0.001$) as men were more likely to develop POAG (55.4%) compared to 28.9% for women. However women were more likely to develop PACG (44.4%) compared to only 18.9% for men. No significant difference was found between gender discrepancy and the development of PXFG. We found no statistically significant difference between both genders regarding other parameters. Mean values of different glaucoma-related parameters for both genders are detailed in (Table 2).

Regarding central corneal thickness (CCT), our results showed the following mean measurements: 538.31 μm (SD = 36.30) in eyes with POAG, 544.45 μm (SD = 28.57) in eyes with PXFG, 506.91 μm (SD = 34.55) in eyes with PACG, and 549.63 μm (SD = 42.9) in the control group. First, we studied the difference between CCT of each glaucoma type and the control group, we found that subjects with PACG had significantly thinner corneas than the control group ($p = 0.021$). No statistically

Table 1 General descriptive for the main three types of glaucoma and control group

	Type of Glaucoma			Control
	Primary Open Angle Glaucoma	Closed Angle Glaucoma	Pseudoexfoliation Glaucoma	
Gender				
Male Frequency (%)	41 (75.9%)	14 (41.2%)	19 (61.3%)	27 (47.4%)
Female Frequency (%)	13 (24.1%)	20 (58.8%)	12 (38.7%)	30 (52.6%)
Age				
Mean (±SD)	64.26 (±9.18)	66.85 (±9.98)	67.8 (±6.93)	54.85 (±10.9)
Eye				
Right Frequency (%)	27 (50%)	18 (52.9%)	16 (51.6%)	28 (49.1%)
Left Frequency (%)	27 (50%)	16 (47.1%)	15 (48.4%)	29 (50.9%)

significant difference was found between CCT of control group and any of POAG or PXFG groups ($p = .702$). Upon comparing mean CCT between glaucoma groups, we found a significant difference between the groups in general ($p < 0.001$), so we performed a post-hoc analysis to find the group differences as shown in (Table 3).

Upon studying the relation between CCT and parameters of optic nerve damage (CDR, MD, and RNFL) in patients with glaucoma, we found that CCT is negatively and significantly correlated with CDR ($p = 0.012$, $r = -0.231$), so that the thinner the cornea, the higher the CDR. We also found a significantly positive correlation between CCT and MD ($p < 0.001$, $r = 0.327$), so that the thinner the cornea the lower the MD (more advanced visual field loss). Finally, we found a positive correlation between CCT and RNFL ($p = .007$, $r = .283$) meaning that the thinner the cornea, the thinner the RNFL. No significant correlation was found between CCT and either IOP or pattern standard deviation (PSD).

We studied factors predicting visual field mean deviation (MD), and found that it is significantly associated with both CDR ($p < 0.001$) and RNFL ($p = 0.003$). Upon analyzing the relation between type of glaucoma and our measured parameters, we found several significant relations; our results are summarized in (Table 2). No statistical significance was found between either the age or laterality of the involved eye (left or right) on one hand and type of glaucoma or other measured parameters on the other hand.

Discussion

This study was done on a Jordanian population, a poorly studied population regarding glaucoma and its risk factors. The mean central corneal thicknesses (CCT) of normal adults and patients with 3 different types of glaucoma was measured by corneal topography. We also established that CCT in patients with PACG is significantly thinner than in other glaucoma types and in the control group. As visual field defect is an important outcome in glaucoma, we found that both cup to disc ratio (CDR) and retinal nerve fiber layer (RNFL) thickness, as measured by Optical Coherence Tomography, are the main factors associated with lower mean deviations on visual field testing. Gender discrepancy in glaucoma type preferences found to be in concordance with some previous reports where men are more likely to develop

Table 2 Gender differences of the mean glaucoma parameters measured in this study among glaucoma patients

	Gender	Mean	Std. Deviation	Std. Error Mean
Intra-ocular Pressure	Male	15.1739	4.49347	0.66253
	Female	15.6724	5.12744	0.95214
Cup to Disc Ratio	Male	0.6234	0.27892	0.03242
	Female	0.5587	0.24368	0.03633
Mean Deviation	Male	−5.5229	5.97786	0.71965
	Female	−6.6430	5.83435	0.88973
Pattern Standard Deviation	Male	3.9250	1.72405	0.21222
	Female	4.2298	1.51917	0.23167
Retinal Nerve Fiber Layer Thickness	Male	77.5424	21.27373	2.47302
	Female	78.3881	19.10243	2.91309
Central Corneal Thickness (CCT)	Male	534.5270	34.14763	3.96958
	Female	525.0444	41.09797	6.12652

Table 3 Relation between type of glaucoma and different parameters

Parameter	Primary Open Angle Glaucoma	Closed Angle Glaucoma	Pseudoexfoliative Glaucoma	Between subject effect p-value	Mean difference (95% CI)	Post-hoc p-value
Intraocular pressure (mmHg)	15.2 (4.3)	13.6 (3.2)*	17.3 (5.8)*	0.049	* 3.7 (0.1–7.2)	*0.04
Cup to disc ratio	0.61 (0.25)	0.72 (0.18)*	0.44 (0.29)*	0.006	* 0.3 (0.8–0.47)	*0.004
Retinal nerve fiber layer thickness (µm)	80.5 (20.8)	70.8 (18.2)	82.2 (20.9)	0.084	–	–
Central corneal thickness (µm)	538.3 (36.3)*	506.9 (34.6)*#	544.5 (28.6)#	< 0.001	* 46.2 (21. 9-70.6) # 36.6 (10. 5-62.7)	* < 0.001 # 0.004
Visual field mean deviation (dB)	–4.9 (5.6)*	–9.0 (6.8)*#	–4.7 (4.4)#	< 0.001	7.3 (3. 5-11.1) #7.5 (3. 5-11.6)	* < 0.001 # < 0.001
Visual field Pattern standard deviation	4.0 (1.7)	4.1 (1.8)	4.1 (1.5)	0.351	–	–

Mean reading for each parameter and its standard deviation are presented. Significant differences between any two readings as analyzed by post-hoc analysis were marked by either (*) or (#)

POAG [14], and women are at higher risk for PACG, likely due to anatomical predisposition [15]. (Fig. 1) shows images for a patient with advanced chronic angle closure glaucoma and with significantly thin central corneal thickness, where the visual field test demonstrating a superior arcuate scotoma splitting fixation and ocular coherence tomography of the retinal nerve fiber layer thickness (OCT RNFL) shows significant thinning.

Previous studies, that were done on western populations, aimed to find the relation between CCT and other parameters, including visual field defects, have mainly included POAG eyes, and they found significantly more advanced visual field defects for lower CCT compared to thicker ones [16, 17]. Here, we studied different types of glaucoma patients and control participants from a Jordanian population, and we found similar correlations where patients with lower CCT had significantly more

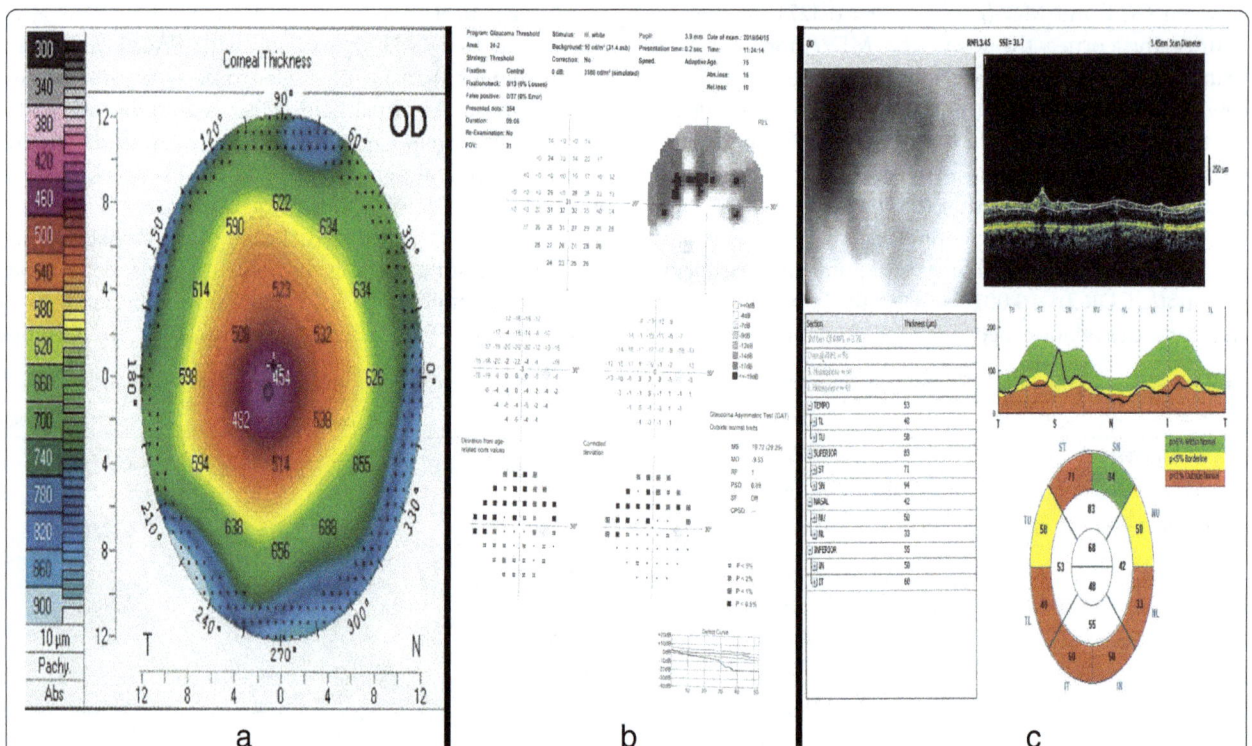

Fig. 1 Imaging in a patient with advanced chronic angle closure glaucoma. **a** Pentacam printout of right eye corneal thickness map showing a central corneal thickness (CCT)of 454 µm, which is significantly thinner than average CCT of 530–550 µm. **b** Threshold 24–2 Visual Field test of the right eye demonstrating a superior arcuate scotoma splitting fixation. **c** Ocular coherence tomography of the retinal nerve fiber layer thickness (OCT RNFL) of the right eye showing significant thinning (Overall RNFL = 58).

advanced visual field defects, and thinner RNFL. We also found that patients with PACG had the lowest CCT compared to POAG, PXFG, and controls. An Iranian study, that included both POAG and PACG patients, found that POAG patients have lower CCT compared to their PACG counterparts [18]. Regarding PXFG, a Caucasian study found a significantly lower CCT in PXFG patients compared to POAG patients [19], this emphasizes the profound difference in CCT in different ethnic groups and the importance of CCT as a risk factor for progression of glaucoma.

The strong relation between CCT and ethnicity is well-studied. A large study that was done on a Chinese population to study the relation between CCT and around 20 variables found that ethnicity is one of the important determinants of CCT [20]. A worldwide meta-analysis found that the average CCT for normal eyes derived from various racial groups, regardless of the device used, was 544 μm [21], a value that is thinner than that for the Jordanian population we studied (550 μm). Comparing CCT values of our Jordanian population with Caucasian ethnicity, the most represented ethnicity in ethnicity-comparing studies [22], Caucasian ethnicity mean CCT was similar to Jordanian's (550 ± 30.5 μm) [23]. On the other hand, African ethnicity has a lower CCT than that for Jordanians (514.77 ± 31.86) [23]. It should be noted that the technique used to measure CCT can affect the results [24], and although the results from commonly used devices mostly correlate, the direct comparison between them might not be accurate [22], so that we will only include studies that used similar techniques for direct value comparison purposes. Regarding CCT difference between different glaucoma types, only PACG eyes have thinner corneas compared to POAG, PXFG, and control eyes, This comes in accordance with what a recent study suggested, where no difference in corneal thickness between POAG, PXFG, and control eyes was found [25].

Other reports generally have results that are comparable to ours, except for a study by Tolesa and Gessesse that was done on Ethiopian patients [26], and found thicker CCT in patients with POAG (520 ± 38.95) compared to PXFG patients (507 ± 35).

Several previous studies have reported the association between larger CDR and glaucomatous progression [27]. Here, we found that patients with larger CDR have worse mean deviation (MD) compared to those with smaller ratios. In Ocular Hypertension Treatment Study [28], they found that cup to disc ratio is also a predictor of the development of POAG in normal subjects. A recent study found that for every 0. 1-unit increase in the CDR, there is an increase in the decay rate of visual field by 23% [29]. We also found that the largest CDR is found in PACG patients, followed by POAG, and finally PXFG.

Similarly, we found that RNFL thickness measured by Optical Coherence Tomography (OCT) is also a good indicator for the severity of visual field loss represented by the mean deviation (MD). In a 12-year study, the risk estimate for moderate and severe visual field defects found to suggest a seven to eight times greater likelihood for future field loss for eyes with initial atrophy [30]. Where previous reports found an association between IOP and MD [30], we think that this effect is indirect through affecting the CDR, as the relation between IOP and MD did not reach significance when we corrected for CDR, probably because these were treated IOP readings.

Several limitations of this study exist. We advice future studies to include only one eye for each included subject (independence of observation) to overcome correlated observation issue as explained in a previous study, although it can be corrected using certain statistical tests [31]. Moreover, a longitudinal approach to follow Middle Eastern patients would provide a better insight on the outcome of different CCT. Although this is a multicenter study, future studies from other Arabian countries should consider including larger sample size to confirm the generalizability of our results.

Conclusion

We found that PACG patients have the thinnest CCT compared to other types of glaucoma, namely POAG and PXFG. We also demonstrated that glaucomatous eyes with thinner corneas will probably have more advanced glaucomatous optic neuropathy. This emphasizes the importance of making CCT measurement a part of standard care in all glaucoma patients since it can predict patients with worse prognosis, and therefore can indicate the need for more aggressive management and earlier diagnosis. Finally, we showed that cup to disc ratio, retinal nerve fiber layer thickness and mean deviation on visual field testing usually are in concordance regarding the severity of glaucoma.

Abbreviations
CCT: Central corneal thickness; CDR: Cup-to-disc ratio; IOP: Intraocular pressure; MD: Visual field mean deviation; OCT: Ocular coherence tomography; PACG: Primary angle closure glaucoma; POAG: Primary open angle glaucoma; PSD: Pattern standard deviation; PXFG: Pseudoexfoliative glaucoma; RNFL: Retinal nerve fiber layer

Acknowledgements
We would like to thank Dr.Doukhi Hunaiti, The University of Jordan for his professional statistical consultation during our statistical analysis review.

Funding
None.

Authors' contributions

Conception and design of the study: SM, SAA. Acquisition of data: FA, MH. Analysis and interpretation of data: SM, SAA. Drafting of the manuscript: SM, SAA. Critical revision of the manuscript: SM, SAA, MH. All authors read and approved the final version to be published.

Competing interests

The authors declare that they have no competing interests

Author details

[1]Ophthalmology, Glaucoma and Anterior Segment Surgeon, University of Jordan Hospital, The University of Jordan, Amman, Jordan. [2]School of Medicine, The University of Jordan, Amman 11942, Jordan. [3]Department of Ophthalmology, University of Jordan Hospital, The University of Jordan, Amman 11942, Jordan.

References

1. Quigley HA, Broman AT. The number of people with glaucoma worldwide in 2010 and 2020. Br J Ophthalmol. 2006;90(3):262–7.
2. Jonasson F, Damji KF, Arnarsson A, Sverrisson T, Wang L, Sasaki H, Sasaki K. Prevalence of open-angle glaucoma in Iceland: Reykjavik eye study. Eye. 2003;17(6):747.
3. Palko JR, Qi O, Sheybani A. Corneal alterations associated with pseudoexfoliation syndrome and glaucoma: a literature review. J Ophthal Vision Res. 2017;12(3):312.
4. Dimasi DP, Burdon KP, Craig JE. The genetics of central corneal thickness. Br J Ophthalmol. 2010;94(8):971–6.
5. Goldmann HA. The glaucoma problem. InTrans. 2nd. Glaucoma Conf; 1957. p. 137–65.
6. Hansen FK, Ehlers N. Elevated tonometer readings caused by a thick cornea. Acta Ophthalmol. 1971;49(5):775–8.
7. Doughty MJ, Laiquzzaman M, Müller A, Oblak E, Button NF. Central corneal thickness in European (white) individuals, especially children and the elderly, and assessment of its possible importance in clinical measures of intra-ocular pressure. Ophthalmic Physiol Opt. 2002;22(6):491–504.
8. La Rosa FA, Gross RL, Orengo-Nania S. Central corneal thickness of Caucasians and African Americans in glaucomatous and nonglaucomatous populations. Arch Ophthalmol. 2001;119(1):23–7.
9. Aghaian E, Choe JE, Lin S, Stamper RL. Central corneal thickness of Caucasians, Chinese, Hispanics, Filipinos, African Americans, and Japanese in a glaucoma clinic. Ophthalmology. 2004;111(12):2211–9.
10. Wang SY, Melles R, Lin SC. The impact of central corneal thickness on the risk for glaucoma in a large multiethnic population. J Glaucoma. 2014;23(9):606.
11. Bechmann M, Thiel MJ, Roesen B, Ullrich S, Ulbig MW, Ludwig K. Central corneal thickness determined with optical coherence tomography in various types of glaucoma. Br J Ophthalmol. 2000;84(11):1233–7.
12. Baarah BT, Shatnawi RA, Khatatbeh AE. Causes of permanent severe visual impairment and blindness among Jordanian population. Middle East Afr J Ophthal. 2018;25(1):25.
13. Al-Zubi K, Sarayrah F, Al-Awaishah M. Glaucoma awareness and knowledge among Jordanian people. Global J Health Sci. 2017;9(8):40.
14. Rudnicka AR, Mt-Isa S, Owen CG, Cook DG, Ashby D. Variations in primary open-angle glaucoma prevalence by age, gender, and race: a Bayesian meta-analysis. Invest Ophthalmol Vis Sci. 2006;47(10):4254–61.

15. Cedrone C, Mancino R, Cerulli A, Cesareo M, Nucci C. Epidemiology of primary glaucoma: prevalence, incidence, and blinding effects. Prog Brain Res. 2008;173:3–14.
16. Lin W, Aoyama Y, Kawase K, Yamamoto T. Relationship between central corneal thickness and visual field defect in open-angle glaucoma. Jpn J Ophthalmol. 2009;53(5):477–81.
17. Jonas JB. Clinical implications of peripapillary atrophy in glaucoma. Curr Opin Ophthalmol. 2005;16(2):84–8.
18. Moghimi S, Zandvakil N, Vahedian Z, Mohammadi M, Fakhraie G, Coleman AL, Lin SC. Acute angle closure: qualitative and quantitative evaluation of the anterior segment using anterior segment optical coherence tomography. Clin Exp Ophthalmol. 2014;42(7):615–22.
19. Kitsos G, Gartzios C, Asproudis I, Bagli E. Central corneal thickness in subjects with glaucoma and in normal individuals (with or without pseudoexfoliation syndrome). Clin Ophthal (Auckland, NZ). 2009;3:537.
20. Pan CW, Li J, Zhong H, Shen W, Niu Z, Yuan Y, Chen Q. Ethnic variations in central corneal thickness in a rural population in China: the Yunnan minority eye studies. PLoS One. 2015;10(8):e0135913.
21. Doughty MJ, Zaman ML. Human corneal thickness and its impact on intraocular pressure measures: a review and meta-analysis approach. Surv Ophthalmol. 2000;44(5):367–408.
22. Belovay GW, Goldberg I. The thick and thin of the central corneal thickness in glaucoma. Eye. Feb. 2018;15:1.
23. Baboolal SO, Smit DP. South African Eye Study (SAES): ethnic differences in central corneal thickness and intraocular pressure. Eye. 2018;32:749–56.
24. Wong AC, Wong CC, Yuen NS, Hui SP. Correlational study of central corneal thickness measurements on Hong Kong Chinese using optical coherence tomography, Orbscan and ultrasound pachymetry. Eye. 2002;16(6):715.
25. Ayala MJ, Pérez-Santonja JJ, Artola A, Claramonte P, Alió JL. Laser in situ keratomileusis to correct residual myopia after cataract surgery. J Refract Surg. 2001;17(1):12–6.
26. Tolesa K, Gessesse GW. Central corneal thickness in newly diagnosed glaucoma patients in south West Ethiopia: a cross-sectional study. BMC Ophthalmol. 2016;16(1):152.
27. Nicolela MT, Drance SM, Broadway DC, Chauhan BC, McCormick TA, LeBlanc RP. Agreement among clinicians in the recognition of patterns of optic disk damage in glaucoma. Am J Ophthalmol. 2001;132(6):836–44.
28. Gordon MO, Beiser JA, Brandt JD, Heuer DK, Higginbotham EJ, Johnson CA, Keltner JL, Miller JP, Parrish RK, Wilson MR, Kass MA. The ocular hypertension treatment study: baseline factors that predict the onset of primary open-angle glaucoma. Arch Ophthalmol. 2002;120(6):714–20.
29. Lee JM, Cirineo N, Ramanathan M, Nouri-Mahdavi K, Morales E, Coleman AL, Caprioli J. Performance of the visual field index in glaucoma patients with moderately advanced visual field loss. Am J Ophthalmol. 2014;157(1):39–43.
30. Quigley HA, Enger C, Katz J, Sommer A, Scott R, Gilbert D. Risk factors for the development of glaucomatous visual field loss in ocular hypertension. Arch Ophthalmol. 1994;112(5):644–9.
31. Sainani K. The importance of accounting for correlated observations. PM&R. 2010;2(9):858–61.

34

The effect of ranibizumab and aflibercept treatment on the prevalence of outer retinal tubulation and its influence on retreatment in neovascular age-related macular degeneration

Attila Kovacs[1], Timea Kiss[1], Ferenc Rarosi[2], Gabor M. Somfai[3,4], Andrea Facsko[1] and Rozsa Degi[1*]

Abstract

Background: We aimed to analyze the differences in the prevalence of outer retinal tubulation (ORT) in neovascular age-related macular degeneration (AMD) treated with anti-vascular endothelial growth factor (anti-VEGF) agents, either aflibercept or ranibizumab. Our further aim was to examine the changes in the frequency of injections of ranibizumab before and after ORT appearance.

Methods: Two hundred thirty six eyes of 230 patients were included in the study (184 eyes treated with ranibizumab by pro re nata regimen (PRN), 52 eyes with aflibercept bimonthly) and followed for 6–24 months. Using optical coherence tomography (OCT), the first appearance of ORT was documented, and fixed time point evaluations were also made every six months to determine the existence of ORT. The number of injections, the presence or absence of subretinal hyperreflective material (SHRM) at treatment initiation and visual acuity were also noted.

Results: The survival analysis with Cox proportional hazard model showed no significant difference between the ranibizumab and aflibercept groups in relation to the development of ORT ($p = 0.79$, hazard ratio 0.92). In the PRN treated ranibizumab group the number of injections showed significant decrease after ORT development ($p = 0.004$). When SHRM was present at treatment initiation the chance of developing ORT was 2.75 and 11.14 times higher in the ranibizumab and aflibercept groups, respectively.

Conclusions: The prevalence of ORT increased over time independently from the chosen anti-VEGF drug. Our results suggest that upon the appearance of ORT a decrease in retreatments can be expected.

Keywords: Outer retinal tubulation, Prevalence, Anti-VEGF, Aflibercept, Retreatment, Subretinal hyperreflective material

Background

Outer retinal tubulation (ORT) is a spectral-domain optical coherence tomography (SD-OCT) biomarker [1], first described by Zweifel et al. [2]. They defined ORTs as hyporeflective, branching tubular structures with hyperreflective borders within the outer nuclear layer of the retina [2]. The "en face" OCT technique can help map these branching networks [3]. ORTs have been observed in many retinal diseases, including exudative age-related macular degeneration (AMD) [2]. Based on histological reports, the border of the outer retinal tubulation consists of photoreceptor inner segment mitochondria and external limiting membrane (ELM), with fluid and photoreceptor outer segments being potentially present in the ovoid hyporeflective lumen of the ORT [4–6]. Adaptive optics scanning laser ophthalmoscopy findings are in correlation with histology reports and show lack of ORT cone

* Correspondence: degirozsa57@gmail.com
[1]Department of Ophthalmology, Faculty of Medicine, University of Szeged, 10-11 Koranyi fasor, Szeged 6720, Hungary
Full list of author information is available at the end of the article

reflectivity which can be due to the loss of cone outer segments and subsequent retinal remodeling [7].

Schaal et al. classified outer retinal tubulations as either open (incomplete closure with curving external limiting membrane at the ends, horizontally elongated shape in cross-section) or closed (completely encircled, oval shape in cross-section) ORTs [4].

ORT can be mistaken for intraretinal cysts, or subretinal fluid but with the recognition of its hyperreflective border and special occurrence in the outer nuclear layer these mistakes can be reduced, leading to a reduction in the rate of anti-VEGF overtreatment in exudative AMD [2].

The ORT prevalence in exudative AMD is low at the time of first diagnosis but over time during anti-VEGF therapy its prevalence increases [8, 9]. The importance of ORT as an OCT biomarker for photoreceptor degeneration is due to its connection with reduced visual acuity [1, 8–10].

It has been also reported that ORTs develop above areas of subretinal hyperreflective material (SHRM) or atrophy [8, 9]. SHRM is a medium- to hyperreflective mass between the neurosensory retinal layers and retinal pigment epithelium on OCT [11]. It usually represents either a type II choroidal neovascular complex or is the consequence of an active choroidal neovascularisation, including subretinal haemorrhage and lipid or fluid exudation [1, 11, 12].

The aim of the present study was to investigate the prevalence of ORTs in eyes with neovascular AMD undergoing treatment either with ranibizumab or aflibercept. Our further aim was to examine the changes in the frequency of injections before and after ORT appearance. We also assessed the presence of subretinal hyperreflective material and its relationship with ORT.

Methods
Ethics, consent
This retrospective study was performed at the Medical Retina Unit of the Ophthalmology Department of University of Szeged, in Hungary. The study was approved by the Institutional Review Board of University of Szeged Albert Szent-Györgyi Clinical Centre (reference number: 3650) and was in accordance with the ethical standards of the Declaration of Helsinki. Since this was a retrospective review of patient data, informed consent was not required. The need for a consent was formally waived by the ethics committee, and this was also in line with the national regulations.

Patients
Treatment-naïve exudative AMD patients were enrolled in the study. For the ranibizumab group enrollment took place between October 2014 to April 2016 while patients in the aflibercept group were enrolled between April 2015 to April 2016.

All patients were over 50 years of age, the mean follow-up period was 16.3 months and 9.2 months (range 6–24 months and 6–12 months) in the ranibizumab and aflibercept groups, respectively.

During each visit a comprehensive ophthalmic examination was carried out including best-corrected visual acuity (BCVA, Early Treatment Diabetic Retinopathy Study (ETDRS) score) assessment, slit-lamp biomicroscopy, dilated funduscopy and SD-OCT examination of the retina (Heidelberg Spectralis, Heidelberg Engineering, Heidelberg, Germany). Eyes with poor quality SD-OCT scans (Q index below 20) or with poor compliance were excluded from the study (14 eyes from the ranibizumab and 3 eyes from the aflibercept group).

Treatment regimen for both ranibizumab (0.5 mg) and aflibercept (2 mg) started with 3 monthly injections. After this initiation phase the ranibizumab group was treated by a pro re nata (PRN) regimen with follow-up visits scheduled monthly. The retreatment criteria for ranibizumab patients consisted of any subretinal or intraretinal fluid on OCT, or new haemorrhage on funduscopy. In the aflibercept group follow-up after the loading phase was scheduled every two months, treatment was given at each follow-up. The above regimens were in accordance with the available treatment guidelines in Hungary at the time of the study.

For SD-OCT imaging a pattern size of 5.8×5.8 mm, $20° \times 20°$ was applied with 25 B-scans, using the "follow-up" mode. By manual review of the scan volumes we determined the first appearance of the ORT in both groups. We also assessed the presence of ORT at fixed time points at baseline, month 6 and 12 in both groups and at months 18 and 24 in the ranibizumab group. Images were assessed by two independent retina specialists, in case of incongruity the images were referred to a third retina specialist to make a decision. During the evaluation of OCT scans we did not differentiate between the above described open (incomplete hyperreflective ring) and closed (complete hyperreflective ring) forms of ORT according to Schaal [4]. Thus, both types of ORT detected on the images were considered an ORT positive case. The criterion of ORT was a hyperreflective ovoid-elongated structure in the outer nuclear layer of the retina with lower reflective content (Fig. 1).

The readers also identified the presence or absence of subretinal hyperreflective material on SD-OCT images at treatment initiation. The criterion for SHRM was a medium- to hyperreflective mass between the neurosensory retinal layers and retinal pigment epithelium, as described by Keane et al. [11] (Fig. 1).

Statistical methods
The BCVA was compared across the two groups using the Mann-Whitney U-test. The survival analysis for

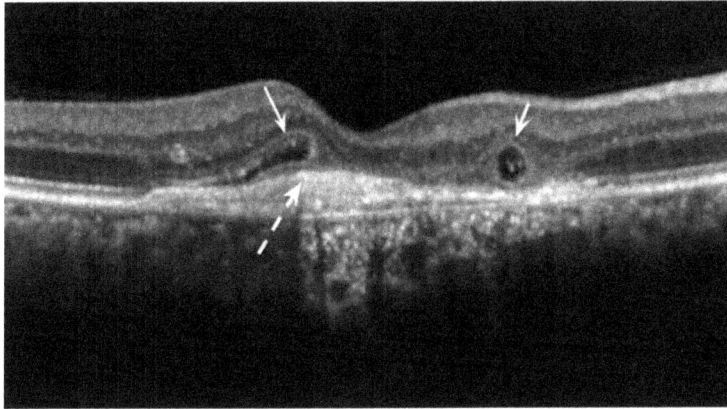

Fig. 1 Outer retinal tubulations and subretinal hyperreflective material on an SD-OCT single B-scan. Open and closed ORTs in cross section (left and right solid arrows) above subretinal hyperreflective material (dash arrow). The definition of ORT was a hyperreflective ovoid-elongated structure in the outer nuclear layer of the retina with lower reflective content

ORT development was analyzed by a Cox proportional hazard model. We analyzed the correlation between the presence of SHRM at treatment initiation with the development of ORT by Chi-square test and calculated relative risks. Where zeros were involved for the computation of relative risk, 0.5 was added to all cells, according to the previous suggestions [13].

The injection rate was calculated only in the PRN treated ranibizumab group due to the fixed 2 month therapeutic regimen of aflibercept. We assessed the injection rate only before and after the appearance of outer retinal tubulation and compared using the the Mann-Whitney U-test. In order to correct bias due to the unequal follow-up time (some patients had a higher number of injections due to the longer follow-up), we divided the follow-up time with the number of injections and calculated with monthly injections.

A p-value of $p < 0.05$ was taken as statistically significant. For the analyses the IBM SPSS Software (Version 22) was used.

Results

In the ranibizumab group we evaluated 184 eyes of 179 patients, with a median age of 74 years (range 51 to 88), while in the aflibercept group there were 52 eyes of 51 patients with a median age of 75 years (range 58 to 87).

The mean baseline best corrected visual acuities in the two groups were (mean ± SD) 59.16 ± 13.9 (median 61) and 53.96 ± 13.54 (median 55.5) ETDRS letters in the ranibizumab and aflibercept group, respectively. There was no significant difference between the two groups (Mann-Whitney U-test $p = 0.083$). The BCVA at the end of the follow-up was 57.19 ± 20.19 (median 63) and 59.46 ± 15.54 (median 64) ETDRS letters in the ranibizumab and aflibercept group, respectively. There

was no significant difference between the two groups (Mann-Whitney U-test $p = 0.69$).

Table 1 shows the number of eyes during the follow-up in the two groups. The number of eyes was reduced over time due to gradual enrollment in the study, thereby not every patient reached the same follow-up time. In the ranibizumab group outer retinal tubulation was observed in 17.4% of cases at baseline, in 33.7% of cases at month 6, in 45.3% of cases at month 12, and in 55.3% and in 60.8% of cases at months 18 and 24, respectively. The ORT prevalence in the aflibercept group was 23.1% at baseline, 40.4% at month 6, and 50% at month 12.

The survival analysis showed no significant difference between the ranibizumab and aflibercept treated groups in terms of ORT development. ($p = 0.79$, hazard ratio 0.92, 95% confidence interval 0.500–1.693) (Fig. 2).

The injection rates showed that the mean injection number per month before the ORT appearance was 0.37 ± 0.17 while after the ORT development it decreased to 0.21 ± 0.17 (Mann-Whitney U-test $p = 0.004$).

The presence of subretinal hyperreflective material at treatment initiation in the two subgroups was 75.5% in the ranibizumab, and 80.8% in the aflibercept group. In

Table 1 Number of eyes reaching the follow-up in the ranibizumab and aflibercept treated groups

Time point	Ranibizumab n (eyes)	Aflibercept n (eyes)
Baseline	184	52
at 6 months	184	52
at 12 months	161	28
at 18 months	103	0
at 24 months	51	0

Table legend: The column with "n" corresponds to the number of eyes reaching the follow-up

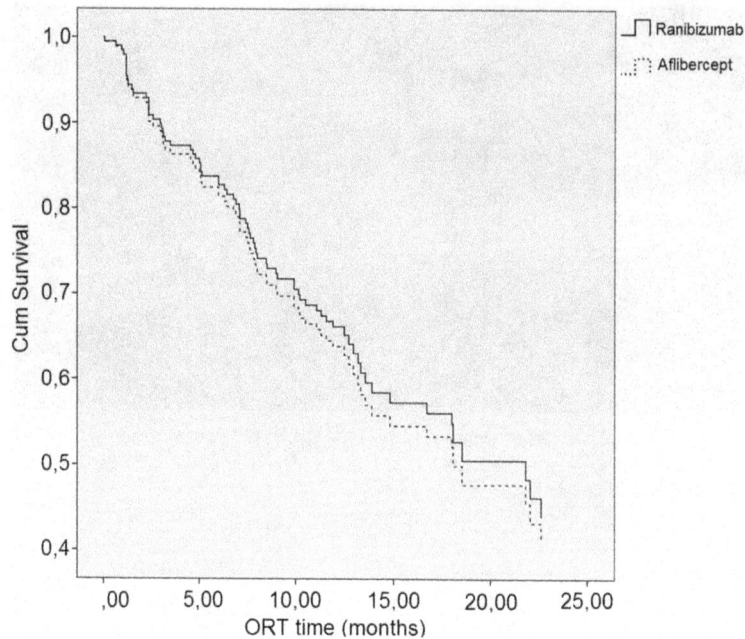

Fig. 2 Cox proportional hazard model of ORT survival in the ranibizumab and aflibercept groups

the ranibizumab treated group ORT developed in 85 eyes of 139 eyes with SHRM (61.15%), while without SHRM (45 eyes) ORTs were found merely in 10 eyes (22.2%) corresponding to a relative risk of 2.75. ($p < 0.01$). In the aflibercept treated group 55.81% of eyes with SHRM developed ORT (24 eyes of 43). No ORT developed in the eyes without SHRM (out of 9 eyes), consistent with a relative risk of 11.14 ($p < 0.01$).

Discussion

Our study found no significant difference between the ranibizumab and aflibercept treated groups according to ORT development. There was a statistically significant reduction in the frequency of injections in the ranibizumab treated group before and after ORT appearance. The presence of SHRM at treatment initiation as a biomarker had a statistically significant correlation with the development of ORT in both groups.

Zweifel first described outer retinal tubulation in 2009 [2]. Later the authors reported ORTs in various retinal disorders like neovascular AMD, geographic atrophy, polypoidal choroidal vasculopathy, non-AMD associated choroidal neovascularisation, and other degenerative retinal disorders (e.g. retinitis pigmentosa, gyrate atrophy, choroideremia, Stargardt disease, pattern dystrophy) [2, 3, 14–19].

The pathogenesis of ORT formation is still not completely clear, though recent reports helped a lot exploring it. Dolz-Marco et al. called the attention on the role of Müller cells in the pathomechanism of ORT development, namely the progressive photoreceptor damage that can result in Müller cell activation which thereby starts to produce glial fibrillary acidic protein, facilitating the formation of ORT [20]. Based on histological examinations it seems that the evolution of ORT starts with ELM and ellipsoid zone disruption [4]. ELM starts to scroll inward at its free edges, representing an initial form of ORT, leading to the development of a formed open ORT. With time the large, open ORTs split, their margins beginning to scroll ending in multiple smaller closed ORTs. During the scrolling process a downward displacement of adjacent inner nuclear layer and outer plexiform layer happens separating each ORT, and causing the appearance of microcystic lesions in the inner nuclear layer. The downward displacement of these layers might be due to the involvement of Müller cells in this scrolling/dragging process as Müller cells are contributing to the constitution of ELM with the inner segments of photoreceptors [4, 15, 20, 21].

Most of the studies in the field focused on exudative AMD and its relationship with ORT. From these reports it is known that ORT is an SD-OCT biomarker, the prevalence of which increases with time and is associated with decreased visual acuity [1, 8, 9]. It has been also reported that ORTs develop adjacent to areas of subretinal hyperreflective material or atrophy [8, 9]. The differential diagnostic importance of outer retinal tubulation lies in the avoidance of overtreatment due to its similarity to intraretinal fluid [2, 8].

In the present study, we evaluated treatment-naïve exudative AMD patients treated with ranibizumab and aflibercept regarding the presence of outer retinal tubulation. Altogether 236 eyes were followed in both groups with no statistical difference between the baseline characteristics of the two groups considering age and BCVA.

The prevalence of ORT continuously increased during the follow-up period, in both groups. In the ranibizumab group its prevalence almost quadrupled at the 24-month follow-up, while there was a doubling in the aflibercept group in 12 months. It is important to note, that in the ranibizumab group the baseline prevalence was lower (17.4% versus 23.1%). Dirani et al. found a similar increasing trend in their study starting with 2.5% at presentation, reaching 41.6% at 4 years of follow-up [8]. In our study the baseline ORT prevalence was higher compared to other reports [8, 9]. The reason behind this could be the more advanced disease state at the time of presentation (due to the real life nature of our retrospective study) and a relative delay in therapy initiation due to country-specific financial difficulties. The poorer baseline BCVA in both groups also supports this idea.

There is one previous article known, describing ORT development in 24 non-treatment-naïve eyes, treated with aflibercept only after receiving at least 6 ranibizumab injection, reporting an initial 97% ORT prevalence which later decreased to 75% [22].

To our knowledge, our study is the first to report results in treatment naïve patients treated with aflibercept and its connection with ORT development. The Cox proportional hazard model analysis suggested that there was no difference between the two in-label therapies ranibizumab and aflibercept in regard to the prevalence of outer retinal tubulation. Lee et al. in the Comparison of AMD Treatment Trials (CATT) study group evaluated the prevalence of ORTs in ranibizumab and bevacizumab treated neovascular AMD patients, and found no difference between the two drugs related to the prevalence of outer retinal tubulation [9].

In the present study we found a statistically significant difference in the monthly injection rate before and after the appearance of outer retinal tubulation in the ranibizumab treated group. Our results suggest that in patients who develop ORT a decrease in the retreatment rate can be expected which may be a very important clinical marker. Although we had a PRN regimen according to the Hungarian guidelines, Lee et al. found no difference between the fixed monthly regimen versus PRN regimen in regards to ORT development in patients treated either with ranibizumab or bevacizumab [9].

We found a statistically significant connection between ORT development and the presence of subretinal hyperreflective material at treatment initiation. When subretinal hyperreflective material was present the chance of developing ORT was 2.75., and 11.14 higher in the ranibizumab and aflibercept groups, respectively, in accordance with the results of Lee et al. in ranibizumab and bevacizumab treated patients [9].

Our findings, in concordance with the above mentioned study results suggest that ORT is independent of the chosen anti-VEGF drug or the dosing regimen of intravitreal anti-VEGF treatment. The appearance of ORT suggests that the clinicians can expect a decrease in the number of injections when following a pro re nata ranibizumab regimen. Our fixed bimonthly treatment with aflibercept did not allow us to analyze the injection rate before and after ORT development in this group. Our study also supports the previously reported higher prevalence of ORT development in the presence of subretinal hyperreflective material at treatment initiation [9].

There is a number of limitations of our study. Namely, the relatively small sample size in the aflibercept group compared to the ranibizumab group, along with the bimonthly follow-up in the aflibercept group. We believe that the number of subjects involved in both groups is comparable with other studies published in the field, while the bimonthly treatment regimen with aflibercept was fixed due to the country-specific guideline regulations. The decreasing number of eyes during the follow-up could also bias the analysis by including patients with increasing disease severity. However, we believe these factors were similar to those in similar studies available in the field. The strength of this report is the comparison of present in-label therapies, ranibizumab and aflibercept in exudative AMD patients in relation to ORT besides the evaluation of the injection rate in association with outer retinal tubulation. We used real life data that makes the study more relevant in the daily clinical practice.

Conclusions

The development of ORT could be a potential biomarker for the treatment prognosis in patients with wet AMD. Its clinical significance lies also in its similarity to activity-related intraretinal fluid. Further studies are needed to explore the nature and development of ORTs employing a comparable dosing and follow-up regimen of all three currently available anti-VEGF drugs ranibizumab, bevacizumab and aflibercept.

Abbreviations

AMD: Age-related macular degeneration; anti-VEGF: Anti-vascular endothelial growth factor; BCVA: Best-corrected visual acuity; CATT: Comparison of AMD Treatment Trials; CNV: Choroidal neovascularisation; ELM: External limiting membrane; ETDRS: Early Treatment Diabetic Retinopathy Study; OCT: Optical coherence tomography; ORT: Outer retinal tubulation; PRN: Pro re nata; SD-OCT: Spectral-domain optical coherence tomography; SHRM: Subretinal hyperreflective material

Acknowledgments

This research received no specific grant from any funding agency in the public, commercial, or not-for-profit sectors.

Funding

No funding was received for this research.

Authors' contributions

AK, RD made the conception and design of the study and analyzed the OCT images, in case of incongruity the final decision was made by AF. AK and TK collected and arranged the data (demographics, visual acuity, injection number and date). FR made the statistical analyzes and also the interpretation of data together with GMS. AK, TK drafted the manuscript. GMS was a major contributor editing it. AF, GMS and RD revised the manuscript. All authors read and approved the final manuscript.

Competing interests

The authors declare that they have no competing interests.

Author details

[1]Department of Ophthalmology, Faculty of Medicine, University of Szeged, 10-11 Koranyi fasor, Szeged 6720, Hungary. [2]Department of Medical Physics and Informatics, Faculty of Medicine, University of Szeged, Szeged, Hungary. [3]Augenzentrum Pallas Kliniken, Olten, Switzerland. [4]Department of Ophthalmology, Faculty of Medicine, Semmelweis University, Budapest, Hungary.

References

1. Schmidt-Erfurth U, Waldstein SM. A paradigm shift in imaging biomarkers in neovascular age-related macular degeneration. Prog Retin Eye Res. 2016;50: 1–24. https://doi.org/10.1016/j.preteyeres.2015.07.007.

2. Zweifel SA, Engelbert M, Laud K, Margolis R, Spaide RF, Freund KB. Outer retinal tubulation: a novel optical coherence tomography finding. Arch Ophthalmol. 2009;127(12):1596–602. https://doi.org/10.1001/archophthalmol. 2009.326.

3. Wolff B, Matet A, Vasseur V, Sahel JA, Mauget-Faÿsse M. En face OCT imaging for the diagnosis of outer retinal tubulations in age-related macular degeneration. J Ophthalmol. 2012;2012:542417. https://doi.org/10.1155/ 2012/542417.

4. Schaal KB, Freund KB, Litts KM, Zhang Y, Messinger JD, Curcio CA. Outer retinal tubulation in advanced age-related macular degeneration: optical coherence tomographic findings correspond to histology. Retina. 2015;35(7): 1339–50. https://doi.org/10.1097/IAE.0000000000000471.

5. Litts KM, Messinger JD, Freund KB, Zhang Y, Curcio CA. Inner segment remodeling and mitochondrial translocation in cone photoreceptors in age-related macular degeneration with outer retinal Tubulation. Invest Ophthalmol Vis Sci. 2015;56(4):2243–53. https://doi.org/10.1167/iovs.14-15838.

6. Litts KM, Messinger JD, Dellatorre K, Yannuzzi LA, Freund KB, Curcio CA. Clinicopathological correlation of outer retinal tubulation in age-related macular degeneration. JAMA Ophthalmol. 2015;133(5):609–12. https://doi. org/10.1001/jamaophthalmol.2015.126.

7. Litts KM, Wang X, Clark ME, Owsley C, Freund KB, Curcio CA, Zhang Y. Exploring photoreceptor reflectivity through multimodal imaging of outer retinal tubulation in advanced age-related macular degeneration. Retina. 2017;37(5):978–88. https://doi.org/10.1097/IAE.0000000000001265.

8. Dirani A, Gianniou C, Marchionno L, Decugis D, Mantel I. Incidence of outer retinal tubulation in ranibizumab-treated age-related macular degeneration. Retina. 2015;35(6):1166–72. https://doi.org/10.1097/IAE.0000000000000439.

9. Lee JY, Folgar FA, Maguire MG, Ying GS, Toth CA, Martin DF, Jaffe GJ, CATT Research Group. Outer retinal tubulation in the comparison of age-related macular degeneration treatments trials (CATT). Ophthalmology. 2014; 121(12):2423–31. https://doi.org/10.1016/j.ophtha.2014.06.013.

10. Faria-Correia F, Barros-Pereira R, Queirós-Mendanha L, Fonseca S, Mendonça L, Falcão MS, Brandão E, Falcão-Reis F, Carneiro AM. Characterization of neovascular age-related macular degeneration patients with outer retinal tubulations. Ophthalmologica. 2013;229(3):147–51. https://doi.org/10.1159/ 000346854.

11. Keane PA, Patel PJ, Liakopoulos S, Heussen FM, Sadda SR, Tufail A. Evaluation of age-related macular degeneration with optical coherence tomography. Surv Ophthalmol. 2012;57(5):389–414. https://doi.org/10.1016/j. survophthal.2012.01.006.

12. Shah VP, Shah SA, Mrejen S, Freund KB. Subretinal hyperreflective exudation associated with neovascular age-related macular degeneration. Retina. 2014; 34(7):1281–8. https://doi.org/10.1097/IAE.0000000000000166.

13. Agresti A. Categorical data analysis. 2nd ed. Gainesville: Wiley; 2002.

14. Hariri A, Nittala MG, Sadda SR. Outer retinal tubulation as a predictor of the enlargement amount of geographic atrophy in age-related macular degeneration. Ophthalmology. 2015;122(2):407–13. https://doi.org/10.1016/j. ophtha.2014.08.035.

15. Hua R, Liu L, Hu Y, Chen L. The occurrence and progression of outer retinal tubulation in Chinese patients after intravitreal injections of ranibizumab. Sci Rep. 2015;7(5):7661. https://doi.org/10.1038/srep07661.

16. Goldberg NR, Greenberg JP, Laud K, Tsang S, Freund KB. Outer retinal tubulation in degenerative retinal disorders. Retina. 2013;33(9):1871–6. https://doi.org/10.1097/IAE.0b013e318296b12f.

17. Iriyama A, Aihara Y, Yanagi Y. Outer retinal tubulation in inherited retinal degenerative disease. Retina. 2013;33(7):1462–5. https://doi.org/10.1097/IAE. 0b013e31828221ae.

18. Giachetti Filho RG, Zacharias LC, Monteiro TV, Preti RC, Pimentel SG. Prevalence of outer retinal tubulation in eyes with choroidal neovascularization. Int J Retina Vitreous. 2016;2(1):6. https://doi.org/10.1186/ s40942-016-0029-8.

19. Jung JJ, Freund KB. Long-term follow-up of outer retinal tubulation documented by eye-tracked and en face spectral-domainoptical coherence tomography. Arch Ophthalmol. 2012;130(12):1618–9. https://doi.org/10. 1001/archophthalmol.2012.1902.

20. Dolz-Marco R, Litts KM, Tan ACS, Freund KB, Curcio CA. The evolution of outer retinal tubulation, a neurodegeneration and gliosis prominent in macular diseases. Ophthalmology. 2017;124(9):1353–67. https://doi.org/10. 1016/j.ophtha.2017.03.043.

21. Preti RC, Govetto A, Filho RGA, Cabral Zacharias L, Gianotti Pimentel S, Takahashi WY, Monteiro MLR, Hubschman JP, Sarraf D. Optical coherence tomography analysis of outer retinal tubulations: sequential evolution and pathophysiological insights. Retina. 2018;38(8):1518–25. https://doi.org/10. 1097/IAE.0000000000001810.

22. Massamba N, Dirani A, Butel N, Fardeau C, Bodaghi B, Ingram A, Lehoang P. Evaluation of outer retinal tubulations in eyes switched from intravitreal ranibizumab to aflibercept for treatment of exudative age-related macular degeneration. Graefes Arch Clin Exp Ophthalmol. 2017;255(1):61–7. https:// doi.org/10.1007/s00417-016-3423-x.

35

Association between genetic variation of complement *C3* and the susceptibility to advanced age-related macular degeneration

Jun Zhang[1†], Shuang Li[1†], Shuqiong Hu[2], Jiguo Yu[1] and Yi Xiang[1*] ⓘ

Abstract

Background: The purpose of this study is to discuss whether genetic variants (rs2230199, rs1047286, rs2230205, and rs2250656) in the *C3* gene account for a significant risk of advanced AMD.

Methods: We performed a meta-analysis using electronic databases to search relevant articles. A total of 40 case-control studies from 38 available articles (20,673 cases and 20,025 controls) were included in our study.

Results: In our meta-analysis, the pooled results showed that the carriage of G allele for rs2230199 and the T allele for rs1047286 had a tendency to the risk of advanced AMD (OR = 1.49, 95% CI = 1.39–1.59, $P < 0.001$; OR = 1.45, 95% CI = 1.37–1.54, P < 0.001). Moreover, in the subgroup analysis based on ethnicity, rs2230199 and rs1047286 polymorphisms were more likely to be a predictor of response for Caucasian region (OR = 1.48, 95% CI = 1.38–1.59, $P < 0.001$; OR = 1.45, 95% CI = 1.37–1.54, P < 0.001). Besides, pooled results suggested that the G allele of rs2230199 could confer susceptibility to advanced AMD in Middle East (OR = 1.62, 95% CI = 1.33–1.97, $P < 0.001$).

Conclusion: In our meta-analysis, *C3* genetic polymorphisms unveiled a positive effect on the risk of advanced AMD, especially in Caucasians. Furthermore, numerous well-designed studies with large sample-size are required to validate this conclusion.

Keywords: Age-related macular degeneration, *C3* gene, Polymorphism, Meta-analysis

Background

Age-related macular degeneration (AMD) is a complex and progressive retinal disorder influenced by family history, aging, race, smoking and diet, which caused irreversible visual impairment in a growing number of elderly persons [1, 2]. The early stage of AMD is characterized by pigmentary abnormalities of the retinal pigment epithelium (RPE) and extracellular deposits called drusen under the retina [3]. As the condition progresses, two advanced forms of this disease are developed: extensive pigment epithelium atrophy (geographic atrophy or dry AMD) or subretinal choroidal neovascular membrane (exudative or wet

AMD). Although constituting only 10–15% of all AMD cases, advanced forms account for nearly 80% of AMD-related blindness in western countries [4]. It has been reported that the prevalence of advanced AMD is estimated at 3% in people aged > 65 years old, rising to 11% in those > 85 years old in developed world [5]. While, the pooled prevalence of advanced AMD is 0.56% among aged 40–79 years in Asian countries [6].

Advanced AMD has been implicated with important risk factors listed above, it is a multifactorial disease which influenced by a combination of environmental and genetic susceptibility [1, 3, 7, 8]. Although the well-defined pathogeny of advanced AMD remains to be unresolved, genetic association studies have provided consequential insights into the molecular basis of advanced AMD. Several genes at chromosomal loci 1q32 and 10q26, involving in inflammation and

* Correspondence: xyxyyanke@126.com
†Jun Zhang and Shuang Li contributed equally to this work.
[1]Department of Ophthalmology, the Central Hospital of Wuhan, Tongji Medical College, Huazhong University of Science and Technology, NO. 26 Shengli Street, Wuhan 430014, Hubei Province, China
Full list of author information is available at the end of the article

complement activation pathway, have been plausible candidate, as supported by the laboratory research in vitro and vivo that inflammation and immune response related proteins were found in drusen [9–11]. So far, the strongest genetic association has been identified on 1q32 with single nucleotide polymorphisms (SNPs) in complement factor H (*CFH*) gene by candidate region and whole genome association analyses [12, 13].

Apart from CFH, the central element of the complement cascade, complement component C3a has been interconnected with the vascular endothelial growth factor expression, geographic atrophy, retinal pigment epithelium deterioration, and progression to choroidal neovascularization [11, 14, 15]. These studies strongly indicated that aberrant regulation or activation of the complement pathway confer susceptibility to the main mechanism of advanced AMD. As the main regulator of the alternative complement pathway, several genetic variants in *C3* gene have been investigated with advanced AMD in different ethnic groups, the pooled results are incompatible and ambiguous. According to the International HapMap Project database, the human *C3* gene is located on chromosome 19 and exhibits nine common genetic SNPs (rs2230199, rs1047286, rs2241394, rs2250656, rs344542, rs2230205, rs339392, rs3745565, and rs11569536). Used for screening the electronic database and manual searching, the most widely condidate polymorphisms of the *C3* gene which at least has been surveyed in three pertinent studies are rs2230199, rs1047286, rs2230205 and rs2250656. In order to better understand the genetic risk of *C3* gene in the relationship with exudative AMD, we performed a meta-analysis to illuminate this association and determine whether the genetic variants of *C3* gene conferred susceptibility to advanced AMD.

Materials and methods
Literature search
A systematic search of electronic database such as PubMed, Embase, CNKI, Cochrane library and Web of Science was conducted with the following keywords: ("AMD" or "maculopathy" or "macular degeneration" or "age-related maculopathy" or "age-related macular degeneration") and ("complement 3" or "complement C3" or "C3" or "complement component 3") and ("variant" or "mutation" or "genetic" or "SNP" or "polymorphism" or "genetic polymorphism" or "genetic variant" or "single nucleotide polymorphism"). Each database was thoroughly scanned and was up to date as of September 1 2018. Our meta-analysis was mainly focused on case-control studies, without any language limitation imposed in the literature searching.

Study selection
Retrieved articles were considered eligible for our meta-analysis when they met the following inclusion

criteria: (1) investigating the disease risk of *C3* polymorphism with advanced AMD; (2) detailed genotyping data for each site could be acquired to estimate the odds ratio (OR) and 95% confidence interval (CI) based on genetic model contrast; (3) individual for all selected samples met the modified version of the age-related eye disease study (AREDS) grading system as described elsewhere. Major exclusion criteria were limited to several items as follow: (1) overlapping subjects in several articles for the same research group; (2) only focused on families' individuals rather than sporadic advanced AMD patients; (3) abstract from conferences, letters, review articles and case reports. When several articles included some of the same samples, the one with largest individuals and thorough genotype information would be winnowed for our meta-analysis.

Data extraction
Data from the retrieved studies were extracted independently by two reviewers (J.Z. and S.L.). The following items obtained from each eligible articles included: the first author, the year of publication, country and ethnicity of subjects, information on study design, sample size, genotyping methods and distribution in case and control groups. Two authors carefully inspected the raw statistics and reached a consensus in all aspects. If any disagreement still existed, the third author (S.H.) would be invited to chew over current controversy and resolve the dispute.

Quality assessment
Quality assessment of the screened studies was also independently conducted by two reviewers (J.Z. and S.L.) in the basis of the HuGENet Handbook [16]. A total of six bias assessment items were refined to investigate the relationship between genes and diseases from this handbook, including bias in selection of cases, bias in selection of controls, bias in genotyping cases, bias in genotyping controls, bias in population stratification, confounding bias, multiple tests, and selective outcome reports. The quality evaluation of every items for extracted articles was defined as "Yes" or "No". Separately, "Unclear" was designated if there was not enough information to make a decision. A series of corrections and judgements were performed independently by another coauthor (S.H.) if debate still lasted in the assessment. Consensus referring all items was achieved after discussion.

Statistical analysis
Allele and genotype frequency of each *C3* polymorphic site were counted between cases and healthy controls. The genetic strength association including pooled ORs and 95% CIs was assessed using different genetic models, including allele model (A vs. a), homozygote model (AA vs. aa), heterozygote model (Aa vs. aa), dominant (AA+Aa

vs. aa), recessive (AA vs. Aa+aa). The heterogeneity assumption between studies was estimated and evaluated by Cochran's Q statistic as well as the I^2 statistic. The result that our P value of Q statistic was less than 0.05 or the I^2 value was greater than 50% suggested apparent heterogeneity, thus a random-effect model was utilized in our model analysis. Otherwise, the fixed-effect model was performed [17]. Sensitivity analyses was conducted to assess the effect of each study and the stability of the pooled ORs by removing included study in turn from the compiled list. Begg's funnel plots [18] and Egger's regression test [19] were furthered to detect the potential publication bias. All statistical analysis using two-sided P values was executed by STATA 12.0 software (StataCorp LP, College Station, Texas, USA). A significant difference was estimated under the level of 0.05. The final results needed to be tested and verified by two authors (J.Z. and S.L.) respectively.

Results

Overall characteristics of selected studies and quality assessment

The flow diagram for literature searching is summarized in Fig. 1. A total of 1201 articles from the five databases (Additional file 1) were filtered by our search method. Of which, 886 studies were excluded for the three aspects: (1) 711 duplicated articles; (2) 83 articles not related to the theme of this investigation; (3) 92 articles mainly referred to abstract, conference, review, and case report. Through our rigorous inspection, 269 ones in the rest of articles were stroke out. Of them, 172 articles were focused on the every stage of AMD but not advanced AMD, 97 articles were not concerned with the association between advanced AMD and $C3$ genetic polymorphism. The other 46 full-text articles were left in our meta-analysis. Seven of them did not have detailed genotype data after cautiously reading the included literatures. Besides, two papers were investigated by the same author and the same batch of patients from Iran [20, 21]. We decided to choose the one which had larger samples size and more comprehensive directions. Finally, 40 case-control studies regarding the association of $C3$ gene with advanced AMD from 38 available publications were generally contained in our current meta-analysis [4, 20, 22–57]. The common characteristics of each article are generally showed in Table 1. As listed in the table, 30 studies from Caucasian region, 7 studies from East Asian group and 3 studies from Middle East have been chosen in our meta-analysis. The genotyping methods for our whole sample are distinct and the results could be validated in different ways.

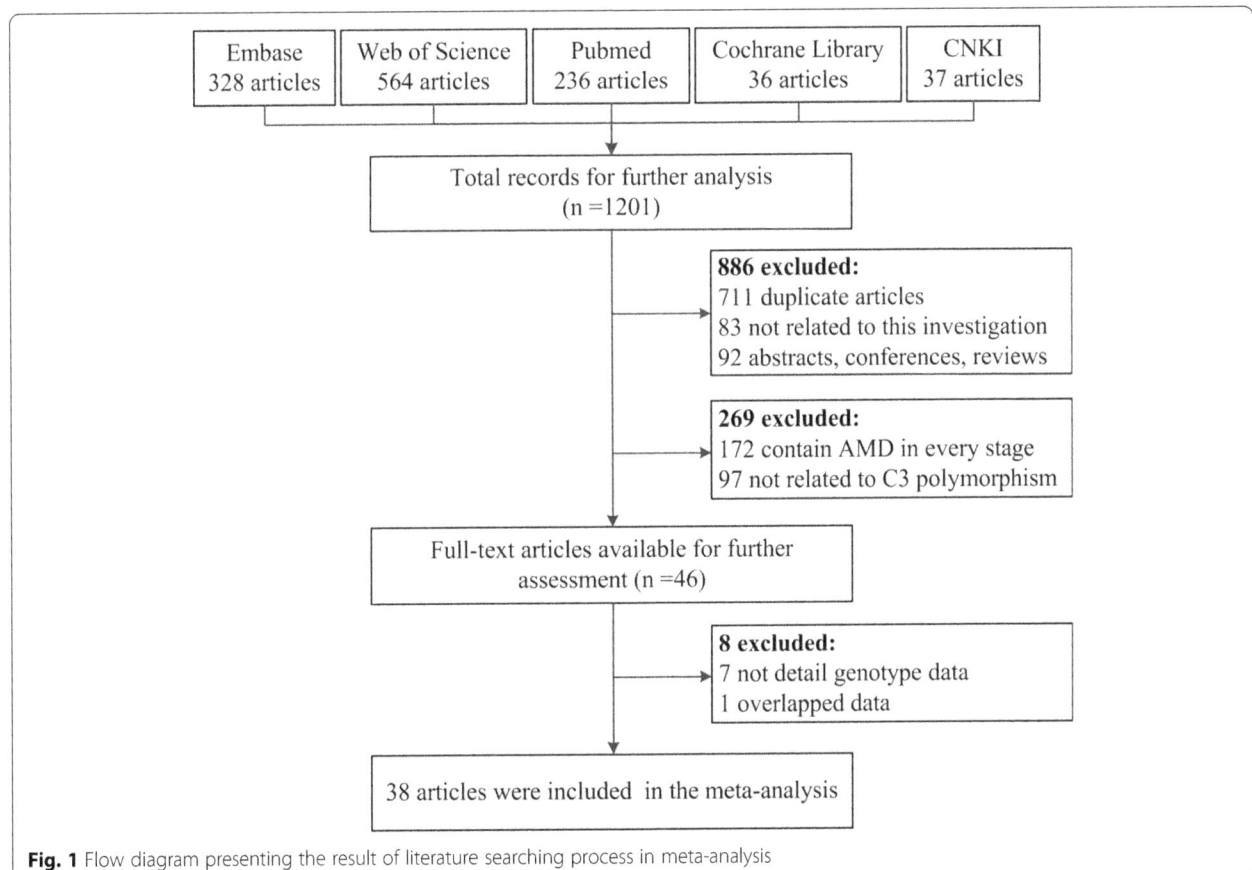

Fig. 1 Flow diagram presenting the result of literature searching process in meta-analysis

Table 1 The General Characteristics of All Studies Included in our Meta-Analysis

Refs	Year	Country	Ethnicity	Case/Control	Mean age of AMD	Mean age of control	Typing teaching	Study design
Yate et al. [54]	2007	UK	Caucasian	603/350	79.4 ± 7.2	75.3 ± 7.8	SNaPshot	Sex-,age-,ethnic-, matched
Yate et al. [54]	2007	Scotland	Caucasian	244/351	77.8 ± 9.2	78.0 ± 8.5	TaqMan	Sex-,age-,ethnic-, matched
Maller et al. [41]	2007	America	Caucasian	1238/934	NA	NA	MALDI-TOF MS	Age-,ethnic-, matched
Edwards et al. [31]	2008	America	Caucasian	444/300	NA	NA	Illumina GoldenGate	Age-,ethnic-, matched
Spencer et al. [50]	2008	America	Caucasian	286/701	76.5 ± 7.7	66.9 ± 8.3	TaqMan	Sex-,age-,ethnic-, matched
Scholl et al. [4]	2009	German	Caucasian	99/612	71.8 ± 7.4	76.2 ± 5.3	MALDI-TOF MS	Sex-,age-,ethnic-, matched
Francis et al. [32]	2009	America	Caucasian	211/187	79	74	Sequencing	Age-,ethnic-, matched
Park et al. [44]	2009	America	Caucasian	898/599	80.6 ± 5.0	77.6 ± 4.3	Illumina GoldenGate	Sex-,age-,ethnic-, matched
Despriet et al. [30]	2009	Netherlands	Caucasian	268/173	78.7 ± 7.7	74.1 ± 6.3	TaqMan	Sex-,age-,ethnic-, matched
Bergeron et al. [22]	2009	America	Caucasian	421/215	64.8	66.5	TaqMan	Sex-,age-,ethnic-, matched
Reynolds et al. [47]	2009	America	Caucasian	120/60	82.0 ± 6.9	79.0 ± 4.4	MALDI-TOF MS	Sex-,age-,ethnic-, matched
Pei et al.[45]	2009	China	East Asian	123/130	70.6 ± 8.2	69.2 ± 10.1	MALDI-TOF MS	Sex-,age-,ethnic-, matched
Cui et al. [29]	2010	China	East Asian	150/161	66.6 ± 8.4	65.7 ± 7.8	PCR-RFLP/ Sequencing	Sex-,age-,ethnic-, matched
Zerbib et al. [56]	2010	France	Caucasian	1080/406	79.0 ± 7.4	67.8 ± 7.7	TaqMan	Sex-,age-,ethnic-, matched
McKay et al. [43]	2010	Northern Ireland	Caucasian	437/436	77.6	74.9	SNaPshot	Sex-,age-,ethnic-, matched
Chen et al. [25]	2010	America	Caucasian	2157/1150	78.6	74.1	Illumina GoldenGate	Sex-,age-,ethnic-, matched
Kopplin et al. [37]	2010	America	Caucasian	377/161	NA	NA	Affymetrix GeneChip	Age-,ethnic-, matched
Liu et al. [39]	2010	China	East Asian	158/220	64.0 ± 6.6	63.0 ± 7.8	SNaPshot	Sex-,age-,ethnic-, matched
Yu et al. [55]	2011	America	Caucasian	1082/221	79.5 ± 5.5	77.0 ± 4.6	MALDI-TOF MS	Sex-,age-,ethnic-, matched
Chen et al. [26]	2011	America	Caucasian	1335/509	70.2 ± 5.1	67.0 ± 4.3	SNaPshot	Sex-,age-,ethnic-, matched
Hageman et al. [33]	2011	America	Caucasian	1132/822	76.5 ± 7.1	76.4 ± 7.3	NA	Sex-,age-,ethnic-, matched
Peter et al. [46]	2011	America	Caucasian	48/1260	NA	NA	TaqMan	Age-,ethnic-, matched
Yanagisawa et al. [53]	2011	Japan	East Asian	420/197	74.0 ± 7.5	72.0 ± 6.0	TaqMan	Sex-,age-,ethnic-, matched
Martinez et al. [42]	2012	Spain	Caucasian	259/191	NA	NA	SNaPshot	Age-,ethnic-, matched
Smailhodzic et al. [49]	2012	Netherlands	Caucasian	197/150	NA	NA	Sequencing	Sex-,age-,ethnic-, matched
Buentello et al. [23]	2012	Mexico	Caucasian	159/152	76.4 ± 8.1	73.5 ± 6.8	PCR-RFLP	Sex-,age-,ethnic-, matched

Table 1 The General Characteristics of All Studies Included in our Meta-Analysis *(Continued)*

Refs	Year	Country	Ethnicity	Case/Control	Mean age of AMD	Mean age of control	Typing teaching	Study design
Tian et al. [51]	2012	China	East Asian	535/469	NA	NA	MALDI-TOF MS	Age-,ethnic-, matched
Losonczy et al. [40]	2012	Hungary	Caucasian	275/106	76.0 ± 7.3	79.1 ± 6.1	PCR-RFLP	Sex-,age-,ethnic-, matched
Cipriani et al. [27]	2012	UK	Caucasian	893/2199	78.6 ± 7.5	NA	Illumina BeadChip	Sex-,age-,ethnic-, matched
Jaouni et al. [36]	2012	Israel	Middle East	317/159	78.1 ± 7.6	70.8 ± 8.2	PCR-RFLP	Sex-,age-,ethnic-, matched
Wu et al. [52]	2013	China	East Asian	165/216	69.4 ± 10	64.5 ± 8.0	TaqMan	Sex-,age-,ethnic-, matched
Helgason et al. [35]	2013	Iceland	Caucasian	1107/2869	NA	NA	Illumina BeadChip	Age-,ethnic-, matched
Helgason et al. [35]	2013	America	Caucasian	1525/1288	NA	NA	Illumina BeadChip	Age-,ethnic-, matched
Contreras et al. [28]	2014	Mexico	Caucasian	273/201	76.0 ± 8.0	65.5 ± 9.8	TaqMan	Sex-,age-,ethnic-, matched
Caire et al. [24]	2014	Spain	Caucasian	154/141	75.4 ± 7.2	78.5 ± 7.2	SNaPshot	Sex-,age-,ethnic-, matched
Liu et al. [38]	2014	China	East Asian	200/275	75.3 ± 7.7	74.3 ± 7.6	TaqMan	Sex-,age-,ethnic-, matched
Hautamaki et al. [34]	2015	Finland	Caucasian	301/119	NA	NA	Sequencing	Age-,ethnic-, matched
Saksens et al. [48]	2016	Netherlands	Caucasian	571/900	76.6 ± 8.5	71.3 ± 6.7	KASP	Sex-,age-,ethnic-, matched
Bonyadi et al. [20, 21]	2017	Iran	Middle East	266/228	76.4 ± 7.6	72.7 ± 6.8	PCR-RFLP	Sex-,age-,ethnic-, matched
Habibi et al. [57]	2017	Tunisia	Middle East	145/207	73.1 ± 8.1	NA	PCR-SSP	Age-,ethnic-, matched

Bias assessment of the included studies

Overall results in Table 2 primarily expound the evaluation of potential sources of bias in our included studies. Overall, the quality of the included studies was consistently absolute. Of the studies, there was no obvious bias in the selection of cases and controls, genotyping controls, population stratification, confounding bias, multiple tests, or selective outcome reports.

Relationship of *C3* gene polymorphisms with advanced AMD susceptibility

Several genetic models for *C3* polymorphisms including rs2230199, rs1047286, rs2230205, rs2250656 were used in our meta-analysis and the combined results are presented in Table 3. Briefly, 36 studies discussed the association of rs2230199 with advanced AMD, 13 studies investigated the relationship between rs1047286 and advanced AMD, 5 studies referred to rs2230205, rs2250656, respectively.

Association between SNP rs2230199 of *C3* gene and advanced AMD

As shown in Table 3, there was a significant association between the rs2230199 SNP and advanced AMD

susceptibility in the overall populations (allelic model: OR = 1.49, 95% CI = 1.39–1.59, $P < 0.001$; homozygote model: OR = 2.33, 95% CI = 1.98–2.74, $P < 0.001$; heterozygote model: OR = 1.53, 95% CI = 1.41–1.64, $P < 0.001$; dominant model: OR = 1.62, 95% CI = 1.51–1.74, $P < 0.001$; recessive model: OR = 1.99, 95% CI = 1.70–2.34, $P < 0.001$). Moreover, the subgroup analysis straitified by ethnicity indicated that rs2230199 conferred obvious susceptibility to advanced AMD in the group of Caucasian in allelic (OR = 1.48, 95% CI = 1.38–1.59, $P < 0.001$) (Fig. 2), homozygote (OR = 2.20, 95% CI = 1.87–2.60, $P < 0.001$), heterozygote (OR = 1.55, 95% CI = 1.43–1.67, $P < 0.001$), dominant (OR = 1.63, 95% CI = 1.51–1.75, $P < 0.001$), recessive (OR = 1.88, 95% CI = 1.59–2.21, $P < 0.001$) models (Table 3). Besides, the allelic comparison yielded a positive correlation in Middle East group (OR = 1.62, 95% CI = 1.33–1.97, $P < 0.001$). However, this relationship was not significant in East Asian group for any genetic models (Table 3).

Association between SNP rs1047286 of *C3* gene and advanced AMD

Significant association between this SNP and advanced AMD was confirmed in the overall populations (allelic

Table 2 Assessment of potential bias in included studies

Year	First author	Bias in selection of cases	Bias in selection of controls	Bias in genotyping controls	Bias in population stratification	Confounding bias	Multiple test and Selective outcome reports
2007	Yate et al. [54]	NO	NO	NO	NO	NO	NO
2007	Maller et al. [41]	NO	NO	NO	NO	NO	NO
2008	Edwards et al. [31]	NO	NO	NO	NO	NO	NO
2008	Spencer et al. [50]	NO	NO	NO	NO	NO	NO
2009	Scholl et al. [4]	NO	NO	NO	NO	NO	NO
2009	Francis et al. [32]	NO	NO	NO	NO	NO	NO
2009	Park et al. [44]	NO	NO	NO	NO	NO	NO
2009	Despriet et al. [30]	NO	NO	NO	NO	NO	NO
2009	Bergeron et al. [22]	NO	NO	NO	NO	NO	NO
2009	Reynolds et al. [47]	NO	NO	NO	NO	NO	NO
2009	Pei et al. [45]	NO	NO	NO	NO	NO	NO
2010	Cui et al. [29]	NO	NO	NO	NO	NO	NO
2010	Zerbib et al. [56]	NO	NO	NO	NO	NO	NO
2010	McKay et al. [43]	NO	NO	NO	NO	NO	NO
2010	Chen et al. [25]	NO	NO	NO	NO	NO	NO
2010	Kopplin et al. [37]	NO	NO	NO	Unclear	NO	NO
2010	Liu et al. [39]	NO	NO	NO	NO	NO	NO
2011	Yu et al. [55]	NO	NO	NO	NO	NO	NO
2011	Chen et al. [26]	NO	NO	NO	NO	NO	NO
2011	Hageman et al. [33]	NO	NO	NO	Unclear	NO	NO
2011	Peter et al. [46]	Yes	NO	NO	Unclear	NO	NO
2011	Yanagisawa et al. [53]	NO	NO	NO	NO	NO	NO
2012	Martinez et al. [42]	NO	NO	NO	NO	NO	NO
2012	Smailhodzic et al. [49]	NO	NO	NO	NO	NO	NO
2012	Buentello et al. [23]	NO	NO	NO	NO	NO	NO
2012	Tian et al. [51]	NO	NO	NO	NO	NO	NO
2012	Losonczy et al. [40]	NO	NO	NO	NO	NO	NO
2012	Cipriani et al. [27]	NO	Yes	NO	NO	NO	NO
2012	Jaouni et al. [36]	NO	NO	NO	NO	NO	NO
2013	Wu et al. [52]	NO	NO	NO	NO	NO	NO
2013	Helgason et al. [35]	NO	NO	NO	NO	NO	NO
2014	Contreras et al. [28]	NO	NO	NO	NO	NO	NO
2014	Caire et al. [24]	NO	NO	NO	NO	NO	NO
2014	Liu et al. [38]	NO	NO	NO	NO	NO	NO
2015	Hautamaki et al. [34]	NO	NO	NO	NO	NO	NO
2016	Saksens et al. [48]	NO	NO	NO	NO	NO	NO
2017	Bonyadi et al. [20, 21]	NO	NO	NO	NO	NO	NO
2017	Habibi et al. [57]	NO	NO	NO	NO	NO	NO

model: OR = 1.45, 95% CI = 1.37–1.54, $P < 0.001$; homozygote model: OR = 2.06, 95% CI = 1.56–2.72, $P < 0.001$; heterozygote model: OR = 1.72, 95% CI = 1.51–1.96, $P < 0.001$; dominant model: OR = 1.76, 95% CI = 1.56–2.00, $P < 0.001$; recessive model: OR = 1.71, 95% CI = 1.30–

2.24, $P < 0.001$). In subgroup analysis stratified by ethnicity, our meta-analysis indicated significant correlation of rs1047286 with advanced AMD in the five genetic models (allelic model: OR = 1.45, 95% CI = 1.37–1.54, $P < 0.001$ (Fig. 3); homozygote model: OR = 2.06, 95% CI =

Table 3 Main Results of Pooled ORs and Analysis of *C3* gene polymorphism with advanced AMD in our Meta-Analysis

Subgroup	No. of studies	No. of patients		Allele model		Homozygote model		Heterozygote model		Dominant model		Recessive model	
		Cases	Control	OR(95% CI)	P	OR(95% CI)	P	OR(95% CI)	P	OR(95% CI)	P	OR(95% CI)	P
C3 rs2230199 (Associated allele vs. Reference allele: G vs. C)													
Overall	36	34,805	29,499	1.49 (1.39,1.59)	< 0.001	2.33 (1.98,2.74)	< 0.001	1.53 (1.41,1.64)	< 0.001	1.62 (1.51,1.74)	< 0.001	1.99 (1.70,2.34)	< 0.001
Caucasian	28	31,372	26,130	1.48 (1.38,1.59)	< 0.001	2.20 (1.87,2.60)	< 0.001	1.55 (1.43,1.67)	< 0.001	1.63 (1.51,1.75)	< 0.001	1.88 (1.59,2.21)	< 0.001
East Asian	5	2122	2388	1.11 (0.56,2.20)	0.76	–	–	1.32 (0.91,1.93)	0.144	1.49 (1.04,2.15)	0.032	5.60 (1.57,19.9)	–
Middle East	3	1311	981	1.62 (1.33,1.97)	< 0.001	–	–	1.07 (0.66,1.73)	0.798	1.49 (0.95,2.34)	0.085	25.5 (3.35,194)	–
C3 rs1047286 (Associated allele vs. Reference allele: T vs. C)													
Overall	13	16,232	16,222	1.45 (1.37,1.54)	< 0.001	2.06 (1.56,2.72)	< 0.001	1.72 (1.51,1.96)	< 0.001	1.76 (1.56,2.00)	< 0.001	1.71 (1.30,2.24)	< 0.001
Caucasian	10	14,688	14,548	1.45 (1.37,1.54)	< 0.001	2.06 (1.56,2.72)	< 0.001	1.72 (1.50,1.96)	< 0.001	1.76 (1.55,2.00)	< 0.001	1.71 (1.30,2.24)	< 0.001
East Asian	3	1544	1674	1.75 (0.49,6.29)	0.388	–	–	2.06 (0.38,11.3)	0.404	2.06 (0.38,11.3)	0.404	–	–
C3 rs2230205 (Associated allele vs. Reference allele: A vs. G)													
Overall	5	3302	2732	0.99 (0.89,1.11)	0.903	1.04 (0.77,1.42)	0.780	1.00 (0.80,1.23)	0.967	1.00 (0.81,1.22)	0.992	1.06 (0.81,1.37)	0.687
Caucasian	1	880	598	0.90 (0.66,1.23)	0.507	0.45 (0.12,1.60)	0.215	0.98 (0.69,1.39)	0.902	0.93 (0.66,1.32)	0.699	0.45 (0.13,1.60)	0.217
East Asian	4	2422	2134	1.01 (0.89,1.14)	0.903	1.10 (0.80,1.51)	0.546	1.01 (0.77,1.32)	0.967	1.04 (0.80,1.33)	0.787	1.10 (0.84,1.43)	0.497
C3 rs2250656 (Associated allele vs. Reference allele: G vs. A)													
Overall	5	3278	2632	0.90 (0.75,1.08)	0.257	0.76 (0.49,1.16)	0.207	0.78 (0.65,0.95)	0.014	0.78 (0.65,0.94)	0.010	0.83 (0.55,1.27)	0.391
Caucasian	1	874	512	0.82 (0.64,1.05)	0.117	0.77 (0.42,1.42)	0.407	0.76 (0.55,1.05)	0.097	0.76 (0.56,1.04)	0.085	0.87 (0.48,1.57)	0.642
East Asian	4	2404	2120	0.92 (0.73,1.16)	0.486	0.74 (0.41,1.37)	0.340	0.80 (0.63,1.02)	0.068	0.79 (0.63,1.00)	0.052	0.80 (0.44,1.45)	0.456

1.56–2.72, P < 0.001; heterozygote model: OR = 1.72, 95% CI = 1.50–1.96, P < 0.001; dominant model: OR = 1.76, 95% CI = 1.55–2.00, P < 0.001; recessive model: OR = 1.71, 95% CI = 1.30–2.24, P < 0.001) (Table 3). This association could not be found in East Asian group for any genetic model (Table 3).

Association between SNP rs2230205 of *C3* gene and advanced AMD

No association between this SNP and advanced AMD was achieved in the overall populations (allelic model: OR = 0.99, 95% CI = 0.89–1.11, P = 0.903; homozygote model: OR = 1.04, 95% CI = 0.77–1.42, P = 0.780; heterozygote model: OR = 1.00, 95% CI = 0.80–1.23, P = 0.967; dominant model: OR = 1.00, 95% CI = 0.81–1.22, P = 0.992; recessive model: OR = 1.06, 95% CI = 0.81–1.37, P = 0.687). Subgroup analysis of Caucasian and East Asian group showed that there was a lack of relationship in any of the genetic models (Fig. 4, Table 3).

Association between SNP rs2250656 of *C3* gene and advanced AMD

The results of meta-analysis showed that there was not a positive association between this SNP and advanced AMD in the overall populations (allelic model: OR = 0.90, 95%

CI = 0.75–1.08, P = 0.257; homozygote model: OR = 0.76, 95% CI = 0.49–1.16, P = 0.207; recessive model: OR = 0.83, 95% CI = 0.55–1.27, P = 0.391). But a weakly protective risk between this SNP and advanced AMD was observed in heterozygote model and dominant model (OR = 0.78, 95% CI = 0.65–0.95, P = 0.014; OR = 0.78, 95% CI = 0.65–0.94, P = 0.010, respectively). In the stratified analysis by ethnicity, there was no association in any of the genetic models. (Fig. 5, Table 3).

Heterogeneity test and sensitivity analysis

Significant heterogeneity between these studies was observed among two SNPs (rs2230199 and rs2250656) (P < 0.1) (Figs. 2, 5). The results of our subgroup analysis confirmed that ethnicity was the primary sources of heterogeneity. Additionally, sensitivity analysis was conducted to evaluate the effect of individual study on the pooled ORs by sequentially omitting each study. The pooled ORs were not affected by removing any study (Fig. 6, the sensitivity analysis of rs2230199; others see Additional file 2: Figures S1-S3).

Publication bias

Publication bias is a potential problem, thus Begg's funnel plots and Egger's regression tests were applied to investigate the publication bias for *C3* genetic polymorphism.

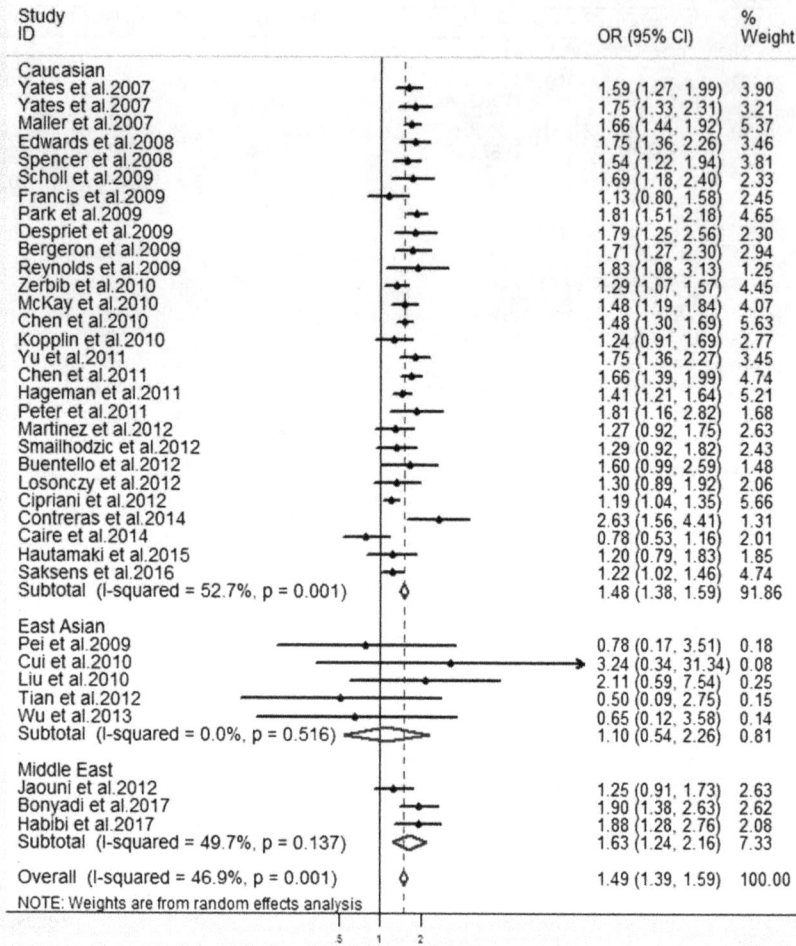

Study ID		OR (95% CI)	% Weight
Caucasian			
Yates et al.2007		1.59 (1.27, 1.99)	3.90
Yates et al.2007		1.75 (1.33, 2.31)	3.21
Maller et al.2007		1.66 (1.44, 1.92)	5.37
Edwards et al.2008		1.75 (1.36, 2.26)	3.46
Spencer et al.2008		1.54 (1.22, 1.94)	3.81
Scholl et al.2009		1.69 (1.18, 2.40)	2.33
Francis et al.2009		1.13 (0.80, 1.58)	2.45
Park et al.2009		1.81 (1.51, 2.18)	4.65
Despriet et al.2009		1.79 (1.25, 2.56)	2.30
Bergeron et al.2009		1.71 (1.27, 2.30)	2.94
Reynolds et al.2009		1.83 (1.08, 3.13)	1.25
Zerbib et al.2010		1.29 (1.07, 1.57)	4.45
McKay et al.2010		1.48 (1.19, 1.84)	4.07
Chen et al.2010		1.48 (1.30, 1.69)	5.63
Kopplin et al.2010		1.24 (0.91, 1.69)	2.77
Yu et al.2011		1.75 (1.36, 2.27)	3.45
Chen et al.2011		1.66 (1.39, 1.99)	4.74
Hageman et al.2011		1.41 (1.21, 1.64)	5.21
Peter et al.2011		1.81 (1.16, 2.82)	1.68
Martinez et al.2012		1.27 (0.92, 1.75)	2.63
Smailhodzic et al.2012		1.29 (0.92, 1.82)	2.43
Buentello et al.2012		1.60 (0.99, 2.59)	1.48
Losonczy et al.2012		1.30 (0.89, 1.92)	2.06
Cipriani et al.2012		1.19 (1.04, 1.35)	5.66
Contreras et al.2014		2.63 (1.56, 4.41)	1.31
Caire et al.2014		0.78 (0.53, 1.16)	2.01
Hautamaki et al.2015		1.20 (0.79, 1.83)	1.85
Saksens et al.2016		1.22 (1.02, 1.46)	4.74
Subtotal (I-squared = 52.7%, p = 0.001)		1.48 (1.38, 1.59)	91.86
East Asian			
Pei et al.2009		0.78 (0.17, 3.51)	0.18
Cui et al.2010		3.24 (0.34, 31.34)	0.08
Liu et al.2010		2.11 (0.59, 7.54)	0.25
Tian et al.2012		0.50 (0.09, 2.75)	0.15
Wu et al.2013		0.65 (0.12, 3.58)	0.14
Subtotal (I-squared = 0.0%, p = 0.516)		1.10 (0.54, 2.26)	0.81
Middle East			
Jaouni et al.2012		1.25 (0.91, 1.73)	2.63
Bonyadi et al.2017		1.90 (1.38, 2.63)	2.62
Habibi et al.2017		1.88 (1.28, 2.76)	2.08
Subtotal (I-squared = 49.7%, p = 0.137)		1.63 (1.24, 2.16)	7.33
Overall (I-squared = 46.9%, p = 0.001)		1.49 (1.39, 1.59)	100.00
NOTE: Weights are from random effects analysis			

Fig. 2 Evaluation of the association between *C3* genetic polymorphism (rs2230199) with advanced AMD

Four symmetrical funnel plots suggested that both tests had no evidence of significant bias (data not shown). Furthermore, as emerged in Table 4, the pooled *P* values for both tests are more than 0.05.

Discussion

AMD is a multifactorial disease, in which complement system mediated inflammation plays a pivotal role. Several pathways including the alternative complement component have been described to be implicated in the development of AMD [54]. As the central element of the complement cascade, *C3* has been a plausible candidate gene since its cleavage product C3a was confirmed in drusen. In our current meta-analysis, 20,673 patients and 20,025 controls from 38 articles were combined to detect the association of *C3* genetic polymorphisms with advanced AMD. We came to the conclusion that two nonsynonymous SNPs rs2230199 and rs1047286 were demonstrated an increased pathogenic effect on advanced

AMD (rs2230199: allelic model: OR = 1.49, 95% CI = 1.39–1.59, *P* < 0.001; homozygote model: OR = 2.33, 95% CI = 1.98–2.74, P < 0.001; rs1047286: allelic model: OR = 1.45, 95% CI = 1.37–1.54, P < 0.001; homozygote model: OR = 2.06, 95% CI = 1.56–2.72, P < 0.001). Moreover, our meta-analysis discovered that SNP rs2250656 decreased the risk of advanced AMD susceptibility, which a protective association was acquired in heterozygote model and dominant model. Obviously, the results of SNP rs2250656 with advanced AMD needed to be validated with larger samples and studies in different ethnicity.

Being consistent with previous studies, the G allele of rs2230199 conferred susceptibility to advanced AMD in Caucasian group. In our meta-analysis, we first confirmed that the G allele of rs2230199 could be linked with AMD in Middle East but not East Asian region, though rather larger population needed to be validated in the future. Besides, our meta-analysis found a novel association between the T allele of

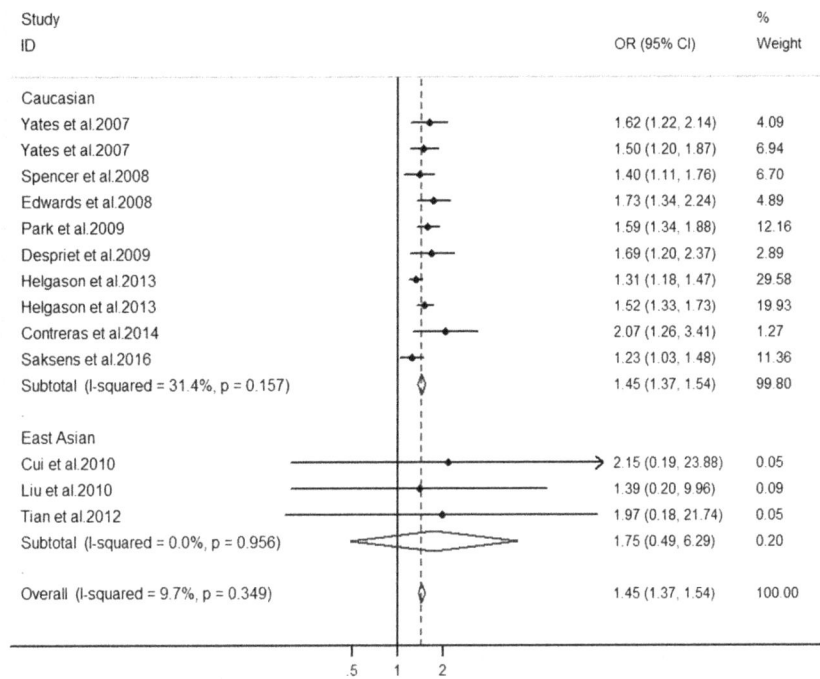

Fig. 3 Assessment of the association between *C3* genetic polymorphism (rs1047286) with advanced AMD

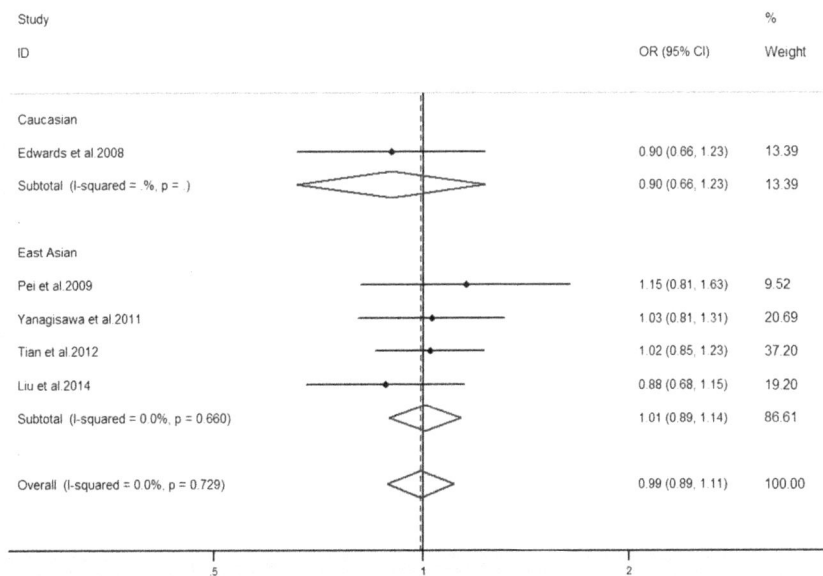

Fig. 4 Estimation of the association between *C3* genetic polymorphism (rs2230205) with advanced AMD

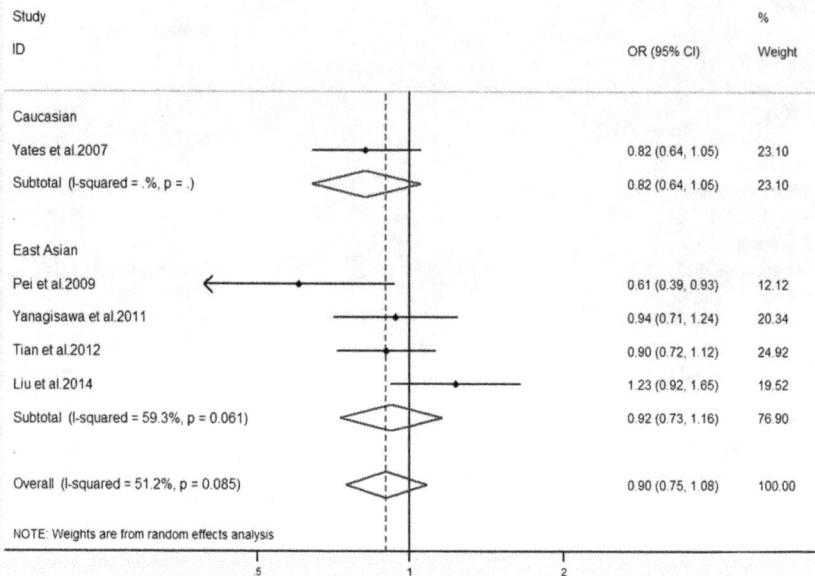

Fig. 5 Evaluation of the association between *C3* genetic polymorphism (rs225065) with advanced AMD

rs1047286 and advanced AMD in Caucasian but not East Asian group.

The common polymorphisms rs2230199 and rs1047286 in the *C3* gene have been identified as genetic risk factors for advanced AMD in Caucasian populations. However, the allele frequencies of rs2230199 vary widely among different ethnicities. Frequencies of the risk G allele at rs2230199 were 25% to 31% in AMD cases and 19% to 21% in controls in Caucasians [29]. Besides, the frequencies of G allele was 14% to 25% in both cases and controls in Middle East region [20, 57]. While, the risk allele were absent in Japanese and rare (< 1%) in Chinese populations

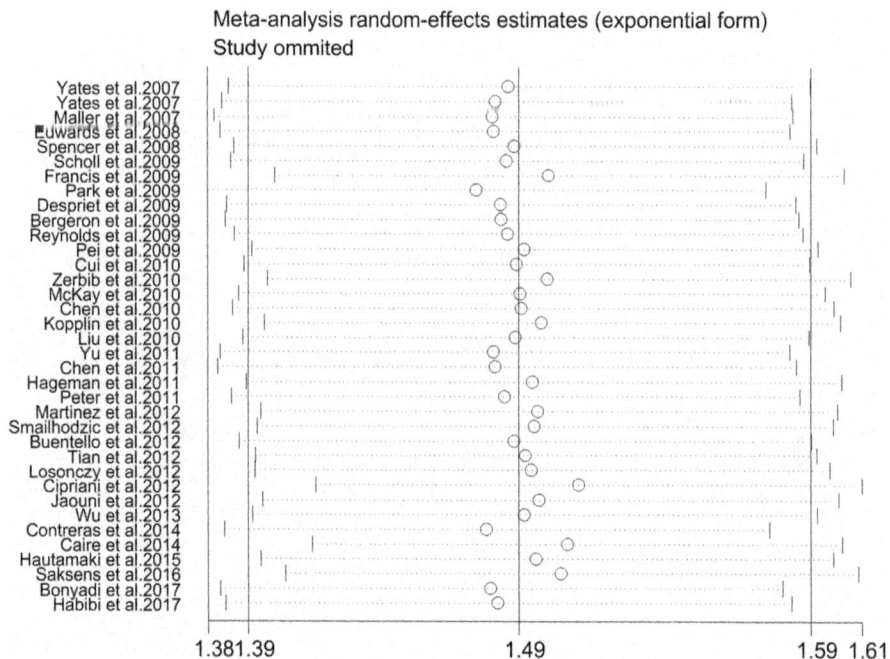

Fig. 6 Evaluation of the sensitivity analysis between *C3* genetic polymorphism (rs2230199) with advanced AMD

Table 4 Bias between *C3* genetic polymorphism with advanced AMD in our Meta-Analysis

Polymorphism	Number of publication	Publication bias	
		Begg's test	Egger's test
rs2230199	36	0.653	0.790
rs1047286	13	0.428	0.124
rs2230205	5	1.000	0.905
rs2250656	5	1.000	0.594

[53]. For rs1047286, frequencies of the risk T allele were 27% to 29% in AMD and 20% to 22% in controls in Caucasians. Cui et al. [29] also foud that rs1047286 was only 0.3% to 1% in both cases and controls and was not significantly associated with advanced AMD in Chinese population. The facts that rs2230199 and rs1047286 did not show tendency to risk of advanced AMD in East East but in Caucasian and Middle East could be explained by the lower minor allele frequencies (< 5%) of this two SNPs, suggesting that the susceptibility to advanced AMD by the variants of rs2230199 and rs1047286 did not transcend ethnic lines. In other words, this difference in the association between different ethnicities may result from other influence factors such as geography, the level of socioeconomic development or race.

The gene for *C3* is located on the short arm of chromosome 19 and consists of 41 exons, which forms 13 functional domains. *C3* is the most abundant complement component and significant *C3* messenger RNA is detected in the neural retina, choroid, RPE, and cultured RPE cells [58]. Cleavage of C3 into C3a and C3b is the central step in complement activation, which amplifies the complement response, resulting in the formation of lytic pores in the cell membrane. Janssen et al. [59] argued that cleaved native *C3* undergoes important structural rearrangements which causes conformational changes exposing binding sites for complement components and drusen including C3 and its activation products was confirmed in the finding that local inflammation and activation of the complement cascade can contribute to the pathogenesis of AMD. Notably, animal studies conducted by Bora et al. [60, 61] have indicated that *C3* deficiency in $C3^{-/-}$ mice prevented the formation of choroidal neovascularization in advanced AMD (wet AMD), indicating that C3 is a pivotal element of this activation process.

In our meta-analysis, four SNPs including rs2230199, rs1047286, rs223205 and rs2250656 were analyzed in the pooled data. Among them, rs2230199 and rs1047286 are located in the first ring of macroglobulin domains, which conduct a prominent function for correct orientation of the thioester-containing domain. The amino acid changes induced by the genetic mutations may alter the configuration of the macroglobulin ring [62]. With evidence supporting a biologic functional effect through the formation of two

electrophoretic allotypes in rs2230199 genetic site (*C3*F and *C3*S), the two alleles showed a differential capacity to bind monocyte- complement receptor. Helgason et al. [35] noted that the G allele in rs2230199 (*C3*F) was associated with the reduction of *C3* gene binding to CFH, which leads to an increase in complement activation. Additionally, rs2230199 variant may alter the net charge of the molecule and influence the position of the thioester-containing domain. Except for advanced AMD, the risk variant of rs2230199 has been previously considered as associated with other immune-mediated conditions, such as IgA nephropathy, systemic vasculitis.

In the current meta-analysis, rs1047286 variant showed significant association with advanced AMD in Caucasian populations. Despriet et al. [30] argued that rs2230199 and rs1047286 variants were in high linkage disequilibrium (LD) (D' = 0.90, r^2 = 0.80), which haplotype analyses suggested that the effect of the *C3* alleles was independent from the established genetic and environmental risk factors. Furthermore, our pooled analysis of neighboring SNPs of rs2230199 indicated that the allele frequency of the variant rs2230205 and rs2250656 was not significantly different between the advanced AMD cases and controls. Pei et al. [45] confirmed that the G allele of rs2250656 variant may be a protective factor for the development of AMD in East Asian. Given that the site of rs2250656 lies near the junction of intron 2 and exon 3, which contain short sequences and regulate the expression of gene and neighboring genes, it may contribute to the low risk for advanced AMD. Obviously, our pooled results were inconsistent with Pei's report, owing to the relative small sample size and distinct environmental elements.

In a previous meta-analysis where a total of 15 independent studies with 5593 cases and 5181 controls were included, Zhang et al. [63] indicated that rs2230199 C > G SNP increased the risk of AMD development and the G allele was a risk factor for AMD in Caucasian but not Asians. Moreover, Yu et al. [64] have implemented a systemic meta-analysis and the overall results suggested a positive association between rs2230199, rs1047286 and AMD susceptibility. Additionally, Despriet et al. [30] have clarified these positive associations for only four available studies. In comparison to previous meta-analyses, our analysis mainly focused on the major form of AMD (advanced AMD) and was involved with a greater number of studies and larger sample size. These would make our pooled ORs more believable, stable, and accurate than before, especially in the association with advanced AMD. Moreover, our present meta-analysis encompassed an acceptable quality evaluation system, minimizing the potential bias.

Considerable efforts have been paid to discuss the potential relationship between *C3* genetic polymorphisms and advanced AMD, some limitations for our present meta-analysis need to be declared. First, heterogeneity among the ethnic groups was discovered when investigating the association of *C3* genetic variants with advanced AMD. However, based on the results of the sensitivity analysis, it is clear that the overall effect was not affected by heterogeneity. Additionally, there was no obvious publication bias detected in the contrast of *C3* gene with advanced AMD. Second, the number of patients and controls was relatively small in each included study; therefore, a great number of samples from different ethnic regions are required for further analysis. Third, the effects of common confounding factors, including sex, age, body mass index, smoking, and diet were not evaluated in the present study because of insufficient data. Fourth limitation is that only three ethnic backgrounds with relatively few studies were taken into consideration, thus further efforts to reduce the incidence of ethnic bias will be needed once raw data become available. Finally, the electronic databases from which we selected eligible studies were listed in English and Chinese; therefore, a language bias may be existed in our meta-analysis.

Conclusion

The present meta-analysis provided a series of evidence-based pooled data for a significant association between rs2230199, rs1047286 and susceptibility to advanced AMD, especially in Caucasians. Additional well-designed work with a larger number of studies in which incorporate different ethnicities together with gene-gene and gene-environment is recommended to better confirm the functional role of the two nonsynonymous polymorphisms.

Acknowledgments
None.

Funding
This work was supported by National Natural Science Foundation Project (81300761) and Key Project of Health and Family Planning Commission of Wuhan Municipality (WX18A08).

Authors' contributions
YX designed the study. JZ and SL collected and checked the available information from eligible articles in this meta-analysis. SH analyzed the data. JY prepared the Fig. 1-6, Additional file 1: Fig. S1-S3 and Table 1-4. JZ and SL wrote the main manuscript text. YX reviewed and revised the manuscript. All authors censored and approved the manuscript.

Competing interests
The authors declare that they have no competing interests.

Author details
[1]Department of Ophthalmology, the Central Hospital of Wuhan, Tongji Medical College, Huazhong University of Science and Technology, NO, 26 Shengli Street, Wuhan 430014, Hubei Province, China. [2]Department of Ophthalmology, the Jingzhou aier eye hospital, Jingzhou, Hubei Province, China.

References

1. Kokotas H, Grigoriadou M, Petersen MB. Age-related macular degeneration: genetic and clinical findings. Clin Chem Lab Med. 2011;49(4):601–16.
2. Klein R, Peto T, Bird A, Vannewkirk MR. The epidemiology of age-related macular degeneration. Am J Ophthalmol. 2004;137(3):486–95.
3. de Jong PT. Age-related macular degeneration. N Engl J Med. 2006; 355(14):1474–85.
4. Scholl HP, Fleckenstein M, Fritsche LG, Schmitz-Valckenberg S, Gobel A, Adrion C, Herold C, Keilhauer CN, Mackensen F, Mossner A, et al. CFH, C3 and ARMS2 are significant risk loci for susceptibility but not for disease progression of geographic atrophy due to AMD. PLoS One. 2009;4(10):e7418.
5. Vingerling JR, Klaver CC, Hofman A, de Jong PT. Epidemiology of age-related maculopathy. Epidemiol Rev. 1995;17(2):347–60.
6. Kawasaki R, Yasuda M, Song SJ, Chen SJ, Jonas JB, Wang JJ, Mitchell P, Wong TY. The prevalence of age-related macular degeneration in Asians: a systematic review and meta-analysis. Ophthalmology. 2010;117(5):921–7.
7. Haddad S, Chen CA, Santangelo SL, Seddon JM. The genetics of age-related macular degeneration: a review of progress to date. Surv Ophthalmol. 2006; 51(4):316–63.
8. Cackett P, Wong TY, Aung T, Saw SM, Tay WT, Rochtchina E, Mitchell P, Wang JJ. Smoking, cardiovascular risk factors, and age-related macular degeneration in Asians: the Singapore Malay eye study. Am J Ophthalmol. 2008;146(6):960–7 e961.
9. Hageman GS, Anderson DH, Johnson LV, Hancox LS, Taiber AJ, Hardisty LI, Hageman JL, Stockman HA, Borchardt JD, Gehrs KM, et al. A common haplotype in the complement regulatory gene factor H (HF1/CFH) predisposes individuals to age-related macular degeneration. Proc Natl Acad Sci U S A. 2005;102(20):7227–32.
10. Johnson PT, Betts KE, Radeke MJ, Hageman GS, Anderson DH, Johnson LV. Individuals homozygous for the age-related macular degeneration risk-conferring variant of complement factor H have elevated levels of CRP in the choroid. Proc Natl Acad Sci U S A. 2006;103(46):17456–61.
11. Nozaki M, Raisler BJ, Sakurai E, Sarma JV, Barnum SR, Lambris JD, Chen Y, Zhang K, Ambati BK, Baffi JZ, et al. Drusen complement components C3a and C5a promote choroidal neovascularization. Proc Natl Acad Sci U S A. 2006;103(7):2328–33.
12. Haines JL, Hauser MA, Schmidt S, Scott WK, Olson LM, Gallins P, Spencer KL, Kwan SY, Noureddine M, Gilbert JR, et al. Complement factor H variant increases the risk of age-related macular degeneration. Science. 2005; 308(5720):419–21.
13. Klein RJ, Zeiss C, Chew EY, Tsai JY, Sackler RS, Haynes C, Henning AK, SanGiovanni JP, Mane SM, Mayne ST, et al. Complement factor H polymorphism in age-related macular degeneration. Science. 2005; 308(5720):385–9.
14. Hageman GS, Luthert PJ, Victor Chong NH, Johnson LV, Anderson DH, Mullins RF. An integrated hypothesis that considers drusen as biomarkers of immune-mediated processes at the RPE-Bruch's membrane interface in aging and age-related macular degeneration. Prog Retin Eye Res. 2001;20(6): 705–32.
15. Johnson LV, Leitner WP, Staples MK, Anderson DH. Complement activation and inflammatory processes in Drusen formation and age related macular degeneration. Exp Eye Res. 2001;73(6):887–96.
16. Little J, Higgins J, Bray M, Ioannidis J, Khoury M, Manolio T, Smeeth L, Sterne J: The HuGENet™ HuGE Review Handbook, version 1.0. 2006.
17. Higgins JP, Thompson SG, Deeks JJ, Altman DG. Measuring inconsistency in meta-analyses. Bmj. 2003;327(7414):557–60.
18. Begg CB, Mazumdar M. Operating characteristics of a rank correlation test for publication bias. Biometrics. 1994;50(4):1088–101.
19. Egger M, Davey Smith G, Schneider M, Minder C. Bias in meta-analysis detected by a simple, graphical test. Bmj. 1997;315(7109):629–34.
20. Bonyadi M, Mohammadian T, Jabbarpoor Bonyadi MH, Fotouhi N, Soheilian M, Javadzadeh A, Moein H, Yaseri M. Association of polymorphisms in complement component 3 with age-related macular degeneration in an Iranian population. Ophthalmic Genet. 2017;38(1):61–6.

21. Bonyadi M, Jabbarpoor Bonyadi MH, Yaseri M, Mohammadian T, Fotouhi N, Javadzadeh A, Soheilian M. Joint association of complement component 3 and CC-cytokine ligand2 (CCL2) or complement component 3 and CFH polymorphisms in age-related macular degeneration. Ophthalmic Genet. 2017;38:1–6.

22. Bergeron-Sawitzke J, Gold B, Olsh A, Schlotterbeck S, Lemon K, Visvanathan K, Allikmets R, Dean M. Multilocus analysis of age-related macular degeneration. European journal of human genetics : EJHG. 2009;17(9):1190–9.

23. Buentello-Volante B, Rodriguez-Ruiz G, Miranda-Duarte A, Pompa-Mera EN, Graue-Wiechers F, Bekker-Mendez C, Ayala-Ramirez R, Quezada C, Rodriguez-Loaiza JL, Zenteno JC. Susceptibility to advanced age-related macular degeneration and alleles of complement factor H, complement factor B, complement component 2, complement component 3, and age-related maculopathy susceptibility 2 genes in a Mexican population. Mol Vis. 2012;18:2518–25.

24. Caire J, Recalde S, Velazquez-Villoria A, Garcia-Garcia L, Reiter N, Anter J, Fernandez-Robredo P, Alfredo G-L. Growth of geographic atrophy on fundus autofluorescence and polymorphisms of CFH, CFB, C3, FHR1-3, and ARMS2 in age-related macular degeneration. JAMA ophthalmology. 2014;132(5):528–34.

25. Chen W, Stambolian D, Edwards AO, Branham KE, Othman M, Jakobsdottir J, Tosakulwong N, Pericak-Vance MA, Campochiaro PA, Klein ML, et al. Genetic variants near TIMP3 and high-density lipoprotein-associated loci influence susceptibility to age-related macular degeneration. Proc Natl Acad Sci U S A. 2010;107(16):7401–6.

26. Chen Y, Zeng J, Zhao C, Wang K, Trood E, Buehler J, Weed M, Kasuga D, Bernstein PS, Hughes G, et al. Assessing susceptibility to age-related macular degeneration with genetic markers and environmental factors. Arch Ophthalmol (Chicago, Ill : 1960). 2011;129(3):344–51.

27. Cipriani V, Leung HT, Plagnol V, Bunce C, Khan JC, Shahid H, Moore AT, Harding SP, Bishop PN, Hayward C, et al. Genome-wide association study of age-related macular degeneration identifies associated variants in the TNXB-FKBPL-NOTCH4 region of chromosome 6p21.3. Hum Mol Genet. 2012;21(18):4138–50.

28. Contreras AV, Zenteno JC, Fernandez-Lopez JC, Rodriguez-Corona U, Falfan-Valencia R, Sebastian L, Morales F, Ochoa-Contreras D, Carnevale A, Silva-Zolezzi I. CFH haplotypes and ARMS2, C2, C3, and CFB alleles show association with susceptibility to age-related macular degeneration in Mexicans. Mol Vis. 2014;20:105–16.

29. Cui L, Zhou H, Yu J, Sun E, Zhang Y, Jia W, Jiao Y, Snellingen T, Liu X, Lim A, et al. Noncoding variant in the complement factor H gene and risk of exudative age-related macular degeneration in a Chinese population. Invest Ophthalmol Vis Sci. 2010;51(2):1116–20.

30. Despriet DD, van Duijn CM, Oostra BA, Uitterlinden AG, Hofman A, Wright AF, ten Brink JB, Bakker A, de Jong PT, Vingerling JR, et al. Complement component C3 and risk of age-related macular degeneration. Ophthalmology. 2009;116(3):474–80 e472.

31. Edwards AO, Fridley BL, James KM, Sharma AK, Cunningham JM, Tosakulwong N. Evaluation of clustering and genotype distribution for replication in genome wide association studies: the age-related eye disease study. PLoS One. 2008;3(11):e3813.

32. Francis PJ, Hamon SC, Ott J, Weleber RG, Klein ML. Polymorphisms in C2, CFB and C3 are associated with progression to advanced age related macular degeneration associated with visual loss. J Med Genet. 2009;46(5):300–7.

33. Hageman GS, Gehrs K, Lejnine S, Bansal AT, Deangelis MM, Guymer RH, Baird PN, Allikmets R, Deciu C, Oeth P, et al. Clinical validation of a genetic model to estimate the risk of developing choroidal neovascular age-related macular degeneration. Human genomics. 2011;5(5):420–40.

34. Hautamaki A, Seitsonen S, Holopainen JM, Moilanen JA, Kivioja J, Onkamo P, Jarvela I, Immonen I. The genetic variant rs4073 A-->T of the Interleukin-8 promoter region is associated with the earlier onset of exudative age-related macular degeneration. Acta Ophthalmol. 2015;93(8):726–33.

35. Helgason H, Sulem P, Duvvari MR, Luo H, Thorleifsson G, Stefansson H, Jonsdottir I, Masson G, Gudbjartsson DF, Walters GB, et al. A rare nonsynonymous sequence variant in C3 is associated with high risk of age-related macular degeneration. Nat Genet. 2013;45(11):1371–4.

36. Jaouni T, Averbukh E, Burstyn-Cohen T, Grunin M, Banin E, Sharon D, Chowers I. Association of pattern dystrophy with an HTRA1 single-nucleotide polymorphism. Arch Ophthalmol (Chicago, Ill : 1960). 2012;130(8):987–91.

37. Kopplin LJ, Igo RP Jr, Wang Y, Sivakumaran TA, Hagstrom SA, Peachey NS, Francis PJ, Klein ML, SanGiovanni JP, Chew EY, et al. Genome-wide association identifies SKIV2L and MYRIP as protective factors for age-related macular degeneration. Genes Immun. 2010;11(8):609–21.

38. Liu K, Lai TY, Chiang SW, Chan VC, Young AL, Tam PO, Pang CP, Chen LJ. Gender specific association of a complement component 3 polymorphism with polypoidal choroidal vasculopathy. Sci Rep. 2014;4:7018.

39. Liu X, Zhao P, Tang S, Lu F, Hu J, Lei C, Yang X, Lin Y, Ma S, Yang J, et al. Association study of complement factor H, C2, CFB, and C3 and age-related macular degeneration in a Han Chinese population. Retina (Philadelphia, Pa). 2010;30(8):1177–84.

40. Losonczy G, Vajas A, Takacs L, Dzsudzsak E, Fekete A, Marhoffer E, Kardos L, Ajzner E, Hurtado B, de Frutos PG, et al. Effect of the Gas6 c.834+7G>a polymorphism and the interaction of known risk factors on AMD pathogenesis in Hungarian patients. PLoS One. 2012;7(11):e50181.

41. Maller JB, Fagerness JA, Reynolds RC, Neale BM, Daly MJ, Seddon JM. Variation in complement factor 3 is associated with risk of age-related macular degeneration. Nat Genet. 2007;39(10):1200–1.

42. Martinez-Barricarte R, Recalde S, Fernandez-Robredo P, Millan I, Olavarrieta L, Vinuela A, Perez-Perez J, Garcia-Layana A, Rodriguez de Cordoba S. Relevance of complement factor H-related 1 (CFHR1) genotypes in age-related macular degeneration. Invest Ophthalmol Vis Sci. 2012;53(3):1087–94.

43. McKay GJ, Dasari S, Patterson CC, Chakravarthy U, Silvestri G. Complement component 3: an assessment of association with AMD and analysis of gene-gene and gene-environment interactions in a northern Irish cohort. Mol Vis. 2010;16:194–9.

44. Park KH, Fridley BL, Ryu E, Tosakulwong N, Edwards AO. Complement component 3 (C3) haplotypes and risk of advanced age-related macular degeneration. Invest Ophthalmol Vis Sci. 2009;50(7):3386–93.

45. Pei XT, Li XX, Bao YZ, Yu WZ, Yan Z, Qi HJ, Qian T, Xiao HX. Association of c3 gene polymorphisms with neovascular age-related macular degeneration in a chinese population. Curr Eye Res. 2009;34(8):615–22.

46. Peter I, Huggins GS, Ordovas JM, Haan M, Seddon JM. Evaluation of new and established age-related macular degeneration susceptibility genes in the Women's Health Initiative sight exam (WHI-SE) study. Am J Ophthalmol. 2011;152(6):1005–13 e1001.

47. Reynolds R, Hartnett ME, Atkinson JP, Giclas PC, Rosner B, Seddon JM. Plasma complement components and activation fragments: associations with age-related macular degeneration genotypes and phenotypes. Invest Ophthalmol Vis Sci. 2009;50(12):5818–27.

48. Saksens NT, Lechanteur YT, Verbakel SK, Groenewoud JM, Daha MR, Schick T, Fauser S, Boon CJ, Hoyng CB, den Hollander AI. Analysis of risk alleles and complement activation levels in familial and non-familial age-related macular degeneration. PLoS One. 2016;11(6):e0144367.

49. Smailhodzic D, Klaver CC, Klevering BJ, Boon CJ, Groenewoud JM, Kirchhof B, Daha MR, den Hollander AI, Hoyng CB. Risk alleles in CFH and ARMS2 are independently associated with systemic complement activation in age-related macular degeneration. Ophthalmology. 2012;119(2):339–46.

50. Spencer KL, Olson LM, Anderson BM, Schnetz-Boutaud N, Scott WK, Gallins P, Agarwal A, Postel EA, Pericak-Vance MA, Haines JL. C3 R102G polymorphism increases risk of age-related macular degeneration. Hum Mol Genet. 2008;17(12):1821–4.

51. Tian J, Yu W, Qin X, Fang K, Chen Q, Hou J, Li J, Chen D, Hu Y, Li X. Association of genetic polymorphisms and age-related macular degeneration in Chinese population. Invest Ophthalmol Vis Sci. 2012;53(7):4262–9.

52. Wu L, Tao Q, Chen W, Wang Z, Song Y, Sheng S, Li P, Zhou J. Association between polymorphisms of complement pathway genes and age-related macular degeneration in a Chinese population. Invest Ophthalmol Vis Sci. 2013;54(1):170–4.

53. Yanagisawa S, Kondo N, Miki A, Matsumiya W, Kusuhara S, Tsukahara Y, Honda S, Negi A. A common complement C3 variant is associated with protection against wet age-related macular degeneration in a Japanese population. PLoS One. 2011;6(12):e28847.

54. Yates JR, Sepp T, Matharu BK, Khan JC, Thurlby DA, Shahid H, Clayton DG, Hayward C, Morgan J, Wright AF, et al. Complement C3 variant and the risk of age-related macular degeneration. N Engl J Med. 2007;357(6):553–61.

55. Yu Y, Reynolds R, Fagerness J, Rosner B, Daly MJ, Seddon JM. Association of variants in the LIPC and ABCA1 genes with intermediate and large drusen

and advanced age-related macular degeneration. Invest Ophthalmol Vis Sci. 2011;52(7):4663–70.

56. Zerbib J, Richard F, Puche N, Leveziel N, Cohen SY, Korobelnik JF, Sahel J, Munnich A, Kaplan J, Rozet JM, et al. R102G polymorphism of the C3 gene associated with exudative age-related macular degeneration in a French population. Mol Vis. 2010;16:1324–30.

57. Habibi I, Sfar I, Kort F, Bouraoui R, Chebil A, Limaiem R, Ayed S, Ben Abdallah T, El Matri L, Gorgi Y. Complement component C3 variant (R102G) and the risk of Neovascular age-related macular degeneration in a Tunisian population. Klin Monatsbl Augenheilkd. 2017;234(4):478–82.

58. Mullins RF, Russell SR, Anderson DH, Hageman GS. Drusen associated with aging and age-related macular degeneration contain proteins common to extracellular deposits associated with atherosclerosis, elastosis, amyloidosis, and dense deposit disease. FASEB J : official publication of the Federation of American Societies for Experimental Biology. 2000;14(7):835–46.

59. Janssen BJ, Christodoulidou A, McCarthy A, Lambris JD, Gros P. Structure of C3b reveals conformational changes that underlie complement activity. Nature. 2006;444(7116):213–6.

60. Bora PS, Hu Z, Tezel TH, Sohn JH, Kang SG, Cruz JM, Bora NS, Garen A, Kaplan HJ. Immunotherapy for choroidal neovascularization in a laser-induced mouse model simulating exudative (wet) macular degeneration. Proc Natl Acad Sci U S A. 2003;100(5):2679–84.

61. Bora PS, Sohn JH, Cruz JM, Jha P, Nishihori H, Wang Y, Kaliappan S, Kaplan HJ, Bora NS. Role of complement and complement membrane attack complex in laser-induced choroidal neovascularization. J Immunol (Baltimore, Md : 1950). 2005;174(1):491–7.

62. Nishida N, Walz T, Springer TA. Structural transitions of complement component C3 and its activation products. Proc Natl Acad Sci U S A. 2006; 103(52):19737–42.

63. Zhang MX, Zhao XF, Ren YC, Geng TT, Yang H, Feng T, Jin TB, Chen C. Association between a functional genetic polymorphism (rs2230199) and age-related macular degeneration risk: a meta-analysis. Gen Mol Res : GMR. 2015;14(4):12567–76.

64. Qian-Qian Y, Yong Y, Jing Z, Xin B, Tian-Hua X, Chao S, Jia C. Nonsynonymous single nucleotide polymorphisms in the complement component 3 gene are associated with risk of age-related macular degeneration: a meta-analysis. Gene. 2015;561(2):249–55.

Permissions

The contributors of this book come from diverse backgrounds, making this book a truly international effort. This book will bring forth new frontiers with its revolutionizing research information and detailed analysis of the nascent developments around the world.

We would like to thank all the contributing authors for lending their expertise to make the book truly unique. They have played a crucial role in the development of this book. Without their invaluable contributions this book wouldn't have been possible. They have made vital efforts to compile up to date information on the varied aspects of this subject to make this book a valuable addition to the collection of many professionals and students.

This book was conceptualized with the vision of imparting up-to-date information and advanced data in this field. To ensure the same, a matchless editorial board was set up. Every individual on the board went through rigorous rounds of assessment to prove their worth. After which they invested a large part of their time researching and compiling the most relevant data for our readers.

The editorial board has been involved in producing this book since its inception. They have spent rigorous hours researching and exploring the diverse topics which have resulted in the successful publishing of this book. They have passed on their knowledge of decades through this book. To expedite this challenging task, the publisher supported the team at every step. A small team of assistant editors was also appointed to further simplify the editing procedure and attain best results for the readers.

Apart from the editorial board, the designing team has also invested a significant amount of their time in understanding the subject and creating the most relevant covers. They scrutinized every image to scout for the most suitable representation of the subject and create an appropriate cover for the book.

The publishing team has been an ardent support to the editorial, designing and production team. Their endless efforts to recruit the best for this project, has resulted in the accomplishment of this book. They are a veteran in the field of academics and their pool of knowledge is as vast as their experience in printing. Their expertise and guidance has proved useful at every step. Their uncompromising quality standards have made this book an exceptional effort. Their encouragement from time to time has been an inspiration for everyone.

The publisher and the editorial board hope that this book will prove to be a valuable piece of knowledge for researchers, students, practitioners and scholars across the globe.

List of Contributors

Jing Cao
Department of pharmacy, Linyi People's hospital of Shandong University, LinYi 276003, China

Tao Wang and Meng Wang
Department of Ophthalmology, Linyi People's hospital of Shandong University, No. 27, Jiefang road, LinYi, Shandong 276003, China

Jee Hye Lee and Choun-Ki Joo
Department of Ophthalmology and Visual Science, Seoul St. Mary's Hospital, The Catholic University of Korea, Seoul, South Korea

Yong Eun Lee
The Ian eye center, Seoul, South Korea

Mihyun Choi, Minji Kang, Jeehye Lee and Choun-Ki Joo
Department of Ophthalmology, College of Medicine, Seoul St. Mary's Hospital, The Catholic University of Korea, 222, Banpo-daero, Seocho-gu, Seoul 06591, Republic of Korea.

Marjorie Z. Lazo
Catholic Institute for Visual Science, College of Medicine, Seoul St. Mary's Hospital, The Catholic University of Korea, Seoul, Republic of Korea

Qing Huang, Yongzhi Huang, Qu Luo and Wei Fan
Department of Ophthalmology, West China Hospital of Sichuan University, Sichuan Province, Chengdu, China

Ling Yeung
Department of Ophthalmology, Chang Gung Memorial Hospital, Keelung, Taiwan
College of Medicine, Chang Gung University, Taoyuan, Taiwan

Nan-Kai Wang, Wei-Chi Wu and Kuan-Jen Chen
College of Medicine, Chang Gung University, Taoyuan, Taiwan
Department of Ophthalmology, Chang Gung Memorial Hospital, No 5, Fu Hsing Street, Kuei Shan, Taoyuan, Taiwan

Yinghong Ji, Xianfang Rong and Yi Lu
Department of Ophthalmology and Eye Institute, Eye and ENT Hospital of Fudan University, Key Laboratory of Myopia of State Health Ministry, and Key Laboratory of Visual Impairment and Restoration of Shanghai, No. 83 Fenyang Road, Shanghai 200031, China

Fei Yuan
Department of Ophthalmology, Zhongshan Hospital of Fudan University, Shanghai, People's Republic of China

Xi Zhang
Department of Ophthalmology, Zhongshan Hospital of Fudan University, Shanghai, People's Republic of China
Department of Ophthalmology, Eye and ENT Hospital of Fudan University, Shanghai, People's Republic of China
Department of Ophthalmology, Myopia Key Laboratory of the Health Ministry, Shanghai, People's Republic of China

Xun Chen, Xiaoying Wang and Xingtao Zhou
Department of Ophthalmology, Eye and ENT Hospital of Fudan University, Shanghai, People's Republic of China
Department of Ophthalmology, Myopia Key Laboratory of the Health Ministry, Shanghai, People's Republic of China

Suk-Gyu Ha, Jungah Huh, Bo-Ram Lee and Seung-Hyun Kim
Department of Ophthalmology, Korea University College of Medicine, Seoul, Korea
Department of Ophthalmology, Korea University Anam Hospital, 73, Inchon-ro, Seongbuk-gu, Seoul 02841, South Korea

Bingqian Liu, Tao Li, Ying Lin, Wei Ma, Xiaohong Chen, Cancan Lyu, Yonghao Li and Lin Lu
State Key Laboratory of Ophthalmology, Zhongshan Ophthalmic Center, Sun Yat-sen University, 54 South Xianlie Road, Guangzhou 510060, Guangdong, China

Yan Wang
Department of Ophthalmology, Shenzhen Hospital of Southern Medical University, Shenzhen, China

Haisong Chen, Zheming Wu, Yun Chen and Manshan He
Guangzhou Aier Eye Hospital, Guangzhou, China

Jiawei Wang
Eye Center of Shandong University, The Second Hospital of Shandong University, Shandong University, Jinan 250000, China

Won Jae Kim and Myung Mi Kim
Department of Ophthalmology, Yeungnam University College of Medicine, 170, Hyeonchung-ro, Nam-gu, Daegu 42415, South Korea

Serkan Demirkan, Güzin Samav, Özgür Gündüz and Ayşe Karabulut
Department of Dermatology and Venerology, Kirikkale University Faculty of Medicine, Yenisehir District, Tahsin Duru Avenue, No:14, Yahsihan, Kirikkale, Turkey

Zafer Onaran, Fatma Özkal and Erhan Yumuşak
Department of Ophtalmology, Kirikkale University Faculty of Medicine, Yenisehir District, Tahsin Duru Avenue, No:14, Yahsihan, Kirikkale, Turkey

Min Wu, Zhu Lin Hu, Dan He, Wen Rong Xu and Yan Li
Department of Ophthalmology, Yunnan Key Laboratory for prevention and treatment of eye diseases, Yunnan Innovation Team for Cataract and Ocular fundus Disease (2017HC010), Yunnan Eye Institute, Yunnan Eye Hospital, The 2nd People's Hospital of Yunnan Province, Kunming, China
Department of Ophthalmology, The 4th Affiliated Hospital of Kunming Medical University, Kunming, Yunnan, China

Norihiko Ishizaki
Department of Ophthalmology, Yao Tokushukai General Hospital, 1-17 Wakakusa-cho, Yao, Japan
Department of Ophthalmology, Osaka Medical College, 2-7 Daigaku-machi, Takatsuki, Osaka 569-8686, Japan

Teruyo Kida, Masanori Fukumoto, Takaki Sato, Hidehiro Oku and Tsunehiko Ikeda
Department of Ophthalmology, Osaka Medical College, 2-7 Daigaku-machi, Takatsuki, Osaka 569-8686, Japan

Xuehan Qian, Nan Wei, Xiaoli Qi, Xue Li, Jing Li, Ying Zhang, Ning Hua, Yuxian Ning and Gang Ding
Department of Strabismus and Pediatric Ophthalmology, Tianjin Medical University Eye Hospital, Tianjin, China

Beihong Liu, Xu Ma and Binbin Wang
Department of Genetics, Center for Genetics, National Research Institute for Family Planning, 12 Dahuisi Road, Haidian, Beijing 100081, China.

Jing Wang
Department of Medical Genetics and Developmental Biology, School of Basic Medical Sciences, Capital Medical University, Beijing, China

Yu Zhang and Yue-guo Chen
Department of Ophthalmology, Peking University Third Hospital, 49 North Huayuan Road, Haidian District, Beijing 100191, China

Azusa Fujikawa, Hirofumi Kinoshita, Makiko Matsumoto, Masafumi Uematsu, Eiko Tsuiki and Takashi Kitaoka
Department of Ophthalmology and Visual Sciences, Graduate School of Biomedical Sciences, Nagasaki University, 1-7-1 Sakamoto, Nagasaki, Nagasaki 852-8501, Japan

Yasser Helmy Mohamed
Department of Ophthalmology and Visual Sciences, Graduate School of Biomedical Sciences, Nagasaki University, 1-7-1 Sakamoto, Nagasaki, Nagasaki 852-8501, Japan
Department of Ophthalmology, EL-Minia University Hospital, EL-Minia, Egypt

Kiyoshi Suzuma
Department of Ophthalmology and Visual Sciences, Graduate School of Medicine Kyoto University, Kyoto, Japan

Cerys J. Evans and Alison J. Hardcastle
UCL Institute of Ophthalmology, London, UK

Lubica Dudakova
Research Unit for Rare Diseases, Department of Paediatrics and Adolescent Medicine, First Faculty of Medicine, Charles University and General University Hospital in Prague, Ke Karlovu 2, 128 08 Prague 2, Czech Republic

Pavlina Skalicka and Petra Liskova
Research Unit for Rare Diseases, Department of Paediatrics and Adolescent Medicine, First Faculty of Medicine, Charles University and General University Hospital in Prague, Ke Karlovu 2, 128 08 Prague 2, Czech Republic
Department of Ophthalmology, First Faculty of Medicine, Charles University and General University Hospital in Prague, Prague, Czech Republic

Gabriela Mahelkova
Department of Ophthalmology, Second Faculty of Medicine, Charles University and Motol University Hospital, Prague, Czech Republic

Ales Horinek
3rd Department of Medicine, Department of Endocrinology and Metabolism, First Faculty of Medicine, Charles University and General University Hospital in Prague, Prague, Czech Republic Institute of Biology and Human Genetics, First Faculty of Medicine, Charles University and General University Hospital in Prague, Prague, Czech Republic

Stephen J. Tuft
Moorfields Eye Hospital, London, UK

Wei Zhang, Jian Song, Yue Zhang, Yingxue Ma, Jing Yang, Guanghui He and Song Chen
Tianjin Eye Hospital, Tianjin Key Lab of Ophthalmology and Visual Science, Tianjin Eye Institute, Clinical College of Ophthalmology Tianjin Medical University, No. 4, Gansu Road, Tianjin 300020, China

Hejun Chen and Xi Shen
Ruijin Hospital Affiliated to Shanghai Jiao Tong University School of Medicine, No. 197 Rui Jin Er Road, Shanghai 200025, China

Xi Zhang
Xinhua Hospital Affiliated to Shanghai Jiao Tong University School of Medicine, No.1665 Kongjiang Road, Shanghai 200092, China

Jin Sun Hwang, Yoon Pyo Lee, Seok Hyun Bae, Ha Kyoung Kim, Kayoung Yi and Young Joo Shin
Department of Ophthalmology, Hallym University Medical Center, Hallym University College of Medicine, 948-1 Daerim1-dong, Youngdeungpo-gu, Seoul 150-950, Korea

Xia Hua
Department of Ophthalmology, the Second Hospital of Tianjin Medical University, Tianjin, China

Yongxiao Dong and Jianying Du
Department of Ophthalmology, the First People's Hospital of Xianyang, Shanxi 712000, China

Jin Yang and Xiaoyong Yuan
Tianjin Eye Hospital, Tianjin Key Lab of Ophthalmology and Visual Science, Clinical College of Ophthalmology, Tianjin Medical University, Tianjin 300020, China

Haeng-Jin Le
Department of Ophthalmology, Seoul National University College of Medicine, Seoul, South Korea
Department of Ophthalmology, Seoul National University Hospital, 101 Daehak-Ro, Jongno Gu, Seoul 110-744, Republic of Korea

Seong-Joon Kim
Department of Ophthalmology, Seoul National University College of Medicine, Seoul, South Korea
Seoul Artificial Eye Center, Seoul National University Hospital Clinical Research Institute, Seoul, South Korea
Department of Ophthalmology, Seoul National University Hospital, 101 Daehak-Ro, Jongno Gu, Seoul 110-744, Republic of Korea

Feng Chen, Dan Cheng, Jiandong Pan, Zhongxu Tian, Fan Lu and Lijun Shen
School of Optometry and Ophthalmology and Eye Hospital of Wenzhou Medical University, Number 270, West Xueyuan Road, Lucheng District, Wenzhou 325000, Zhejiang, China

Chongbin Huang and Xingxing Cai
Neonate Department, Yueqing Maternal and Child Health Hospital, Yueqing, China

Meng-su Tang and Li-wei Ma
Department of Ophthalmology, the Fourth Affiliated Hospital of China Medical University, No. 11 Xinhua Road, Heping District, Shenyang 110004, Liaoning Province, China

Shu-qi Zhang
Department of Ophthalmology, the 463 Hospital of the Chinese People's Liberation Army, Shenyang 110021, Liaoning Province, China

So Min Ahn, Suk Yeon Lee, Seong-Woo Kim, Jaeryung Oh and Cheolmin Yun
Department of Ophthalmology, Korea University College of Medicine, 123, Jeokgeum-ro, Danwon-gu, Ansan-si, Gyeonggi-do, Seoul, South Korea

Soon-Young Hwang
Department of Biostatistics, Korea University College of Medicine, Seoul, South Korea

Jay Chhablani, Raja Narayanan, Abhilash Goud and Annie Mathai
Smt. Kanuri Santhamma Retina Vitreous Centre, L.V.Prasad Eye Institute, Kallam Anji Reddy Campus Banjara Hills, Hyderabad 500034, India

Rayan Alshareef
Department of Ophthalmology, McGill University, Montreal, Quebec, Canada

David Ta Kim
Department of Surgery, Division of Ophthalmology, Faculty of Medicine and Health Sciences, Université de Sherbrooke, Sherbrooke, Quebec, Canada

Seung Wan Nam and Kyu Yeon Cho
Department of Ophthalmology, Samsung Medical Center, Sungkyunkwan University School of Medicine, Seoul, South Korea

Dong Hui Lim
Department of Ophthalmology, Samsung Medical Center, Sungkyunkwan University School of Medicine, Seoul, South Korea
Department of Preventive Medicine, Graduate School, The Catholic University of Korea, Seoul, South Korea
Department of Ophthalmology, Samsung Medical Center, #81 Irwon-ro, Gangnam-gu, Seoul 06351, South Korea

Tae-Young Chung
Department of Ophthalmology, Samsung Medical Center, Sungkyunkwan University School of Medicine, Seoul, South Korea
Department of Ophthalmology, Samsung Medical Center, #81 Irwon-ro, Gangnam-gu, Seoul 06351, South Korea

Hye Seung Kim and Kyunga Kim
Biostatistics and Clinical Epidemiology Center, Research Institute for Future Medicine, Samsung Medical Center, Seoul, South Korea

Junwon Jang and Sungeun E. Kyung
Department of ophthalmology, University of Dankook, Dankook University Hospital, 359 Manghang-Ro, Dongnam-Gu, Cheonan-City, Chungchungnam-Do, South Korea

Xudong Peng, Guiqiu Zhao, Jing Lin, Jianqiu Qu, and Cui Li
Department of Ophthalmology, The Affiliated Hospital of Qingdao University, NO. 16 Jiangsu Road, Qingdao 266003, Shandong Province, China

Yingxue Zhang
Department of Biochemistry, Immunology and Microbiology, Wayne State University School of Medicine, 540 E. Canfield Avenue, Detroit, MI 48201, USA

Saki Omatsu, Kazuyuki Hirooka, Eri Nitta and Kaori Ukegawa
Department of Ophthalmology, Kagawa University Faculty of Medicine, 1750-1 Ikenobe, Miki, Kagawa 761-0793, Japan

Jing Dong
Department of Ophthalmology, The First Hospital of Shanxi Medical University, Taiyuan 030001, Shanxi, People's Republic of China

Yaqin Zhang, Haining Zhang, Zhijie Jia, Suhua Zhang, Bin Sun and Xiaogang Wang
Department of Ophthalmology, Shanxi Eye Hospital, No. 100 Fudong Street, Taiyuan 030002, Shanxi, People's Republic of China

Yongqing Han
Department of Ophthalmology, Affiliated Hospital of Inner Mongolia University for the Nationalities, Tongliao 028007, Inner Mongolia, People's Republic of China

Sana' Muhsen
Ophthalmology, Glaucoma and Anterior Segment Surgeon, University of Jordan Hospital, The University of Jordan, Amman, Jordan

Feras Alkhalaileh and Mohammad Hamdan
School of Medicine, The University of Jordan, Amman 11942, Jordan

Saif Aldeen AlRyalat
Department of Ophthalmology, University of Jordan Hospital, The University of Jordan, Amman 11942, Jordan

Attila Kovacs, Timea Kiss, Andrea Facsko and Rozsa Degi
Department of Ophthalmology, Faculty of Medicine, University of Szeged, 10-11 Koranyi fasor, Szeged 6720, Hungary

Ferenc Rarosi
Department of Medical Physics and Informatics, Faculty of Medicine, University of Szeged, Szeged, Hungary

Gabor M. Somfai
Augenzentrum Pallas Kliniken, Olten, Switzerland
Department of Ophthalmology, Faculty of Medicine, Semmelweis University, Budapest, Hungary

Jun Zhang, Shuang Li, Jiguo Yu and Yi Xiang
Department of Ophthalmology, the Central Hospital of Wuhan, Tongji Medical College, Huazhong University of Science and Technology, NO, 26 Shengli Street, Wuhan 430014, Hubei Province, China

Shuqiong Hu
Department of Ophthalmology, the Jingzhou aier eye hospital, Jingzhou, Hubei Province, China

Index